1990 YEAR BOOK OF DERMATOLOGY®

The 1990 Year Book® Series

Year Book of Anesthesia®: Drs. Miller, Kirby, Ostheimer, Roizen, and Stoelting

Year Book of Cardiology®: Drs. Schlant, Collins, Engle, Frye, Kaplan, and O'Rourke

Year Book of Critical Care Medicine®: Drs. Rogers and Parrillo

Year Book of Dentistry®: Drs. Meskin, Ackerman, Kennedy, Leinfelder, Matukas, and Rovin

Year Book of Dermatology®: Drs. Sober and Fitzpatrick

Year Book of Diagnostic Radiology®: Drs. Bragg, Hendee, Keats, Kirkpatrick, Miller, Osborn, and Thompson

Year Book of Digestive Diseases®: Drs. Greenberger and Moody

Year Book of Drug Therapy®: Drs. Hollister and Lasagna

Year Book of Emergency Medicine®: Dr. Wagner

Year Book of Endocrinology®: Drs. Bagdade, Braverman, Halter, Horton, Kannan, Korenman, Molitch, Morley, Odell, Rogol, Ryan, and Sherwin

Year Book of Family Practice®: Drs. Rakel, Avant, Driscoll, Prichard, and Smith

Year Book of Geriatrics and Gerontology®: Drs. Beck, Abrass, Burton, Cummings, Makinodan, and Small

Year Book of Hand Surgery®: Drs. Dobyns, Chase, and Amadio

Year Book of Hematology®: Drs. Spivak, Bell, Ness, Quesenberry, and Wiernik

Year Book of Infectious Diseases®: Drs. Wolff, Barza, Keusch, Klempner, and Snydman

Year Book of Infertility: Drs. Mishell, Paulsen, and Lobo

Year Book of Medicine®: Drs. Rogers, Des Prez, Cline, Braunwald, Greenberger, Wilson, Epstein, and Malawista

Year Book of Neonatal and Perinatal Medicine: Drs. Klaus and Fanaroff

Year Book of Neurology and Neurosurgery®: Drs. Currier and Crowell

Year Book of Nuclear Medicine®: Drs. Hoffer, Gore, Gottschalk, Sostman, Zaret, and Zubal

Year Book of Obstetrics and Gynecology®: Drs. Mishell, Kirschbaum, and Morrow

Year Book of Occupational and Environmental Medicine: Drs. Emmett, Brooks, Harris, and Schenker

Year Book of Oncology: Drs. Young, Longo, Ozols, Simone, Steele, and Weichselbaum

Year Book of Ophthalmology®: Drs. Laibson, Adams, Augsburger, Benson, Cohen, Eagle, Flanagan, Nelson, Reinecke, Sergott, and Wilson

Year Book of Orthopedics®: Drs. Sledge, Poss, Cofield, Frymoyer, Griffin, Hansen, Johnson, Springfield, and Weiland

Year Book of Otolaryngology–Head and Neck Surgery®: Drs. Bailey and Paparella

Year Book of Pathology and Clinical Pathology®: Drs. Brinkhous, Dalldorf, Grisham, Langdell, and McLendon

Year Book of Pediatrics®: Drs. Oski and Stockman

Year Book of Plastic, Reconstructive, and Aesthetic Surgery: Drs. Miller, Bennett, Haynes, Hoehn, McKinney, and Whitaker

Year Book of Podiatric Medicine and Surgery®: Dr. Jay

Year Book of Psychiatry and Applied Mental Health®: Drs. Talbott, Frances, Frances, Freedman, Meltzer, Schowalter, and Yudofsky

Year Book of Pulmonary Disease®: Drs. Green, Loughlin, Michael, Mulshine, Peters, Terry, Tockman, and Wise

Year Book of Speech, Language, and Hearing: Drs. Bernthal, Hall, and Tomblin

Year Book of Sports Medicine®: Drs. Shephard, Eichner, Sutton, and Torg, Col. Anderson, and Mr. George

Year Book of Surgery®: Drs. Schwartz, Jonasson, Peacock, Shires, Spencer, and Thompson

Year Book of Urology®: Drs. Gillenwater and Howards

Year Book of Vascular Surgery®: Drs. Bergan and Yao

1990

The Year Book of DERMATOLOGY®

Editors

Arthur J. Sober, M.D.

Associate Professor of Dermatology, Harvard Medical School, and Associate Chief of Dermatology, Massachusetts General Hospital

Thomas B. Fitzpatrick, M.D., Ph.D.

Edward Wigglesworth Professor, Department of Dermatology, Harvard Medical School, and Massachusetts General Hospital

Mosby Year Book

St. Louis Baltimore Boston Chicago London Philadelphia Sydney Toronto

Mosby Year Book

Dedicated to Publishing Excellence

Editor-in-Chief, Year Book Publishing: Nancy Gorham
Sponsoring Editor: Rebecca A. Ede
Manager, Medical Information Services: Edith M. Podrazik
Senior Medical Information Specialist: Terri Strorigl
Assistant Director, Manuscript Services: Frances M. Perveiler
Associate Managing Editor, Year Book Editing Services: Elizabeth Fitch
Production Coordinator: Max F. Perez
Proofroom Supervisor: Barbara M. Kelly

Mosby-Year Book, Inc.
11830 Westline Industrial Drive
St. Louis, MO 63146

Editorial Office:
Mosby-Year Book, Inc.
200 North LaSalle St.
Chicago, IL 60601

International Standard Serial Number: 0093-3619
International Standard Book Number: 0-8151-7912-X

Contributing Editors

Joseph C. Alper, M.D.
Associate Professor of Medicine (Dermatology), Brown University
Jeffrey D. Bernhard, M.D.
Associate Professor of Medicine (Dermatology), University of Massachusetts Medical School
Jessica L. Fewkes, M.D.
Assistant Professor of Dermatology, Harvard Medical School
Thomas J. Flotte, M.D.
Assistant Professor of Pathology, Harvard Medical School
Richard W. Gange, M.D.
Associate Professor of Dermatology, Harvard Medical School
Richard A. Johnson, M.D.
Clinical Instructor in Dermatology, Harvard Medical School
Richard Masters, M.D.
Assistant Clinical Professor, Harvard Medical School
Samuel L. Moschella, M.D.
Clinical Professor of Dermatology, Harvard Medical School
Peter E. Pochi, M.D.
Professor of Dermatology, Boston University
Arthur R. Rhodes, M.D., M.P.H.
Associate Professor of Dermatology and Medicine, University of Pittsburgh
Nicholas A. Soter, M.D.
Professor of Dermatology, New York University
Robert S. Stern, M.D.
Associate Professor of Dermatology, Harvard Medical School
Martin A. Weinstock, M.D., Ph.D.
Assistant Professor of Medicine (Dermatology), Brown University

Table of Contents

The material in this volume represents literature reviewed up to November 1989.

Journals Represented

Year Book Medical Publishers subscribes to and surveys nearly 850 U.S. and foreign medical and allied health journals. From these journals, the Editors select the articles to be abstracted. Journals represented in this YEAR BOOK are listed below.

APMIS: Acta Pathologica, Microbiologica et Immunologica
Acta Dermato-Venereologica
Acta Odontologica Scandinavica
American Family Physician
American Journal of Clinical Pathology
American Journal of Dermatopathology
American Journal of Diseases of Children
American Journal of Emergency Medicine
American Journal of Industrial Medicine
American Journal of Medicine
American Journal of Ophthalmology
American Journal of Pathology
American Journal of Sports Medicine
American Journal of Surgical Pathology
American Surgeon
Annales de Dermatologie et de Venereologie
Annals of Allergy
Annals of Clinical Biochemistry
Annals of Internal Medicine
Annals of Plastic Surgery
Archives of Dermatological Research
Archives of Dermatology
Archives of Internal Medicine
Archives of Pathology and Laboratory Medicine
Archives of Surgery
Arthritis and Rheumatism
Brain—Journal of Neurology
British Journal of Cancer
British Journal of Dermatology
British Journal of Plastic Surgery
British Medical Journal
Canadian Medical Association Journal
Cancer
Cleveland Clinic Journal of Medicine
Clinica Chimica Acta
Clinical Nephrology
Clinical Pharmacology and Therapeutics
Clinical Radiology
Clinical and Experimental Allergy
Clinical and Experimental Dermatology
Contact Dermatitis
Cutis
Dermatologica
Diseases of the Colon and Rectum
Gastrointestinal Radiology
General Hospital Psychiatry
Genitourinary Medicine
Hautarzt

Head and Neck Surgery
Histopathology
Human Pathology
International Journal of Cancer
International Journal of Dermatology
International Journal of Leprosy and Other Mycobacterial Diseases
Journal of Acquired Immune Deficiency Syndromes
Journal of Allergy and Clinical Immunology
Journal of Clinical Oncology
Journal of Clinical Pathology
Journal of Cutaneous Pathology
Journal of Dermatologic Surgery and Oncology
Journal of Dermatology
Journal of Emergency Medicine
Journal of Infectious Diseases
Journal of Investigative Dermatology
Journal of Medical Genetics
Journal of Occupational Medicine
Journal of Pathology
Journal of Pediatrics
Journal of Reproductive Medicine
Journal of Urology
Journal of the American Academy of Dermatology
Journal of the American Medical Association
Journal of the National Cancer Institute
Lancet
Leprosy Review
Les Nouvelles Dermatologies
Medical Journal of Australia
Medicine
Modern Pathology
New England Journal of Medicine
Pediatric Infectious Disease Journal
Pediatrics
Plastic and Reconstructive Surgery
Postgraduate Medical Journal
Presse Medicale
Quarterly Journal of Medicine
Reviews of Infectious Diseases
Scandinavian Journal of Plastic and Reconstructive Surgery
Seminars in Dermatology
Transplantation
Western Journal of Medicine
Zeitschrift Für Hautkrankheiten

Trends in Dermatology: Ozone Depletion and the Dermatologist: Need We Prepare for the Consequences of a UVB "Holocaust"* in the Next Decades?

THOMAS B. FITZPATRICK, M.D., PH.D.
Edward Wigglesworth Professor, Department of Dermatology, Harvard Medical School, and Massachusetts General Hospital

"In many respects, the atmosphere may be considered an extension of the biosphere. Its composition is changing rapidly at the present time, for a variety of reasons linked ultimately to pressures exerted by an expanding population and the aspirations of this population for an enhanced quality of life. The human species is now a force of consequence for change on a global scale. Its presence is evident from pole to pole, from the depths of the ocean to the heights of the stratosphere."†—Micheal B. McElroy, Prof. of Atmospheric Sciences, Harvard University

"The aspirations of [the] population for an enhanced quality of life" include refrigeration, which is possible at the present time only with the use of chlorofluorocarbons (CFCs). There is a serious question whether developing countries will be able to afford the alternatives for these gaseous pollutants. Developing nations need CFCs that are cheap, stable materials for refrigeration and air-conditioning equipment. Not only are CFCs not being cut back in the Third World countries as they are now in some large countries (the United States and the United Kingdom), but in fact it is said that at the present time a new factory for producing CFCs is being built in China.

What will this mean for all of us if there is no diminution of the production of CFCs? These inert gases migrate through the atmosphere where they can remain for more than 75 years. Ozone molecules are destroyed by chlorine, which is formed from the breakdown of CFCs by exposure to stratospheric solar ultraviolet radiation. As ozone molecules in the stratosphere are decreased, more ultraviolet B (UVB) passes through (i.e., is not filtered) and a higher UVB intensity is present on the earth's surface.

Three statements can be made about this problem of ozone depletion:

Statement 1: Ozone depletion by CFCs is now, in 1990, a certainty. Stratospheric ozone is a filter of a special, very tiny portion (less than 3%) of the sun's emission: ultraviolet radiation. In fact, the ozone filter selectively screens a particular region of the ultraviolet radiation known as UVB (290–320 nm). Any decrease in the stratospheric ozone filter will result in an increase in the total intensity of UVB radiation at the surface of the earth.

Statement 2: Ultraviolet B is harmful to all living things. Although not ionizing radiation such as the x-ray, UVB is without any known beneficial effects for living things and can be regarded as selectively destructive

*Literally, destruction by fire. Greek *holos* = whole; *kostos* = burnt.
†Presented at the Stated Meeting of American Academy of Arts and Sciences, in Cambridge, Mass, Oct 12, 1988.

radiation to DNA in cell nuclei at all levels of organization from plankton to humans. Deoxyribonucleic acid is altered in such a manner that repetitive "hits" on the DNA target by photons lead to irreversible damage to the biosphere, listed here in order of importance to humans:

Indirect Effects on Humans:
1. On *zooplankton*, which are important in the aquatic food chain; a decrease will seriously affect the supply of fish for human consumption.
2. On *phytoplankton*, which fix carbon dioxide; a reduction will lead to an increase in global warming by the "greenhouse" effect.
3. On the *quality of life*, for humans, which will be markedly changed with increased UVB reaching ground level; this is because UVB increases the production of trophospheric ozone, degrading the air quality, as has already happened in Los Angeles and other cities.

Direct Effects on Humans:
1. On *keratinocytes* and *melanocytes*; alteration will result in skin cancers, especially fatal malignant melanoma (See Tables 1 and 2.)
2. On special *white cells* in the blood circulating through the skin, *T lymphocytes;* these cells are important in immunity, and damage to them will seriously reduce the defenses against viral infections such as herpes simplex.
3. On the *eye*; this will lead to the development of cataracts and intraoclular malignant melanoma.

The UVB effects on cells are dose-dependent, cumulative, and irreversible.

Statement 3: A global ban on CFCs is required. Ozone depletion by CFCs is a global problem: Unless every nation bans production there will be no diminution of stratospheric CFCs; there are no national boundaries in the stratosphere.

Certain investment strategies involved: if we cannot make safe alternatives to CFCs that can be purchased cheaply by developing countries, do we need to prepare now to adapt to increased UVB levels? Plants and animals cannot adapt except over years, and this is the critical and urgent problem for our society.

How can humans adapt to high levels of UVB? (1) By staying out of the sun—an unrealistic alternative; or (2) by using topical and potential oral UVB sun-protective medications. There is, however, very poor compliance at present in the use of the available, highly effective, topical UVB-protective chemicals in lotions and ointments. There are no effective oral drugs that can protect the skin against the effects of UVB.

Ultraviolet Radiation and Melanoma: The Serious Effects of Ozone Depletion

In the past two decades there have been several reviews (see the Bibliography) of the role of sunlight in the pathogenesis of skin cancer, including malignant melanoma (MM) of the skin. Since the National Academy of Sciences assessment of the problem in 1982, much new data have become available. An EPA publication, an excellent 129-page critical review of the problem, concludes that "solar radiation plays a role in CMM [cutaneous malignant melanoma] development."

Some of the conclusions on which the EPA based its decision in the affirmative for the role of sunlight in the pathogenesis of human melanoma include the following:

1. Whites have a higher incidence of melanoma than brown or black persons.

2. Whites who tan poorly or not at all have more melanoma than whites who tan well. This is supported by large case-control studies from Western Australia (C. D. J. Holman's group) showing that the inability to tan (skin phototype I) is the most important *pigmentary* trait associated with the risk of melanoma.

3. The incidence of melanoma has been rising in cohorts in a manner consistent with changes in patterns of exposure, particularly with respect to increasing intermittent, intense, sun exposure of certain anatomical sites. Consistent with this fact is a higher incidence in higher social classes (professional) and in indoor workers.

4. Immigrants who move to sunny climates (e.g., Israel, Australia, California) have higher rates of melanoma than populations who remain in their country of origin. "Immigrants develop rates approaching those of prior (but native born) immigrants to the adopted country; this is particularly accentuated in individuals arriving at or just before the age of puberty (10 to 14 years)."

5. A recent study demonstrated a strong relationship between the levels of measured UVB and the incidence of melanoma.

6. In xeroderma pigmentosum there is a 2,000-fold increased risk of melanoma by age 20.

7. The type and site of origin of MM is related to age and sex. Every one agrees that one form of melanoma is clearly related to prolonged exposure to sunlight: lentigo maligna melanoma (LMM), which occurs almost invariably on skin sites in which there is marked dermatoheliosis (sun-damaged skin). Also, the incidence of LMM increases progressively with age, except for an early peak at 60 to 69 years, but superficial spreading melanoma (SSM) reaches a peak at 50 to 59 years and then declines. More than 80% of LMM occurs on the head and neck, whereas SSM, which occurs on the trunk and lower limbs (in females), increases in incidence from age 20 to 29 (females) and 30 to 39 (males).

8. By using predictions of UVB from a NASA model and a database for cutaneous MM developed by the EPA, a dose-response relationship for melanoma mortality was developed. It is estimated that a 1% change in ozone would result in a 0.8%to 1.5% change in cutaneous MM mortality.

Evolution of Knowledge Regarding Stratospheric Ozone Depletion Leading to Increased UVB

1971: Senator William Proxmire calls for a study of ozone depletion resulting from a contemplated fleet of military supersonic transports (SSTs).

TABLE 1.—Sun-Induced Skin Cancers in Humans: Factors in the Dose Response

	BASAL/SQUAMOUS CELL	MALIGNANT MELANOMA
AGE ONSET	Higher incidence over 55 years Incidence increases with age in the most exposed areas (face and neck)	Higher incidence in young and middle-aged adults Decreased incidence rates for SSM in migrants after age 15 to Australia and Israel
SEX	Male > female	Females have a higher incidence in Northern Europe
LATITUDE GRADIENT	Incidence directly related to measured UVB	Incidence directly related to measured UVB
OCCUPATION	Outdoor	Indoor "white collar" professional
EXPOSURE PATTERN	Prolonged repeated exposures: - farmers - construction workers	Intermittent intense exposures: - "weekenders" - charter flights to sunny climates

		Severe sunburn in childhood and sun exposure in childhood increases susceptibility to melanoma later in life
	HOST FACTORS	
SKIN COLOR	White persons with light skin Rare in pigmented (brown, black) persons High incidence of squamous cell carcinoma in blacks with albinism	White persons with light skin Rare in pigmented (brown, black) persons Melanoma is rare in blacks with albinism
SKIN PHOTOTYPE (SPT)	Increased incidence in SPT I and II (sunburn easily)	Increased incidence in SPT I and II (sunburn easily)
SITES OF PRE-DILECTION	Face, neck, and forearms (habitually exposed areas)	Trunk (upper back in both males and females)

HOST FACTORS (Cont'd)

	BASAL/SQUAMOUS CELL	MALIGNANT MELANOMA
		Higher incidence in legs of females
		Clark's dysplastic nevus is known to occur on the upper back of males and females, and is present on the legs of females more than in males; this may explain the paradox of melanoma arising in sites that are not habitually exposed areas.
		In populations with brown and black skin color, lesions occur in acral areas: on the soles, palms, toes, fingers, and nail bed and mucosae.
IMMUNO-SUPPRESSION	Renal transplant patients have aggressive SCC in UV-exposed skin	Renal transplant patients have an increased incidence of MM

ALTERED CELL SENSITIVITY TO UVR		
1. Precursor lesions	Solar keratosis	Lentigo maligna Clark's melanocytic nevus ("dysplastic" nevus) ? Common acquired nevomelanocytic nevi Congenital nevomelanocytic nevus
	Epidermodysplasia verruciformis	?VIRUS + SUN
	nevus + Human Papilloma Virus	---PRECURSOR
2. DNA repair defect	Xeroderma pigmentosum (RECESSIVE TRAIT)	Xeroderma pigmentosum (RECESSIVE TRAIT)
HUMAN MODEL	Basal cell nevus syndrome (autosomal dominant)	Familial melanoma with Clark's melanocytic (dysplastic) nevus (probably autosomal dominant)
ANIMAL MODEL	UVB=induced SCC (mice)	UVB-induced melanoma in opposum

TABLE 2.—Sun-Induced Skin Cancers: Statistics (U.S. 1989)

	BASAL/SQUAMOUS CELL	MALIGNANT MELANOMA
MAGNITUDE OF THE PROBLEM (yearly)	500,000 NEW PATIENTS	29,000 NEW PATIENTS
SEVERITY OF THE PROBLEM (yearly)	1,600 DEATHS Disfigurement Disability	6,000 DEATHS Mortality Increasing 3.0% per year!

1973–1974: An hypothesis that changed the course of the next two decades in our thinking about ozone depletion was proposed by Prof. F.S. Rowland and Mario Molina in *Nature: Chlorofluorocarbons (CFCs) drift into the stratosphere, are bombarded with ultraviolet, and release chlorine; this then destroys ozone: One atom of chlorine destroys up to 100,000 molecules of ozone.* They called for a ban on CFC production, but Congress (with pressure from Dupont) delayed action, waiting for confirmation of the Rowland-Molina hypothesis.

1975–1979: Several succesive committees of the National Academy of Sciences assess the problem with a team of scientists, epidemologists, and dermatologists.

1976: All nonessential aerosol sprays containing CFCs were banned in the United States following publication of a National Academy of Sciences report. This publication concluded that nonmelanoma skin cancer was directly related to ultraviolet radiation, and that ultraviolet radiation could play a role in the etiology of MM.

Few countries mimicked the U.S. action, however, and the Environmental Protection Agency dismissed the ozone depletion hypothesis as another "environmental scare." Dupont did not start to make safe alternatives. Uncertainty prevailed—National Academy of Sciences estimates of ozone losses ranged from 2% to 20%.

1984: The CFC problem suddenly became clarified by a single event: A continent-sized hole in the ozone shield of Antarctica was discovered, with a decrease in the ozone layer by as much as 67%. Most important was the discovery, by specially modified spy planes, of high concentrations of chlorine monoxide—the reaction product of chlorine and ozone molecules. The source of the chlorine was CFCs.

1985: The U.S. Secretary of the Interior responded by advising people to stay indoors, or let them wear hats, use sunscreens and sunglasses! To these hasty and inconsiderate remarks, the Senate quickly responded with a resolution to phase out CFCs and halons.

1987: The Montreal Protocol, adopted by many but not *all* nations, called for a freeze in production in July 1989, at 1986 production levels, followed by a 20% cut in four years and a 30% cut in 1988.

1989: Twelve European Community countries, in a surprising turnaround, voted to phase out all CFC production by the end of the present century and to cut production by 85% as soon as possible. Today in Germany, the sale of refrigerators is helped by proclaiming that they are "50% CFC free." But what about China and other developing countries that cannot afford the expensive alternatives to CFCs? The ban must be total and global, or the ozone depletion will continue.

Summary and Conclusions

The history of the ozone depletion leading to a UVB increase includes the efforts of a dozen dermatologists who have served on several committees of the National Academy of Sciences and the EPA and who have delved into this problem. I have been involved since 1971 when Senator Proxmire of Wisconsin called me to testify at the U.S. Capitol regarding the skin cancer question in relation to an increase of UVB.

The skin is a major human target of UVB, and the word *cancer* has emotional appeal to stir up the scientific community and the public. As a matter of fact, skin cancer is the least important of the effects of stratospheric perturbation. The effects on ecosystems are far more devastating, but not easy to measure. It was skin cancer that was most known, but knowledge of skin cancer statistics was fragmentary, as the problem had not been studied by epidemiologists and statisticians. Certainly, there was little belief by almost anyone that UVB was implicated in MM: It occurs in the wrong site, in young people, and the epidemiology is not at all similar to that of nonmelanoma cancer, which is known to be related to sunlight exposure.

In 1971 there was, in fact, a great deal of uncertainty about the ozone depletion hypothesis itself—the question then was supersonic transports emitting nitric oxide into the stratosphere, causing destruction of ozone. But only modeling systems were available.

Now after two decades, we have much new data on skin cancer and facts regarding ozone depletion not by SSTs but by industrial chemicals—chlorofluorocarbons and halons.

There are now these factual statements to be made:

1. The widely used CFCs and halons cause destruction of ozone in the stratosphere, leading to an increase in UVB at the earth's surface.
2. Study of nonmelanoma and melanoma skin cancer by a team of epidemiologists and statisticians supported by the National Academy of Sciences and the E.P.A. has shown that there has been a dramatic increase in the incidence of skin cancer (melanoma and nonmelanoma) in white people in the past three decades.
3. Ultraviolet radiation causes skin cancer: UVB is clearly an action spectrum for nonmelanoma skin cancer (Table 3), and is a putative action spectrum for malignant melanoma in mammals.
4. There is an intense global effort to ban the production fo CFCs and to develop safe alternatives for these highly essential compounds that have so many uses in our society, especially in refrigeration, a vital service in developing countries, with health implications.

TABLE 3.—Ozone Depletion and Nonmelanoma Skin Cancer*

1. **Squamous cell carcinoma will increase by 2% to 5% for each 1% depletion of ozone.**

2. **Basal cell carcinoma will increase by 1% to 3% for each 1% depletion of ozone.**

**An Assessment of the Risks of Stratospheric Modification,* U.S. Environmental Protection Agency, October 1986.

The dermatologist is the primary physician for the management of the patient with skin cancer and for this reason needs to be involved in the ozone depletion problem on a national and international level.

Bibliography

Fitzpatrick TB, Sober AJ: Sunlight and skin cancer. *N Engl J Med* 313:818–820, 1985.

Grobecker AJ (ed): *Climactic Impact Assessment Program (CIAP): Impacts of Climate Change on the Biosphere.* Washington, DC, Dept of Transportation, CIAP Monograph 5, DOT, TSWT-75-55, 1975.

Hoffman JS, Longstreth JD (eds): *Ultraviolet Radiation and Melanoma with a Special Focus on Assessing the Risks of Stratospheric Ozone Depletion.* Washington, DC, EPA 400/1-87/001D, December 1987.

Ley RD, et al: Ultraviolet radiation-induced malignant melanoma in *Monodelphis domestica. Photochem Photobiol* 50:1–5, 1989.

National Academy of Sciences (NAS): *Halocarbons: Effects on Stratospheric Ozone.* Washington, DC, National Academy Press, 1976.

National Academy of Sciences (NAS): *Protection of Depletion of Stratospheric Ozone by Chlorofluorocarbons.* Washington, DC, National Academy Press, 1979.

National Academy of Sciences (NAS): *Causes and Effects of Stratospheric Ozone Reduction: An Update.* Washington, DC, National Academy Press, 1979.

Tucker MA, et al: Sunlight exposure as risk factor for intraocular malignant melanoma. *N Engl J Med* 313:789–792, 1985.

Urbach F (ed): *The Biologic Effects of Ultraviolet Radiation: With Emphasis on the Skin.* New York, Pergamon Press, 1969.

Part of this material was presented at a public hearing, Jan. 25, 1990, Stratospheric Ozone Depletion and H.R. 2699; The Stratospheric Ozone Protection Act of 1989, U.S. House of Representatives, Committee on Energy and Commerce, Subcommittee on Health and the Environment, Chairman, Henry A. Waxman. Table 1 was prepared with the help of Arthur J. Sober, M.D.

Statistics of Interest to the Dermatologist

MARTIN A. WEINSTOCK, M.D., PH.D.
Assistant Professor of Medicine (Dermatology), Brown University

TABLE 1.—New Cases of Selected Reportable Infectious Diseases in the United States

	1939	1949	1959	1969	1979	1989‖
AIDS	—	—	—	—	—	34,340
Anthrax	54	54	12	4	0	0
Congenital rubella	—	—	—	31	62	3
Congenital syphilis	—	—	—	—	—	243
Diphtheria	24,053	7,969	934	241	59	2
Gonorrhea	182,314*	317,950	240,254	534,872	1,004,058§	689,922§
Hansen's disease	—	41	44	98	185	169
Leptospirosis	—	17	83	89	94	98
Measles	403,317	625,281	406,162	25,826	13,597	16,236
Meningococcal infections	1,972	3,519	2,180	2,951	2,724	2,595
Plague	1	3	4	5	13	4
Rocky Mountain spotted fever	559	570	199	498	1,070	619
Rubella	—	—	—	57,686	11,795	373
Smallpox	9,877	49	0	0	0	0
Syphilis (primary and secondary)	—	41,942	9,799	19,130	24,874§	42,600§
Toxic shock syndrome	—	—	—	—	—	376
Tuberculosis	103,922†‡	134,865†‡	57,535‡	39,120‡	27,669	21,520
Tularemia	2,291	1,179	459	149	196	144
U.S. population (millions)	130.9	148.7	176.5	201.4	220.1	247.1

—, Data not available.
*Data are for fiscal year.
†Includes newly reported inactive cases.
‡Reporting criteria changed in 1975.
§Civilian cases only.
‖For 52 weeks ending December 31, 1988. Sources:
Centers for Disease Control: Annual summary 1984: Reported morbidity and mortality. *MMWR* 33:124–129, 1986.
Centers for Disease Control: *MMWR* 38:891, 1990.

TABLE 2.—Geographic Distribution of the Acquired Immune Deficiency Syndrome (AIDS)

Number of Cases	
Africa	38,248
United States	113,211
America, excluding the United States	21,328
Asia	494
Europe	28,576
Oceania	1,742
World Total	203,599

Countries Reporting 100 or More Cases

Africa	
Angola	104
Burkina Faso	555
Burundi	2,355
Central African Republic	662
Congo	1,250
Ivory Coast	1,010
Ethiopia	236
Ghana	921
Kenya	6,004
Malawi	2,586
Rwanda	1,806
Senegal	269
South Africa	310
Sudan	113
Uganda	7,375
Tanzania	4,158
Zaire	4,636
Zambia	1,892
Zimbabwe	1,148
Americas	
Argentina	377
Bahamas	350
Bermuda	122
Brazil	8,064
Canada	3,130
Chile	149
Colombia	471
Costa Rica	113
Dominican Republic	1,028
French Guiana	150
Guadeloupe	133
Haiti	2,215
Honduras	344
Jamaica	121
Mexico	2,683
Peru	210
Trinidad and Tobago	456
United States	113,211
Venezuela	419
Asia	
Japan	108
Europe	
Austria	332
Belgium	563
Denmark	494
France	8,025
West Germany	4,220
Greece	249
Ireland	108
Italy	4,663
Netherlands	1,044
Norway	139
Portugal	333
Spain	3,965
Sweden	346
U. K.	2,717
Yugoslavia	101
Oceania	
Australia	1,562
New Zealand	154

Note—These data represent all cases reported to the World Health Organization from the onset of the AIDS epidemic to December 31, 1989. The accuracy and timelines of the reports are depend on the responsible agency in each reporting country.

Source:

Weekly Epidemiological Record 65:1–2, 1990.

TABLE 3.—Acquired Immunodeficiency Syndrome (AIDS) in the United States

Adult/Adolescent Exposure Category	Male 1988 No.	Male 1988 (%)	Male 1989 No.	Male 1989 (%)	Females 1988 No.	Females 1988 (%)	Females 1989 No.	Females 1989 (%)	Totals 1988 No.	Totals 1988 (%)	Totals 1989 No.	Totals 1989 (%)	Cumulative total* No.	Cumulative total* (%)
Male homosexual/bisexual contact	18,130	(64)	19,652	(63)	—		—		18,130	(57)	19,652	(57)	70,083	(61)
Intravenous (IV) drug use (female and heterosexual male)	5,828	(21)	6,139	(20)	1,752	(53)	1,831	(50)	7,580	(24)	7,970	(23)	24,212	(21)
Male homosexual/bisexual contact and IV drug use	2,129	(8)	2,138	(7)	—		—		2,129	(7)	2,138	(6)	8,117	(7)
Hemophilia/coagulation disorder	295	(1)	286	(1)	5	(0)	9	(0)	300	(1)	295	(1)	1,062	(1)
Heterosexual contact†	605	(2)	782	(3)	998	(30)	1,172	(32)	1,603	(5)	1,954	(6)	5,630	(5)
Receipt of blood transfusion, blood components, or tissue‡	524	(2)	467	(2)	345	(11)	301	(8)	869	(3)	768	(2)	2,830	(2)
Other/undermined§	809	(3)	1,508	(5)	181	(6)	313	(9)	990	(3)	1,821	(5)	3,842	(3)

Adult/adolescent subtotal	28,320	(100)	30,972	(100)	3,281	(100)	3,626	(100)	31,601	(100)	34,598	(100)	115,786	(100)
Pediatric (<13 Years Old) Exposure Category														
Hemophilia/coagulation disorder	39	(12)	25	(7)	—		1	(0)	39	(7)	26	(4)	106	(5)
Mother with/at risk for HIV infection	237	(71)	273	(81)	231	(89)	274	(90)	468	(79)	547	(85)	1,614	(81)
Receipt of blood transfusion, blood components, or tissue	47	(14)	25	(70)	19	(7)	15	(5)	66	(11)	40	(6)	212	(11)
Undetermined	11	(3)	12	(4)	11	(4)	15	(5)	22	(4)	27	(4)	63	(3)
Pediatric subtotal	334	(100)	335	(100)	261	(100)	305	(100)	595	(100)	640	(100)	1,995	(100)
Total	28,654		31,307		3,542		3,931		32,196		35,238		117,781	

*Includes 3 patients known to be infected with HIV-2.

†Pattern II transmission is observed in areas of central, eastern, and southern Africa and in some Caribbean countries. In these countries most of the reported cases occur in heterosexuals, and the male-to-female ratio is approximately 1:1. Intravenous drug use and homosexual transmission either do not occur, or occur at a low level.

‡Includes 6 transfusion recipients who received blood screened for HIV antibody and 1 tissue recipient.

§"Other" refers to 2 health-care workers who seroconverted to HIV and contracted AIDS after occupational exposure to HIV-infected blood. "Undetermined" refers to patients whose mode of exposure to HIV is unknown, i.e., patients under investigation; patients who died, were lost to follow-up, or refused interview; and patients whose mode of exposure to HIV remains undetermined after investigation.

Source:

Centers for Disease Control, *HIV/AIDS Surveillance Report,* January 1–22, 1990.

TABLE 4.—Incidence Rate of Melanoma, United States Whites

1987	11.2 per 100,000 population
1982	9.4 per 100,000 population
1977	8.0 per 100,000 population
1970	4.5 per 100,000 population

Note.—Incident cases are those that are newly diagnosed. Estimates are age-adjusted and based on surveillance of cancer morbidity among approximately 10% of the United States population.

Sources:

1987 Annual Cancer Statistics Review. Bethesda, Md, National Cancer Institute, 1988. NIH Publication No. 88–2789.

Cutler SJ, Young JL: *Third National Cancer Survey: Incidence Data.* Bethesda, Md, National Cancer Institute, 1975, NIH Publication No. 75:787.

Surveillance, Epidemiology, and End Results Program, unpublished data.

TABLE 5.—Malignant Melanoma 5-Year Survival Rate, United States

Year of Diagnosis	All Stages	Stage I
1979–1984	80%	90%
1970–1973	69%	83%
1960–1964	63%	79%
1950–1954	49%	71%

Source:

1987 Annual Cancer Statistics Review. Bethesda, Md, National Cancer Institute, 1988.

TABLE 6.—Melanoma Deaths, United States

	Number of Deaths
Year	Melanoma
1989	6,300*
1986	5,673
1976	4,181
1966	2,716
1956	1,786

*Estimate.

Sources:

McKay FW, Hanson MR, Miller RW: Cancer mortality in the United States: 1950–1977. *Natl Cancer Inst Monogr* 59:222, 1982.

National Center for Health Statistics: *Vital Statistics of the United States, 1986;* vol II, Mortality, Part A. Washington DC, United States Government Printing Office, 1988. Dept. of Health and Human Services. PHS Publication No. 88–1122.

Silverberg E, Lubera JA: Cancer Statistics, 1990. *CA* 40:9–26, 1990.

TABLE 7.—Mycosis Fungoides 5-Year Survival Rate by Age and Race, All Stages, United States

	Race	
Age	White	Black
<50	84%	65%
50–59	77%	47%
60–69	63%	48%
<70+	40%	34%

Note.—Excludes patients with previous malignancies.

Source:

Weinstock MA, Horm, JW: Population based estimate of survival and determinants of prognosis in patients with mycosis fungoides. *Cancer* 62:1658, 1988.

TABLE 8.—Contact Dermatitis in North America: Patch Test Results From the North American Contact Dermatitis Research Group, August 1987–July 1989

			% of positive tests relevant		
	N	% Positive	Present	Past	Total
Nickel sulfate, 2.5% pet.	2,308	7.3	49	38	87
Potassium dichromate, 0.25% pet.	2,431	1.9	61	8	69
Benzocaine 5% pet.	2,442	1.3	25	34	59
Rosin 20% pet.	2,433	1.8	26	23	49
Diazolidinyl urea 1% pet.	2,444	1.3	54	4	58
Paraphenylenediamine 1% pet.	2,389	3.6	49	16	65
Imidazolidinyl urea 2% aq.	2,448	1.1	55	0	55
Cinnamic alcohol 5% pet.	2,382	3.9	44	11	55
Benzoyl peroxide 1% pet.	2,429	1.9	11	15	26
Wool wax alcohol (lanolin) 30% pet.	2,437	1.6	73	10	83
Carba mix 3% pet.	2,416	2.5	64	12	76
Neomycin sulfate 20% pet.	2,420	2.3	41	30	71
Thiuram mix 1% pet.	2,372	4.4	79	9	88
Formaldehyde 1% aq.	2,388	3.7	54	4	58
Ethylenediamine dihydrochloride 1% pet.	2,430	1.9	12	35	47
Epoxy resin 1% pet.	2,431	1.9	57	20	77
Quaternium 15 2% pet.	2,378	4.1	60	9	69
Para-tert.-butylphenol formaldehyde resin 1% pet.	2,446	1.2	54	0	54
Black rubber mix (PPD Mix) 0.6%	2,446	1.2	50	4	54
Thimerosal 0.12 pet.	2,350	5.4	14	25	39
Balsam of Peru 25% pet.	2,383	3.9	33	14	47
Diaminodiphenyl-methane 0.5% pet.	2,433	1.8	20	6	26
Mercaptobenzothiazole	2,441	1.4	79	6	15

Source:

Nethercott JR: North American Contact Dermatitis Research Group, personal communication.

TABLE 9.—Contact Dermatology in Belgium.
Proportion of Positive Patch Tests to Standard Chemicals in 1,086 Patients Tested in 1989*

1. Nickel sulfate, 34%
2. Fragrance mix, 10%
3. Cobalt chloride, 10%
4. Balsam of Peru, 9.5%
5. Potassium dichromate, 7%
6. Colophony, 7%
7. Paraphenylenediamine, 5%
8. Wool alcohols, 5%
9. Neomycin sulfate, 4%
10. Thiuram derivatives, 3%
11. Cl + Me-isothiazolinone, 3%
12. Para-tertiary-butyl phenol-formaldehyde resin, 2%
13. Ethylenediamine hydrochloride, 2%
14. Parabens, 2%
15. PPD (black rubber) mix, 1%
16. Benzocaine, 1%
17. Epoxy resin, 1%
18. Sterosan vioform, 1%
19. Formaldehyde, 1%
20. Mercaptobenzothiazole*, 1%
21. Mercapto mix, 1%
22. Primin, 0.2%
23. Quaternium 15, 0.2%

*Of the patients tested, 607 had at least 1 positive reaction.
Note.—Tests were done according to ICDRG and EECDRG guidelines. (See Andersen KE, Burrows D, Cronin E, et al: Recommended changes to standard series. *Contact Dermatitis* 19:389, 1988.) Carba mix has been withdrawn and mercaptobenzothiazole has been added to the standard series.
Source:
Doons-Goossens A: University of Sitarie Ziekenhuizen, Leuven, Belgium, personal communication.

TABLE 10.—Contact Dermatitis, Italy (GIRDCA* Data): Proportion of Positive Patch Tests to Standard Chemicals Among 24,130 Patients With at Least 1 Positive Patch Test, 1984–1988

1. Nickel sulfate, 33%
2. Potassium dichromate, 10.5%
3. Cobalt chloride, 9%
4. Fragrance mix, 7%
5. Balsam of Peru, 5%
6. Ethylenediamine hydrochloride, 4.5%
7. Diaminodiphenylmethane, 4%
8. Paraphenylenediamine, 3.5%
9. Thiuram mix, 3%
10. PPD (black rubber) mix, 2.2%
11. Carba mix, 2.2%
12. Colophony, 2%
13. Neomycin sulfate, 2%
14. Para-tert-butyl phenolformaldehyde resin, 1.6%
15. Benzocaine, 1.6%
16. Formaldehyde, 1.5%
17. Parabens, 1.5%
18. Ammoniated mercury, 1.3%
19. Wool alcohols, 1.3%
20. Mercapto mix, 1%
21. Epoxy resin, 1%
22. Mercaptobenzothiazole, 1%
23. Quinoline mix, 0.7%
24. Imidazolydinylurea, 0.6%
25. Quaternium 15, 0.6%
26. Turpentine peroxides, 0.3%

*GIRDCA: Gruppo Italiano Ricerca Dermatiti da Contatto e Ambientali.

Sources:

Sertoli A, Gola M: *Semin Dermatol* 8:120–126, 1989.

Sertoli A, Personal communication.

TABLE 11.—Nonfederal Dermatologists by Age and Sex, January 1, 1988

	Sex		
Age Group	Males	Females	Total
younger than 35	774	565	1,339
35–44	1,858	469	2,327
45–54	1,416	161	1,577
55–64	799	58	857
65 and older	594	30	624
Total	5,441	1,283	6,724

Source:

Physician Characteristics and Distribution in the U.S., 1988. Chicago, American Medical Association, 1988.

TABLE 12.—Distribution of Dermatologists per Million Population in the United States (Actual Number in Parentheses)

State	1968		1978		1988	
Alabama	12	(41)	14	(52)	20	(80)
Alaska	4	(1)	0	(0)	10	(5)
Arizona	17	(28)	27	(62)	27	(91)
Arkansas	12	(23)	15	(33)	19	(45)
California	26	(507)	34	(737)	39	(1,067)
Colorado	17	(33)	21	(56)	25	(83)
Connecticut	23	(68)	28	(88)	38	(123)
Delaware	13	(7)	15	(9)	20	(13)
District of Columbia	47	(38)	45	(31)	60	(37)
Florida	17	(100)	27	(230)	33	(394)
Georgia	12	(52)	20	(100)	24	(147)
Hawaii	24	(18)	26	(23)	30	(32)
Idaho	7	(5)	13	(11)	15	(15)
Illinois	16	(179)	18	(203)	24	(273)
Indiana	10	(52)	13	(71)	17	(93)
Iowa	12	(34)	15	(44)	23	(66)
Kansas	6	(14)	11	(26)	14	(35)
Kentucky	7	(21)	15	(51)	19	(72)
Louisiana	16	(57)	22	(85)	30	(132)
Maine	8	(8)	11	(12)	13	(15)
Maryland	12	(46)	24	(101)	36	(165)
Massachusetts	26	(142)	26	(153)	38	(223)
Michigan	18	(153)	19	(176)	26	(238)
Minnesota	21	(75)	21	(85)	26	(110)
Mississippi	8	(18)	10	(23)	11	(30)
Missouri	16	(74)	18	(86)	22	(110)
Montana	9	(6)	18	(14)	19	(15)
Nebraska	8	(12)	13	(21)	14	(22)
Nevada	14	(6)	21	(13)	20	(20)
New Hampshire	16	(11)	25	(21)	26	(27)
New Jersey	19	(134)	22	(164)	30	(233)
New Mexico	10	(10)	18	(22)	25	(37)
New York	29	(531)	28	(500)	38	(674)
North Carolina	12	(58)	19	(107)	25	(162)
North Dakota	9	(6)	15	(10)	28	(19)
Ohio	15	(160)	16	(173)	24	(258)
Oklahoma	14	(35)	14	(40)	16	(51)
Oregon	26	(51)	25	(60)	31	(84)
Pennsylvania	18	(214)	19	(222)	26	(315)
Rhode Island	18	(16)	28	(26)	35	(35)
South Carolina	5	(14)	11	(33)	20	(68)
South Dakota	7	(5)	12	(8)	16	(11)
Tennessee	9	(36)	14	(62)	20	(96)
Texas	14	(156)	18	(229)	22	(372)
Utah	13	(13)	18	(23)	24	(41)
Vermont	14	(6)	12	(6)	24	(13)
Virginia	14	(64)	20	(103)	25	(145)
Washington	14	(43)	23	(84)	27	(121)
West Virginia	9	(16)	13	(24)	13	(24)
Wisconsin	15	(64)	19	(88)	24	(113)
Wyoming	6	(2)	7	(3)	6	(3)
Total	18	(3,490)	21	(4,650)	28	(6,724)

Note.—includes professionally active nonfederal dermatologists on January 1 of the indicated year.

Sources:

Distribution of Physicians, Hospitals, and Hospital Beds in the U.S., 1967. Chicago, American Medical Association, 1968.

Physician Distribution and Medical Licensure in the U.S., 1977. Chicago, American Medical Association, 1979.

Physician Characteristics and Distribution in the U.S., 1988. Chicago, American Medical Association, 1988.

TABLE 13.—Dermatology Trainees in the United States

Year Residency to Be Completed	Number of Physicians
1992	315
1991	292
1990	281

Source:
Stluka TH: American Academy of Dermatology, personal communication.

TABLE 14.—Diplomates Certified by the American Board of Dermatology

Year	Average Number Per Year
1989	288
1988	264
1983–1987	270
1973–1977	265
1963–1967	102
1953–1957	76
1943–1947	56
1933–1937	77
Total 1933 through 1989	8,080

Source:
Livingood CS: American Board of Dermatology, personal communication.

TABLE 15.—Enrollment in Health Maintenance Organizations (HMOs) in the United States

Year	Number of HMOs	Number Enrolled	% of Population
1989	590	32,492,784	13.1
1988	643	31,366,031	12.8
1987	662	28,587,119	11.8
1986	595	23,663,626	9.8
1985	393	18,893,607	7.9
1984	305	15,128,500	6.4
1979	215	8,226,053	3.7

Sources:
Group Health Association of America, personal communication.
Interstudy, personal communication.
U.S. Bureau of the Census: *Statistical Abstract of the United States: 1989*, ed 109. Washington DC, 1989.
U.S. Bureau of the Census: *Statistical Abstract of the United States: 1982–1983*, ed 103. Washington DC, 1982.

TABLE 16.—Outpatient Visits to U.S. Dermatologists by Diagnosis*

Diagnosis	Proportion of All Visits Attributed to This Diagnosis		
	1985	1980	1975
Acne vulgaris	19%	28%	22%
Eczematous dermatitis*	9%	9%	11%
Warts†	9%	9%	8%
Skin cancer	6%	5%	6%
Benign neoplasms of the skin	5%	3%	3%
Psoriasis‡	5%	5%	3%
Fungal infections of the skin	4%	4%	3%
Hair disorders	3%	4%	1%
Bacterial infections of the skin	2%	1%	2%

Note.—All data are estimates on a probability sample survey of office-based nonfederally employed physicians in the continental United States.

*Contact dermatitis, atopic dermatitis, and related disorders (ICD codes 691 and 692).

†Excludes visits for condylomata.

‡Excludes visits for psoriatic arthritis.

Source:

Gagnon RD, National Ambulatory Medical Care Survey, personal communication.

TABEL 17—Dermatologic Procedures Performed by General Internists

	Punch Biopsy	Electrosurgical or Cyrosurgical Removal of Skin Lesions
	% Who Perform Procedure	
Location of Practice		
Rural	50%	39%
Small city (<25,000)	32%	32%
Large city (>25,000)	18%	22%
Year of MD degree		
Before 1972	16%	21%
1972 or later	29%	27%
Overall	22%	24%
Mean number done during previous year	8.6	35.4

Source:

Wigton RS, Nicolas JA, Blank BA: Procedural skills of the general internist: A survey of 2,500 physicians. *Ann Intern Med* 111:1023, 1989. The survey was mailed in December 1986.

TABLE 18—Results of the American Academy of Dermatology Skin Cancer Screening Program

		Diagnosis Suspected			
Year	No. Screened	Precancerous Lesions	Basal Cell Carcinoma	Squamous Cell Carcinoma	Malignant Melanoma
1989	78,486	21,887	6,266	761	593
1988	67,124	14,494	4,457	474	435
1987	41,649	9,136	2,798	302	257
1986	41,486	10,366	3,049	398	262
1985	32,000	2,479	1,056	163	97
Total	260,745	58,362	17,626	2,098	1,644

Source:

American Academy of Dermatology, personal communication.

TABLE 19.—Leading Dermatology Journals

Journal	IIMPACT FACTOR 1988	1983	1978	NO. OF ARTICLES PUBLISHED* 1988
Journal of Investigative Dermatology	3.5	2.8	2.0	240
Archives of Dermatology	2.0	1.9	1.9	194
Journal of the American Academy of Dermatology	1.8	1.7	†	289
British Journal of Dermatology	1.8	1.9	1.2	212
Contact Dermatitis	1.0	0.5	0.3	251
American Journal of Dermatopathology	0.9	1.1	†	70
Archives of Dermatological Research	0.8	1.1	1.0	107
Acta Dermato-venereologica	0.8	0.8	1.1	112
Dermatologica	0.8	0.7	0.6	121
Journal of Cutaneous Pathology	0.8	0.6	0.5	61
International Journal of Dermatology	0.7	0.6	0.3	174
Clinical and Experimental Dermatology	0.6	0.6	0.3	105
Photodermatology	0.6	†	†	45
Journal of Dermatological Surgery and Oncology	0.6	0.6	†	121
Hautarzt	0.5	0.3	0.6	140

Notes.—This table lists in order the 15 dermatology journals with the highest 1988 "impact factor." The 1988 impact factor of a journal is the average number of instances (per article) in which an article published by the journal in 1987 or 1986 was cited in 1988 by any journal indexed by the Institute for Scientific Information. The 1983 "impact factor" is the average number of times an article from 1982 or 1981 was cited in 1983. The 1978 "impact factor" is similarly defined.

*Includes orginal articles, technical notes, and review articles.

†not available.

Sources:

Garfield E: *SCI Journal Citation Reports: A Bibliometric Analysis of Science Journals in the ISI Database.* Philadelphia, Institute for Scientific Information 1989, 1984, and 1979.

Institute for Scientific Information, personal communication.

1 Acne and Related Disorders

Acne in Schoolchildren: No Longer a Concern for Dermatologists
Rademaker M, Garioch JJ, Simpson NB (Glasgow Royal Infirmary)
Br Med J 298:1217–1220, May 6, 1989 1–1

Because experience with recruitment for clinical research suggested that the severity of acne may have decreased, the prevalence and severity of this disease were examined in a random selection of schoolchildren in Glasgow who represented all socioeconomic groups. Children completed questionnaires and underwent facial examinations by 2 physicians; severity was assessed by an established scoring system.

In boys the prevalence of acne at age 12 years was 40%, increasing to 95% at age 16; the prevalence in girls was 61% at 12 years and 83% at 16. Grades of acne of 1 or higher, on a scale of 0–10, were found in only 1.8% of boys and 0.3% of girls; minimal (grade 0.05 to 0.375) acne was the most common. The source of advice on treatment usually was the student's family, with 15% of boys and 17% of girls visiting the family physician solely for acne treatment. Of these, only 5 students had seen a dermatologist.

A comparison of these results with those from 20 years earlier showed that acne has decreased in prevalance and severity. Wider use of over-the-counter preparations and better treatment by general practitioners probably account for this decline. Other than being a source of education for primary health care workers, the dermatologist has only a small role in acne management for school-aged children.

▶ The title of this article suggests an unsettling ambiguity that is not clarified until one reads the entire article. What the authors have concluded from their population survey, in spite of no really adequate comparison database, is that the severity of acne is less than it used to be (in Glasgow schoolchildren), with also an "apparent" (but actually much less so) decline in prevalence. They attribute all of this to better self-care, self-medication, advice from druggists, and to treatment by nondermatologist physicians, hence an explanation for the authors' somewhat misleading article title.—P.E. Pochi, M.D.

Clinical Markers of Androgenicity in Acne Vulgaris
Sheehan-Dare RA, Hughes BR, Cunliffe WJ (The Gen Infirmary, Leeds, England)
Br J Dermatol 119:723–730, December 1988 1–2

The pathogenesis of acne vulgaris is incomplete, although it is known that androgenic stimulation of sebaceous glands is necessary for its development. Because most patients with acne attending dermatology clinics do not have other features of androgenicity (e.g., hirsutism, menstrual irregularity, or amenorrhea), the relationship between acne severity and clinical markers of hyperandrogenism was studied in 268 females aged 12–44 years. They were divided into 3 groups by acne severity: physiologic or no acne, moderate acne, and severe acne. The data were analyzed using one-way analysis of variance and chi square tests.

Of the 268 patients, 190 had not received hormonal therapy; 5 of 77 who were in the physiologic acne range had no acne, 68 had moderate acne, and 45 had severe acne. No significant differences in age at menarche or incidence of menstrual irregularity or amenorrhea were observed among the 3 groups. Reports of excessive body hair or clinical hirsutism were similarly low in all 3 groups. No significant correlation was found between acne and hirsute grades. Female pattern androgenic alopecia was found in 2 patients with moderate acne. Male pattern androgenic alopecia grade 2a was observed in similar proportions in all 3 groups.

Of 78 women who had received hormonal therapy, 62 had taken oral contraceptives and 16 had antiandrogen therapy. Of the 78, 26 had physiologic, 24 moderate, and 28 severe acne. The mean age at menarche was similar to that in women not receiving hormonal therapy. Compared with those not receiving hormonal therapy, menstrual irregularities and excessive body hair before hormonal therapy were similar in frequency.

There was no correlation between acne severity and clinical markers of androgenicity. Further, most women with acne had no abnormality in other androgen target organs, indicating that the increased sebaceous gland activity occurring in acne is not a result of hyperandrogenemia; other factors may be operative. A possible explanation may be an abnormal response of the pilosebaceous unit to normal circulating androgens.

▶ The results of this study confirm the general impression of most dermatologists, namely, that women with acne do not frequently exhibit other androgenic manifestations. This report found no differences in the incidence of such clinical signs among 3 groups of women with acne varying from "physiologic" to severe, but there was no non-acne control group in which a lower prevalence of hirsutism, irregular menses, and so on might have been encountered.—P.E. Pochi, M.D.

Acne Vulgaris and Malignancy

Sheehan-Dare RA, Cunliffe WJ, Simmons AV, Child JA, McKinney PA, Cartwright RA (Gen Infirmary; St James Univ Hosp; Univ of Leeds, England)

Br J Dermatol 119:669–673, November 1988 1–3

If persons with acne, by virtue of increased exposure or responsiveness to *Propionibacterium acnes*, have enhanced immune function, it would be expected that individuals in whom malignant disease develops during adolescence or early adulthood would have less acne or less severe acne than normal persons. The frequency and severity of acne were investigated in 70 patients with lymphomas and leukemias, Hodgkin's disease, non-Hodgkin's lymphoma, acute myeloid leukemia, acute lymphoblastic leukemia, and chronic granulocytic leukemia. The mean age at diagnosis was 23.4 years. Seventy matched controls were studied for comparison.

A history of acne was less common among patients than among matched controls, and physical examination showed fewer patients than controls with acne. Also, fewer patients than controls had received treatment prescribed by a medical practitioner for their acne.

These findings suggest that there is a reduced incidence of acne, or its more severe forms, among patients with lymphomas and leukemias. Therefore, increased exposure or response by *P. acnes,* as appears to occur with acne, may confer protection against malignant disease.

▶ Shuster's provocative hypothesis, advanced in 1976, that *P. acnes* (which is identical to *Corynebacterium parvum,* an experimental immunoadjuvant) might protect against the development of infections and neoplasms, and that this protection might be enhanced in individuals with acne in whom *P. acnes* is usually more abundant, led the authors of this report to examine patients with lymphomas and leukemias in an effort to determine whether acne was or had been less prevalent in this group. The only "positive" finding was that these cancer patients had been treated previously for acne somewhat less frequently than had noncancer subjects. This information was gleaned from questionnaires, with a further inherent weakness admitted to the authors, i.e., that there was no information of any socioeconomic differences between the 2 groups that might have prompted professional care to be sought by one group and not by another.

A corollary of this putative association, and only barely and obliquely hinted at by the authors at the conclusion of their article, is the effect chronic antibiotic therapy for acne or other conditions would have, or for that matter even the short-term severe reduction of *P. acnes* as a result of oral isotretinoin treatment. These intriguing issues are deserving of further inquiry.—P.E. Pochi, M.D.

Prior X-Ray Therapy for Acne Related to Tumors of the Parotid Gland

Preston-Martin S (Univ of Southern California, Los Angeles)

Arch Dermatol 125:921–924, July 1989 1–4

An epidemiologic case-control study of tumors of the parotid gland was conducted to test the hypothesis that the development of these tumors is related to radiation exposure during previous x-ray treatment for acne. The study population consisted of patients with a histologically confirmed tumor of the parotid gland, as identified by the University of Southern California Cancer Surveillance Program. Of 531 eligible patients with parotid tumors diagnosed from 1976 through 1984, 430 completed interviews with the investigators. The control population consisted of neighborhood persons who were matched individually for sex, race, and age. After exclusions for various reasons, the data of 408 case-control pairs were analyzed. Of the 408 patients, 269 had benign tumors of the parotid gland and 139 had malignant tumors. None of the controls had a parotid tumor.

Malignant tumors of the parotid gland were strongly associated with radiation treatment to the head 5 or more years before diagnosis. For benign tumors, the association with previous irradiation was less strong and not statistically significant. Radiation treatment had been administered as early as 1929 and as recently as 1975. Patients had undergone a median of 12 x-ray treatments, and controls a median of 8. A dose-response analysis confirmed that the risk for malignant parotid tumors was increased with an increasing number of x-ray treatments.

Clinicians who still use irradiation in the treatment of acne, as well as those who care for patients with a history of radiation therapy for acne, should be aware of the additional risk for the development of parotid gland tumors associated with such treatment.

▶ This population-based study confirms the results of earlier reports showing that x-ray treatment of acne increases the risk of parotid gland tumors. Such neoplasms result only from ionizing radiation. Although the use of superficial x-ray therapy for acne has declined in the past 20–25 years to nearly zero usage now, the latent period before a tumor appears may be decades, so that dermatologists will still be seeing many patients who have received x-ray treatment in the past. The history is most important in this regard, not only because of the complication of parotid tumor development discussed in this report, but also because of the possible development of thyroid tumors and, of course, skin malignancies.—P.E. Pochi, M.D.

Azelaic Acid for the Treatment of Acne: A Clinical Comparison With Oral Tetracycline

Hjorth N, Graupe K (Univ of Copenhagen; Schering Aktiengesellschaft, Berlin)

Acta Derm Venereol (suppl) 143:45–48, 1989 1–5

The therapeutic effect of azelaic acid cream on acne has been attributed to its antimicrobial activity. The efficacy of azelaic acid cream was compared with that of orally administered tetracycline in 2 randomized, multicenter studies. The first study included 333 patients who had mostly papulopustular acne with a severity grade of II/III; the second study included 261 patients with acne conglobata or nodulocystic or papulopustulosa nodosa acne. The tetracycline-treated groups in both studies received a dosage of 1 g/day at first and then gradually lesser amounts, as well as the cream base of the azelaic acid. In the groups given azelaic acid in both studies, the dosage was 20% azelaic acid cream twice daily, as well as placebo capsules.

After 5 months, patients with moderate acne given azelaic acid and those given tetracycline had similar reductions in the median number of inflamed lesions and in total lesion count and in percentage reduction in lesion count. Time-response relationships were similar with both treat-

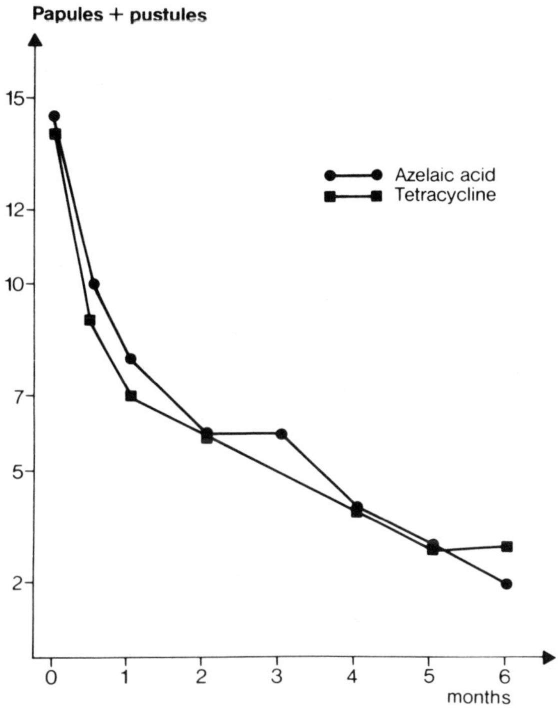

Fig 1–1.—Reduction of inflamed facial papules and pustules during treatment of severe acne. The numbers given at each visit are median values. *Circles* indicate treatment with azelaic acid (n = 126); *squares*, treatment with tetracycline (n = 135). (Courtesy of Hjorth N, Graupe K: *Acta Derm Venereol* (suppl) 143:45–48, 1989.)

ments. In patients with more severe acne, the magnitude of response and time course (Fig 1–1) were similar to those in the other study. Azelaic acid was generally well tolerated.

In inflammatory acne, the 20% azelaic acid cream is therapeutically effective, with results similar to those achieved with orally administered tetracycline. For lesions on the back, a combination of topical and systemic treatment is advisable.

▶ This study, comparing topical azelaic acid and oral tetracycline in acne, is similar in many respects to one reported previously (1). The results obtained were also similar, whereby azelaic acid and tetracycline were shown to be equally effective. The findings of the present study are even more impressive, as they involved nearly 600 acne patients in a multicenter investigative trial and showed an 85% reduction in facial inflammatory lesions with both modalities. However, one drawback, shared with the earlier study, is that there was no placebo group included, so that the actual improvement attributable to the active drug moieties could not be determined.—P.E. Pochi, M.D.

Reference

1. Bladon PT, et al: *Br J Dermatol* 114:493, 1986.

A Comparative Study of Benzoyl Peroxide and Clindamycin Phosphate for Treating Acne Vulgaris

Swinyer LJ, Baker MD, Swinyer TA, Mills OH Jr (Univ of Utah; Owen Labs, Fort Worth, Tex; Robert Wood Johnson Med School, New Brunswick, NJ)
Br J Dermatol 119:615–622, November 1988 1–6

The efficacy of benzoyl peroxide was compared with that of 1% clindamycin phosphate in the treatment of 60 patients with mild to moderate acne vulgaris. The skin surface parameters of oiliness, erythema, peeling, and dryness were evaluated. The patients were randomly assigned to either treatment, and returned for follow-up 2, 4, 8, and 12 weeks after initial evaluation. All 60 patients completed the 12-week study; none missed any visits.

Both treatments reduced the number of comedones; however, results with benzoyl peroxide were significantly better at 2-, 8-, and 12-week evaluations (Fig 1–2). Both treatments effectively reduced inflamed lesions, but the results were not significantly different; benzoyl peroxide tended to be more effective. Total lesions in both groups were reduced beginning with the fourth week. Significant differences between treatment groups were not seen until week 12, by which time benzoyl peroxide therapy had reduced the total number of lesions by 59.8%, whereas clindamycin had reduced the total by 34.3%. There were no adverse effects with either treatment. Oiliness remained constant with clindamycin, but decreased significantly with benzoyl peroxide. There were no differences in erythema between groups. Peeling was significantly less among patients given clindamycin. Dryness was also significantly less in the clindamycin-treated group at weeks 2, 4, and 8, but there was no significant difference between groups at week 12.

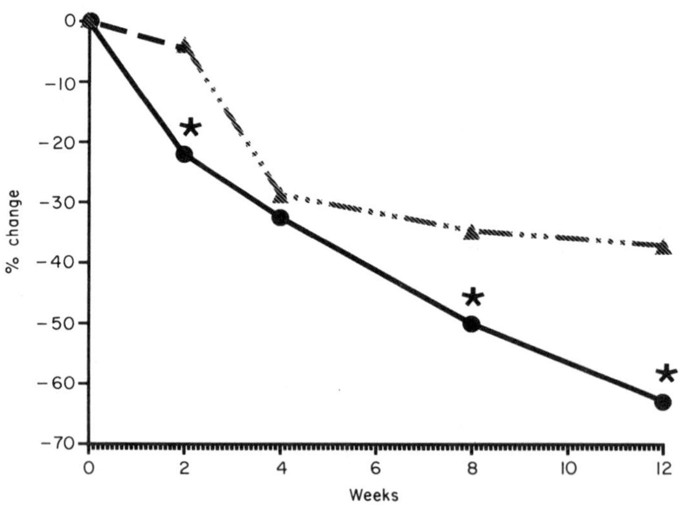

Fig 1–2.—Mean percentage change from baseline in numbers of noninflamed lesions in acne patients treated with benzoyl peroxide *(circles)* or clindamycin phosphate *(triangles)*. *Significant difference between the 2 treatments (Courtesy of Swinyer LJ, Baker MD, Swinyer TA, et al: *Br J Dermatol* 119:615–622, November 1988.)

Both benzoyl peroxide and clindamycin phosphate significantly reduced lesion counts in patients with mild to moderate acne vulgaris over 12 weeks. However, benzoyl peroxide produced a significantly greater reduction. Clindamycin phosphate had a milder effect on the skin surface.

▶ The outcome of this study speaks for itself. In the article's introduction, the authors make note of a plethora of reports on the effect of benzoyl peroxide and topical antibiotics in acne. But probably none among them include a study of patients using both benzoyl peroxide and clindamycin phosphate, something that is surely done frequently in clinical practice, particularly when one considers that the mechanism of the antibacterial action of each drug is different.— P.E. Pochi, M.D.

A Double-Blind Clinical Trial With a Lotion Containing 5% Benzoyl Peroxide and 2% Miconazole in Patients With Acne Vulgaris

Mesquita-Guimarães J, Ramos S, Tavares MR, Carvalho MR (Faculty of Medicine and Hosp S João, Porto, Portugal)

Clin Exp Dermatol 14:357–360, September 1989 1–7

Both benzoyl peroxide alone and a miconazole-benzoyl peroxide combination applied topically are effective against acne vulgaris. In a controlled, randomized, double-blind study the effectiveness of a lotion containing 5% benzoyl peroxide and 2% miconazole was compared with that of a control preparation containing only 2% benzoyl peroxide in patients with inflammatory or comedonal acne. The lotions were applied once a day for the first week and then twice daily through day 45.

The 2 lotions had similar effects in patients with comedonal acne. In patients with inflammatory acne, the combination lotion was significantly more effective at day 30, with a 66% reduction in number of lesions, than the single-ingredient lotion, with which the reduction was 37%. A difference remained at day 45, but it was no longer significant. Adverse effects, including erythema, itching, and moderate exfoliation, were similar with both regimens.

These results suggest that combination treatment has a therapeutic role in acne vulgaris. Imidazole compounds reduce lipase activity and act against *Propionibacterium acnes* and *Staphylococcus* organisms in vitro. A synergistic effect has been reported when benzoyl peroxide and miconazole are used together.

▶ This is yet another, and probably not the last, article to be published on the benzoyl peroxide-miconazole treatment of acne. Several previously published studies have similarly purported to show that the combination is superior to benzoyl peroxide alone, but not very convincingly so. Although this was a double-blind controlled study, only 15 acne patients comprised each of the 2 treatment groups. The finding that the benzoyl peroxide-miconazole combination was statistically superior to benzoyl peroxide alone at 30 days but not at 45 days raises serious questions as to the validity of the claimed benefit.—P.E. Pochi, M.D.

Erythromycin Resistant Propionibacteria in Antibiotic Treated Acne patients: Association With Therapeutic Failure

Eady EA, Cove JH, Holland KT, Cunliffe WJ (Univ of Leeds; Leeds Gen Infirmary, England)

Br J Dermatol 121:51–57, July 1989 1–8

Erythromycin is a second-line drug for use in patients with acne who fail to respond to tetracycline therapy, but resistant isolates of cutaneous propionibacteria have been found in several countries. Microbiologic studies were done in 51 patients given erythromycin in an oral dosage of 500 mg twice daily and in 53 given topical therapy with clindamycin 1%. The patients had been treated for 4 months or longer. Most of those given erythromycin also were using benzoyl peroxide topically, and many clindamycin-treated patients were taking oral drugs as well.

Erythromycin-resistant propionibacteria were isolated from the skin in 47% of erythromycin- or clindamycin-treated patients and in 3% of untreated controls. Patients who responded to the oral form of erythromycin carried resistant organisms less often than those who did not respond or who relapsed. Most resistant isolates were *Propionibacterium acnes* or *Proprionibacterium granulosum.*

Either erythromycin orally or clindamycin topically promotes the development of resistant propionibacteria. The isolates in the present study were phenotypically indistinguishable from most erythromycin-resistant bacteria whose resistance results from methylation of 23S ribosomal RNA.

▶ This article describes one of a series of investigations in recent years by Eady and colleagues that have addressed the problem of the frequent development of erythromycin-resistant strains of *P. acnes* in acne patients treated with oral erythromycin or topical clindamycin. In this study the highest incidence of resistance occurred in patients clinically unresponsive to erythromycin, or in whom the acne had relapsed during drug treatment. The authors' recommendation that oral erythromycin treatment of acne be limited to those patients who have never received the drug (presumably for any purpose) seems unduly restrictive. But their admonition that patients are best treated for no longer than 6 months to permit replacement of the developing resistant organisms by sensitive strains is more reasonable. In fact, it has been my clinical experience that a substantial percentage of patients who respond satisfactorily to oral erythromycin have a relapse of their acne before this time.—P.E. Pochi, M.D.

Incidence of Chloracne Among Chemical Workers Potentially Exposed to Chlorinated Dioxins

Bond GG, McLaren EA, Brenner FE, Cook RR (Dow Chemical Co, Midland, Mich; Dow Chemical USA, Midland, Mich; Dow Chemical Pacific Ltd, Wanchai, Hong Kong)

J Occup Med 31:771–774, September 1989 1–9

Choracne is the only proven consequence of overexposure to chlorinated dioxins. The incidence of chloracne was evaluated in 2,192 chemical workers potentially exposed to chlorinated dioxins during the period 1940–1982.

Among the 2,072 workers with available company medical records, 15.9% had chloracne. The condition developed over a considerable time span, peaking between 1964 and 1979. The incidence was highest among the youngest workers and among those who worked in the production of chlorinated phenols rather than with products derived from those materials. The risk of chloracne increased with total duration of exposure, the highest exposure intensity to 2,3,7,8-tetra-chlorodibenzo-*p*-dioxin (TCDD), and the cumulative dose of exposure to either TCDD or hexa- to octachlorinated dioxins.

The risk of chloracne development in these chemical workers was associated with age at first exposure to dioxin contaminants and with several measures of acute and cumulative exposure to these materials.

▶ This pedestrian account of chloracne in chemical plant workers exposed to chlorinated phenols and derivative compounds cited an incidence of its occurrence in 1 of 6 workers. Little new information emerges from this report on chloracne, a skin disorder most dermatologists have never encountered.— P.E. Pochi, M.D.

An Epidemiological Study of Rosacea

Berg M, Lidén S (Karolinska Sjukhuset, Stockholm)

Acta Derm Venereol (Stockh) 69:419–423, 1989 1–10

The clinical types, prevalence, etiology, and pathogenesis of rosacea were studied in a nonselected population of 809 office workers. Rosacea was diagnosed in 81 patients, for a prevalence of 10%, (table), and most

Age and Sex Distribution of the 81 Individuals (of 809) With Either the Erythematotelangiectatic (ET) or the Papulopustular (PP) Type of Rosacea

Age	ET		PP		Both types	
(years)	Women *n* (%)	Men *n* (%)	Women *n* (%)	Men *n* (%)	Women *n* (%)	Men *n* (%)
–29	1 (3)	0	0	0	1 (3)	0
30–39	10 (9)	5 (5)	0	0	10 (9)	5 (5)
40–49	25 (15)	6 (5)	11 (7)	0	36 (22)	6 (5)
50–59	11 (9)	4 (5)	1 (1)	3 (3)	12 (10)	7 (8)
60–	3 (9)	1 (5)	0	0	3 (9)	1 (5)
total	50 (11)	16 (5)	12 (3)	3 (1)	62 (14)	19 (5)

(Courtesy of Berg M, Lidén S: *Acta Derm Venereol* (Stockh) 69:419–423, 1989.)

patients had a rather mild form of disease. Rosacea was of an erythematotelangiectatic type in 81% of the patients and of a papulopustular type in 19%. Unilateral lesions were noted in 11 patients. Although 17% of patients with rosacea were impaired by sunlight, 26% were improved. In patients with rosacea, 27% had migraine and 42% had a tendency to flush, compared to 13% with migraine and 16% with a tendency to flush in the comparison group. Persons with good pigmentation ability had a tendency to a decreased occurrence of rosacea. The frequency of eye complaints was similar in individuals with and without rosacea.

Rosacea was more prevalent among women; 14% of women and only 5% of men had this disease. Unilateral rashes were not unusual. Flushing and the regulatory mechanism of the blood vessels appear to play a role in the pathogenesis of rosacea.

▶ The population studied by Berg and Lidén is a fair complexioned one with a higher frequency of solar-induced telangiectasias and erythema than would be found in patients with a higher average skin type. Even if all of the erythematotelangiectatic cases were eliminated, a 2% frequency in this normal population would suggest a high prevalence in the population at large. The variable and conflicting response to sunlight has been noted by others; some find sunlight therapeutic, and others find it provocative. Does this suggest that more than 1 type of rosacea exists? Should patients with the erythematotelangiectatic form who worsen with solar exposure be evaluated for lupus erythematosus?—A.J. Sober, M.D.

Rosacea: A Histopathological Study of 75 Cases

Ramelet A-A, Perroulaz G (Centre Hospitalier Universitaire Vaudois, Lausanne, Switzerland)

Ann Dermatol Venereol 115:801–806, 1988 1–11

Rosacea is a common, poorly defined disorder of unknown etiology and variable clinical presentation. Most available studies of rosacea were done to determine whether *Demodex folliculorum* has a role in its etiology. The records of and biopsy materials from 75 patients with confirmed rosacea were reviewed retrospectively. Only those patients for whom the clinical diagnosis agreed with the histopathologic findings were included.

During a 10-year period, rosacea was diagnosed in 41 men aged 23–72 years and 34 women aged 32–68 years. On average, there were 4 tissue sections available per patient. Tissue blocks from 7 patients with granulomatous rosacea were serially sectioned and examined for residual hair follicles, degenerated collagen fibers, and *Demodex* mites. All slides were assessed for degree of elastotic degeneration, vasodilatation, inflammatory infiltration, and the presence of *D. folliculorum*.

All 75 specimens showed elastotic degeneration and vasodilation, ranging in degree from slight to moderate to marked (Fig 1–3). Inflammatory infiltration also occurred consistently. In 62 specimens the infiltrates consisted primarily of lymphohistiocytes. In 6 instances mostly polynuclear neutrophils were found in the infiltrates. Epithelioid infiltrates unrelated to

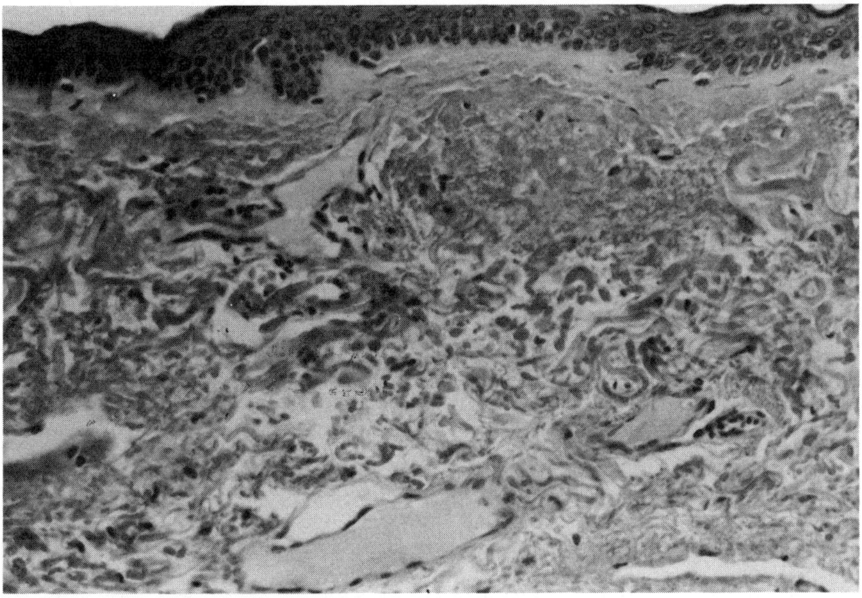

Fig 1–3.—Elastotic degeneration and vasodilatation. (Courtesy of Ramelet A-A, Perroulaz G: *Ann Dermatol Venereol* 115:801–806, 1988.)

a follicle were present in 4 specimens, and those surrounding a follicle-related necrosis in 3. *Demodex* mites were found in only 2 samples, but no follicles were involved. *Demodex* was not found in any of the 7 patients with granulomatous rosacea. The number and appearance of hair follicles were normal for the sites from which the specimens had been removed.

The findings of this histologic study of rosacea point to elastotic degeneration as the initial disease process, followed by vasodilatation and inflammation. The *Demodex* mite does not appear to have a major role in the etiology of rosacea.

▶ This study is of note because the textbook histopathologic description of rosacea is quite nonspecific, and rosacea is usually characterized as an inflammatory disorder of the dermis. The condition affects the central third of the face, thus large biopsy series are lacking; this study's report on 75 patients is noteworthy. The earliest pathophysiologic change in rosacea appears to be instability of the vasculature and manifests with flushing and blushing and subsequently with fixed dilated vessels (telangiectasias). This feature was reflected histopathologically by the presence of vasodilation in all 75 biopsy specimens. Elastotic degeneration, an early feature of all cases, raises the concern that ultraviolet damage may play a role in rosacea. This study appears to exclude *Demodex* as a factor for either rosacea "vulgaris" or granulomatous rosacea. (See also the report by Marks and Harcourt-Webster.)—A.J. Sober, M.D.

Reference

1. Marks R, Harcourt-Webster J-N: *Arch Dermatol* 100:683, 1969.

Unilateral Demodectic Rosacea

Shelley WB, Shelley ED, Burmeister V (Med College of Ohio, Toledo; Univ of Illinois, Peoria)

J Am Acad Dermatol 20:915–917, May 1989 1–12

The 2 mites *Demodex folliculorum* and *Demodex brevis* are present universally in healthy skin and are thought to be harmless. Recent evidence, however, suggests that the mites may occasionally be pathogenic. One patient had chronic dermatitis of the cheek until *Demodex* mites were eliminated.

Man, 36, had been treated without success for rosaceal dermatitis of the right cheek of 4 years' duration. Solar exposure, sweating, and shaving exacerbated the condition. Scrapings of the area showed numerous hair follicle mites in both adult and larval forms. Many follicles were infected with the mites. No *Demodex* organisms were found on unaffected areas of his face. Treatment with 250 mg of metronidazole 3 times a day for 8 months brought improvement, but the patient had a relapse when the drug was discontinued. Crotamiton cream applied daily for 1 month returned the patient's skin to normal except for persistent telangiectasia, which was treated with tetracycline.

Metronidazole controlled this patient's inflammation but did not eliminate the organisms because the drug is not miticidal. Only a miticidal preparation such as crotamiton, which can be tolerated long term, cures the eruption. The dermatitis appears to result from heavy colonization of the mites.

▶ A basic inconsistency in this article is the proposed etiologic role of *Demodex* in this patient who responded to oral metronidazole and relapsed upon its discontinuation. Metronidazole has no direct activity against *Demodex,* thus if metronidazole's effect is therapeutic, such action must be directed against a consequence of the *Demodex* infestation, e.g., counteracting *Demodex*-induced inflammation. (See Abstract 1–11, which fails to find evidence for a *Demodex* etiology in a large series of rosacea cases.) A basic problem may be that rosacea-like eruptions may have diverse etiologies, such as being steroid-induced and the like. Also, it may represent a symptom complex rather than a single disease. In the present case the authors found temporal evidence for the involvement of *Demodex* in a unilateral rosacea-like eruption. The patient received corticosteroids during the 4 years of the eruption, but we are not told the duration of use and whether the steroids were fluorinated.—A.J. Sober, M.D.

Skin Problems in Workers Using Visual Display Terminals: A Study of 201 Patients

Berg M (Karolinska Hosp, Stockholm)

Contact Dermatitis 19:335–341, November 1988 1–13

Skin problems have been reported in visual display terminal (VDT) operators, usually rosacea or a rosacea-like dermatitis. To investigate the possibility that such problems are actually associated with certain physical factors connected with VDT use, studies were made in 201 affected patients.

Of these, 18% claimed that their condition improved overnight and 21% that it improved over the weekend. Twenty-five patients had skin problems mainly on the side of the face commonly turned toward the VDT. Half of the patients had rosacea, but their subjective skin symptoms were generally more severe than those in ordinary cases of rosacea. These patients reported severe pain, itching, and burning. The others had primarily common facial dermatoses, e.g., seborrheic eczema, acne vulgaris, and atopic dermatitis. Skin types did not differ significantly from those of a control population. Eighteen percent had nonspecific skin problems, such as redness and itching.

Attempts to correlate skin problems with the VDTs' electrostatic field strength were unsuccessful because of difficulties in eliminating it. Migraine-like headaches were reported by 40% of patients. At an average follow-up of 8 months, two thirds of the patients had fewer skin complaints.

The 18% of patients with nonspecific skin problems most closely resemble previously reported patients. Follow-up analysis suggested that most patients improve with time, even without treatment.

▶ The latest on this is Berg's thesis published as a supplement to *Acta Dermato-Venereologica* (1). He concludes: "Most patients referred for dermatological examination suspected of having skin disease related to work with VDU's had ordinary facial skin disorders, and half of them had rosacea. Two thirds of them improved without pharmacological therapy in spite of continued work with VDU's. . . . The occurrence of skin disease in VDU-exposed people is entirely coincidental from an epidemiological point of view. An increase in subjective sensations in the skin in people with such work is registered. . . ." This comment would be longer, but my face is beginning to itch. . . .—J.D. Bernhard, M.D.

Reference

1. Berg M: *Acta Derm Venereol (Stockh)* Suppl 150:3–40, 1989.

2 Bacterial and Miscellaneous Infections

Topical Mupirocin Treatment of Impetigo Is Equal to Oral Erythromycin Therapy

Mertz PM, Marshall DA, Eaglstein WH, Piovanetti Y, Montalvo J (Univ of Miami; Dept of Public Health of the City of San Juan, Puerto Rico)
Arch Dermatol 125:1069–1073, August 1989 2–1

Systemic antimicrobial therapy has been much more effective than topically applied antimicrobials in the treatment of skin infections. Mupirocin is a topical antimicrobial with confirmed effectiveness in the treatment of primary skin infections, impetigo, and pyoderma. The effects of topical mupirocin were compared with those of oral erythromycin ethylsuccinate in the treatment of impetigo in 53 clinically and bacteriologically assessable patients, mostly children, each with 1–5 primary impetigo lesions.

All had positive cultures of *Staphylococcus aureus, Streptococcus pyogenes,* or both. Twenty-eight patients aged 6 months to 32 years (mean, 5.7 years) received topical treatment with mupirocin ointment, and 25 patients aged 10 months to 9 years (mean, 5 years) were treated orally with erythromycin. Pretreatment cultures indicated 44 pathogens in the 28 mupirocin-treated patients and 37 pathogens in the 25 erythromycin-treated patients. Lesions were examined clinically and cultured bacteriologically on days 0, 3, and 8, the last day of treatment, and 1 week thereafter.

Cures were achieved in 26 of the 28 mupirocin-treated patients (93%) and in 24 of the 25 erythromycin-treated patients (96%). At the end of the treatment period *S. aureus* was eradicated in 88% of the mupirocin-treated patients and in 37% of the erythromycin-treated patients. The difference was statistically significant. *Streptococcus pyogenes* was eradicated in 89% of the mupirocin-treated patients and in 72% of the erythromycin-treated patients. In the latter group 2 patients had recurrence of *S. aureus* infection at follow-up, and 1 had a recurrence of *S. pyogenes.* None of the mupirocin-treated patients had bacterial recurrences.

Topically applied mupirocin is as effective as orally administered erythromycin in the treatment of cutaneous bacterial infection.

▶ At last, a topical agent that works well against localized impetigo. This article also illustrates the high rate of staph resistance to erythromycin. Erythromycin should not be used when staph infection is suspected and perhaps should not have been used as the comparative agent in this study.—R.S. Stern, M.D.

Topical 2% Mupirocin Versus 2% Fusidic Acid Ointment in the Treatment of Primary and Secondary Skin Infections
Gilbert M (Hôp de L'Enfant-Jésus, Quebec)
J Am Acad Dermatol 20:1083–1087, June 1989 2–2

Mupirocin is the first exclusively topical antibiotic for the treatment of skin infections that has only minimal systemic absorption. It exerts a bactericidal effect against a broad range of gram-positive organisms. Topical mupirocin (Bactroban, 2%) in the treatment of primary and secondary skin infections was compared with fusidic acid (Fucidin) ointment in a double-blind, randomized trial. Of 70 patients, 35 were given mupirocin and 35, fusidic acid, to apply to the affected area 3 times a day for 7 days. *Staphylococcus aureus* and *Streptococcus* species were the most common pathogens.

Of 34 evaluable patients treated with mupirocin, a clinical cure was achieved in 18 and significant improvement was noted in 15. Similarly, of 35 patients treated with fusidic acid, a clinical cure was achieved in 18 and significant improvement in 15. Bacteriologic cure rates were 97% and 87%, respectively. No adverse effects were noted with either treatment.

Topical 2% mupirocin is as effective and safe as topical fusidic acid in the treatment of primary and secondary skin infections. Because it is a novel molecule not related to any available antibiotic, it can be used safely without concern for cross-resistance to other antibiotics. Topical 2% mupirocin is a superior agent for the treatment of superficial skin infections, particularly in a hospital setting.

▶ We have mupirocin; maybe we should have fusidic acid ointment, which to my knowledge is not available in the United States.—R.S. Stern, M.D.

Treatment of Impetigo and Ecthyma: A Comparison of Sulconazole With Miconazole
Nolting S, Strauss WB (Westfälischen Wilhelms Univ, Münster, West Germany; Syntex Research, Palo Alto, Calif)
Int J Dermatol 27:716–719, December 1988 2–3

A previous study of superficial skin infections in children indicated that as many as 98% of the *Staphylococcus aureus* organisms cultured from pyodermal lesions are resistant to penicillin and other antibiotics. The topical form of the antifungal agent sulconazole nitrate works against gram-positive bacteria and other pathogens in vitro. A randomized, double-blind clinical trial compared the antibacterial efficacy and safety of sulconazole nitrate 1% cream with that of miconazole nitrate 2% cream in 80 patients aged 1–74 years with impetigo or ecthyma. Miconazole nitrate is effective against *S. aureus* and streptococci.

Sixty-six patients had impetigo and 14 had ecthyma. They were assigned randomly to 14 days of treatment with either sulconazole or miconazole. Bacterial cultures were taken from all pyodermal lesions that yielded group A β-hemolytic streptococci or pathogenic staphylococci. Cultures were again taken and evaluated on days 4, 7, and 14.

Bacterial cultures from 26 of 32 sulconazole-treated impetigo patients and from 17 of 34 miconazole-treated impetigo patients were negative by day 4. Bacterial cultures from all 32 sulconazole-treated patients and from 32 miconazole-treated patients (94%) were negative by day 7. On day 14 the bacterial culture from 1 miconazole-treated impetigo patient was still positive.

Bacterial cultures from 4 of 8 sulconazole-treated patients with ecthyma and from 2 of the 6 miconazole-treated patients with ecthyma were negative by day 4. Cultures from 7 of the 8 sulconazole-treated patients and from 5 of the 6 miconazole-treated patients were negative by day 7. Bacterial cultures from all 14 patients with ecthyma were negative by day 14.

Both creams promptly relieved the pyodermal signs, and both were considered safe and effective in the treatment of impetigo and ecthyma. Sulconazole reversed the culture results faster than miconazole did and was clearly superior to miconazole in reducing the severity of the impetigo crusts. The difference between the 2 treatments did not reach statistical significance.

▶ Sulconazole and miconazole are effective topical antifungal agents and appear to have additional antibacterial activity as well. Before their widespread use in treatment of impetigo/ecthyma, their efficacy should be compared with that of mupirocin (Bactroban), which has been shown to cure or improve 85% of skin infections when applied 3 times daily for at least 5 days (1). The antibacterial activity of sulconazole and miconazole may make them excellent therapeutic choices for *S. aureus* infections or streptococcal superinfected dermatophytosis.—R.A. Johnson, M.D.

Reference

1. Orecchio RM, et al: *Curr Ther Res* 39:82, 1986.

Quantitative Cultures of Biopsy Specimens From Cutaneous Cellulitis

Duvanel T, Auckenthaler R, Rohner P, Harms M, Saurat JH (Hôp Cantonal Universitaire, Geneva)

Arch Intern Med 149:293–296, February 1989 2–4

Cutaneous cellulitis is a generic term for infections involving the dermis and hypodermis. When it involves a lower limb, cutaneous cellulitis is often mistaken for deep venous thrombosis, accounting for up to 30% of false diagnoses of the latter condition. The microbiologic features of cutaneous cellulitis were studied by using quantitative cultures of infected tissue.

Twenty-five patients with untreated cutaneous cellulitis were studied prospectively. The infection involved a lower limb in all but 1 patient, in whom an upper limb was involved. Two full-thickness, 6-mm punch biopsy specimens were obtained from each patient: 1 from the center of the lesion and the other from the periphery. One third of each specimen was used for microbiologic study, one third for histologic study, and one third for electron microscopy study. Only the results of gram stain of histologic slides were reviewed.

Three central and 6 peripheral specimens among a total of 50 contained pathogens. Of 7 needle aspiration cultures, 2 contained pathogens. The density of microorganisms was low in all but 2 cases, in which densities reached 3.2×10^6 colony-forming units per g of tissue near the edge of an ulcer. The low density of microorganisms was at odds with the intensity of the inflammation, suggesting that some factor other than infection might be involved. Because 72% of the patients had some form of lymphatic failure, it may be that lymphatic failure has a role in the etiology of inflammation.

▶ Unfortunately, little mention (other than lymphatic failure) was made in this report as to the coexistence of chronic diseases, such as diabetes mellitus or hematologic malignancy, or of immunocompetence in these patients. In a recent study of the influence of underlying disease on cellulitis (1) the utility of cellulitis needle aspirates was examined in 87 patients (mean age, 44 years). More than half had underlying diseases or conditions, including intravenous drug abuse (18), diabetes mellitus (17), hematologic malignancies (6), and cardiovascular disorders (5). Needle aspirate cultures were positive in 26 of the 46 patients with underlying disease (57%) but in only 7 of the 41 patients without underlying disease (17%). Of diabetes with cellulitis 70.5% had positive aspirate cultures. All 6 patients with hematologic malignancies had positive aspirates; 3 of these also had positive blood cultures with the same organism. Of intravenous drug abusers 39% had positive aspirate cultures, 2 of whom were also bacteremic. *Staphylococcus aureus* was the infectious agent in 33% of patients with cellulitis; group A streptococcus was present in 27%. Other organisms (40%) isolated from aspirate cultures were *Pasteurella multocida, Escherichia coli, Proteus mirabilis, Clostridium septicum,* group B streptococcus, *Acinetobacter, Enterobacter, Hemophilus influenzae,* and *Pseudomonas aeruginosa.*—R.A. Johnson, M.D.

Reference

1. Kielhofner MA, et al: *Arch Intern Med* 148:2451, 1988.

Streptococcal Cause of Erysipelas and Cellulitis in Adults: A Microbiologic Study Using a Direct Immunofluorescence Technique

Bernard P, Bedane C, Mounier M, Denis F, Catanzano G, Bonnetblanc J-M
(CHU Dupuytren, Limoges, France)

Arch Dermatol 125:779–782, June 1989 2–5

The bacteriologic diagnosis of erysipelas and cellulitis is often disappointing. With a direct immunofluorescent (DIF) technique using commercially available antibodies, *Streptococcus* organisms (groups A, C, D, and G) were sought in skin biopsy specimens of 42 adults, 27 with erysipelas and 15 with cellulitis involving the lower limb in all but 1 case.

In situ detection of streptococci was achieved by DIF in 26 of 37 patients with bacteriologic or serologic evidence of streptococci infection, for an estimated sensitivity of 0.7. Streptococcal pathogens were grouped in 19 of 27 patients with erysipelas, including group A in 13, group B in 1, group C in 1, and group G in 4 (table). Similarly, 10 of 15 patients with cellulitis were grouped as follows: group A in 9 and group B in 1. The combined data, including conventional cultures, DIF studies, and serologic findings, identified *Streptococcus* organisms, particularly *Streptococcus pyogenes* A, as the cause of bacterial infection in 26 of 27 patients with erysipelas and 11 of 15 with cellulitis.

The DIF technique is a valuable method for detecting in situ streptococci in erysipelas or cellulitis involving the lower limbs in adults. Erysipelas or cellulitis in adults is almost always caused by streptococci, particularly group A streptococcus.

▶ In adults with cellulitis but without underlying diseases, yields of cultures of aspirates, biopsy specimens, and blood are uniformly low, i.e., 25% (1, 2). Most of these patients respond to empirical treatment that covers either *S. aureus* or group A streptococcus. Bernard and coworkers' study of DIF in detecting the infectious bacteria in erysipelas and cellulitis is promising for future clinical application. Although DIF detected streptococcal antigens in 19 of 27 patients with erysipelas, in only 8 of them were the DIF results confirmed by culture of the same type of streptococcus (further confirmation was provided by maximal antistreptolysin O and antistreptodornase titers). In 2 of the 19 patients, DIF was positive for group A streptococcus, and the culture of a cutaneous sample isolated *S. aureus*. In that the DIF technology is not too difficult, this diagnostic method may prove to be practical in the clinical pathology laboratory of a community hospital.—R.A. Johnson, M.D.

References

1. Ginsberg MB: *South Med J* 74:530, 1981.
2. Hook EW, et al: *Arch Intern Med* 146:295, 1986.

Bacteriologic Investigation in Erysipelas

Patient No./ Age, y/Sex	Bacteriology of Cutaneous Samples	DIF	Antibody Titer, IU/mL*	
			ASO	**ASD**
1/F/84	*Streptococcus pyogenes* (A)	A (2+)	320	160
2/F/72	*S pyogenes* (A)	A (3+)	640	320
3/F/55	*S pyogenes* (A); *Staphylococcus aureus*	A (1+)	320	1280
4/F/65	*S pyogenes* (A)	...	640	5120
5/F/78	...	A (2+)	<50	320
6/F/86	*Pseudomonas aeruginosa*	A (3+)	400	1280
7/F/78	*P aeruginosa; Streptococcus faecalis* (D)	A (3+)	80	160
8/F/77	*S aureus*	A (2+)	1280	80
9/F/81	*S aureus*	A (1+)	80	160
10/M/84	*S faecalis* (D); *P aeruginosa; Proteus mirabilis*	A (1+)	320	<50
11/F/42	...	A (2+)	<50	<50
12/M/45	...	A (2+)	160	160
13/F/76	...	A (1+)	160	2560
14/M/80	*Streptococcus* B3†	...	160	160
15/M/71	*Streptococcus equissimilis* (C)	C (1+)	1600	<50
16/M/73	*Streptococcus* G; *S aureus*	G (1+)	1280	640
17/M/25	*Streptococcus* G†	G (1+)	320	160
18/F/93	*Streptococcus* G; *S aureus*	G (3+)	<50	<50
19/F/79	*Streptococcus* G	G (1+)	320	80
20/M/64	...	...	640	320
21/F/82	*S aureus*	...	160	640
22/F/78	*Staphylococcus epidermidis*	...	1280	160
23/M/64	...	...	<50	320
24/F/65	...	...	320	<50
25/M/57	...	...	1280	<50
26/F/29	...	...	320	80
27/M/59	...	...	80	160

Abbreviations: DIF, direct immunofluorescence detection of groups A, C, D, and G streptococci; *ASO,* antistreptolysin; *ASD,* antistreptodornase.

*Data are maximal titers obtained in each patient.

†In blood cultures only.

(Courtesy of Bernard P, Bedane C, Mounier M, et al: *Arch Dermatol* 125:779–782, June 1989.

***Staphylococcus aureus* Skin Carriage and Development of Peritonitis in Patients on Continuous Ambulatory Peritoneal Dialysis**

Sesso R, Draibe S, Castelo A, Sato I, Leme I, Barbosa D, Ramos O (Escola Paulista de Medicina, São Paulo, Brazil)

Clin Nephrol 31:264–268, May 1989 2–6

Peritonitis remains a major complication of continuous ambulatory peritoneal dialysis. *Staphylococcus aureus* is the most frequent causative agent of peritonitis in Brazil. Forty-three patients receiving continuous ambulatory peritoneal dialysis were followed for more than 15 months to assess the role of skin carriage of *S. aureus*. Eleven patients changed to hemodialysis during the study period. Two of 4 deaths were caused by *S. aureus* sepsis.

Sixteen patients (37%) were chronic carriers of *S. aureus* in the nares or the exit site of the catheter; 12 others were intermittent carriers. Fifty episodes of peritonitis occurred in 422 patient-months of observation. *Staphylococcus aureus* caused 16 episodes in 15 patients, all of whom were carriers. The 8 patients studied had the same phage type of peritoneal isolates and the skin. Half of the 21 episodes of catheter exit-site infection were caused by *S. aureus*.

An epidemiologic relationship between *S. aureus* carriage and peritonitis in patients receiving continuous ambulatory peritoneal dialysis was confirmed. When *S. aureus* infection is prevalent, eradication of carriage is warranted before peritoneal dialysis is undertaken. Oral administration of rifampin reportedly is effective in eradicating carriage in patients colonized at both nasal and extranasal sites.

▶ In patients with chronic placement of tubes through the skin or within the hypodermis, infection is common and begins with *S. aureus* nasal colonization followed by infection of the exit site of the catheter. Individuals infected with HIV have a 47% incidence of *S. aureus* nasal carriage, compared to 27% in non-HIV-infected controls (1); low-dose oral clindamycin has been used successfully as prophylaxis in this group at risk for life-threatening invasive *S. aureus* infection (2, 3). Rifampin is particularly effective against *S. aureus* nasal carriage because of the high concentration achieved in nasal secretions (4). Mupirocin (Bactroban) may also prove to be an effective topical agent applied to the nose and exit site of the catheter as prophylaxis for deeper *S. aureus* infection.— R.A. Johnson, M.D.

References

1. Ganesh R, et al: *Lancet* 2:558, 1989.
2. Klempner MS, et al: *JAMA* 260:2682, 1988.
3. Rolston KVI: *JAMA* 261:1444, 1989.
4. McAnally TP, et al: *Antimicrob Agents Chemother* 25:422, 1984.

Septic Scarlet Fever Due to *Streptococcus pyogenes* Cellulitis

Shaunak S, Wendon J, Monteil M, Gordon AM (Medway Hosp, Gillingham; Charing Cross and Westminster Med School, London; All Saint's Hosp, Chatham, England)

Q J Med 69:921–925, November 1988 2–7

Streptococcus pyogenes cellulitis associated with scarlet fever, severe toxemia, and septicemia is rarely seen in the postantibiotic era. Scarlet fever caused by *S. pyogenes* serotype M1/T1/OF− cellulitis was diagnosed in 3 previously healthy adults aged 34, 39, and 57 years. All 3 had a rash typical of scarlet fever. None had a history of sore throat, and no streptococci were isolated from throat cultures.

Despite prompt treatment with large doses of benzylpenicillin and surgical débridement in 2 patients, bacteremia, acute renal failure, adult respiratory distress syndrome, and disseminated intravascular coagulation developed in all of them. The punctate erythema was followed by desquamation of the skin over the face and trunk, as well as the palms, soles, and tongue. Immunoglobulin levels were low in 2 patients and high in 1. Two patients died. Autopsy of 1 patient showed an enlarged liver and spleen and subendocardial petechial hemorrhages typical of scarlet fever.

These cases emphasize the severity of *S. pyogenes* serotype M1/T1/OF− cellulities associated with scarlet fever. With the reemergence of highly virulent streptococci, a high index of suspicion and early referral may reduce the grave prognosis of this illness.

▶ Scarlet fever is an acute infection of the tonsils or skin caused by an erythrogenic exotoxin-producing strain of group A β-hemolytic *S. pyogenes* (uncommonly by exotoxin-producing *Staphylococcus aureus),* manifested by a characteristic toxigenic exanthem. In addition to pharyngitis and impetigo, other infections caused by this streptococcus include erysipelas, necrotizing fasciitis, myositis, puerperal fever, and bacteremia. When the infecting streptococcus produces the erythrogenic toxin, these infections can also be associated with a scarlatiniform exanthem. In 2 recent reports of toxic shocklike syndrome caused by *S. pyogenes* (1, 2), 22 additional patients were reported with necrotizing fasciitis, with or without myositis, and an associated high morbidity rate and mortality rate of 35%. Apparently, such serious streptococcal infections were much more common at the beginning of the century. These authors suggest that much more virulent group A streptococci producing the pyrogenic toxin A associated with scarlet fever has reappeared in their community.—R.A. Johnson, M.D.

References

1. Cone LA, et al: *N Engl J Med* 317:146, 1987.
2. Stevens DL, et al: *N Engl J Med* 321:1, 1989.

Cutaneous Pathology in Toxic Shock Syndrome

Vuzevski VD, van Joost Th, Wagenvoort JHT, Michiels Dey JJ (Univ Hosp Rotterdam/Dijkzigt; Erasmus Univ Rotterdam)

Int J Dermatol 28:94–97, March 1989 2–8

Toxic shock syndrome is characterized by fever, headache, skin eruption, subcutaneous edema, and mucous membrane hyperemia with prodromes of myalgia, vomiting, diarrhea, and pharyngitis. Most patients initially have diffuse scarlatiniform erythroderma followed by fine desquamation of the skin, peeling of the palms and soles, and loss of hair and nails during convalescence.

Woman, 25, had fever, hypotension, emesis, myalgia, diarrhea, and peritonitis-like symptoms 1 day after right-sided mastitis developed during an uneventful postpartum period. Multiple skin punch biopsy specimens were obtained 5 days after disease onset, at the time of overt diffuse intravascular coagulation and erythroderma. On examination of the biopsy specimens with light microscopy, the epidermis appeared slightly hyperplastic and spongiotic. Some epidermal cells showed intercellular edema. Necrosis of the keratinocytes was the most prominent feature in different layers of the epidermis. Eosinophilic necrotic keratinocytes were noted in all epidermal layers. Necrotic areas were often invaded by numerous neutrophils and eosinophils. The papillary dermis showed moderate diffuse edema. There were striking vascular changes, including a lymphocytic infiltrate, endothelial cell vacuolization and thrombi, mostly in the capillaries and arterioles of the papillary and reticular dermis. With direct immunofluorescence staining, conspicuous granular depositions of IgM, C3, and complement factor C1q were noted in the walls of the dermal capillaries. Electron microscopy showed cellular enlargement in the endothelial cells of capillaries and arterioles, hypertrophy of the Golgi apparatus, an increase of granular endoplasmic reticulum and ribosomes, and a large number of dense bodies. These histopathologic findings and those reported previously in the literature were compared (table).

Careful assessment of lesional skin biopsy specimens during the evolution of toxic shock syndrome can substantially establish the distinct histopathologic features of this disease. These features, in conjunction with the other hallmarks of toxic shock syndrome, enable its differentiation from other severe acute toxic skin eruptions.

▶ This article presents a well-illustrated review of the pathology of toxic shock syndrome and an examination of the literature. Despite the number of clinical cases, the number of descriptions of the pathology of this entity in the skin is quite small. This case is unique for the presence of intracapillary thrombi.—T.J. Flotte, M.D.

Data From the Literature on the Cutaneous Pathology in 11 Patients With Toxic Shock Syndrome

Authors (cases Relevant for Survey)	Skin Biopsy*	Epidermis	Dermis
Fisher et al., 1981 Case 4 and 5	Day 3 and 4 of acute illness	†	Perivascular lymphocytic infiltrate (confirmed by EM)* sparing papillary dermis
Abdul-Karim et al., 1981	Day 4 of acute illness	Intraepithelial edema, subepithelial blister	Perivascular mononuclear inflammatory cell infiltrate
	Day 8	?	Perivascular infiltrate with lymphocytes, histiocytes, and occasional eosinophils and plasma cells
Chesney et al., 1981	?	Mild hyperkeratosis	Perivascular lymphocytes and neutrophilic infiltration
Tofte et al., 1981	? Late-onset rash	?	Lymphocyte cuffing of the vessels. Some luminal polymorph nuclear cells
Paris et al., 1982	?	?	Perivasculitis
Larkin et al., 1982	?	?	Perivascular lymphocytic infiltration
Elbaum et al., 1984 (1 case)	Day 3 of acute illness (from vesicular lesions)	Parakeratosis, subepithelial blister containing mononuclears	Perivascular infiltrates of lymphocytes and eosinophils

	Day 4 of acute illness (from erythematous macular lesion)	Parakeratosis with intact granular layer	Perivascular infiltrates of lymphocytes and eosinophils
Hurwitz and Ackerman, 1985			
Case 1	Day 2 of acute illness (from sunburn-like rash)	Slight spongiosis, few necrotic keratinocytes, invasion neutrophils	Perivascular infiltrates of lymphocytes, neutrophils, and rare eosinophils
Case 2	Day 7 of acute illness (from sunburn-like rash)	Prominent spongiosis, necrotic keratinocytes	Perivascular and slightly interstitial predominantly lymphocytic infiltrate
Case 5	Day 2 following onset rash (from erythematous rash)	Slight spongiosis, necrotic keratinocytes	Perivascular mixed cell infiltrate with lymphocytes, neutrophils, and histiocytes principally around the blood vessels
Vuzevski et al. (present report)	Day 5 of acute illness = sunburn-like rash with purpura	Slight spongiosis, necrotic keratinocytes, invasion of neutrophils and eosinophils, intraepidermal cleavage	Perivascular infiltrate of lymphocytes, histiocytes, plasma cells, intracapillary thrombi

*Data of the day of skin biopsy (as far as detailed by the authors).
†? = No exact details provided by the authors.
(Courtesy of Vuzevski VC, van Joost Th, Wagenvoort JHT, et al: *Int J Dermatol* 28:94–97, March 1989.)

Cutaneous Manifestations of Infection with *Corynebacterium* Group JK
Dan M, Somer I, Knobel B, Gutman R (Edith Wolfson Med Ctr, Holon, Israel)
Rev Infect Dis 10:1204–1207, November–December 1988 2–9

Increasingly, *Corynebacterium* group JK is recognized as a pathogen in patients with prosthetic devices, indwelling catheters, valvular defects, and granulocytopenia. The clinical manifestations of this infection are diverse.

Man, 36, after cytotoxic chemotherapy for promyelocytic leukemia, had bone marrow suppression. Progressive weakness, gingival bleeding, and fever developed, and he was treated with amikacin, mezlocillin and cloxacillin. Fever persisted, with blood cultures negative for any organism. His condition deteriorated; amphotericin B therapy was begun, and a 2 × 2 cm area of subcutaneous induration with a small central erosion appeared in the left groin. Blood cultures became positive for "diphtheroids," and vancomycin therapy was begun. The original lesion increased in size, becoming swollen and erythematous with the central erosion deeply ulcerated; new, similar lesions appeared. Nevertheless, the patient gradually improved. The identity of the organism was confirmed as *Corynebacterium* group JK, sensitive only to vancomycin. No further lesions developed after 1-year follow-up.

Granulocytopenic hosts not uncommonly have skin and soft tissue manifestations of *Corynebacterium* group JK septicemia, whereas they are rarely seen in patients with endocarditis. Primary lesions are usually the portal of entry into the bloodstream for the organism and are commonly found at sites of bone marrow biopsy, intravascular catheter insertion, and perianal fissures. Secondary lesions can develop as a papular rash, soft tissue abscess, or necrotic soft tissue lesions.

▶ *Corynebacterium* group JK, gram-positive diphtheroids are commensal cutaneous bacteria of healthy individuals. In hospitalized patients they occur in highest concentration in the perineal, inguinal, and axillary areas, carriage increasing with increasing age, male gender, previous antibiotic therapy, duration of hospital stay, and presence of an underlying malignancy. *Corynebacterium* group JK sepsis occurs in granulocytopenic patients, beginning as a focus of infection at a break in the mucocutaneous surface. This focus commonly occurs at a needle puncture site, whether in venipuncture, bone marrow aspiration, or indwelling catheterization, or at a break in the perineal or inguinal skin. The focal infection extends to become a site of minimally inflammatory cellulitis, from which the organism enters the bloodstream. As in the case presented, the cellulitis can be multifocal and progress to necrosis and ulcer formation. Most commonly, septicemia is the presenting manifestation of *Corynebacterium* group JK invasion rather than the cutaneous infection.—R.A. Johnson, M.D.

Gram-Negative Folliculitis
Poli F, Prost C, Revuz J (Hôp Henri-Mondor, Créteil, France)
Ann Dermatol Venereol 115:797–800, 1988 2–10

Gram-negative bacterial (GNB) folliculitis, first described in the United States in 1968, has been widely reported since then. Until now, no case reports had appeared in the French literature, suggesting that the condition may not have been recognized earlier. Six patients with GNB folliculitis were treated during a recent 12-month period. Four men and 2 women aged 22–54 years (mean age, 32.8 years) were first seen with acne vulgaris of the face that was resistant to treatment. The patients had been treated for a mean of 10.8 years with oral tetracycline and topical tretrinoin or benzoyl peroxide. Pus samples were collected from 2 to 10 pustules, as well as from the perinasal region, and were cultured for GNB.

Various GNB were isolated, including *Enterobacter cloacae, Escherichia coli,* and *Proteus mirabilis.* However, only a few pustules per patient contained gram-negative bacteria. Four patients were treated with antibiotics that were active in vitro against the specific bacteria. The lesions cleared within 2 weeks. Two patients were treated with isotretinoin alone in oral doses of 1 mg/kg/day. Their lesions cleared after 2–3 months of treatment. Although isotretinoin has no antibacterial activity, it induces environmental changes that are unfavorable to GNB.

Gram-negative bacterial folliculitis appears to result from an imbalance in the cutaneous and mucosal flora thought to be caused by long-term tetracycline use. At present, the prevalence of GNB folliculitis is probably underestimated, particularly in France. More cases of GNB folliculitis will probably be reported once the condition becomes better known and better recognized.

▶ Gram-negative folliculitis has discovered France (or vice versa). There is nothing especially distinctive about this report of 6 individuals with this disorder, except that in 1 of them the isolated gram-negative organism was *Streptococcus faecalis.* Mon Dieu!—P.E. Pochi, M.D.

Infection-Induced Panniculitis

Patterson JW, Brown PC, Broecker AH (Med College of Virginia, Richmond; Univ of Rochester, New York)
J Cutan Pathol 16:183–193, August 1989 2–11

Panniculitis caused by infection is well known. To determine to what extent the microscopic features of panniculitis from infection overlap with those of primary forms of panniculitis, histopathologic studies were made in 15 patients (table).

Special staining identified the organisms in 14 patients. In 6 of these the causative agent was confirmed by cultures. In another case culture of a lesion was positive despite negative special staining. Gram-positive or gram-negative bacteria caused the panniculitis in 8 patients, atypical mycobacteria in 2, *Nocardia* in 2, and fungi in 3. Most patients were predisposed to immunosuppression, but at least 2 had no other major medical problems.

Microscopic Features in Cases of Infectious Panniculitis

Case number	Organism in tissue	Special subcutaneous features
1	Gram positive cocci	Mixed panniculitis; few epithelioid cells; abscesses absent
2	Gram negative bacilli (*Klebsiella*)	Mixed panniculitis; foamy macrophages; abscesses absent
3	Gram positive cocci	Erythema nodosum-like; foamy macrophages
4	Gram positive cocci (*Staph., Strep.*)	Mixed panniculitis; organisms visible as basophilic masses on H&E staining
5	Gram positive cocci (*Staph.*)	Mixed panniculitis
6	Gram positive cocci	Erythema nodosum-like; absence of vascular proliferation and hemorrhage
7	Gram positive cocci (botryomycosis)	Mixed panniculitis; plasma cells and giant cells; absent microcysts and abscesses; grains visible on H&E staining
8	*Pseudomonas* sp. (not seen in tissue)	Mixed panniculitis; small vessel vasculitis; absent vascular proliferation and abscesses
9	*Nocardia* sp.	Nodular vasculitis-like; absent microcysts and abscesses
10	*Nocardia* sp.	Mixed panniculitis; absent hemorrhage, vascular proliferation, microcysts, abscesses
11	Atypical mycobacteria	Mixed panniculitis; epithelioid and giant cells; foamy macrophages; absent necrosis
12	Atypical mycobacteria	Mixed panniculitis; epithelioid and giant cells; foamy macrophages; fibrosis
13	*Candida* sp.	Mixed panniculitis; giant cells; foamy macrophages; fibrosis; absent microcysts, necrosis
14	*Candia* sp.	Mixed panniculitis; some plasma cells and neutrophils; fibrosis; absent necrosis and abscesses
15	*Fusarium* sp.	Erythema nodosum-like; small vessel vasculitis; absent hemorrhage and microcysts; organisms visible on H&E staining

Abbreviations: H & E, hematoxylin and eosin; *sp,* species.
Unless otherwise indicated, a case showed hemorrhage, a predominantly neutrophilic infiltrate with some lymphocytes and macrophages, vascular proliferation, fat microcysts, necrosis or sweat gland necrosis, and neutrophilic abscesses.
(Courtesy of Patterson JW, Brown PC, Broecker AH: *J Cutan Pathol* 16:183–193, August 1989.)

Some variability in microscopic findings and some overlap with established forms of panniculitis were noted. Three specimens resembled acute, neutrophilic erythema nodosum. There was evidence of vasculitis in septicemias from *Pseudomonas, Nocardia,* and *Fusarium.* However, there were several distinctive features associated with infectious panniculitis of diverse causes. These included epidermal changes, e.g., acanthosis and parakeratosis; dermal edema with a diffuse or perivascular neutrophilic infiltrate; and mixed septal-lobular panniculitis with neutrophilic infiltration, vascular proliferation and hemorrhage, and necrosis.

Physicians should suspect infection in virtually any patient with panniculitis, especially if the patient is immunosuppressed. The microscopic features delineated in this study should arouse even greater suspicion of an infectious process.

▶ This paper presents a very interesting study of panniculitis. The authors have attempted to identify the histologic characteristics that are associated with a true infectious panniculitis. This is a particularly important approach because the area of panniculitis is still very poorly understood. The ability to segregate those lesions that are clearly infectious would be of enormous benefit to both the pathologist and the dermatologist who are responsible for the patient's care. This approach to panniculitis and this paper both deserve careful study.— T.J. Flotte, M.D.

Primary and Secondary Syphilis, 20 Years' Experience: 2. Clinical Features

Mindel A, Tovey SJ, Timmins DJ, Williams P (Univ College and Middlesex School of Medicine, London)

Genitourin Med 65:1–3, February 1989 2–12

Studies on the recent epidemiology of early syphilis have shown an increased incidence of early syphilis among homosexual men. The clinical features of primary and secondary syphilis were reviewed retrospectively in the records of 946 patients with primary syphilis and 854 with secondary syphilis.

Among 946 patients with primary syphilis, 182 of the 184 heterosexual men and 467 of the 728 homosexual men had chancres on the penis; 249 homosexual men had chancres in the perianal or anal region. Chancres at sites other than the genital or anorectal areas were uncommon. Of the 29 women with genital chancres, 22 were affected on the vulva or vagina and 6 on the cervix. Lymphadenectomy was more frequently associated with genital chancres than with chancres at other sites. In homosexual men, 316 of the 418 genital chancres had enlarged draining lymph nodes, compared with only 104 of the chancres at the perianal site.

The clinical features of the 3 groups of patients with secondary syphilis were similar, with most patients having a rash and lymphadenopathy (table). However, heterosexual men more often had histories of chancres and lymphadenopathy than did homosexual men.

Clinical Features of Secondary Syphilis in 3 Groups

	Heterosexual men	*Homosexual men*	*Women*
History of chancre	24/71 (34)	159/692 (23)	7/57 (12)
Chancre still present	25/74 (34)	198/710 (28)	10/57 (18)
Rash	72/74 (97)	654/700 (93)	49/56 (88)
Lymphadenopathy	56/72 (78)	407/653 (62)	27/55 (49)
Mucus patches			
Genital	4/72 (6)	27/700 (4)	4/58 (7)
Oral	16/73 (22)	112/688 (16)	11/57 (19)
Fever	4/72 (6)	38/692 (6)	3/58 (5)
Malaise	10/73 (14)	89/700 (13)	7/58 (12)
Condylomata lata			
Genital	3/73 (4)	29/692 (4)	5/56 (9)
Perianal	7/73 (10)	104/685 (15)	5/57 (9)
Alopecia	5/72 (7)	24/695 (4)	3/57 (5)

Percentages are in parentheses.

(Courtesy of Mindel A, Tovey SJ, Timmins DJ, et al: *Genitourin Med* 65:1–3, February 1989.)

The main difference in the clinical features of primary syphilis between homosexual and heterosexual men was the considerable preponderance of anal chancres observed in homosexual men. The clinical features of secondary syphilis do not appear to have changed much in modern times.

▶ The results of this 20-year retrospective study of syphilis are old news. In the United States, the incidence of syphilis in homosexual men has actually decreased markedly during the past 5 years because of the HIV epidemic and safer sexual practices. The overall incidence of syphilis has, however, increased in association with the epidemic of "crack" cocaine use. Currently, the major concern about primary syphilis and other genital ulcers, such as chancroid and genital herpes, is the associated increased risk for HIV infection.—R.A. Johnson, M.D.

A Prospective Study of Tick Bites in an Endemic Area for Lyme Disease

Costello CM, Steere AC, Pinkerton RE, Feder HM Jr (Middlesex Mem Hosp, Middletown, England; Univ of Connecticut, Farmington; Tufts Univ)

J Infect Dis 159:136–139, January 1989 2–13

As a result of increased public awareness of Lyme disease in regions where ixodid ticks are endemic, more persons who find ticks attached to themselves now consult their physicians. The question then arises whether they should be treated immediately with prophylactic antibiotics, or whether they should be treated only if symptoms of Lyme disease develop.

A double-blind, placebo-controlled, clinical trial was carried out in a 6-month period; 56 patients aged 5–85 years with *Ixodes dammini* tick bites participated. Each was asked to bring in the tick, attached or not, for identification and analysis. Sixteen patients had a tick removed by their physicians, 32 brought the tick with them, and 8 gave a history of a tick bite within the previous 72 hours. Twenty-seven of the 48 ticks brought in were already desiccated and could not be examined. Six of the 21 evaluable ticks carried *Borrelia burgdorferi.* Twenty-seven patients were treated with penicillin and the other 29 were given placebo.

Three patients in each group had been bitten by infected ticks. One of the 29 patients given placebo experienced erythema migrans, headache, malaise, and fatigue 14 days after the tick bite. The tick she brought in had been desiccated and could not be examined. Treatment with doxycycline for 10 days led to complete resolution of her symptoms, and she had no sequelae. None of the 27 patients in the penicillin-treated group had symptoms of Lyme disease, but 1 had an allergic reaction to the penicillin. Serologic studies did not reveal seroconversion, but 5 patients had positive IgG antibody titers to *B. burgdorferi.*

The study population was too small for any definitive conclusions to be made as to the advisability of prophylactic antibiotic therapy after a tick bite. However, the risk of acquiring Lyme disease from a recognized tick bite appears to be less than the infection rate in ticks.

▶ The authors report that the risk of asymptomatic seroconversion or symptomatic infection by *B. burgdorferi* following a known ixodid tick bite was only 3%, which was the same as the rate of drug reaction to the penicillin chemoprophylaxis. In that the incidence of *B. burgdorferi* infection in the collected *I. dammini* ticks was 29%, at first impression the rate of infection in individuals bitten by tick seems quite low. In that previous studies have shown a high rate of spirochetal infection (up to 90%) attributable to *I. dammini* in certain highly endemic areas on the northeast coast, in comparison to a low rate of 3% for *Ixodes pacificus* infections in California, the chance of Lyme borreliosis developing after an ixodid tick bite probably varies considerably with the rate of tick infection. In West Germany, 17% of biting ticks were infected with *B. burgdorferi,* but less than 1% of children bitten had symptomatic infections. Possible reasons for the low rate of infectivity include low infectivity of certain strains of *B. burgdorferi,* too brief a period of tick attachment, too few spirochetes transmitted, and/or natural resistance to infection in certain individuals. Within hyperendemic geographic areas it would appear reasonable to use chemoprophylaxis for *B. burgdorferi* infection in some individuals at risk because of residence or occupation, or in those immunocompromised by HIV infection.—R.A. Johnson, M.D.

Treatment of Multiple Subcutaneous *Nocardia asteroides* Abscesses With Ciprofloxacin and Doxycycline

Bath PMW, Pettingale KW, Wade J (King's College School of Medicine and Dentistry, London)

Postgrad Med J 65:190–191, March 1989 2–14

Cotrimoxazole is the usual treatment of choice for infections caused by *Nocardia asteroides*. Treatment for cotrimoxazole-resistant strains is less well established. A patient with nocardiosis was treated with oral ciprofloxacin and doxycycline.

Woman, 73, had diffuse lymphoblastic non-Hodgkin's lymphoma, histologic grade 2 and clinical stage 4. She was treated initially with radiotherapy and combination chemotherapy without experiencing complete remission. Her histology changed to plasmacytoid lymphoma with plasma paraprotein. Multiple painful, fluctuant, subcutaneous masses affecting the right axilla, right arm, and left thigh developed. Initial treatment with chlorambucil and prednisolone was stopped, and treatment with cotrimoxazole and benzylpenicillin was begun when pus from the axillary mass revealed gram-positive branching rods compatible with *Nocardia* or *Actinomyces* species. The remaining abscesses were drained surgically. Benzylpenicillin was stopped after 10 days when culture of the pus revealed *N. asteroides.* The patient became pancytopenic, and treatment with cotrimoxazole was stopped after 7 days. Intravenous cefuroxime and amikacin were begun. After 7 days in vitro sensitivities indicated that the *Nocardia* was sensitive to ciprofloxacin, doxycycline, amoxicillin-clavulanic acid, amikacin, and cefuroxime. The *Nocardia* was resistant to sulfamethoxazole, trimethoprim, cotrimoxazole, and amoxicillin. After oral treatment with ciprofloxacin and doxycycline was begun, the patient became pain free, and 2 abscesses stopped draining after 10 weeks. The third abscess healed after 4 months of treatment. Intermittent diarrhea was the only complication. Treatment was expected to continue for a total of 9 months.

Oral ciprofloxacin and doxycycline were used successfully to treat multiple subcutaneous nocardial abscesses in this immunocompromised patient. The treatment is relatively inexpensive and is not associated with any significant side effects.

▶ The treatment of choice for nocardiosis is the trimethoprim-sulfonamide combination (cotrimoxazole) containing 80 mg of trimethoprim and 400 mg of sulfamethoxazole. The usual adult dose is 2 tablets twice daily. Because the patient became pancytopenic and cotrimoxazole was implicated—and the antibiotic sensitivity studies of the isolated *N. asteroides* indicated susceptibility to both ciprofloxacin and doxycycline—the patient was treated with both of these agents. Ciprofloxacin, one of the quinolones developed during the past decade, has an extended antibacterial spectrum that covers gram-positive cocci, including methicillin-resistant, coagulase-positive and coagulase-negative staphylococci, *Pseudomonas aeruginosa, Hemophilus influenzae, Neisseria,* mycobacteria, *Legionella, Chlamydia,* mycoplasmas, *Rickettsia,* and *Brucella.* The features of ciprofloxacin that make it an outstanding new antimicrobial agent include its rapid absorption after oral administration, an extended half-life that permits dosing every 12 hours, excellent penetration into most body tissues and fluids, ease of administration at home without need for frequent outpatient or home visits or inpatient admission, and its unique property of efficacy of oral administration against *P. aeruginosa* (1). Although anaphylactoid reactions have been reported (2), the incidence of adverse cutaneous reactions with ciprofloxacin is less than 1%.—R.A. Johnson, M.D.

References

1. Gentry LO, et al: *Arch Intern Med* 149:2579, 1989.
2. Davis H, et al: *Ann Intern Med* 111:1041, 1989.

Effects of Intradermal Gamma-Interferon in Cutaneous Leishmaniasis

Harms G, Zwingenberger K, Chéhadé AK, Talhari S, Racz P, Mouakeh A, Douba M, Näkel L, Naiff RD, Kremsner PG, Feldmeier H, Bienzle U (Landesinstitut für Tropenmedizin, Berlin; Université d'Alep, Syria; Centro de Dermatologia Tropical e Venereologia "Alfredo da Matta," Manaus, Brazil; Bernhard-Nocht-Institut für Tropenmedizin, Hamburg, West Germany; Instituto Nacional de Pesquisa da Amazonia, Manaus)
Lancet 1:1287–1292, June 10, 1989 2–15

Healing of cutaneous leishmaniasis depends on an effective cell-mediated immune response. Because intracellular parasites in macrophages are a promising target for interferon (IFN) therapy, treatment with recombinant IFN gamma (IFN-γ) was evaluated in patients with lesions caused by *Leishmania braziliensis guyanensis* and *Leishmania tropica*. Thirteen pairs of lesions were studied in each diagnostic group, 1 of each pair being treated by perilesional injection of IFN-γ.

After 3 weeks 12 of 13 lesions caused by *L. braziliensis guyanensis* were smaller compared with 6 control lesions. Only 4 treated lesions were free of parasites. Nine of 13 lesions caused by *L. tropica* resolved completely after IFN-γ injection. Acute inflammation occurred in some treated patients with *L. tropica* lesions, but there were no other adverse effects.

Perilesional injection of IFN-γ can clear lesions in many cases of American cutaneous leishmaniasis or Oriental cutaneous leishmaniasis. Current studies may show whether IFN-γ treatment is comparable with conventional treatment with glucantime, and whether IFN-γ can be an effective adjunct in accelerating healing, thereby minimizing the sequelae of cutaneous leishmaniasis.

▶ The role of immunotherapy in cutaneous leishmaniasis is currently being assessed. Vaccine therapy as prepared and advocated by Convit and his colleagues is presently being used in WHO field trials and has been reported as promising (1). The cost/benefit of intradermal IFN-γ therapy has to be considered when one compares its effectiveness with the currently used intralesional or systemic high-dose pentavalent antimonial therapies. The potential role of γ interferon as part of a combined therapy with other currently used drugs needs to be explored, especially in the more therapeutic-resistant expressions of cutaneous leishmaniasis such as the chronic lupoid, the recidive, the mucocutaneous, and disseminated anergic forms.—S.L. Maschella, M.D.

Reference

1. Convit J, et al: *Lancet* 1:401, 1987.

Combination Therapy (Monomycine and Methyluracil) in Leishmaniasis Cutis

Hossain MZ (The Sechenov 1st Moscow Med Inst, USSR)
Int J Dermatol 27:720–722, December 1988 2–16

Cutaneous leishmaniasis is endemic in the Asiatic part of Russia. Although many forms of therapy have been proposed, no simple, effective treatment is available. The antibiotic monomycine has been reported to be effective in the treatment of cutaneous leishmaniasis. A combination of monomycine and methyluracil was tested, the latter agent being added because of its reported ability to reduce monomycine toxicity.

Fifty patients with acute ulcerative cutaneous leishmaniasis were treated with 250,000 units of monomycine injected intramuscularly every 8 hours and 0.5 g of methyluracil taken orally twice daily for 10 days. All patients had a history of sandfly bites during a visit to Uzbekistan, a known endemic area of cutaneous leishmaniasis. Thirty patients had multiple lesions; the total number of lesions in the 50 patients was 136.

Fifteen patients had complete resolution of the lesions after 21 days, 10 had complete healing after 27 days, and the remaining 25 were cured after 30 days. Thus all ulcers healed within 30 days of inititation of treatment, and all lesions healed without disfigurement or scarring. Only a faint erythema was observed at the sites of the original lesions. During a follow-up period of 12 months, none of the patients had experienced a recurrence of cutaneous leishmaniasis. Both drugs were well tolerated.

▶ The results obtained by the authors seem to be "extraordinary." It appears that the aminoglycoside, paromomycin, has been used systemically for cutaneous leishmaniasis in the USSR. In Israel 72% of patients were clinically cured after treatment with 15% paromomycin and 12% methylbenzethomine chloride in a soft paraffin base (1). The current mainstay of therapy is intralesional sodium stibogluconate (2) for solitary lesions and parenteral pentavalent antimonials in higher doses (similar to those used in visceral leishmaniasis) and for longer periods in refractory cases or cases with multiple lesions. The second-line drug, especially in resistant or mucocutaneous or disseminated anergic disease, is systemic amphotericin B.—S.L. Moschella, M.D.

References

1. El-On J: *J Invest Dermatol* 87:284, 1986.
2. Kellum RE: *J Am Acad Dermatol* 15:620, 1988.

3 Bullous Diseases

The Usefulness of Immunofluorescent Tests in Pemphigus Patients in Clinical Remission

David M, Weissman-Katzenelson V, Ben-Chetrit A, Hazaz B, Ingber A, Sandbank M (Beilinson Med Ctr, Petah Tiqva, Israel; Tel Aviv Univ, Israel)

Br J Dermatol 120:391–395, March 1989 3–1

The autoantibodies of pemphigus vulgaris can be demonstrated in the epidermis by the direct immunofluorescent test (DIF) and in serum by the indirect immunofluorescent test (IIF). The DIF is considered a highly reliable diagnostic test, but it has not been used as a prognostic indicator of relapse, as the test may remain positive for many years after pemphigus vulgaris has regressed clinically. Although the serum antibody titer is usually proportional to the severity of pemphigus vulgaris, the IIF test is not considered reliable enough for assessing disease severity. Epidermal and circulating autoantibody levels as determined by DIF and IIF were measured in patients with pemphigus vulgaris in clinical remission to determine the prognostic validity of these tests.

The study included 13 men aged 59–78 years and 11 women aged 32–87 years with a confirmed diagnosis of pemphigus vulgaris. The average duration of disease was 6.1 years, and all patients had been in clinical remission for 6 months to 4 years; all were receiving maintenance corticosteroid therapy. Follow-up was every 2 months for a total of 20 months. Each patient had 2 DIF tests and 2 IIF tests, performed 6 months apart. Eight patients had negative DIF test results, 7 of which were again negative at follow-up. Six patients had weakly positive DIF tests, and 10 patients had strong positive fluorescence. Seventeen patients had negative and 7 had positive IIF tests; the latter 7 patients also had positive DIF tests. During the 20-month follow-up period, 1 of the 8 patients with negative DIF tests relapsed, compared with 2 of the 6 patients with weakly positive DIF tests and 5 of the 10 patients with strongly positive DIF tests. Deposits of C_3 were also detected in 5 of the 10 patients with strongly positive DIF tests.

The DIF test appears to be useful for identifying immunologic activity in patients who are clinically in remission. Serum titers did not change significantly between tests. The IIF test seems to be a less sensitive indicator of clinical disease progression.

▶ The observation that some patients with positive DIF tests detected on clinically normal-appearing skin during control of pemphigus vulgaris experienced relapse while receiving maintenance corticosteroid therapy led the authors to conclude that a positive DIF test was of predictive value for future relapse. This prognostic aspect of the DIF test needs to be confirmed.—N.A. Soter, M.D.

Endemic Pemphigus Foliaceus (Fogo Selvagem): II. Current and Historic Epidemiologic Studies

Diaz LA, Sampaio SAP, Rivitti EA, Martins CR, Cunha PR, Lombardi C, Almeida FA, Martins Castro R, Macca ML, Lavrado C, Filho GH, Borges P, Chaul A, Minelli L, Empinotti JC, Friedman H, Campbell I, Labib RS, Anhalt GJ (Johns Hopkins Univ; Universidale de São Paulo, Brazil; Escola Paulista de Medicina, São Paulo; Hosp Adhemar de Barros, São Paulo; Hosp Adventista do Penfigo, Mato Grosso, Brazil; et al)

J Invest Dermatol 92:4–12, January 1989 3–2

Pemphigus foliaceus, or Fogo Selvagem, an endemic form of pemphigus, is a common skin disorder in Brazil. It is characterized by superficial cutaneous blisters and erosions. Mucosal surfaces are rarely involved. The Brazilian form of Fogo Selvagem is serologically identical to that seen in North America and Europe but differs in its epidemiology, the frequency of familial cases, and the age distribution among affected persons.

The disease presently is limited to the states of Goias, Mato Grosso do Sul, Parana, São Paulo, and Minas Gerais but appears to be spreading toward the northwest and west. Young peasants and children of either sex or any race exposed to the local ecology in rural areas of endemic states are at highest risk for Fogo Selvagem. The disease occurs only rarely in urban centers.

It is hypothesized that a black fly, *Simulium pruinosum,* may be the precipitating vector for Fogo Selvagem. Significant numbers of family units consisting of multiple, genetically related persons are affected. However, the immunogenetics of the disorder have not yet been studied.

Clinical examination of the skin and serologic screening for pemphigus autoantibodies are specific parameters that may increase the possibility of identifying the etiologic agents responsible for precipitating the autoantibody formation that leads to this autoimmune skin disorder.

▶ The pemphigus foliaceus antigen complex has been identified as the 160-kD glycoprotein desmoglein and the 50-kD plakoglobulin (1, 2). The pemphigus foliaceus antibody is predominantly IgG4 (3). That IgG4 also has been noted in filariasis and *Hymenoptera* venom reaction perhaps represents supporting evidence for the role of the blackfly in the etiology of Fogo Selvagem.—N.A. Soter, M.D.

References

1. Eyre RW, Stanley JR: *J Clin Invest* 81:807, 1988.
2. Korman NJ, et al: *N Engl J Med* 321:631, 1989.
3. Rock B, et al: *N Engl J Med* 320:1463, 1989.

The Pathogenic Effect of IgG4 Autoantibodies in Endemic Pemphigus Foliaceus (Fogo Selvagem)

Rock B, Martins CR, Theofilopoulos AN, Balderas RS, Anhalt GJ, Labib RS, Fu-

tamura S, Rivitti EA, Diaz LA (Johns Hopkins Univ; Univ of São Paulo; Med College of Wisconsin, Milwaukee; Scripps Clinic and Research Found, La Jolla)
N Engl J Med 320:1463–1469, June 1, 1989 3–3

Fogo Selvagem is an autoimmune blistering skin disease caused by IgG autoantibodies to a desmosome-associated glycoprotein. The IgG subclasses involved in this disease were studied in the serum of 29 patients and the skin lesions of 18 patients with active disease.

The predominant disease autoantibodies present in the serum from all patients were of the IgG4 subclass. There was a preferential deposition of IgG4 autoantibodies on the keratinocyte surface of the skin lesions in all patients examined. Serum fractions containing IgG4 autoantibody were transferred to neonatal mice, and the disease was reproduced clinically, histologically, and immunologically in these animals. The IgG4 autoantibodies were detected on the keratinocyte surface of the skin lesions of these mice.

Autoantibodies of the IgG4 subclass appear to be involved in the pathogenesis of Fogo Selvagem. Previously, IgG4 has been considered to be a protective antibody. This is clearly not the case in this condition. Antibodies of the IgG4 subclass may be involved in other autoimmune conditions.

▶ The detection of elevated serum levels of IgG4 and the demonstration of IgG4 deposited on keratinocytes in lesional skin of patients with endemic pemphigus foliaceus, coupled with the development of the cutaneous disease in neonatal mice after subcutaneous injection of IgG4, suggests new pathogenetic mechanism in this disorder. Such studies should be extended to patients with the sporadic form of pemphigus foliaceus.—N.A. Soter, M.D.

Bullous Pemphigoid Antigen Concentration in Normal Human Skin in Relation to Body Area and Age

Hamm G, Wozniak K-D (Martin-Luther-Universität Halle-Wittenberg, Halle, East Germany)
Arch Dermatol Res 280:416–419, November 1988 3–4

The variations in bullous pemphigoid antigen expression in normal human skin in relation to different body regions and to age were studied in 6 cadavers. Two sera with bullous pemphigoid antibodies were tested with 36 specimens of normal human skin and the amount of bullous pemphigoid antigen was estimated by end point titer determinations using indirect immunofluorescence technique.

In terms of body region the greatest expression of antigen was found in plantar sites, whereas the least expression was seen in flexural arm specimens. The highest end point titers were found in the oldest individuals and the lowest in the youngest.

Quantitative differenes of expression of bullous pemphigoid antigen exist depending on the body region from which the biopsy specimen is taken and the age of the donor. This is important to know in connection with indirect immunofluorescence assays for bullous pemphigoid antibodies on human skin.

▶ Bullous pemphigoid antigen, a 230-kD protein that is a normal constituent of the dermoepidermal junction, is associated with hemidesmosomes and is produced by keratinocytes (1–3). This study demonstrates that amounts of bullous pemphigoid antigen are related to age, with lower amounts in infants and higher amounts in those older than 75 years.—N.A. Soter, M.D.

References

1. Stanley JR, et al: *J Invest Dermatol* 82:108, 1984.
2. Westgate GE, et al: *J Invest Dermatol* 86:218, 1985.
3. Mueller S, et al: *J Invest Dermatol* 92:33, 1989.

Treatment of Bullous Pemphigoid With Topical Clobetasol Propionate
Westerhof W (Univ of Amsterdam)
J Am Acad Dermatol 20:458–461, March 1989 3–5

Bullous pemphigoid is a blistering skin disease of unknown etiology. The principal treatment has been systemic steroids, but severe reactions have led to a search for alternative treatment. Topical corticosteroid therapy for bullous pemphigoid was investigated in 10 patients who applied clobetasol propionate cream to the lesions twice daily. New blisters were counted daily. Treatment was continued for an additional 2 weeks after all lesions healed. A less potent topical corticosteroid cream—betamethasone dipropionate—was then substituted. Later, a still lower potency corticosteroid cream—triamcinolone acetonide—replaced betamethasone dipropionate; finally, treatment was stopped altogether. Pituitary adrenal function was determined 1 month after discharge while the patients were receiving betamethasone dipropionate.

All patients responded well to clobetasol propionate treatment. No new blisters developed after treatment began. Complete healing of all lesions was achieved within a mean of 10 days. At follow-up, 7 of 10 patients were in remission, with a duration of 1–10 months. After 4 months 1 patient required reinstitution of clobetasol propionate. Two patients died of unrelated causes. There were no systemic or local side effects with treatment.

The treatment regimen resulted in rapid healing of bullous lesions without adverse effects. Use of a highly potent topical corticosteroid in the long-term treatment of bullous pemphigoid warrants further study in a larger group of patients.

▶ High-potency topical corticosteroid preparations in addition to the concomitant use of systemically administered medications have achieved a place in the treatment of selected lesions in forms of pemphigus and bullous pemphigoid.

Although this paper reports on the sole use of a high-potency topical corticosteroid, the extent of disease may be a limiting factor with this therapeutic approach.—N.A. Soter, M.D.

Clinical Correlations of Linear IgA Deposition at the Cutaneous Basement Membrane Zone

Peters MS, Rogers RS III (Mayo Clinic and Found, Rochester, Minn)

J Am Acad Dermatol 20:761–770, May 1989 3–6

Linear IgA bullous dermatosis comprises a heterogeneous group of subepidermal vesiculobullous diseases defined by the direct immunofluorescence finding of a homogeneous linear pattern of IgA deposition at the basement membrane zone. The specificity of this finding in the diagnosis of primary bullous disease was evaluated. The results of all direct immunofluorescence studies of skin specimens obtained from patients at 1 center during a 5-year period were reviewed.

Of 4,642 specimens submitted, 44 specimens from 42 patients had linear IgA deposition at the basement membrane zone, with or without other immunoglobulins. Of these patients, 36 (86%) had primary subepi-

Linear IgA at the Cutaneous Basement Membrane Zone

Group	Linear IgA	No. of patients
Subepidermal bullous disease with linear IgA without IgG (20 patients)		
A_1	Linear IgA bullous dermatosis	10
A_1	Chronic bullous disease of childhood	2
A_2	Cicatricial pemphigoid	8
Subepidermal bullous disease with linear IgA and IgG (16 patients)		
B_1	Bullous pemphigoid	5
B_1	Epidermolysis bullosa acquisita	1
B_2	Cicatricial pemphigoid	10
Linear IgA without primary bullous disease (6 patients)		
C	Discoid lupus erythematosus	4
C	Urticaria	1
C	Varicella-zoster infection	1
Total number of patients		42

(Courtesy of Peters MS, Rogers RS III: *J Am Acad Dermatol* 20:761–770, May 1989.)

dermal bullous disease, and 20 of them had linear IgA without IgG at the basement membrane zone. Ten of these had clinical adult linear IgA bullous dermatosis, 2 had chronic bullous disease of childhood, and 8 had cicatricial pemphigoid. Sixteen had linear IgA and IgG at the basement membrane zone, 10 with clinical cicatricial pemphigoid, 5 with bullous pemphigoid, and 1 with epidermolysis bullosa acquisitia. Patients with cicatricial pemphigoid who had linear IgA without IgG at the basement membrane zone had a higher frequency of mucosal and ocular involvement than those with both immunoglobulins at the basement membrane zone (table).

The direct immunofluorescence finding of linear IgA deposition at the basement membrane zone correlates with primary subepidermal bullous disease in a high percentage of patients but reflects a heterogeneous group of blistering disorders.

▶ Linear deposition of IgA is a sign, not a diagnostic entity. In addition to the disease listed in this paper, linear IgA deposits have been noted in bullous systemic lupus erythematosus. See Maurice et al.'s review of the immunofluorescence findings in 279 patients with primary bullous disease (1).—A.J. Sober, M.D.

Reference

1. Maurice PDL, et al: *Clin Exp Dermatol* 11:352, 1986.

Epidermolysis Bullosa Simplex Superficialis: A New Variant of Epidermolysis Bullosa Characterized by Subcorneal Skin Cleavage Mimicking Peeling Skin Syndrome

Fine J-D, Johnson L, Wright T (Univ of Alabama, Birmingham; Birmingham VA Med Ctr)

Arch Dermatol 125:633–638, May 1989 3–7

A variant of epidermolysis bullosa simplex—epidermolysis bullosa simplex superficialis—is characterized by skin cleavage just below the level of the stratum corneum. It appears to be an autosomal dominant trait, differing from other autosomal dominant forms of epidermolysis bullosa simplex by milia, atrophic scarring, and involvement of oral or ocular surfaces, or both.

In 2 of 7 cases a second, more focal cleft was found within the lower third of the epidermis. In some cases the stratum corneum was almost totally separated from the rest of the epidermis. Electron microscopy showed focal homogenization of the stratum corneum in some areas.

Epidermolysis bullosa simplex superficialis and peeling skin syndrome have in common only the same level of skin cleavage; it is by no means clear that the latter is a variant of epidermolysis bullosa simplex.

▶ This paper nicely illustrates a new variant of epidermolysis bullosa simplex. The major differential diagnosis for this entity is peeling skin syndrome. However, there seem to be significant differences in age of onset, distribution, morphological features, mode of inheritance, clinical presentations, and seasonal variations.—T.J. Flotte, M.D.

Autosomal Recessive Epidermolysis Bullosa Simplex: Generalized Phenotypic Features Suggestive of Junctional or Dystrophic Epidermolysis Bullosa, and Association With Neuromuscular Diseases

Fine J-D, Stenn J, Johnson L, Wright T, Bock H-GO, Horiguchi Y (Univ of Alabama, Birmingham; Yale Univ; Univ of Mississippi, Jackson)

Arch Dermatol 125:931–938, July 1989 3–8

Epidermolysis bullosa simplex is characterized by rather localized, recurrent, intraepidermal blisters that develop after minor mechanical trauma to the skin. Mucous membranes and other organs are rarely involved. In almost all cases, this form of epidermolysis bullosa is transmitted as an autosomal dominant disorder. An autosomal recessive form of the disease characterized by cutaneous features more representative of junctional or dystrophic epidermolysis bullosa was diagnosed in 2 patients, both of whom had associated muscular dystrophy. Four additional patients with autosomal recessive epidermolysis bullosa simplex with similar findings were encountered.

The patients were a black male infant, a 6-year-old boy who was the infant's fourth cousin, and a 43-year-old white man and his twin sister. The latter patients' parents were first cousins of Russian heritage. All 4 patients had generalized cutaneous findings that included milia, atrophic scarring, nail dystrophy, and scalp alopecia. These presentations have traditionally been attributed to either junctional or dystrophic epidermolysis bullosa. In addition, both children had associated congenital muscular dystrophy, and the woman had congenital myasthenia gravis that had been treated by thymectomy. Both children had marked growth retardation, anemia, and oral erosions or ulcerations.

Immunofluorescence mapping studies, monoclonal antibody studies, and transmission electron microscopic examinations were performed on skin biopsy specimens obtained from the 2 children and the man. The findings were indicative of skin cleavage within or above the level of the basal keratinocytes, confirming the presence of epidermolysis bullosa simplex rather than the junctional or dystrophic form.

Thus there exists an autosomal recessive form of epidermolysis bullosa simplex that may be associated with skin presentations more indicative of the junctional or dystrophic form than of the simplex form. Furthermore, patients with this form of epidermolysis bullosa simplex may have more generalized disease activity and congenital neuromuscular disorders.

▶ This very interesting paper can be interpreted in at least 2 different ways. The authors chose to present these patients as having a scarring form of epidermolysis bullosa simplex. From a histologic vantage point, this is correct. My own inclination, however, is to look upon these patients as having a different disease, perhaps a new subset of epidermolysis bullosa. I think that the uniform association with neuromuscular disease supports this. Of course, the proof will be when the gene product of this group of disorders is determined.—T.J. Flotte, M.D.

Studies on Two Siblings With Recessive Dystrophic Epidermolysis Bullosa (Hallopeau-Siemens) and the Plasminogen Activator and Its Inhibitor in the Lesion

Kaneko F, Tsukinaga I, Ando M, Ohkawara A, Oguchi H, Oikawa K, Nagai M (Hokkaido Univ, Sapporo; Nagai Skin Clinic, Aza Inuyama, Inuyama, Japan)

Dermatologica 178:156–163, 1989 3–9

The mechanism of blistering in recessive dystrophic epidermolysis bullosa (RDEB) is unclear, but recent evidence suggests that the increased activity of a protease or defects in protease inhibitors are involved. The relationship between plasminogen activator and its inhibitors to the formation of blisters was examined in 2 siblings with RDEB. A girl, 13 years old, and her brother, 10 years old, were born with bullous lesions. The girl was treated unsuccussfully with vitamin E and diphenylhydantoin administered orally and with topical antibiotic ointments. Both had severe blistering and erosions.

Hematologic findings included hyperfibrinogenemia, hyper-γ globulinemia and marked thrombocytosis. Immunofluorescent examination revealed strong deposits of plasminogen, fibrin degradation products, and α_1-antitrypsin around the blisters, with little α_2-macroglobulin present. Because these results indicated high plasminogen activity in the lesions, the patients were treated twice daily with topical application of 0.5% to 1% of the strong plasminogen activator inhibitor camostat mesylate (N,N-dimethylcarbonylacetate *p*-(*p*-guanidinobenzoyloxy)phenylacetate methane sulfonate, FOY 305). After 2 weeks of application, eroded lesions quickly dried and improved, unlike lesions treated with bacitracin ointment.

Plasminogen activator was produced by the degraded tissues and their infiltrates. This finding and the therapeutic success of a strong plasminogen activator inhibitor indicate that plasminogen activator in the lesions is important in the development of blisters in RDEB.

▶ This paper presents potentially important news for patients with RDEB. Of course, the study needs to be repeated with many more controls in order to show that the effects seen in these 2 patients are not a "fluke." Remember the vitamin E story with RDEB several years back?—J.C. Alper, M.D.

Recurrent Erythema Multiforme

Huff JC, Weston WL (Univ of Colorado)

Medicine 68:133–140, May 1989 3–10

In a recent prospective clinical analysis of erythema multiforme (EM), 22 patients who had more than 1 episode of EM were identified. Such patients may have a distinct clinical subset of this disease. The patients had an average age of 29 years and an average of 12 previous episodes of EM, each episode lasting approximately 3 weeks. The average length of time between episodes was 4.9 months.

Patients had an average of 188 EM skin lesions at the time of examination. The isomorphic phenomenon, lesions appearing at sites of skin trauma, occurred in 19 patients. Photodistribution of skin lesions occurred in 15. Grouping of lesions over the elbows and knees was noted in 7 patients, and nailfold involvement was observed in 7.

Evidence indicates that herpes simplex virus is associated with recurrent EM. Each of the patients had a history of herpes simplex virus infections preceding at least 1 of the earlier EM episodes. Sera from each patient had antibodies to herpes simplex virus detectable by enzyme immunoassy. However, the virus was not isolated from the throat at the time of EM or from an EM skin lesion in any of the patients. All 11 patients tested at the time of their next herpes simplex infection had positive viral cultures for herpes simplex virus taken from the suspected recurrent herpes lesion. Eight EM skin samples were assessed by indirect immunofluorescence with a monoclonal antibody to common herpes simplex virus glycoprotein gB, and all had positive staining of keratinocytes. Only a third of the patients with a single episode of EM had a history of possible herpes lesions preceding EM. In all patients with recurrent EM, herpes simplex virus should be considered the most likely cause.

▶ This is a very fine review of the problem of recurrent EM. The authors conclude that recurrent EM is most probably caused by herpes simplex virus infection, and for this reason corticosteroids are not indicated (they don't help). In contrast to drug-induced major forms of EM, these patients are generally afebrile and not systemically ill. If therapy is necessary, acyclovir reportedly is helpful in eliminating recurrent episodes.— R. Masters, M.D.

4 Collagen Vascular Disease

Outcome in Systemic Lupus Erythematosus: A Prospective Study of Patients From a Defined Population

Jonsson H, Nived O, Sturfelt G (Univ of Lund)

Medicine 68:141–150, May 1989 4–1

Present knowledge of the outcome of systemic lupus erythematosus (SLE) stems principally from studies of racially mixed populations, and few prospective longitudinal studies have been done. Epidemiologic methodology was used to study the prospective outcome of SLE in a Caucasian cohort in Sweden.

All adult SLE patients in a defined population of approximately 160,000 were followed prospectively, beginning in 1980. The study sample included 86 patients, all of whom underwent clinical examination and blood sampling at 2-month intervals. The prevalence of symptomatic secondary Sjögren's syndrome was estimated by questionnaire; if patients were symptomatic, researchers sought diagnostic verification with rose bengal staining or lip biopsy, or both. Functional impairment was classified according to Steinbrocker's method. Patients with major flares were assigned to 1 of 2 groups on the basis of whether they had subsequent flares during the study period.

The incidence of the disease was 4 cases per 100,000 adults per year. By the end of 1986, point prevalence was 42 cases per 100,000 population at risk. Five-year survival in the prospective group was 97%. Patients had a normal rate of employment. Ninety-eight percent of patients had musculoskeletal involvement, and 77% had mucocutaneous involvement (table). Immunologic studies showed a 73% frequency of positive anti-dsDNA and a 10% frequency of rheumatoid factor positivity. The median frequency of American Rheumatism Association criteria was 6. Men had more serositis and renal symptoms than women; 16% of the patients were men. After the diagnosis year, disease flares were constant at 0.2 flares per year per patient. Patients with renal disease had little functional impairment. Prolonged glucocorticoid treatment was associated with both morbidity and mortality.

The low mortality, low frequency of serious complications, and normal employment rates could be attributable at least in part to efficient identification of patients. Findings of late morbidity and mortality associated with glucocorticoid treatment suggest a conservative approach in the treatment of quiescent SLE.

Cumulative Organ System Involvement in the Study Group

Manifestation	Entire study group (n=86)	Patients diagnosed 1979–1986 (n=50)	Patients diagnosed before 1979 (n=36)
Mucocutaneous	77	74	81
Malar rash	43	34	56
Discoid lupus	23	24	22
Photosensitivity	52	50	54
Oral ulcers	13	12	14
Musculoskeletal	98	96	100
Arthritis	98	96	100
Myositis	3	2	6
Serositis	62	54	72
Glomerulonephritis	30	24	39
Neuropsychiatric	47	40	56
Epilepsy	5	6	3
Psychosis	8	8	8
Cerebral infarction	8	6	11
Hematologic	49	42	58
Leukopenia	42	38	47
Thrombocytopenia	10	6	17
Hemolytic anemia	2	2	3

Numbers are percentages.
(Courtesy of Jonsson H, Nived O, Sturfelt G: *Medicine* 68:141–150, May 1989.)

▶ In this study of patients with SLE, 18 of 86 (21%) experienced cutaneous vasculitis, although the methods of documentation of this diagnosis were not mentioned. Of patients with photosensitivity, 41% had anti-Ro (SSA) and 26% anti-La (SSB) antibodies, in contrast to 48% and 6%, respectively, of those without photosensitivity. During flares, involvement of the skin was considered a minor manifestation and was not further discussed.—N.A. Soter, M.D.

Subacute Cutaneous Lupus Erythematosus: Clinicopathologic Findings in Thirteen Cases

Herrero C, Bielsa I, Font J, Lozano F, Ercilla G, Lecha M, Ingelmo M, Mascaró JM (Hosp Clinico, Barcelona)
J Am Acad Dermatol 19:1057–1062, December 1988 4–2

Subacute cutaneous lupus erythematosus is a distinct clinical, serologic, and genetic subset of lupus erythematosus. Among 167 patients with lupus erythematosus seen during a 3-year period, 13 (7%) had subacute cutaneous lupus erythematosus.

The cutaneous features consisted of a widespread and symmetric, slightly desquamative annular pattern (85%) (table) usually located on sun-exposed areas. Vesicular-bullous lesions were present on the active margins (38%), and the lesions regressed without atrophic scarring. About 70% of the patients had some evidence of systemic involvement,

Dermatologic Features

Features	Patients No.	%
Annular lesions	11	85
Papulosquamous lesions	2	15
Discoid lupus erythematosus	0	0
Periungual telangiectasia	5	38
Livedo reticularis	0	0
Nonscarring alopecia	4	33
Raynaud's phenomenon	3	23
Mucous membrane ulcers	5	38

(Courtesy of Herrero C, Bielsa I, Font J, et al: *J Am Acad Dermatol* 19:1057–1062, December 1988.)

and 46% met American Rheumatism Association criteria for systemic lupus erythematosus. Antinuclear antibodies were present in 54% of patients. Antibodies to the Ro antigen were present in 60% and to the double-stranded DNA in 15%. None of the patients had positive titers of anti-RNP or anti-Sm antibodies. The HLA-DR3 phenotype was evident in 82% of patients. Histologic examination showed vacuolar degeneration of the basal layer, with no thickening of the basement membrane, and a perivascular lymphocytic infiltrate. Noteworthy was the presence of abundant epidermal colloid bodies in 63% of cases; focal areas of severe epidermal necrosis in 54% corresponded to the active border of the annular lesions.

The clinical and immunologic features of these patients with subacute cutaneous lupus eythematosus are similar to those described by most authors. However, the epidermal alterations evident on histologic examination have not been emphasized previously. It is possible that only widespread annular or gyrate cutaneous lesions with active, scaly, vesicular, or crusty borders may be associated with subacute cutaneous lupus erythematosus.

▶ The authors emphasize the extent of epidermal alterations in skin biopsy specimens obtained from patients with subacute cutaneous lupus erythematosus and suggest a correlation with the clinical appearance of the lesion. To confirm this hypothesis, both time-course studies of lesion evolution and careful correlative studies of different morphological portions in a single lesion should be performed.—N.A. Soter, M.D.

Correlation of Anti-Ro Antibody With Photosensitivity Rash in Systemic Lupus Erythematosus Patients

Mond CB, Peterson MGE, Rothfield NF (Univ of Connecticut)

Arthritis Rheum 32:202–204, February 1989 4–3

The significance of anti-Ro antibodies in patients with systemic lupus erythematosus (SLE) is controversial. Sera from 131 patients with SLE were tested by counterimmunoelectrophoresis for the presence of anti-Ro antibody to determine the relationship of anti-Ro antibodies to specific manifestations of the disease.

Fifteen percent of the patients tested positive for anti-Ro antibody. Age, sex, and the total number of revised criteria met did not differ significantly between patients who were positive and those who were negative for anti-Ro antibody. The antibody was not significantly related to the presence of renal disease or to other SLE criteria; however, anti-Ro was present in significantly more patients with a photosensitivity rash than in those who had no rash.

A significant association between anti-Ro antibody and photosensitivity rash in SLE patients was noted. However, no significant relationship was found between anti-Ro and other SLE criteria or between anti-Ro and demographic variables.

▶ Photosensitivity was defined in this study as an eruption resulting from an unusual reaction to sunlight determined by the patient's history or physician's observation. For the dermatologist, a more precise characterization of the photosensitivity would have been of value inasmuch as a variety of types of photosensitivity occur in patients with lupus erythematosus.—N.A. Soter, M.D.

Phototests in Patients With Various Forms of Lupus Erythematosus

Wolska H, Blaszczyk M, Jablońska S (Warsaw School of Medicine, Warsaw, Poland)

Int J Dermatol 28:98–103, March 1989 4–4

Light hypersensitivity in lupus erythematosus (LE) is well documented, but information on the photsensitivity test in patients with LE is scarce. Responses on exposure to ultraviolet B, 290–320 nm, were tested in 227 patients with discoid LE, discoid disseminated LE, systemic LE, or suba-

TABLE 1.—Persistence of Erythema as Related to Ultraviolet Dose in Patients With Long-Lasting Erythema

LE Subset (No. of Cases)	No. of Patients with Prolonged Erythema	Prolonged Erythema After 1 MED	Prolonged Erythema After ≥2 MED
SLE (67)	55	21 (38.2%)	34 (61.8%)
SCLE (24)	24	13 (54.2%)	11 (45.8%)
DDLE (21)	17	8 (47.1%)	9 (52.9%)
DLE (90)	51	15 (29.4%)	36 (70.6%)

(Courtesy of Wolska H, Błaszczyk M, Jabłońska S: *Int J Dermatol* 28:98–103, March 1989.)

TABLE 2.—Reproduction of Skin Lesions After Single Exposure to ~0.025–0.145 J/cm³ of Ultraviolet B

LE Subset	No. of Patients Observed	No. of Patients with Induced Lesions (%)
SLE	67	16 (23.9%)
SCLE	24	15 (62.5%)
DDLE	21	9 (42.8%)
DLE	90	9 (10%)

(Courtesy of Wolska H, Błaszczyk M, Jabłońska S: *Int J Dermatol* 28:98–103, March 1989.)

cute cutaneous LE. The minimal erythema dose and its distribution, persistence of erythema, and photoreproduction of lesions were evaluated.

Patients differed considerably from controls in reactivity to ultraviolet B. There were significant differences between patients with various LE forms, even after a single ultraviolet exposure. A lowered minimal erythema dose, compared with controls, was noted most often in patients with systemic LE and least frequently in patients with discoid LE. Prolonged persistence of erythema induced by 1–2 minimal erythema dose was a constant finding in subacute cutaneous LE. It was noted in more than 80% of patients with systemic LE and discoid disseminated LE, and in 56.7% of patients with discoid LE. Photoreproduction of lesions after a single exposure to ultraviolet B was observed most often in patients with subacute cutaneous LE and least often in those with discoid LE (Tables 1 and 2).

Results of photosensitivity tests varied widely in relation to the various types of LE in a large group of patients.

▶ These investigators have drawn on their wide experience with LE to document the results of phototesting in 227 patients. Other investigators in much smaller series have not demonstrated consistently lowered minimal erythema doses of ultraviolet B, although the persistence of erythema for abnormally long periods has been a common finding. In this paper both a lowered minimal erythema dose and persistent erythema were frequent (using unblinded evaluation of erythema). Ro antibodies were noted in only 5 of 17 subacute cutaneous lupus erythematosus patients; the authors point out that this could result from use of an immunodiffusion assay.—R.W. Gange, M.D.

Bullous Systemic Lupus Erythematosus

Fleming MG, Bergfeld WF, Tomecki KJ, Tuthill RJ, Norris M, Benedetto EA, Weber LA (Cleveland Clinic Found)

Int J Dermatol 28:321–326, June 1989 4–5

Observations were made in a patient with bullous systemic lupus and a second patient with lesions of bullous systemic lupus associated with drug-induced lupus erythematosus—a previously unreported association. The first patient had asymptomatic vesicles and bullae on sun-exposed areas of the face, neck, and arms. Direct immunofluorescence study of perilesional skin showed granular deposits of immunoglobulins and complement components at the dermoepidermal junction. The lesions were controlled by dapsone. The second patient had a bullous eruption after antihypertensive treatment that included hydralazine and reserpine. When those drugs were withdrawn, the skin returned to normal, but joint symptoms persisted and antinuclear antibody remained positive.

The mechanism of blister formation in bullous systemic lupus erythematosus is uncertain. Immune complexes appear to be present, but they also are found in the skin of patients lacking bullae. Possibly, the immune complexes of bullous lupus activate complement more readily. Bullous systemic lupus generally is treated with systemic steroids, but steroids do not consistently prevent or eliminate the lesions. Dapsone often is effective, but the disease may recur.

▶ The potential complexity of the mechanisms of bulla formation in lupus erythematosus is enhanced by the observation that antibodies to type VII procollagen, a component of the basal lamina anchoring the fibril complex of the basement membrane zone that is identical to the acquired epidermolysis bullosa antigen (1), are occasionally detected in sera of patients with bullous lupus erythematosus (2).—N.A. Soter, M.D.

References

1. Woodley DJ, et al: *J Invest Dermatol* 88:525, 1987.
2. Gammon WR, et al: *J Invest Dermatol* 84:472, 1985.

Cutaneous Necrosis Associated With the Lupus Anticoagulant

Frances C, Tribout B, Boisnic S, Drouet L, Piette AM, Piette JC, Blétry O, Wechsler B, Godeau P (Groupe Hospitalier Pitié-Salpêtrière, Paris; Hôp Saint Louis, Paris: Hôp Foch, Suresnes, France)

Dermatologica 178:194–201, 1989 4–6

Extensive cutaneous necrosis associated with a lupus anticoagulant is unusual. This disease affected the limbs of 3 women aged 20–45 years with benign systemic lupus erythematosus. All were otherwise in good general health.

The lesions appeared suddenly as extremely painful, rapidly spreading cutaneous necrosis with a purpuric border on the thighs and legs, as well as, in 1 patient, on the arm (Fig 4–1). All 3 patients had a circulating anticoagulant and positive results of VDRL tests without anticardiolipin antibodies. Skin biopsy findings included a thrombosing microangiitis affecting the dermal vessels. Direct immunofluorescence was positive, showing intravascular deposits of fibrin, IgA, IgM, IgG, and Clq, without deposits at the dermoepidermal junction. Other causes of cutaneous ne-

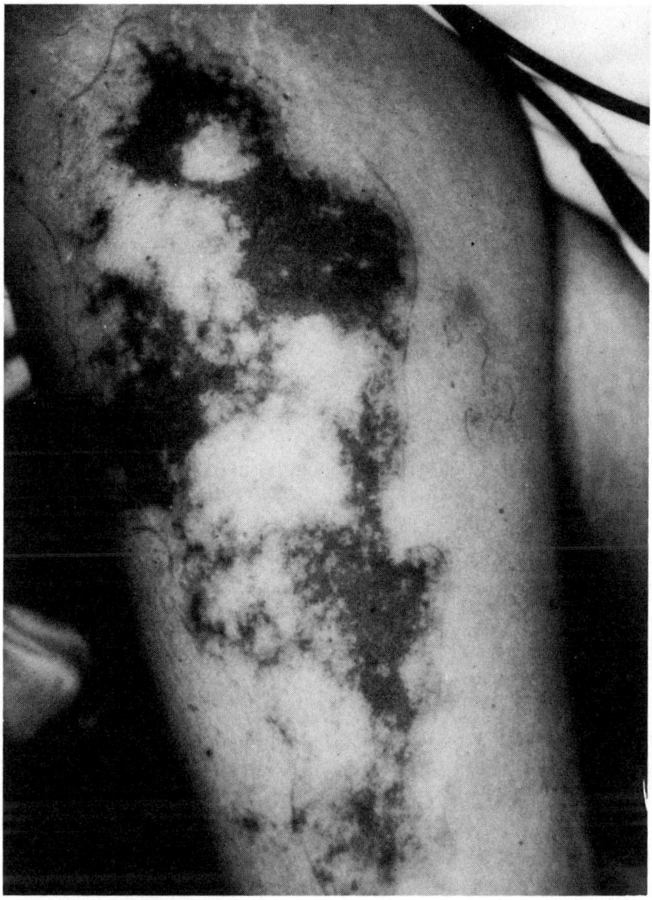

Fig 4–1.—Reticulate necrotic plaques on the legs. (Courtesy of Frances C, Tribout B, Boisnic S, et al: *Dermatologica* 178:194–201, 1989.)

crosis were absent. All 3 patients were treated successfully with pulse methylprednisolone therapy and plasmapheresis.

Cutaneous necrosis associated with lupus anticoagulant resembles that observed in congenital protein C deficiency. This favors the hypothesis of an interaction between the lupus anticoagulant and protein C-S complex. The lupus anticoagulant may have an inhibitory effect on thrombomodulin or protein S.

▶ The lupus anticoagulant is an antiphospholipid antibody composed of IgG or IgM, or both. It is found in patients with antiphospholipid antibody syndrome (1), which itself occurs with lupus erythematosus.

This report annotates the observation that in patients with systemic lupus erythematosus and a lupus anticoagulant extensive areas of purpura and necrosis may develop. Erythematous and violaceous macules on the fingertips that demonstrate thrombi without vasculitis of the dermal blood vessels in skin biopsy specimens also have been reported (2).—N.A. Soter, M.D.

References

1. Hughes GRV, et al: *J Rheumatol* 13:486, 1986.
2. Grob JJ, et al: *J Am Acad Dermatol* 15:211, 1986.

The Spectrum of Livedo Reticularis and Anticardiolipin Antibodies

Asherson RA, Mayou SC, Merry P, Black MM, Hughes GRV (St Thomas' Hosp, London)

Br J Dermatol 120:215–221, February 1989 4–7

Livedo reticularis is characterized by a lattice-like pattern of dilated superficial veins often induced by cold. It has been frequently associated with CNS complications. In a 2-year period, 65 patients were first seen with livedo reticularis. They were assessed for clinical features of CNS disease, venous and arterial thrombosis, Raynaud's syndrome, fetal loss, and cardiac valvular lesions. Researchers also evaluated the platelet count, antinuclear antibodies, and anticardiolipin antibodies (a-Cl). In some patients the lupus anticoagulant also was measured. Patients were separated into a-Cl positive- and a-Cl-negative groups.

There were 28 a-Cl-positive patients, of which 25 were women. Of the 37 a-Cl-negative patients, 33 were women. There was a greater percentage of CNS complications in the a-Cl-positive group, which were statistically significant for cerebrovascular accidents and transient ischemic attacks. They were significant at the 2% level for chorea, but not significant for epilepsy, migraine, or psychiatric disease. The a-Cl-positive group also had more occurrences of venous thrombosis, valvular heart lesions, thrombocytopenia, and fetal loss. At the 5% level or less, the following were significant: thrombocytopenia, thrombosis, valvular heart lesions, and fetal loss. Raynaud's syndrome occurred more often among a-Cl-negative patients.

Patients with livedo reticularis and a-Cl positivity have a signficantly higher risk of cerebrovascular disease than do such patients who are a-Cl negative. The latter may have a higher risk for Raynaud's syndrome.

▶ Antiphospholipid antibodies delineate a syndrome characterized by venous and arterial thromboses, thrombocytopenia, and recurrent fetal loss. This syndrome occurs in patients with lupus erythematosus and other autoimmune disorders, with certain infectious diseases, and as a primary idiopathic syndrome (1–3). This study suggests that patients with livedo reticularis and associated connective tissue disorders should be assessed for the presence of a-Cls.—N.A. Soter, M.D.

References

1. Hughes GRV, et al: *J Rheumatol* 13:486, 1986.
2. Macworth-Young CG, et al: *Ann Rheum Dis* 48:362, 1989.
3. Alarcon-Segovia D, et al: *J Rheumatol* 16:482, 1989.

Raynaud Syndrome in Childhood

Duffy CM, Laxer RM, Lee P, Ramsay C, Fritzler M, Silverman ED (Hosp for Sick Children, Toronto; Wellesley Hosp; Women's College Hosp; Univ of Toronto; Univ of Calgary)

J Pediatr 114:73–78, January 1989 4–8

When Raynaud's syndrome (RS) occurs in childhood, it is usually caused by an underlying connective tissue disease. Criteria are available to help distinguish primary RS from secondary RS (Raynaud's phenomenon) but there are none to predict which patients with RS alone might have a connective tissue disorder.

Twenty-seven patients with childhood onset of RS were studied to determine the prevalence of primary RS and to evaluate the predictive role of antinuclear antibody, nailfold capillary microscopy, and photoelectric plethysmography in such patients. In addition to antinuclear antibodies, serologic studies included rheumatoid factor, anti-dsDNA, and anti-ribonucleoprotein. Nailfold capillary microscopy was performed to determine overall avascularity of the nail bed and the number of enlarged loops (Fig 4–2). To assess digital blood flow, 16 patients underwent photoelectric plethysmography.

The mean age at onset of RS was 11.7 years; 52% had definite and 15% had probable connective tissue disease, and 33% had primary RS. All patients with either definite or probable connective tissue disease had a positive reaction to antinuclear antibody, whereas those with primary RS did not. Nailfold capillary scores also differed significantly between both connective-tissue-disease groups and the primary RS group. All patients had reduced photoelectric plethysmography scores, but differences between groups were not significant.

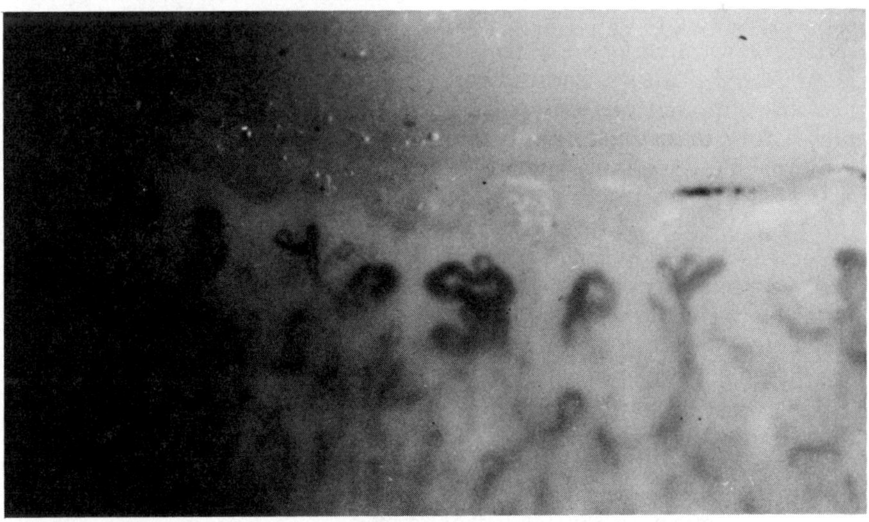

Fig 4–2.—Enlarged and extremely enlarged loops with severe avascularity. (Courtesy of Duffy CM, Laxer RM, Lee P, et al: *J Pediatr* 114:73–78, January 1989.)

Primary RS is more common in children than has been thought. Both antinuclear antibody and nailfold microscopy can differentiate between primary RS and RS with probable or definite connective tissue disease; photoelectric plethysmography is not useful for this purpose.

▶ Although this study suggests that nailfold capillary microscopy and the presence of antinuclear antibody can distinguish between children with primary RS and RS with concomitant connective tissue disorders, the authors properly suggest that further studies are required to predict which children with RS will have connective tissue disorders.—N.A. Soter, M.D.

Hand Warming as a Treatment for Raynaud's Phenomenon in Systemic Sclerosis

Goodfield MJD, Rowell NR (Gen Infirmary at Leeds, England)

Br J Dermatol 119:643–646, November 1988 4–9

Ninety-five percent of patients with systemic sclerosis have Raynaud's phenomenon at some time during their illness. All of the many vasodilatory drugs used to treat this condition result in some degree of symptomatic improvement, although improvement is less in systemic sclerosis than in primary Raynaud's phenomenon. Clinical improvement, however, is associated with little improvement in blood flow. The vasodilatory effect of simple hand warming was evaluated in patients with systemic sclerosis.

Twelve patients with Raynaud's phenomenon resulting from systemic sclerosis warmed their hands for 5 minutes in hand-hot water every 4 hours throughout the day during alternate weeks of a 6-week study. Significantly fewer and shorter attacks of Raynaud's phenomenon occurred during periods of warming than during periods of nonwarming. Eleven patients preferred the warming periods; the other patient was unable to decide which he preferred. Patients reported going outside more often during warming periods, although this difference was not statistically significant. Blood flow was increased significantly in the 8 patients in whom it was measured.

Simple hand warming appears to be effective in the management of patients with Raynaud's phenomenon caused by systemic sclerosis.

▶ Immersion of the hands in hot water (35° C) is a simple maneuver in the treatment of Raynaud's phenomenon associated with systemic sclerosis. This technique should be evaluated in other forms of Raynaud's phenomenon.—N.A. Soter, M.D.

Post-Irradiation Morphoea

Colver GB, Rodger A, Mortimer PS, Savin JA, Neill SM, Hunter JAA (Royal Infirmary, Edinburgh; Western Gen Hosp, Edinburgh; St George's Hosp, Tooting, England; Westminster Hosp, London)

Br J Dermatol 120:831–835, June 1989 4–10

Radiation-induced morphea was mentioned in early dermatology textbooks, but current texts only briefly note this complication. However, because it may be confused with a sclerotic recurrence of the original tumor, awareness of this potential complication is important. Nine women aged 39–85 years with morphea after radiation therapy were observed.

Morphea started in the radiation-exposed zone in all patients but extended slowly beyond it in 4. Radiation-induced morphea did not appear to be related to the total radiation dose, as it developed with doses both less than 20 Gy and more than 69 Gy. Morphea was also not related to the severity of the acute radiation reaction, because in 5 of the 9 patients erythema was only mild or moderate, with small areas of desquamation in 2 of the 5 patients.

Although radiation-induced morphea is not debilitating, dermatologists and radiation oncologists should be aware of its appearance, so as not to confuse it with local tumor recurrence.

▶ Morphea is a puzzle indeed. Possible clues to its etiology are its association with lichen sclerosus et atrophicus, some autoimmune diseases such as vitiligo, and a putative relationship to infection with *Borrelia burgdorferi*. This observation of the development of morphea in irradiated sites *and* the spread of the process to sites that had not been irradiated is baffling. Lichen sclerosis et atrophicus has been observed in the postmastectomy field of radiation (1). The authors remark that radiation fibrosis progressing to fibroblast proliferation occurs in the lung (radiation pneumonitis) and in the kidney (radiation nephritis.)

We have seen a patient recently with breast cancer treated with radiation in whom a morphea-like plaque developed in the area that had been irradiated, but we regarded it as a result of fibrosis from the irradiation. The patient complained of the induration of the skin. This was, in fact, morphea developing in an area *beyond* the site of irradiation.—T.B. Fitzpatrick, M.D., Ph.D.

Reference

1. Yates VM, et al: *Arch Dermatol* 121:1044, 1985.

Antibodies to the *Borrelia burgdorferi* Flagellum in Patients With Scleroderma, Granuloma Annulare, and Porphyria Cutanea Tarda

Halkier-Sørensen L, Kragballe K, Hansen K (Marselisborg Hosp, Aarhus, Denmark; Statens Seruminstitut, Copenhagen)

Acta Derm Venereol (Stockh) 69:116–119, April 1989 4–11

Cutaneous Lyme borreliosis generally includes erythema chronicum migrans, lymphadenosis benigna cutis, and acrodermatitis chronica atrophicans. However, in recent years, *Borrelia burgdorferi* has been associated with other cutaneous disorders. Sera from 175 patients, including 64 with localized scleroderma (morphea), 74 with systemic sclerosis, 16 with granuloma annulare, and 21 with porphyria cutanea tarda, were tested with a new, highly sensitive and specific *B. burgdorferi* flagellum enzyme-linked immunosorbent assay. The control groups included 297 normal healthy volunteers and 30 patients with other skin diseases.

The distribution of individual antibody values and median antibody levels did not differ significantly between controls and patients with scleroderma, granuloma annulare, and porphyria cutanea tarda.

No serologic evidence of an etiologic association between *B. burgdorferi* infection and scleroderma, granuloma annulare, or porphyria cutanea tarda was found. If a skin disorder resembles a *Borrelia* infection, the presence of a positive antibody titer should be evaluated in association with the clinical findings, histologic picture, IgG (or IgM) titer kinetics, and a definite treatment response.

▶ Fibrotic plaques resembling morphea or lichen sclerosis et atrophicus are seen in patients with acrodermatitis chronica atrophicans, a complication of longstanding *Borrelia* infection. Whereas acrodermatitis chronica atrophicans occurs with some frequency in Northern Europe, it is only rarely diagnosed in the United States. In a study from Vienna, Aberer and coworkers (1) reported that 8 of 15 patients with morphea had specific IgG or IgM antibodies to *B. burgdorferi,* that *B. burgdorferi* was cultured from a lesional biopsy specimen of a seropositive patient, that spirochetes were identified in histologic section of morphea-like lesions, and that seropositive patients responded to penicillin therapy. In the present study, Halkier-Sørensen and coworkers, using a *B. burgdorferi* flagellum enzyme-linked immunosorbent assay, did not find serologic evidence that *B. burgdorferi* was associated with either morphea (localized scleroderma) or progressive systemic sclerosis, granuloma annulare, or porphyria cutanea tarda.

It seems likely that morphea and lichen sclerosis et atrophicus are tissue reaction patterns that may be caused by *Borrelia* infection in some cases. The likelihood of morphea or lichen sclerosis et atrophicus being *Borelia* associated depends on the geographic locale. In Northern Europe (e.g., Vienna or Stockholm) and in certain localities in the United States where the incidence of Lyme borreliosis is high, oral treatment of morphea or lichen sclerosis et atrophicus with doxycycline, 100 mg twice daily for 1 month, seems judicious. Where endemicity is low, such treatment, although innocuous, may not be justified.— R.A. Johnson, M.D.

Reference

1. Aberer E, et al: *Acta Derm Venereol (Stockh)* 67:225, 1987.

Antibodies to Ro/SSA Detected by ELISA: Correlation With Clinical Features in Systemic Scleroderma

Bell S, Krieg T, Meurer M (Ludwig-Maximilians-Univ, Munich, West Germany)
Br J Dermatol 121:35–41, July 1989 4–12

Circulating autoantibodies against nuclear and nucleolar antigens, which are found in systemic scleroderma, may help in classifying cases. A new ELISA was used to detect anti-Ro/SSA antibodies in sera from 114 patients with systemic scleroderma.

The Ro/SSA antibody was found in 37% of cases. Serologic results could not be related to major organ involvement, but sicca syndrome and polymyositis were more frequent in antibody-positive patients. The Ro/SSA antibody correlated with antinuclear antibody detected by indirect immunofluorescence using HEp-2 cells as substrate. Rheumatoid factor was more frequent in Ro/SSA-positive patients. Nearly one third of patients with Ro/SSA antibody and 1 of 12 antibody-negative patients had HLA-DR3.

The presence of serum Ro/SSA antibody in patients with scleroderma correlates with the presence of both sicca syndrome and polymyositis.

▶ The detection of serum antibodies to Ro/SSA in patients with scleroderma and concomitant sicca syndrome and polymyositis perhaps suggests broader associations between antibodies and specific clinical manifestations among connective tissue disorders as well as associations with HLA.—N.A. Soter, M.D.

Interleukin-2 in Scleroderma: Correlation of Serum Level With Extent of Skin Involvement and Disease Duration

Kahaleh MB, LeRoy EC (Med Univ of South Carolina, Charleston)

Ann Intern Med 110:446–450, March 15, 1989 4–13

The pathogenesis of scleroderma is unknown, but evidence suggests the presence of a cell-mediated immune mechanism in the disease. Interleukin-2 could be a factor in the pathogenesis of scleroderma. Sera from 47 patients with scleroderma, 20 patients with rheumatoid arthritis, and 14 matched controls were cultured with an interleukin-2-dependent cytotoxic T cell line. The serum level was determined by an enzyme-linked immunosorbent assay.

Cytotoxic T cell line cells did not grow when cultured in Roswell Park Memorial Institute medium supplemented with fetal calf serum. When recombinant human interleukin-2 was added to cells at 25, 50, and 75 units per mL, a stepwise proliferative response in sera was noted in 9 of 20 patients with rheumatoid arthritis and 41 of 47 patients with scleroderma. Mitogenic activity was absent in sera from controls. In sera from patients with scleroderma, a positive correlation was noted between serum level and the skin progression index.

The presence of interleukin-2 in sera from scleroderma patients strongly indicates a role for T cell activation in this disease. The relationship between serum levels and progression of disease suggests that the T cell process may be involved in this progression. Apparently, interleukin-2 inhibitor is present in normal healthy sera but not in scleroderma sera; however, the nature of the inhibitor is unknown.

▶ Serum levels of interleukin-2 should be measured in a variety of cutaneous disorders in which there is T cell activation. It would then be possible to determine the range of cutaneous changes associated with abnormal levels of this cytokine.—N.A. Soter, M.D.

Isotretinoin in the Treatment of Systemic Sclerosis
Maurice PDL, Bunker CB, Dowd PM (Middlesex Hosp, London)
Br J Dermatol 121:367–374, September 1989 4–14

Reportedly, vitamin A derivative, isotretinoin, can inhibit collagen synthesis by fibroblasts and theoretically might be effective in patients with systemic sclerosis. Thirteen patients with systemic sclerosis were treated with isotretinoin, 1 mg/kg daily.

Nine patients completed 6–14 months of treatment; all showed improvement in the cutaneous manifestations of the disease, such as decreased sclerosis, tethering, and edema (Fig 4–3). Symptoms relating to systemic involvement by systemic sclerosis did not improve with isotretinoin. Most patients experienced the well-recognized mucocutaneous side effects of isotretinoin, which required withdrawal of 3 patients from the study within 3 months. None of the laboratory parameters reflecting disease activity indicated any consistent change during treatment. In addition, serum levels of type III procollagen aminopropeptide, the amino-terminal peptide released from type III procollagen during its conversion into collagen, did not show a consistent decline during treatment despite clinical improvement in the skin.

Isotretinoin can improve several of the cutaneous manifestations of

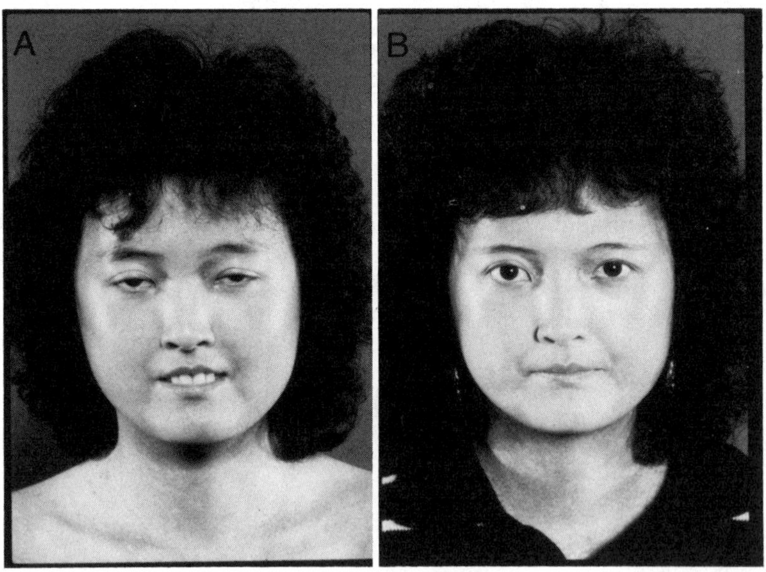

Fig 4–3.—Patient's face, **A**, before and **B**, after 11 months treatment with isotretinoin, showing the reduction in swelling and sclerosis. (Courtesy of Maurice PDL, Bunker CB, Dowd PM: *Br J Dermatol* 121:367–374, September 1989.)

systemic sclerosis. Its mode of action remains unclear, but a preferential suppression of the synthesis of type I collagen may be implicated.

▶ The observation of clinical improvement in the skin of patients with systemic sclerosis after the oral administration of isotretinoin in this open study should be confirmed in a double-blind, placebo-controlled study. Also, it would be important to examine topical tretinoin preparations.—N.A. Soter, M.D.

Cutaneous Changes of Dermatomyositis Precede Muscle Weakness

Rockerbie NR, Woo TY, Callen JP, Giustina T (Univ of Michigan; Calgary Gen Hosp, Alta)

J Am Acad Dermatol 20:629–632, April 1989 4–15

Cutaneous lesions in dermatomyositis may precede, occur simultaneously, or occur after the onset of muscle weakness. Some investigators have suggested that about a third of all patients with dermatomyositis have skin involvement before the onset of muscle weakness. Others suggest a prevalence of about 20%. The case reports of 38 females and 12 males aged 2–83 years at the time of diagnosis, were reviewed to assess the chronologic relationship between onset of skin disease and onset of muscle weakness.

Onset of cutaneous lesions ranged from 51 months before to 14 months after onset of muscle weakness. The onset of muscle weakness and skin involvement coincided within 2 months in 62% of the patients. It could also be inferred that skin involvement was present as the initial feature in 56% of the patients, whereas 16% had muscle weakness as the initial feature. Only 1 patient had muscle weakness for longer than 1 year before the onset of skin involvement. Of the 50 patients, 40 had Gottron's papules and a heliotrope rash on initial examination. There was no association between the clinical course, age, and sex, and the degree of discordance between skin and muscle involvement.

These data suggest that a finding of the characteristic eruption of dermatomyositis in the absence of muscle weakness should not preclude the diagnosis of dermatomyositis. These patients should be investigated further, and follow-up should be actively pursued.

▶ The message is clear: Skin lesions may precede muscle involvement by as much as 51 months (1 patient). Therefore, patients with cutaneous lesions consistent with dermatomyositis should be followed closely.—R. Masters, M.D.

Cyclosporin in Juvenile Dermatomyositis

Heckmatt J, Hasson N, Saunders C, Thompson N, Peters AM, Cambridge G, Rose M, Hyde SA, Dubowitz V (Hammersmith Hosp, London; Middlesex Hosp, London; Harefield Hosp, Middlesex, England)

Lancet 1:1063–1066, May 13, 1989 4–16

Steroids have greatly improved the prognosis of patients with juvenile dermatomyositis, but high doses are associated with a risk of serious complications. The use of cyclosporine was evaluated in 14 patients with juvenile dermatomyositis, all of whom were chronically ill and dependent on prednisolone. Other immunosuppressive agents had failed or caused unacceptable side effects. Patients had been ill for 3 years on average, and all but 2 had serious complications.

Maintenance serum drug levels ranged from 60 to 300 ng/mL. All patients improved, and the dose of prednisolone was decreased from 14 mg to 3 mg daily on average; 6 patients ceased using steroids. Two nonambulant patients became able to walk. Patients have received cyclosporine for an average of 1 year. The goal is to taper treatment after 6–18 months of cyclosporine therapy alone. The dose was lowered in a hypertensive patient because of renal dysfunction.

Cyclosporine is useful in patients with juvenile dermatomyositis who have become dependent on steroids and have failed to respond to other immunosuppressive drugs. For patients not responding adequately to prednisolone, cyclosporine is a relatively nontoxic alternative to cyclophosphamide or methotrexate.

▶ Although the beneficial therapeutic response of patients with juvenile dermatomyositis to the administration of cyclosporine was encouraging, the renal side effects and potential for the development of hematologic malignant conditions should not be dismissed cavalierly. A controlled clinical trial also is needed.—N.A. Soter, M.D.

Plasma Exchange Therapy in Dermatomyositis: A Retrospective Study of 21 Patients

Lok C, Herson S, Roujeau JC, Revuz J, Gérard A, Godeau P (Hôp Henri-Mondor, Créteil; Hôp de la Pitié-Salpêtrière, Paris; Centre Hospitalier Régional de Nancy, France)

Ann Dermatol Venereol 116:219–224, 1989 4–17

Dermatomyositis and polymyositis are disorders of the striated muscles that differ in their specific cutaneous presentation. Both disorders are commonly treated with prednisone in doses of 1–2 mg/kg/day. Methotrexate is added when prednisone is poorly tolerated or when corticosteroids fail to relieve symptoms. Several studies have reported good results with plasma exchange therapy when conventional therapy was ineffective. The case reports of all patients with dermatomyositis who were treated with plasma exchange during a 6-year study period at 8 centers in France were reviewed retrospectively.

The patient population included 7 males and 14 females aged 2.5–72 years (mean, 42.5 years) who underwent 234 plasma exchanges. Sixteen patients were children younger than 15 years. Dermatomyositis was initially acute in 17 patients, subacute in 3, and chronic in 1. Plasma exchange was initiated in 18 patients after prednisone proved ineffective (4 patients) or because of an increase in muscle weakness (14). Each patient received a mean of 11 plasma exchange treatments over a mean of 11 weeks.

Plasma exchange therapy failed in 6 of the 21 cases. Three of the 6 patients died, 1 of complications directly attributable to plasma exchange. The other 15 patients had moderate to major improvement in muscle strength. Serum creatine phosphokinase levels, which were elevated in 12 patients, returned to normal in 10 after completion of plasma exchange.

Although the etiology of dermatomyositis is unknown, some of the proposed hypotheses on the physiopathogenicity of the disease justify the use of plasma exchange. The data from this record review suggest that plasma exchange might indeed be effective in the treatment of dermatomyositis. However, because of the retrospective nature of this study, controlled, randomized clinical trials of plasma exchange are indicated.

▶ This is a retrospective study and the authors conclude that a controlled randomized study is indicated. Plasma exchange has been helpful in some patients in reducing creatine phosphokinase levels, increasing muscular strength (except for the pharyngolaryngeal muscles in this series), and, in previous reports, when muscle biopsies have been done, decreasing histologic evidence of inflammation.

There was 1 death secondary to phlebitis at the femoral puncture site followed by pulmonary embolism, and another death caused by septicemia.

In addition to, or as part of, a controlled randomized study, we need long-term follow-up of results.— R. Masters, M.D.

5 Atopic Dermatitis

Minor Clinical Features of Atopic Dermatitis: Evaluation of Their Diagnostic Significance

Mevorah B, Frenk E, Wietlisbach V, Carrel C-F (Univ of Lausanne, Switzerland)

Dermatologica 177:360–364, December 1988 5–1

Because there is no specific clinical or biological marker for atopic dermatitis, its diagnosis is based on history and clinical presentation. Consequently, the diagnostic criteria for atopic dermatitis vary somewhat among schools. In an effort to standardize the diagnostic criteria, 23 basic and minor features of atopic dermatitis have been proposed. The significance of 7

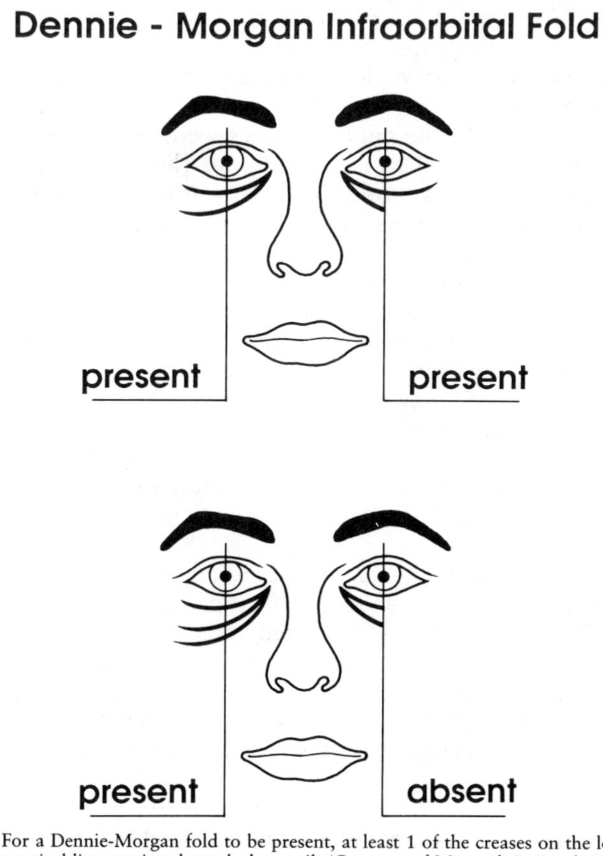

Fig 5–1.—For a Dennie-Morgan fold to be present, at least 1 of the creases on the lower eyelid had to go beyond a vertical line passing through the pupil. (Courtesy of Mevorah B, Frenk E, Wietlisbach V, et al: *Dermatologica* 177:360–364, December 1988.)

Incidence of 8 Minor Features of AD

Minor features	AD (n=105)		Controls (n=113)		Significance
	n	%	n	%	
Infraauricular fissure	51	49.5	13	11.5	***
Wool intolerance	74	77.9	44	41.5	***
White dermographism	43	41.7	15	13.5	***
Nipple eczema	16	15.2	2	1.8	***
Cheilitis	53	50.5	31	27.4	***
Pityriasis alba	36	34.6	18	15.9	***
Anterior neck folds	54	51.4	46	40.7	NS
Dennie-Morgan infraorbital fold	53	50.5	58	51.3	NS

(Courtesy of Mevorah B, Frenk E, Wietlisbach V, et al: *Dermatologica* 177:360–364, December 1988.)

minor features selected arbitrarily from that list plus 1 other feature not on the list was evaluated. The 8 features were nipple eczema, cheilitis, Dennie-Morgan infraorbital fold, pityriasis alba, anterior neck folds, wool intolerance, white dermographism, and infra-auricular fissuring.

The series included 105 patients (median age, 8.5 years) who had the typical clinical presentation of AD atopic dermatitis and 113 controls (median age, 16 years). The minor features were evaluated subjectively as being present or absent. Because there is no clear-cut description of the Dennie-Morgan infraorbital fold, for this feature to be present at least 1 of the creases on the lower eyelid had to go beyond a vertical line passing through the pupil (Fig 5–1).

Nipple eczema, cheilitis, pityriasis alba, wool intolerance, white dermographism, and infra-auricular fissuring were significantly more frequent in patients with atopic dermatitis than in the controls (table). However, anterior neck folds and the Dennie-Morgan infraorbital fold were seen about as often in the patients as in the controls. Thus 6 of the 8 minor features studied are valuable diagnostic clues in atopic dermatitis; the other 2 minor features are of no diagnostic use. Another 2 other minor features of atopic dermatitis—keratosis pilaris and palmoplantar hyperlinearity—have already been shown to have no diagnostic significance.

▶ This study examines children with "classic criteria" atopic dermatitis and a slightly older control group in an effort to determine the usefulness of the minor criteria of Hanifin and Rajka often cited in published reports. The study determined that anterior neck folds and the Dennie-Morgan infraorbital fold had no diagnostic usefulness. A weakness of this study is that the authors did not clearly state the "classic criteria" for their cases of indubitable atopic dermatitis. Perhaps they thought the criteria were so obvious.—A.R. Rhodes, M.D., M.P.H

Unilateral Eruption of Endogenous Eczema After Hemiparesis

Troilius A, Möller H (Lund Univ; Malmö Gen Hosp, Sweden)

Acta Derm Venereol (Stockh) 69:256–258, June 1989 5–2

Symmetric distribution of eczematous eruption is characteristic of endogenous eczema. Endogenous eczema with a unilateral distribution was seen in 5 patients.

All 5 had history of cerebrovascular insult. After hemiparesis, endogenous eczema—nummular eczema, atopic eczema, or pompholyx—developed on the neurologically healthy side (Fig 5–2). In none of the 5 was the eczema associated with seborrheic dermatitis. Furthermore, none had signs of sympathetic disturbance.

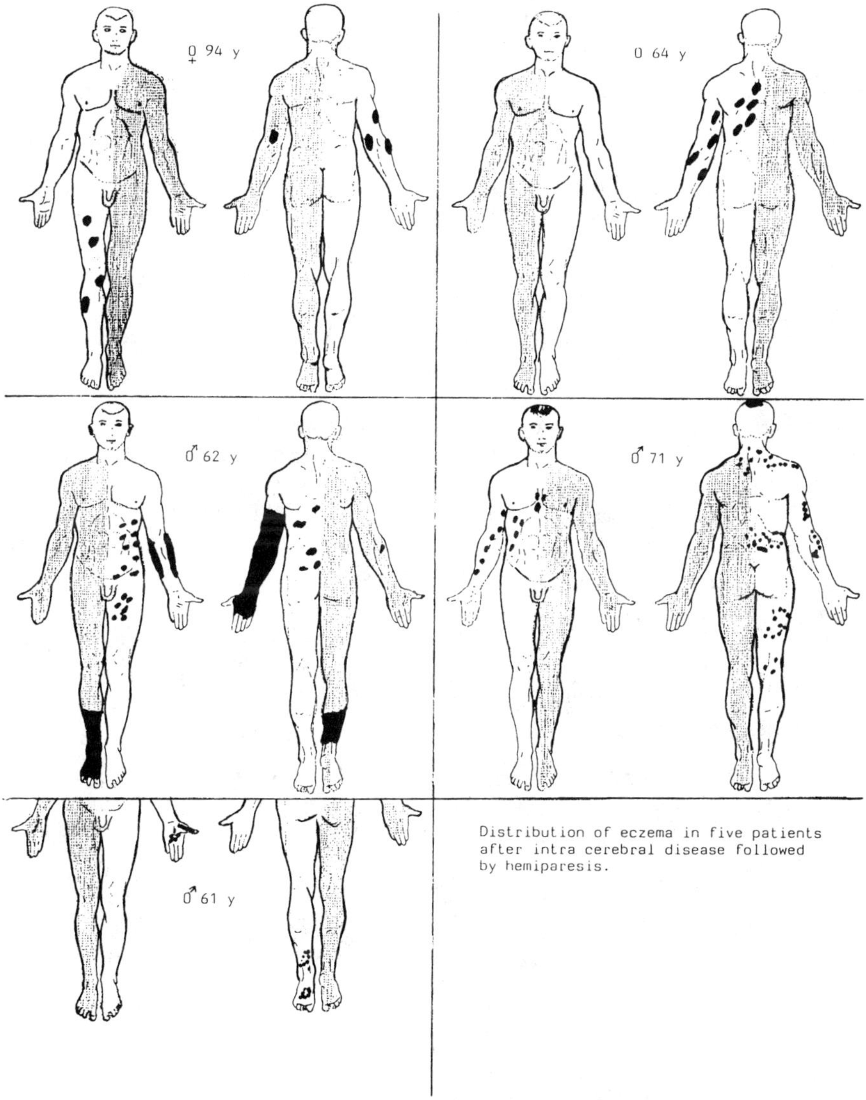

Fig 5–2.—Distribution of eczema in 5 patients after intracerebral disease followed by hemiparesi' (Courtesy of Troilius A, Möller H: *Acta Derm Venereol (Stockh)* 69:256–258, June 1989.)

The etiology of endogenous eczema developing unilaterally on the normal side of a hemiparetic patient is unknown.

▶ If endogenous eczema is "the itch that rashes," perception of itch and ability to scratch may play some role in which eczema may localize in the predisposed after the stress of a cerebrovascular accident.—J.D. Bernhard, M.D.

Epidemiology of Different Types of Hand Eczema in an Industrial City
Meding B, Swanbeck G (Univ of Göteborg; Sahlgren's Hosp, Göteborg)
Acta Derm Venereol [Stockh] 69:227–233, June 1989 5–3

A study was made of the prevalence of various types of hand eczema in an industrial city, as well as the age of onset, duration, continuity of symptoms, and extent of involvement. Questionnaires were sent to 20,000 randomly selected individuals aged 20–65. Of these 1,385 persons who considered themselves to have had hand eczema within the previous 12 months were invited for dermatologic examination.

Hand eczema was confirmed in 1,238 individuals. It was twice as common in women as in men, and the highest prevalence occurred in women aged 20–35 years. Irritant dermatitis was the most common diagnosis (35%), followed by atopic hand eczema (22%) and allergic contact dermatitis (19%). Onset of hand eczema at younger ages was common, particularly in women. The average duration of hand eczema was 11.6 years (range, 0–63 years). The duration of hand eczema correlated significantly with the extent of involvement. The extent of involvement was highest for atopic hand eczema, followed by allergic contact dermatitis. Continuity of symptoms was noted in 23% of the patients, particularly in men and those with high scores of involvement. Atopic hand eczema appeared to be most unfavorable, with an early onset, a long duration, a high frequency of continuous symptoms, and extensive involvement.

Hand eczema is a long-lasting disease with a relapsing course. The long duration suggests that dermatologic care does not appear to be as beneficial as expected.

▶ The authors identify 7 different types of hand eczema: allergic contact dermatitis, irritant dermatitis, atopic hand eczema, hyperkeratotic dermatitis of the palms, pompholyx, and unclassified. [The interchangeability of the terms "eczema" and "dermatitis" is interesting in this context. For fellow quibblers, this is consistent with our own bias, which holds that (1) both terms are useful, (2) "eczema" is a type of "dermatitis," (3) all dermatitis is not eczema, and (4) "faced with two terms for the same thing, one tends to cast about for a distinction." (1)].

Although we agree that hand eczema is a long-lasting disease and that many conventional treatment approaches may not be as good as we imagine, we have seen more than a few patients experience durable remissions with PUVA treatment. Unfortunately, most seem to require some level of regular maintenance treatment, but some do not. Some may need treatment only once every

2–3 weeks to maintain a remission, and some are able to enjoy treatment breaks of 6 months or more. For some patients the opportunity to regain the use of their hands and to return to work outweighs the established relative risks of PUVA treatment. And work may not be the only issue: hand eczema can be a major, if not an insurmountable, impediment to physical intimacy and emotional well-being.—J.D. Bernhard, M.D.

Reference

1. Quine WS: *Quiddities.* Cambridge, Harvard University Press, 1987.

Hand Eczema: An Evaluation of the Frequency of Atopic Background and the Difference in Clinical Pattern Between Patients With and Without Atopic Dermatitis

Svensson Å (Central Hosp, Kristianstad, Sweden)

Acta Derm Venereol (Stockh) 68:509–513, 1988 5–4

Hand eczema is a common disease and 1 that appears to occur even more frequently in patients with an atopic constitution. Patients with long-lasting hand eczema were studied prospectively to determine its association with atopic dermatitis and to examine clinical differences between patients with and without atopic dermatitis. A consecutive group of 63 patients entered the study. All had chronic or chronically recurring hand eczema for at least 6 months. A scoring system was used to define clinically the presence of atopic dermatitis; patch tests also were administered to all patients.

Twenty-nine patients had atopic dermatitis. Of the 34 patients without atopic dermatitis, 6 had current or previous atopic disease. Of the 20 patients with a serum IgE level of >80 kU/L, 15 had atopic dermatitis; 10 with and 10 without atopic dermatitis had positive patch test reactions. Neither the pattern of contact allergy nor the localization of eczema differed between patients with positive and negative patch tests. Palmar hyperlinearity appeared to be significantly more common in patients with atopic dermatitis.

▶ Among the features that suggest atopy: hyperlinear palms, more frequent involvement of the hypothenar region, and more frequent involvement on the dorsal part of the hands. Otherwise, it would appear that hand eczema in patients with and without the atopic diathesis is more alike than different.—J.D. Bernhard, M.D.

Increased Prevalence of Atopic Dermatitis in Kawasaki Disease

Brosius CL, Newburger JW, Burns JC, Hojnowski-Diaz P, Zierler S, Leung DYM (Harvard Med School; Brown Univ)

Pediatr Infect Dis J 7:863–866, December 1988 5–5

An apparent increase in the prevalence of atopic dermatitis was noted in children with Kawasaki disease. Because atopic dermatitis is associated with immunoregulatory abnormalities similar to those found in acute Kawasaki disease, its prevalence among children with Kawasaki disease was investigated.

Eighty-three patients with Kawasaki disease were matched with 83 controls who had innocent heart murmurs. Parents of both groups contributed data via telephone interview. Serum IgE concentrations were determined retrospectively from frozen sera of 44 unselected Kawasaki disease patients and 27 controls who underwent cardiac catheterization.

Of children with Kawasaki disease, 11% also had atopic dermatitis, compared with only 1% of controls. The prevalence of atopic dermatitis was 9 times more in children with Kawasaki disease than in controls, and their serum IgE concentrations were also significantly higher.

These findings suggest a strong association between atopic dermatitis and Kawasaki disease, indicating that host immunoloigic factors may play a significant role in the pathogenesis of the heart disorder. Further studies are needed to confirm the association between atopic dermatitis and Kawasaki disease.

▶ This excellent study demonstrates a significant association between atopic dermatitis and Kawasaki disease. Additional studies are required to corroborate this finding. Host immunologic factors may play an important role in the pathogenesis of this mysterious disease.—A.R. Rhodes, M.D., M.P.H.

Treatment of Itching in Atopic Eczema With Antihistamines With a Low Sedative Profile

Doherty V, Sylvester DGH, Kennedy CTC, Harvey SG, Calthrop JG, Gibson JR (Western Infirmary, Glasgow; Bristol Royal Infirmary; Wellcome Research Labs, Beckenham, England)

Br Med J 298:96, Jan 14, 1989 5–6

The mechanism in antihistamines that relieves itching in patients with atopic eczema is controversial. Some authorities believe it is the sedative effect, but clinical supporting data are not available. New-generation antihistamines with low sedative profiles make better evaluation of this hypothesis possible.

Forty-nine patients with atopic eczema were randomized to receive acrivastine, terfenadine, or placebo for 10 days. Patients received concomitant topical treatment with clobetasone butyrate ointment and aqueous cream as a soap substitute. They were evaluated initially and after 7 days and 14 days.

Both acrivastine and terfenadine were more effective than placebo for all variables assessed. No significant differences between treatment with acrivastine and treatment with terfenadine were detected. Both active agents significantly reduced itching compared with placebo. Because these treatments had low sedative profiles, the belief that antihistamines reduce itching through sedation alone should be examined.

▶ It has been the impression of many that antihistamines are only slightly helpful in the management of atopic dermatitis, possibly related to the sedative effect. In this well-conducted randomized, double-blind, placebo-controlled study, 2 nonsedating antihistamines were determined to be more useful than placebo. Unfortunately, the benefit was not striking. The antihistamines studied are still quite expensive and may not be worth the cost.—A.R. Rhodes, M.D., M.P.H

UVB Phototherapy of Atopic Dermatitis

Jekler J, Larkö O (Univ of Göteborg; Sahlgren's Hosp, Göteborg, Sweden)

Br J Dermatol 119:697–705, December 1988 5–7

Atopic dermatitis is a cosmetically troublesome disease and the accompanying pruritus causes much discomfort. Previous studies have shown that atopic dermatitis tends to subside before adulthood in most patients. However, a recent Swedish study has shown that in at least 40% of patients, it persists into adulthood. Because most patients improve in the summer months, the therapeutic effectiveness of ultraviolet B radiation (UVB) was assessed in 2 paired-comparison studies, 1 in which UVB was compared with placebo and the other in which 2 UVB treatment regimens were compared with each other. In study group I, 17 patients were irradiated with UVB on 1 side of the body and with placebo (visible light) on the other. In study group II, 25 patients were treated with UVB on both sides of the body, 0.8 minimum erythema dose (MED) vs. 0.4 MED.

In study I, 13 UVB-treated body halves improved considerably, whereas only 1 patient improved with placebo treatment. The disease was assessed for severity based on the degree of pruritus, lichenification, scaling, xerosis, vesiculation, excoriations, and erythema, and the results of overall evaluation. The total score, pruritus score, and overall evaluation score were significantly better on the UVB-treated body halves than on those treated with placebo. In study II, 15 of 25 patients healed or improved considerably on the 0.8 MED side compared with improvement in 16 patients on the 0.4 MED side. No statistically significant differences between these dosage regimens were found. Side effects in both studies, which included burning and dryness, were tolerable and mild.

Irradiation with UVB 3 times a week was effective in the treatment of atopic dermatitis. Doses of 0.4 MED were as effective as those of 0.8 MED but caused fewer side effects.

▶ Quite low doses of UVB were effective in this study, during which continued topical steroid usage was permitted. Although the latter was claimed to be greater on the placebo-treated side, steroid use was not assessed quantitatively by weighing the tubes.—R.W. Gange, M.D.

A Double-Blind Comparison of the Efficacy of Betamethasone Dipropionate Cream Twice Daily Versus Once Daily in the Treatment of Steroid Responsive Dermatoses

English JSC, Bunker CB, Ruthven K, Dowd PM, Greaves MW (St John's Hosp for Diseases of the Skin, London; Middlesex Hosp, London; Kirby Warrick Pharmaceuticals, Suffolk, England)

Clin Exp Dermatol 14:32–34, January 1989 5–8

The side effects of topical corticosteroids increase with the potency of the steroids used, but the optimal frequency of application has not been well studied. Whether once-daily application of a potent topical steroid in the treatment of eczema and psoriasis is as effective as twice-daily application was investigated.

Sixty-three patients with eczema and 34 patients with psoriasis were randomly assigned to treatment for 3 weeks with 0.05% betamethasone dipropionate cream applied twice daily or once daily with base cream applied at night. All patients were assessed weekly for their response to treatment. Each patient was also asked to keep a daily diary of progress. The amount of cream used was determined by weighing the returned tubes at the end of the study.

Eighty-five of the 97 patients completed the study. There were no statistically significant differences in any of the parameters measured between once-daily and twice-daily application of betamethasone dipropionate cream. Analysis of the diaries showed no statistically significant difference in the speed of onset of relief of symptoms in the patients with psoriasis. However, patients with eczema noticed improvement of symptoms more quickly with the twice-daily regimen.

Betamethasone dipropionate cream used once daily in the morning in conjunction with an emollient base used at night is as effective as twice-daily application of the active corticosteroid. However, for patients with eczema, twice-daily application of an active steroid is recommended for the first 3–4 days of treatment, with reduction to once-daily application as soon as symptoms subside.

▶ Once is enough.—J.D. Bernhard, M.D.

6 Contact Dermatitis

Tendency to Irritation: Sensitive Skin

Maibach HI, Lammintausta K, Berardesca E, Freeman S (Univ of California, San Francisco)

J Am Acad Dermatol 21:833–835, October 1989 6–1

Earlier studies used the minimal erythema dose as an indicator of the cutaneous response to irritants and inflammatory agents. More recently, transepidermal water loss, dielectric constant, and laser Doppler velocimetry have been used to examine other features of skin function for assessing damage. Use of transepidermal water loss resulted in a correlation between patients with and without a history of dermatologic disease and responses to an irritant. Transepidermal water loss and laser Doppler velocimetry have indicated enhanced responses in black compared with white persons. The clinical observation of relapse after "healing" of hand dermatitis has been confirmed by results that suggest functional aberration of the skin in some persons. Others have identified persons who have sensory irritation without skin findings ("stingers") by double-blind methods. The issue of sensitive skin can be addressed by contemporary methods. The biologic data suggest the validity of the concept of sensitive skin.

▶ Cosmeticians think they know what sensitive skin is. Patients certainly think they do. Some have acne, some have contact allergy, and some have irritation, dryness, or itching. After enough work like this, at least dermatologists will know what *we* mean by "sensitive skin."—J.D. Bernhard, M.D.

Patch Testing With a Standard Series: Results in 12,026 Patients

Enders F, Przybilla B, Ring J, Burg G, Braun-Falco O (Ludwig-Maximilians Univ. München, West Germany)

Hautarzt 39:779–786, December 1988 6–2

Contact dermatitis is one of the most common skin disorders. The number of confirmed contact allergens has become so great that not all can be included in routine patch testing. However, only few of the known allergens are of major clinical importance. The standard series used in routine patch testing contains 27 of the most prevalent allergens. An attempt was made to identify which allergens in a standard series most commonly caused positive reactions; data were broken down by age and by sex.

Between 1977 and 1983, 12,026 patients underwent patch testing with a standard series of allergens; 4,494 (37.4%) had positive reactions to 1 or more allergens in the series. The average number of positive reactions for all patients was 1.85; for all men, 1.87; and for all women, 1.83. The most common positive reactions were to nickel sulfate, fragrance mixes, balsam of Peru, cobalt chloride, potassium dichromate, and wool alcohols. Compared with men, women had significantly more positive reactions to nickel sulfate, cobalt chloride, wool alcohols, and parabens, and significantly fewer positive reactions to potassium dichromate, PPD mix, and epoxy resin. Younger patients had significantly more positive reactions to nickel sulfate and cobalt chloride; middle-aged patients had more positive reactions to potassium dichromate, paraphenylenediamine, formaldehyde, and thiuram mix; and elderly patients had more positive reactions to balsam of Peru, wool alcohols, local anesthetics of the caine group, neomycin sulfate, benzocaine, colophony, clioquinol, mafenide, parabens, and gentamicin sulfate.

The greater incidence of positive reactions to nickel sulfate and cobalt chloride among younger women was attributable to fashion trends in costume jewelry. The greater incidence of positive reactions to epoxy resin, formaldehyde, PPD mix, and thiuram mix in men was associated with professional exposure in various industrial settings.

▶ Skeptics argue that the value of patch testing is diminished by the universe of allergens that must exist but are not included on the "standard tray" (or trays). The logical fallacy in this argument resides in placing more emphasis on what might be missed than on what might be found! One important contribution of large studies such as this one is the demonstration that a fairly limited number of "common" allergens account for a fairly substantial portion of positive reactions, and that certain demographic groups are prone to react to different antigens.—J.D. Bernhard, M.D.

Prevalence and Relevance of Allergic Reactions in Patients Patch Tested in North America: 1984 to 1985

Storrs FJ, Rosenthal LE, Adams RM, Clendenning W, Emmett EA, Fisher AA, Larsen WG, Maibach HI, Rietschel RL, Schorr WF, Taylor JS (North American Contact Dermatitis Group)

J Am Acad Dermatol 20:1038–1045, June 1989 6–3

The North American Contact Dermatitis Group (NACDG) attempts to review constantly the performance of all allergens to present an effective tool in the diagnosis of allergic contact dermatitis. The computerized data obtained by 10 dermatologists from 9 geographical areas who performed patch testing on patients with suspected allergic contact dermatitis from 1984 to 1985 were evaluated. In all, 1,199 patients were patch tested with 32 "standard" allergens, 707 patients with 19 "vehicle and preservative" allergens, and 613 patients with 10 "special study" allergens.

The most common allergens on the standard tray were nickel, *p*-phenylenediamine, quaternium-15, neomycin, thimerosal, formaldehyde, cinnamic aldehyde, ethylenediamine, potassium dichromate, and thiuram mix. Compared with the data of the NACDG in 1972, these allergens were also commonly positive at that time (table, pp 74 & 75). On the vehicle and preservative tray, the most common allergens were ammoniated mercury, 2-bromo-2-nitropropane-1,3-diol (Bronopol), diazolinidyl urea, captan, and chloroxylenol, and DMDM hydantoin. These findings illustrate the increasing importance of formaldehyde and formaldehyde releasers. Diaminodiphenyl methane in 0.5% petrolatum was the most common allergen on the special study tray. Cinnamic aldehyde was best presented at 1% concentration; relevant positive reactions would have been missed with lower concentrations.

These data illustrate the importance of maintaining a dynamic patch testing system to be diagnostically effective.

▶ One of the few applications of computers to clinical medicine that is not a "schlimmbesserung," (an "improvement" that makes things worse). This is a beautiful example of how much can be learned from cooperative efforts, and how much computers can help in a field in which memory and books can go only so far. We hope that work such as this will also lead to software developments that will help the dermatologist to assess "relevancy" of positive patch test results in the office.—J.D. Bernhard, M.D.

Reproducibility of Patch Test Results: Comparison of TRUE Test and Finn Chamber Test Results

Gollhausen R, Przybilla B, Ring J (Dermatologische Klinik und Poliklinik der Ludwig-Maximilians-Univ München, West Germany)
J Am Acad Dermatol 21:843–846, October 1989 6–4

A newly developed patch test, the TRUE test, yields results concordant with those of the Finn Chamber method. To evaluate the reproducibility of patch test results, duplicate patch tests with 12 allergens were applied simultaneously to either side of the back in 63 patients using the TRUE Test. When positive results occurred on only 1 side, it was considered nonreproducible. The same 12 allergens mixed with petrolatum were applied to the upper back according to the Finn Chamber technique. The reproducibility of both test results was compared in 76 other patients.

The concordance of positive reactions between the 2 tests was 57%, somewhat lower than in recently published reports. The low reproducibility of patch testing results indicates the need for improved methods. The relevance of patch test results should be viewed in the light of the patient's medical history.

▶ One can only hope that standardization of all materials in patch tests will improve their accuracy and our ability to interpret them. This paper, and the 2 that surrounded it in a special issue of the *Journal of the American Academy of Dermatology* (October 1989) describe important steps in that direction. Standardization of test materials will certainly be followed by even further refinement in

Comparison of NACDG Results: 1984–1985 and 1972

Allergens	1984-1985 Total tallied	1984-1985 Allergic	1984-1985 Reactivity (%)	1972 Total tested	1972 Allergic	1972 Reactivity (%)
Balsam of Peru 25% petrolatum	1122	37	3.3	NR		
Benzocaine 5% petrolatum	1135	40	3.5	1200	54	4.5
Benzoyl peroxide 1% petrolatum	1115	20	1.8	NT		
Black rubber paraphenylene diamine mix (PPD mix 0.6% petrolatum)	1140	16	1.4	NT		
Caine mix less benzocaine 3% petrolatum	1117	22	2.0	NT		
Carba mix 3% petrolatum	1135	38	3.3	NT		
Cinnamic alcohol 5% petrolatum	1046	28	2.7			
Cinnamic aldehyde 2% petrolatum	1048	62	5.9	NT		
Dibucaine 1% petrolatum	1009	8	0.8	1200	32	2.7
Cyclomethycaine sulfate 1% petrolatum	1012	8	0.8	NT		
Epoxy resin 1% petrolatum	1129	21	1.9	NT		
Ethylenediamine dihydrochloride 1% petrolatum	1120	66	5.9	1200	85	7.1
Eugenol 4% petrolatum	1016	14	1.4	NT		
Formaldehyde 2% water	1144	70	6.1	1200	43	3.6
Hydroxycitronellal 4% petrolatum	1049	16	1.5	NT		

Imidazolidinyl urea 2% water	1134	17	1.5	NT		
Isoeugenol 4% petrolatum	1012	24	2.4	NT		
Lanolin alcohol (wool wax alcohol) 30% petrolatum	135	14	1.2	1200	37	3.1
Mercapto mix 1% petrolatum	1132	30	2.6	NT		
Mercaptobenzothiazole 1% petrolatum*	1141	33	2.9	1200	58	4.8
Neomycin sulfate 20% petrolatum	1131	75	6.6	1200	71	5.9
Nickel sulfate 2.5% petrolatum	1123	109	9.7	1200	131	11.0
Oak moss 5% petrolatum	1038	20	1.9	NT		
Para-tertiary-butylphenol formaldehyde resin 1% petrolatum	1129	9	.9	NT		
Potassium dichromate 0.5% petrolatum	1138	59	5.2	1200	91	7.6
p-Phenylenediamine 1% petrolatum	1138	79	6.9	1200	97	8.1
Quaternium-15 2% petrolatum	1129	76	6.7	NT		
Quaternium-15 2% water	1103	43	3.9	NT		
Rosin (colophony) 20% petrolatum	1132	22	1.9	NT		
Tetracaine 1% petrolatum	1014	8	.8	NT		
Thimerosal 0.1% petrolatum	1137	70	6.2	1200	91	7.6
Thiuram mix 1% petrolatum†	1137	44	3.9	1200	50	4.2

Abbreviation: NT, not tested.
*Mercaptobenzothiazole 2% in 1972.
†Thiram 2% in 1972, not thiuram mix.
(Courtesy of Storrs FJ, Rosenthal LE, Adams RM, et al: *J Am Acad Dermatol* 20:1038–1045, June 1989.)

assessment criteria (e.g., what is the standard definition of a 1+ reaction?) in a completely uniform test system. And then we might hope that some of the important controversies in patch testing may be resolved. Our favorite is the angry ("eczema begets eczema"), excited, aroused, crazy, hyperirritable vs. silent back syndrome(s) (1). If this one ever gets settled, we hope what one of our patients told us doesn't turn out to be true: "My back's not crazy, doc, your head is."—J.D. Bernhard, M.D.

Reference

1. Kligman AM, Gollhausen R: *Br J Dermatol* 115:93, 1986.

Intradermal Testing in Doubtful Cases of Contact Allergy to Metals
Möller H (Lund Univ, Malmö, Sweden)
Contact Dermatitis 20:120–123, February 1989 6–5

Patch test reactions to chromate, cobalt, and nickel are difficult to interpret. However, accuracy is important because positive patch test reactions may have important socioeconomic consequences for patients. Patients with patch test reactions to chromium, cobalt, and nickel that were difficult to interpret were retested with an intracutaneous test.

During a 3-year period, 1,670 patients underwent standard patch testing for the diagnosis of contact dermatitis; 66 of them then underwent supplemental intracutaneous testing with chromate, cobalt, and nickel. Of these 66 patients, 49 were retested because the patch test was difficult to read. In 22 of the 49 patients more than 1 metal was involved. Ten patients were retested because of negative results to a patch test despite a positive history of metal allergy; 7 were retested because of a previously diagnosed metal allergy.

Of 1,670 patch-tested patients, 350 (21%) had contact allergy to 1 or more metal salts. Of the 49 patients with doubtful patch test results, chromate was implicated in 27, cobalt in 19, and nickel in 32. Intracutaneous testing confirmed a metal allergy in 24 instances and rejected it in 54 instances. Intracutaneous testing confirmed a metal allergy in only 3 of 10 patients who had negative results to a patch test despite a positive history of metal allergy. Of the 7 patients with a previously diagnosed contact allergy to metal, only 4 still had the allergy. None of the patients had adverse reactions to intracutaneous testing, probably because only weak solutions were used.

Intracutaneous testing is a harmless procedure that is useful for clarifying doubtful patch test results to metals.

▶ Sometimes the "poritis" caused by these metals in routine patch testing is clear-cut. When it is not, other methods may be helpful in establishing whether true allergic sensitivity is present.—J.D. Bernhard, M.D.

Distribution of Lost-Work-Time Claims for Skin Disease in California Agriculture: 1978–1983

O'Malley MA, Mathias CGT (Natl Inst for Occupational Safety and Health, Cincinnati)
Am J Ind Med 14:715–720, December 1988 6–6

Agricultural workers comprise the occupational group at highest risk for skin diseases. In an effort to identify which subsets of agricultural workers are at especially high risk, examination was made of the distribution of 2,722 claims for lost work time attributable to a skin condition reported to the state of California between 1978 and 1983. California is not representative of agriculture nationwide, but it was selected for study because it keeps detailed employment information and because it accounts for approximately a third of the total number of agricultural workers in the United States.

All claims for skin disease reported to the Supplementary Data Systems, a national workers' compensation database operated by the US Bureau of Labor Statistics, were analyzed by Standard Industrial Classification codes and source of illness. Because claims without lost time are not reported, only skin diseases that involved lost time from work were included.

The 2,722 claimants for lost work time because of skin diseases ranged in age from 14 to 84 years (median, 27.8 years). Most claimants (77.6%) were men. Skin diseases were attributed to exposure to plants in 52.1% of the workers, to chemical exposure in 20.4%, and to food products in 12.5%. The remaining 15% were coded as miscellaneous or nonclassifiable.

The forestry subdivisions reported the highest rate of dermatitis caused by exposure to plants, but this group had not filed any claims for other sources of exposure. For chemical exposures, the highest rate of claims occurred in the horticultural specialties subdivision, but that group also had a significant claims rate for plant-related skin diseases. The vegetables and melon production subdivision had the highest rates of claims for disease attributed to food products but had nearly equally high claims rates for exposure to plants and chemicals.

Although exposures to pesticides and other agricultural chemicals are significant sources of skin disorders in agricultural workers, the role of other major sources of skin diseases in the complex agricultural environment should not be overlooked.

▶ Agriculture may have the highest risk of occupational skin disease in California, but that does not appear to be the case in Worcester, Massachusetts.—J.D. Bernhard, M.D.

Contact Dermatitis in Children

Rademaker M, Forsyth A (Belvidere Hosp, Glasgow)
Contact Dermatitis 20:104–107, February 1989 6–7

Limited clinical data are available on patch testing in young children because allergic contact dermatitis often is not considered as a potential diagnosis in this age group. Furthermore, the level of reactivity and sensitization potential in children is controversial. During a 7-year period,

5,986 patients underwent patch testing for contact dermatitis, 125 of whom were children younger than 12 years of age. Most of the children with atopic dermatitis had a recent history of atypical flare.

Sixty of the 125 children (48%) had 124 positive reactions, which were considered relevant in 55 (table). No relevance could be determined

Positives According to Age

	Age of children (years)							
	≤5	6	7	8	9	10	11	Total
No. children	8	8	12	9	20	30	38	125
+ve patch tests	4	4	6	4	13	10	19	60
−ve patch tests	4	4	6	5	7	20	19	65
balsam of Peru	–	–	–	–	3	1	–	4
benzoic acid	2	1	1	2	2	–	6	14*
benzyl alcohol	–	–	1	–	–	–	–	1
Bismarck Brown	–	–	–	–	1	–	–	1
butylated hydroxytoluene	–	–	2	–	–	–	–	2
carba-mix	1	–	–	–	–	–	–	1
CBS	–	1	–	1	–	–	1	3
cinnamaldehyde	1	–	3	1	1	–	6	12*
cinnamon	1	–	–	–	–	–	1	2*
cinnamyl alcohol	–	–	1	–	–	–	–	1*
chocolate	–	2	–	–	1	–	–	3*
chrome	1	–	–	–	3	1	1	6
clothing (own)	–	–	1	–	–	1	–	2
cobalt	1	–	–	–	1	3	2	7
colophony	–	–	–	–	1	–	1	2
cosmetic (own)	–	–	1	–	–	–	2	3
essence of chocolate	–	1	–	–	1	1	1	4*
ethylenediamine	–	–	–	1	–	–	–	1
eugenol	–	–	–	–	2	–	–	2
formaldehyde	–	–	–	–	–	2	–	2
fragrance-mix	–	–	–	–	2	–	3	5
glutamic acid	1	–	–	–	–	–	–	1*
isoeugenol	–	–	–	–	2	2	–	4
lanolin	–	–	–	–	1	–	–	1
MBTS	–	1	–	–	–	–	–	1
mercapto-mix	–	1	–	–	1	1	1	4
mercury	–	–	1	–	–	–	–	1
musk ambrette	–	–	–	–	–	–	1	1
neomycin	1	–	–	1	–	1	1	4
nickel	1	1	–	–	5	4	7	18
oak moss absolute	–	–	1	–	–	–	2	3
quinoline	–	–	1	–	–	–	–	1
sorbic acid	–	–	1	1	–	–	1	3*
tartrazine	1	–	–	–	–	–	–	1*
TETD	–	–	–	–	–	–	1	1
thimerosal	–	–	1	–	1	–	–	2
total +ves	11	8	15	7	28	17	38	124

*Contact urticaria.

(Courtesy of Rademaker M, Forsyth A: *Contact Dermatitis* 20:104–107, February 1989.)

in the other 5 children. The most common allergens were metals, fragrances, and rubber compounds. Forty children also were tested for contact urticaria against food additives and fragrances; 42 positive reactions were identified in 20 children.

Contact dermatitis in children younger than 12 years of age is not uncommon. Patch testing in this age group proved rewarding. None of the children was sensitized by the testing.

▶ Particularly worth thinking about in the atopic child who continues to worsen despite treatment and expectations.—J.D. Bernhard, M.D.

Patch Testing in Prurigo Nodularis

Zelickson BD, McEvoy MT, Fransway AF (Mayo Clinic and Found, Rochester, Minn)

Contact Dermatitis 20:321–325, May 1989 6–8

Prurigo nodularis is a chronic pruritic papulonodular eruption of unknown cause. Prompted by histologic observations of increased mast cells in prurigo nodularis and history of contact sensitivity in some patients, 32 patients with prurigo nodularis were patch tested for sensitivity to a standard battery of 26 allergens and additional appropriate allergens.

Twenty-five patients had relevant positive reactions. Fragrance, phenylmercuric acetate, potassium dichromate, nickel sulfate, "-caine mix," formaldehyde, ragweed, and neomycin were the frequently reactive allergens. Eleven patients had significant traceable allergen exposure, and 10 had a history of atopy. Biopsy findings in 11 patients were consistent with prurigo nodularis, and 4 of these had coexisting dermatitis. Eleven patients with positive reactions were followed for a mean of 9.5 years (range, 5–14 years). Six had persistent disease, and 5 had resolution or marked improvement of their nodular prurigo, including 3 who noted marked improvement with avoidance of contact allergens.

Prurigo nodularis possibly can occur as a direct result of allergic contact factors. Screening for contact sensitivity may be helpful in managing this refractory dermatosis, particularly if there is coexistent dermatitis.

▶ Because contact allergy may be only 1 of several provocative factors in prurigo nodularis, the follow-up observation that 3 patients with positive patch tests improved with avoidance of contact allergens, 2 patients had persistent disease despite allergen avoidance, and 2 cleared completely without avoiding contact allergens is not entirely surprising. That should in no way blunt the authors' suggestion that patch testing be considered in evaluation of patients with this often dramatically distressing and treatment-resistant disorder. It should also remind us that *idiopathic* is one of the most dangerous words in medicine, because it fosters intellectual surrender before the diagnostic battle even starts.—J.D. Bernhard, M.D.

Contact Sensitivity to Topical Medicaments

Goh CL (Middle Road Hosp, Singapore)

Int J Dermatol 28:25–28, January–February 1989 6–9

Medicament sensitivity is a common cause of allergic contact dermatitis. The pattern of this sensitivity varies from 1 country to another depending on availability of the medication and prescribing habits of physicians. The epidemiology of medicament sensitivity was examined in

Prevalence of Contact Sensitivity to Common Medicaments

Medicament	Women (n = 838)	Men (n = 847)	Total (n = 1685)
Neomycin 25%	74 (8.8%)	58 (6.8%)	132 (7.8%)
Proflavine HCl 0.5%	35 (4.2%)	84 (9.9%)	119 (7.1%)
Clioquinol 3%	30 (3.6%)	43 (5.1%)	73 (4.3%)
Colophony 20%	19 (2.3%)	36 (4.3%)	55 (3.3%)
Wool alcohol 30%	22 (2.6%)	24 (2.8%)	46 (2.7%)
Caine-mix 7%	11 (1.3%)	11 (1.3%)	22 (1.3%)
Fragrance mix 8%	12 (1.4%)	7 (0.8%)	19 (1.1%)
Ethylenediamine HCl 1%	10 (1.2%)	7 (0.8%)	17 (1.0%)
Chlorocresol 1%	12 (1.4%)	5 (0.6%)	17 (1.0%)
Parabens mix 15%	7 (0.8%)	9 (1.1%)	16 (0.9%)
Balsam of peru 25%	12 (1.4%)	24 (2.8%)	16 (0.9%)
Ammoniated mercury 5%	4 (0.5%)	3 (0.4%)	7 (0.4%)
Formalin 2% aq	3 (0.4%)	4 (0.5%)	7 (0.4%)
Promethazine 2%	5 (0.6%)	2 (0.2%)	7 (0.4%)
Chlorhexidine diacetate 0.5% aq	1 (0.1%)	4 (0.5%)	5 (0.3%)
Thimerosal 0.1%	2 (0.2%)	3 (0.4%)	5 (0.3%)
Cetrimide 0.1% aq	0 (0.0%)	4 (0.5%)	4 (0.2%)
Benzoyl peroxide 1%	3 (0.4%)	0 (0.0%)	3 (0.2%)
Gentamicin sulphate 20%	3 (0.4%)	0 (0.0%)	3 (0.2%)
Chloramphenicol 1%	1 (0.1%)	2 (0.2%)	3 (0.2%)
Undecylanic acid as is	0 (0.0%)	3 (0.4%)	3 (0.2%)
Monobenzyl ether of hydroquinone 1%	0 (0.0%)	2 (0.2%)	2 (0.1%)
Resorcinol 1%	1 (0.1%)	1 (0.1%)	2 (0.1%)
Potassium iodide 25%	1 (0.1%)	1 (0.1%)	2 (0.1%)
Triclosan 2%	0 (0.0%)	1 (0.1%)	1 (0.1%)
Nitrofurazone 0.2%	0 (0.0%)	1 (0.1%)	1 (0.1%)
Bismuth subnitrate as is	0 (0.0%)	1 (0.1%)	1 (0.1%)
Benzalkonium Cl 0.1%	0 (0.0%)	1 (0.1%)	1 (0.1%)
Phenyl mercuric nitrate 0.05% aq	1 (0.1%)	0 (0.0%)	1 (0.1%)

Vehicles for allergens: petrolatum unless otherwise stated.
(Courtesy of Goh CL: *Int J Dermatol* 28:25–28, January–February 1989).

1,685 patients patch tested at a contact dermatitis clinic in Singapore between 1985 and 1986.

A total of 379 (22.5%) had medicament sensitivity. The prevalence was 22.1% in women and 22.8% in men (table). The rate appeared to rise with age, being 17.9% for patients less than 40 years of age and 34% for patients more than 39 years old. Prevalence differences in Chinese, Malay, Indian, and other patients were not significant. Common sensitizers included neomycin, proflavine, clioquinol, colophony, and wool alcohol. Significantly more men than women were sensitive to proflavine. Most dermatitis occurred on the limbs, with 44.3% on the upper and 43% on the lower limbs. Facial dermatitis was more common among women.

The risk of allergic contact dermatitis to medications can be decreased if the prevalence of contact sensitivity is monitored regularly. Strong sensitizers should be substituted, and allergen replacement should be considered.

▶ The fly in the ointment might even be the active ingredient.—J.D. Bernhard, M.D.

Identification of Cross-Reaction Patterns in Allergic Contact Dermatitis From Topical Corticosteroids

Coopman S, Degreef H, Dooms-Goosens A (Univ Hosp; Katholieke Univ Leuven, Belgium)

Br J Dermatol 121:27–34, July 1989 6–10

Allergic contact dermatitis caused by corticosteroids is apparently much more common than previously thought. Examining possible cross-allergy patterns between corticosteroids is essential for the further understanding of corticosteroid sensitization. Whether cross-allergic reactions among corticosteroids occur between all substances, some of them, or not at all remains to be determined. Cross-section patterns were identified in allergic contact dermatitis caused by topical corticosteroids.

Associated positive patch test results (APPR) for corticosteroids reported in the literature and in patch test series were analyzed. The 2 hypotheses explored were that the parameters that can preferentially explain associated APPR among corticosteroids are structural variations in the A- and B-rings of the molecule or in the D-ring or C_{20}-, C_{21}-side chain (table). Positive patch tests to corticosteroids occurred about 6 to 7 times more often in well-defined groups of structurally related substances than among corticosteroids of different groups. An analogous substitution pattern on the steroid D-ring or the carbon side chain appears to have a significant effect on the association of positive patch test results. This is not true of other structural variables, such as the presence of a double bond in the steroid A-ring or fluoride substitutions on the B-ring.

Group Definition Under Hypothesis 2

Corticosteroid group	C_{16} substitution	Carbon chain at the ester of C_{17} and/or C_{21}	Type
A	–	⩽acetate or thioesters	hydrocortisone tixocortol pivalate
B	-OH ± 16, 17-cis ketalation	⩽acetate	triamcinolone acetonide
C	$-CH_3$	–	betamethasone
D	⊢	> acetate	hydrocortisone-17-butyrate
	$-CH_3$ or $=CH_2$	⩾acetate	clobetasone-17-butyrate

A, cloprednol, cortisone, cortisone acetate, fludrocortisone, hydrocortisone, hydrocortisone acetate, methylprednisolone acetate, prednisolone, prednisolone acetate, prednisone, tixocortol pivalate. **B**, amcinonide, budesonide, desonide, fluocinolone acetonide, fluocinonide, halcinonide, triamcinolone acetonide, triamcinolone alcohol. **C**, betamethasone, betamethasone sodium phosphate, dexamethasone, dexamethasone sodium phosphate, fluocortolone. **D**, Alclometasone dipropionate, betamethasone valerate, betamethasone dipropionate, clobetasol-17-propionate, clobetasone-17-butyrate, hydrocortisone-17-valerate.

(Courtesy of Coopman S, Degreef H, Dooms-Goosens A: *Br J Dermatol* 121:27–34, July 1989.)

The findings are important factors in selection of a topical steroid for the future treatment of a corticosteroid-sensitive patient.

▶ It is hard to imagine a better example of medical nemesis. One practical implication: Some patients with steroid "nonresponsive" dermatoses may indeed be responding—in the wrong way.—J.D. Bernhard, M.D.

Contact Dermatitis From Topical Imidazole Antifungals: 15 New Cases

Jelen G, Tennstedt D (Hôp Civil, Saverne, France; Univ de Louvain, Belgium; French Contact Dermatitis Research Group)

Contact Dermatitis 21:6–11, July 1989 6–11

Although a recent 10-year review identified only 19 reported episodes of contact dermatitis from imidazole antifungals, 15 such patients have been seen in a 12-year period, suggesting that the condition is probably underreported. All 15 patients had been treated for tinea cruris, tinea pedis, tinea corporis, and dermatitis. Each underwent patch testing with the ICDRG standard series, the antifungal creams, each of the constituents of the antifungal creams, and the vehicles.

Sensitization to a constituent of the vehicle occured in 1 patient; in the other 14 sensitization was found to the imidazole derivatives. In 8 patients, all of the patch tests in the standard series were negative; the other 7 patients reacted to 1 or more allergens in the standard series. Four patients had positive reactions to Daktacort ointment, a combination product containing miconazole plus hydrocortisone. However, in all 4 patients the contact allergy was caused by the miconazole component, not by hydrocortisone.

Cross-reactions between the various imidazole derivatives were observed in 9 patients. Cross-sensitivity occurred particularly between miconazole, isoconazole, and econazole, as their chemical structures are very similar. Contact dermatitis caused by topical imidazole antifungals appears to be rare.

▶ Work-up Step 1: Patch test with the patient's own medication!—J.D. Bernhard, M.D.

Allergic Contact Dermatitis Caused by Transdermal Hyoscine

Gordon CR, Shupak A, Doweck I, Spitzer O (Israeli Naval Hyperbaric Inst, Haifa, Israel)

Br Med J 298:1220–1221, May 6, 1989 6–12

Hyoscine is often administered transdermally to prevent motion sickness and there have been few reports of delayed hypersensitivity. However, of 164 naval crewmen treated for seasickness with transdermal hyoscine, 16 had symptoms of allergic contact dermatitis. All 16 men had erythema and pruritus at the site of the patch. Erythema was evident within 24–48 hours of application of the patch; pruritus began within hours and lasted for several days. When a patch was placed behind the other ear, the patient had the same local reaction. Lesions regressed when patches were removed. Total resolution took up to 2 weeks. All lesions were confined to the site of application. In all patients the reaction reappeared when a new patch was applied. No reactions were observed when placebo patches containing all components except for hyoscine were applied.

Delayed hypersensitivity may be a complication of drugs given transdermally. When new transdermal treatments are evaluated, the possibility of delayed hypersensitivity should be excluded. Such hypersensitivity may develop even after several months of repeated application.

▶ Considering the circumstances—continuous application of a chemical to a thin-skinned site under occlusion—one might fear that failure of allergic contact hypersensitivity to develop ought to be the reportable event.—J.D. Bernhard, M.D.

A Review of 79 Cases of Eyelid Dermatitis

Nethercott JR, Nield G, Holness DL (Univ of Toronto)

J Am Acad Dermatol 21:223–230, August 1989 6–13

Contact dermatitis, the most common eruption of the eyelids, has been attributed to various contactants. Eyelid dermatitis may also be related to underlying diseases such as atopic dermatitis or seborrheic dermatitis. Patch tests were used to assess 79 patients with eyelid dermatitis and 1,012 with dermatitis at other sites.

Of the patients with eyelid dermatitis, 89% were women; only the eyelids were involved in 78.5% of patients. Of the patients with eyelid dermatitis, 46% had allergic contact dermatitis, 15% had irritant contact dermatitis, and 23% had atopic dermatitis. Dermatitis was work related in only 13% of the patients. Compared with the patients who did not have eyelid dermatitis, those affected had more positive reactions to patch tests for cinnamic alcohol, diazolidinyl urea, and neomycin sulfate, and less frequent positive reactions to cobalt and nickel.

Using epicutaneous testing with 1 of 2 screening trays and an aimed tray for perfume allergies, it was possible to elicit relevant positive responses to patch tests and to establish an allergic basis for eyelid dermatitis in almost half of the patients in this series. Many contactants may be the allergen in patients with eyelid dermatitis.

▶ Diazolidinyl urea is a relatively new cosmetic preservative. The high frequency of reactions to it (18%) in the eyelid dermatitis group indicates that we may well see more of such reactions before the cosmetic companies begin to use less of it. The only compounds with a higher frequency of positive reactions in the eyelid dermatitis group were formaldehyde 2% aqueous and cinnamic alcohol 1%. Further, 16% of patients with eyelid dermatitis had a variety of dermatoses other than allergic contact, irritant contact, and atopic dermatitis. Perhaps some of these had "winter dermatitis of the eyelids," which we seem to see a fair amount of in patients whose sensitivity to dry, cold, winter air seems to zero in for that locale.—J.D. Bernhard, M.D.

Contact Lens Intolerance: Allergic Conjunctivitis?

Podmore P, Storrs FJ (Altnagelvin Area Hosp, Londonderry, Northern Ireland; Oregon Health Sciences Univ, Portland)

Contact Dermatitis 20:98–103, February 1989 6–14

Approximately 10% of all contact lens wearers have contact lens intolerance. To determine whether contact lens intolerance is caused by allergic contact conjunctivitis, irritant contact conjunctivitis, or some other unrelated irritants, 20 patients with contact lens intolerance were patch tested to a contact lens solution battery and a contact lens components battery. Patches were read on removal after 48 hours and again after 96 hours. Patients also were tested for contact urticaria to contact lens solution batteries that were placed on intact and scratched skin for 30 minutes.

Eight patients had positive delayed reactions, 6 had contact urticaria reactions, and 9 had no positive reactions. Of the 6 patients with contact urticaria, 5 were allergic to sorbic acid; 2 of these were using a sorbic acid-containing solution. Both were symptomatic and had marked conjunctival injection; 1 also had corneal neovascularization. The sixth patient was allergic to papain and was using a papain-containing solution. Among the positive reactions that persisted for 96 hours, the mercuric compounds were implicated most frequently (table). Two patients had reactions to the acrylate in their contact lenses.

The 9 patients who had no reactions on testing were thought to have either irritant or perhaps allergic contact dermatitis from an untested al-

Positive Delayed Reactions

thimerosal	0.1% pet.	2 positives
phenyl mercuric nitrate	0.05% pet.	3 patients
ammoniated mercury	1% pet.	2 patients
benzethonium chloride	0.1% aq.	2 patients
hydroxyethyl methacrylate	2% pet.	1 patient
triethylene glycol diacrylate	2% pet.	1 patient

(Courtesy of Podmore P, Storrs FJ: *Contact Dermatitis* 20:98–103, February 1989.)

lergen. Giant papillary conjunctivitis also was considered as a cause. Contact lens intolerance could not be attributed conclusively to an allergic reaction in nearly half of the patients.

▶ Eyelid dermatitis may or may not be present as well.—J.D. Bernhard, M.D.

Condoms as a Source of Latex Allergen and Cause of Contact Urticaria
Turjanmaa K, Reunala T (Univ Central Hosp; Univ of Tampere, Finland)
Contact Dermatitis 20:360–364, May 1989 6–15

Condoms are made of rubber latex, the proteins of which can sensitize atopic persons and cause contact urticaria. The effects of 16 different brands of condoms on 46 patients with latex-glove contact urticaria (LGCU) were examined to determine the occurrence of latex allergen in condoms and study the symptoms caused by contact with condoms.

Twenty-nine patients with LGCU had histories of condom use, and 7 (24%) of these had had local swelling or pruritus, or both, during intercourse. Prick tests on the 16 different brands of condom showed that 4 brands caused positive reactions in 52% to 67% of patients, whereas 12 brands were not as allergenic and 1 brand was totally negative. High-pressure liquid chromatography in 1 highly allergenic brand showed protein fractions similar to those eluted from a latex glove.

In addition to rubber gloves and balloons, condoms should be considered as a possible source of latex. Patients with LGCU may experience symptoms from condoms and should be advised to avoid using them.

Allergic Reactions to Rubber Condoms
Rademaker M, Forsyth A (Belvidere Hosp, Glasgow)
Genitourin Med 65:194–195, June 1989 6–16

Contact dermatitis to rubber compounds is common; the responsible allergen usually is an additive rather than rubber latex itself. Awareness of AIDS has increased the use of rubber condoms, thus increasing the number of contact reactions. A new, "hypoallergenic" condom, which is washed in 5% aqueous ammonia solution for 24 hours, was evaluated in 50 rubber-sensitive patients. Most had reacted to wearing rubber gloves. Fifty control patients had routine patch testing.

Twenty-six rubber-sensitive patients reacted to the condoms; 16 reacted to the new condom, 4 to ordinary condoms, and 6 to both. Thirty patients were allergic to thiuram-mix. Four controls had irritant reactions to the new, washed condom; 2 reacted to the ordinary condom.

Washing rubber condoms in ammonia is not sufficient to avoid reactions in those sensitized to rubber accelerators. Nonrubber condoms of sheep gut or polyurethane are available in some countries, but their imperviousness to viral particles is unknown.

▶ These 2 articles are important contributions to the differential diagnosis of intercourse-related pruritus. This is a critical problem, (with localized and generalized variants), whose spectrum ranges from contact dermatitis and contact urticaria to anaphylactic shock. Lest the condom be unjustly accused, other factors must be considered as well. In one case a woman who complained of severe itching after contact with her husband was shown to be sensitive to his sweat and semen, as confirmed by intradermal testing (1).—J.D. Bernhard, M.D.

Reference

1. Freeman S: *Contact Dermatitis* 14:110, 1986.

Anaphylaxis Produced by Rubber Glove Contact: Case Reports and Immunological Identification of the Antigens Involved

Morales C, Basomba A, Carreira J, Sastre A (Hosp La Fe, Valencia, Spain; Alergia-Inmunología Abelló, Madrid)

Clin Exp Allergy 19:425–430, July 1989 6–17

Natural latex sensitization is fairly uncommon. Although previous studies demonstrated specific sensitivity to latex in patients with contact urticaria after contact with rubber gloves, the allergens involved in the IgE-mediated response have not been identified. During a 7-year period, 6 patients reported anaphylactic reactions after contact with rubber gloves. Symptoms included contact urticaria, angioedema, rhinoconjunctivitis, asthma, and hypotension. The patients (5 females, 1 male; aged 17–33 years) underwent skin-prick, provocation, and patch testing with 25 common contactants. Total serum IgE levels also were determined.

All 6 patients had immediate positive reactions to skin-prick testing with glove washing samples and with extracts from natural latex and serum latex. The provocation test, which consisted of applying unwashed pieces of rubber gloves directly over the skin, was positive in all 6. However, washed rubber glove pieces gave negative results. Furthermore, patch testing did not cause any immediate or late reactions to the standard contactants tested. Thus the chemicals used in glove manufacturing were not implicated in the skin sensitivity reactions. Most patients had specific IgE to allergens present in glove washings. Immunoblotting showed that at least 4 soluble polypeptides from natural latex were able to bind specific human IgE. All symptoms could be avoided if the rubber gloves were thoroughly washed with water before use.

The anaphylactic reactions observed after contact with rubber gloves may have been mediated by IgE. Water-soluble and thermostable proteins, rather than chemicals used in glove manufacturing, appeared to be responsible for the observed severe hypersensitivity reactions. These proteins can be removed from the gloves by careful washing.

▶ Why washing rubber gloves in water should be more effective in preventing some reactions than washing condoms in ammonia remains something of a mystery.—J.D. Bernhard, M.D.

Passive Transfer of Contact Sensitivity to Colophony as a Complication of an Allogenic Bone-Marrow Transplant

Olaguibel J, Almodovar A, Giner A, Serrano G, Martinez J, Basomba A (Hosp La Fe; Hosp General, Valencia, Spain)

Contact Dermatitis 20:182–184, March 1989 6–18

The complications associated with successful bone marrow transplantation are well known; however, passive transfer of contact sensitivity has not been reported previously.

Woman, 29, was admitted with pancytopenia of unknown cause. Examination of the bone marrow aspirate revealed grade II marrow aplasia. She underwent allogeneic bone marrow transplantation with marrow donated by her brother. The graft material was HLA identical but ABO incompatible. The brother's previous medical history was negative except for a history of patch-test-confirmed allergic dermatitis from colophony. The bone marrow engraftment was successful, and the patient had no significant complications. One year after transplantation the patient was hospitalized with acute abdominal pain. On the third day after readmission, acute eczema was noted at the site of insertion of the blood catheter. The patient had no history of eczema, contact dermatitis, or other skin disorders. Standard patch testing and a patch test with the tape that held the catheter in place revealed 3+ positive reactions to colophony and to the tape.

The donor's known sensitivity to colophony and the absence of a history of contact dermatitis in the patient before bone marrow grafting suggest that the sensitivity to colophony was passively acquired through the marrow transplantation.

▶ Perhaps donor sensitivities should be routinely noted before bone marrow transplantation.—J.D. Bernhard, M.D.

Hyposensitization to Poison Ivy After Working in a Cashew Nut Shell Oil Processing Factory

Reginella RF, Fairfield JC, Marks JG Jr (Milton S Hershey Med Ctr, Hershey, Pa; Pennsylvania State Univ)
Contact Dermatitis 20:274–279, April 1989 6–19

Allergic contact dermatitis occurs in some individuals exposed to cashew nut shell oil (CNSO). The cashew nut tree, poison ivy, and poison oak are in the same botanical family, Anacardiaceae, and share chemicals that cause allergic contact dermatitis. Interestingly, in workers at a CNSO-processing factory hyposensitization to urushiol, the allergen in poison ivy and oak, occurred through the workers' exposure to CNSO.

Nineteen adults underwent patch tests to urushiol to determine their sensitivity to that allergen after working in a CNSO-processing plant. Ten of the 13 adults with a preemployment history of poison ivy sensitivity had CNSO dermatitis. After working in the factory for several months, 9 of 13 previously sensitive employees reported decreased sensitivity or no sensitivity to poison ivy on oak. When tested with urushiol extract, 10 of the 13 previously sensitive workers tested negatively and 3 tested positively, including 2 with minimal reactions.

Hyposensitization to poison ivy and oak can occur after development of hardening to CNSO. Whether the mechanism of hyposensitization in the workers is a cellular or humoral response is not known.

▶ "Hardening" after repeated exposure to an environmental or topical allergen or irritant is a curious phenomenon that may involve specific immunologic and/or "other" mechanisms. It is not unheard of in industrial situations and also can be seen in milder cases of solar urticaria and polymorphic light eruption.—J.D. Bernhard, M.D.

Topical Prevention of Poison Ivy/Oak Dermatitis

Epstein WL (Univ of California, San Francisco)
Arch Dermatol 125:499–501, April 1989 6–20

The treatment of poison ivy/oak dermatitis is fairly well accepted and standardized among dermatologists, but methods of prevention are still debated. An organoclay preparation was assessed in a double-blind trial for topical protection against experimental poison ivy/oak.

Test materials were given in spray cans containing fluorocarbon aerosols and either organoclay, bentonite, kaolin, or silicone. By direct comparison in the same patient, organoclay proved more effective than bentonite, kaolin, or silicone in 16 of 17 trials. When assessed globally against control responses to urushiol, the organoclay preparation provided 95.3% protection against topical urushiol applications, ranging from 4.75 to 0.0475 nmol. In the same system, bentonite, kaolin, and silicone provided 29.6%, 37.9%, and 32.9% protection, respectively.

Organoclay was significantly superior as a topical preventive agent against experimental urushiol dermatitis than conventional preparations of bentonite, kaolin, or silicone. Organoclay merits further clinical investigation.

▶ Organoclay is a quaternary ammonium salt of sodium bentonite. If it proves as effective in the field as it has in the laboratory (relatively low exposure doses of uroshiol in highly sensitive subjects) it will be a "godsend." Further testing as an investigational new drug before FDA approval means that it will not be coming by overnight mail. When it does, we hope its aerosol is not an ozone depleter.—J.D. Bernhard, M.D.

Isothiazolinone Preservative: Cause of a Continuing Epidemic of Cosmetic Dermatitis

De Groot AC, Herxheimer A (Carolus & Willem-Alexander Hosp, Hertogenbosch, The Netherlands; Charing Cross and Westminster Med School, London)

Lancet 1:314–316, Feb 11, 1989 6–21

Many cosmetics and toiletries are preserved with a mixture of methylisothiazolinone and methylchloroisothiazolinone. These ingredients should be suspected in cosmetic allergy, especially when products are designed to be left on the skin.

For cosmetic use the most common isothiazolinone preservative is kathon CG. When 119 patients with proven cosmetic-related allergic contact dermatitis were patch tested with various cosmetic ingredients, 28% reacted to kathon CG, making it by far the most important allergic ingredient. Occasional manufacturers have exceeded recommended use levels, but most allergic reactions to kathon CG have been traced to products complying with recommendations. Products that are washed off, for example, shampoo, rarely cause a reaction. Approximately half of the patients become sensitized by using products on normal skin, particularly on the face and around the eyes. The remainder have preexisting conditions that are exacerbated by kathon CG.

The use of kathon CG in cosmetics, especially of the "leave-on" type, should be abandoned. At present, most reports of sensitivity have come from in Europe. Kathon CG has not been considered safe for use in "leave-on" cosmetics in the United States. Further research to find substitutes for kathon CG is warranted. The efficacy of lower concentrations might also be investigated. Low concentrations of kathon CG in rinse-off products carry no appreciable risk of contact allergy; these products need not be modified.

▶ Given our usual suppositions about immunologic hypersensitivity, the possible difference in safety between "rinse-off" and "leave-on" cosmetics is interesting. How well different individuals rinse off the "rinse-offs" may vary and may be a factor we should question our contact dermatitis patients about.—J.D. Bernhard, M.D.

Urticarial Papular and Plaque Eruptions: A Noneczematous Manifestation of Allergic Contact Dermatitis

Goh CL (Natl Skin Ctr, Singapore)
Int J Dermatol 28:172–176, April 1989 6–22

Allergic contact dermatitis can present with noneczematous eruptions; in some cases the eruptions are erythematous, urticarial, and papular, with or without a target appearance.

Woman, 60, experienced intense itching of the hairline and scalp 24 hours after using permanent waving lotion on her hair. Erythematous urticarial papules and plaques appeared along the hairline and scalp (Fig 6–1) 3 days later; on the following day the eruptions appeared on her trunk and extremities. Some lesions appeared target-like. The woman had no history of respiratory tract infection nor was she taking medication. She had had generalized eruptions 10 years previously after wearing costume jewelry. The blood count and liver function tests were normal, and hepatitis B surface marker and collagen disease markers were negative. Biopsy of a target-like lesion revealed upper dermal edema and both superficial and deep perivascular infiltration of neutrophils, eosinophils, histiocytes, and lymphocytes, but the epidermis was normal. Treatment with oral prednisolone resolved the eruptions after 2 weeks. On patch testing, the patient was found to

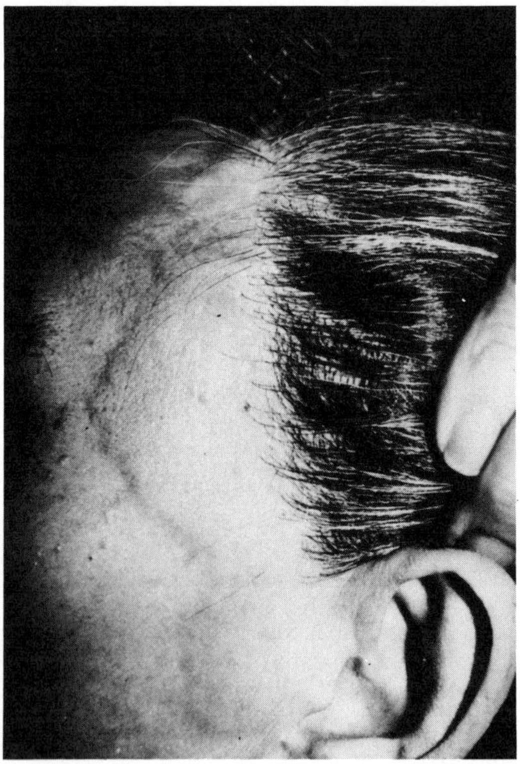

Fig 6–1.—Urticarial lesions along the hairline associated with contact dermatitis to a permanent wave lotion. (Courtesy of Goh CL: *Int J Dermatol* 28:172–176, April 1989.)

be allergic to neomycin, nickel sulfate, and lanolin. She also had a +1 reaction to permanent waving lotion, but a prick test with the lotion was negative. The components of the permanent waving lotion could not be determined, but circumstantial evidence suggested that the eruptions were associated with a contact allergy to the lotion.

These eruptions appear to have different morphological, histologic, and evolutionary characteristics from erythema multiforme. Because the eruptions seem to follow allergic contact dermatitis, the term *urticarial papular and plaque eruptions of contact allergy* is proposed describe the condition. The mechanism of the eruptions is unknown.

▶ The distinction between whatever this is and true erythema multiforme is not trivial. We don't know if it really deserves a name, but the name Goh suggests seems a bit cumbersome (NUPP??). It is also important to think about the difference between noneczematous manifestations of contact dermatitis that occur at the site of contact (such as contact urticaria) and those that may occur as a secondary hypersensitivity reaction at sites not coming into direct contact with the allergen. Alexander Fisher has at least 2 chapters on noneczematous contact dermatitis, including erythema multiforme-like eruptions and "systemic contact dermatitis" in the recent third edition of *Contact Dermatitis* (1).—J.D. Bernhard, M.D.

Reference

1. Fisher A: *Contact Dermatitis,* ed 3. Philadelphia, Lea & Febiger, 1986.

7 Pharmacology and Drug Therapy

Treatment of Hyperhidrosis Manuum by Tap Water Iontophoresis
Dahl JC, Glent-Madsen L (Odense Univ Hosp, Denmark)
Acta Derm Venereol [Stockh] 69:346–348, 1989 7–1

To determine the effectiveness of tap water iontophoretic treatment of emotional hyperhidrosis, a double-blind study under controlled conditions was carried out in 8 women and 3 men with verified palmar hyperhidrosis. All 11 received 15 minutes of active treatment on 1 hand and placebo treatment on the other hand 1–5 times per week.

Patients reported a good subjective effect after 6–12 treatments. When treated with a median current of 4 milliamperes (mamp), there was a median 38% reduction of sweat on the treated hand compared to sweat production before treatment and a median 32% reduction compared with that on the untreated hand, both significant decreases. After 6 patients received maintenance treatment with a median current of 10 mamp every second week for 3 months, sweat production was reduced by a median of 81%. No side effects were observed.

Tap water iontophoresis provides effective local treatment of emotional hyperhidrosis of the hand. Prevention of contact with electrodes may prevent side effects such as erythema, bullae, or burns. The number of treatments, the median current applied, and the iontophoretic device used may influence results.

▶ I don't know. All the studies I read say that iontophoresis works, but when I try it on my patients I never get the same benefits as reported in the literature. Do 2 types of hyperhidrosis exist: emotional and physical? Maybe I only see the physical ones, or maybe the device in this study is more effective. Also, my patients are more bothered by axillary hyperhidrosis than palmar. I wish that a really effective, *long-term* solution would be found for this very distressing disease.—J.C. Alper, M.D.

Treatment of Hyperhydrosis Using Iontophoresis: Principle, Equipment, Methodology, and Results in 93 Cases
Desnos P, Henriet JP, Vigneron JL, Corson N, Munoz MH, Bonerandi JJ (Hôp Sainte-Marguerite, Marseille, France)
Nouv Dermatol 7:551–554, September–October 1988 7–2

In France, hyperhydrosis affects an estimated 12% of the population older than 15 years. Potassium permanganate or aluminum chloride hexahydrate baths are effective only in the treatment of mild to moderate hyperhydrosis. Until recently, surgical sympathectomy was the only effective treatment available for the more severe conditions.

In the United States, iontophoresis in the treatment of palmar and plantar hyperhidrosis is well established, but in France the equipment for ion therapy has only recently become available. Iontophoresis involves placing the involved hands or feet in tanks filled with tap water. An electric current is run between the epidermis and a set of electrodes. The recommended electric current of 20 milliamperes is obtained by adjustment of a potentiometer. The mechanism of action of iontophoresis is not known, but the electric current may act directly on secretory cells.

Between 1983 and 1988, 61 females and 32 males aged 7–62 years (median, 29 years) underwent iontophoresis in the treatment of hyperhidrosis of the extremities. Seventy patients had essential hyperhidrosis, 22 had hyperhidrosis in the presence of acrocyanosis, and 1 had hyperhidrosis as a complication of a posttraumatic shoulder algodystrophy. A total of 39 patients had a family history of the disorder. Of the 93 patients, 58 had hyperhidrosis of all 4 extremities, 12 of the hands only, and 23 of the feet only. All patients were treated according to a standard protocol that prescribed sessions on days 1, 2, 4, 8, 12, 15, 22, and 36. From then on, treatment was given on demand as needed.

Iontophoresis significantly improved hyperhidrosis in 86 of the 93 patients (92.5%). One was only minimally improved after 7 treatments, and 6 patients discontinued treatment because they could not tolerate it. After only 4 treatments, 60 patients were much improved. Neither sex, age, nor duration of symptoms affected the outcome. However, plantar hyperhidrosis improved more slowly than palmar hyperhidrosis. Minimal side effects included the appearance of blisters in patients who pushed down too hard on the metal grids. All side effects resolved spontaneously without treatment.

▶ My comments are the same as those following Abstract 7–1.—J.C. Alper, M.D.

Comparative Efficacy of 12% Ammonium Lactate Lotion and 5% Lactic Acid Lotion in the Treatment of Moderate to Severe Xerosis

Rogers RS III, Callen J, Wehr R, Krochmal L (Mayo Clinic and Found, Rochester, Minn; Univ of Louisville; Bristol-Myers Co, Buffalo)

J Am Acad Dermatol 21:714–716, October 1989 7–3

Previous studies have shown that 12% ammonium lactate lotion is effective in the treatment of xerosis and ichthyosis. To compare the safety and efficacy of 12% ammonium lactate lotion with those of 5% lactic acid lotion in the treatment of moderate to severe xerosis, 33 women and 8 men aged 18–70 years (mean, 47.4 years) with at least grade 4 xerosis on the lateral aspects of both legs took part in a double-blind, multicenter study.

Patients applied 12% ammonium lactate lotion to 1 leg and 5% lactic acid with 2.5% sodium pyrrolidone carboxylic acid lotion to the other leg twice daily for 3 weeks. All medications were supplied and administered in a blinded fashion. The severity of xerosis was evaluated on a 0- to 6-point scale before treatment and 3, 7, 14, and 21 days after the start of treatment. No medication was applied during an additional 21-day regression phase. Patients were told not to use any other topical products on the legs for 2 weeks before the study and during the 2 phases of the study. Ivory soap was used for bathing during all phases of the study.

Both medications resulted in a significant improvement in dry skin severity over time. Improvement was evident by day 3 of treatment and maintained throughout the study. However, the 12% ammonium lactate lotion was significantly more effective than the 5% lactic acid lotion on days 7 and 21 during the active treatment phase, and on days 28, 35, and 42 during the regression phase. The degree of benefit with the 12% lotion became more apparent during the regression phase. Two patients were dropped from the study because of adverse effects: dryness in 1 patient and pruritus and irritation in the other patient related to the use of the 5% lactic acid lotion. Seven patients complained of tingling, stinging, burning, pruritus, or irritation. Thus 12% ammonium lactate lotion is significantly more effective than 5% lactic acid lotion in reducing the severity of xerosis.

▶ I think most of us who care for patients with dry skin knew the results of this study before it was done; we gave up using 5% lactic acid several years ago. It's nice to see 12% ammonium lactate withstand a well-done clinical study, however. What I can't figure at all is why the patients were all bathed with Ivory soap! The results of the study might have been even better with a more reasonable, less drying variety of soap.—J.C. Alper, M.D.

Alpha Hydroxy Acids: Procedures for Use in Clinical Practice

Van Scott EJ, Yu RJ (Temple Univ. Philadelphia)

Cutis 43:222–228, March 1989 7–4

α-Hydroxy acids and α-keto acids applied topically in low concentrations are useful in the treatment of a number of conditions caused by, or associated with, hyperkeratinization. These acid solutions appear to reduce the thickness of the hyperkeratotic stratum corneum by reducing corneocyte cohesion, perhaps through a mechanism that interferes with ionic bonding. Because so many dermatologic conditions are either caused by, or associated with, excessive corneocyte cohesion, these acids have been used in the treatment of such conditions as dry skin, ichthyosis, and follicular hyperkeratosis, among others, that are characterized by stratum corneum retention.

When applied topically in concentrations of 70% and greater, α-hydroxy acids and α-keto acids cause epidermolysis, thus providing a new, alternative treatment for seborrheic keratoses, age spots, actinic keratoses, and common warts. These conditions not only involve distinct epidermal hyperplasia, but they are also characterized by stratum corneum retention. α-Hydroxy acids were also used in the treatment of acne. In concentrations of 5% to 10%, the acid solution can be applied twice daily at home. Topical application of a 70% solution as an office procedure has also been used in the last 2 years. Good results have been obtained with various α-hydroxy acid concentrations in the treatment of keratoses and wrinkles. A cream containing 5% to 15% glycolic acid was applied twice daily at home. In addition, a 70% glycolic acid solution was applied to the face as an office procedure every 1–6 weeks.

Although these experiences did not involve controlled comparative trials, the initial experience with α-hydroxy acids and α-keto acids suggests that extensive and varied clinical trials should be initiated to assess the validity of some of these applications.

▶ The α-hydroxy acids appear to be a new type of topical chemotherapy for the treatment of benigh and premalignant epithelial growths. Dr. Van Scott's experience suggests that these agents may well be valuable alternatives to cryosurgery, phenol, and other acids in the treatment of many common epidermal proliferative disorders.—R.S. Stern, M.D.

Safety of Pregnancy After Discontinuation of Isotretinoin

Dai WS, Hsu M-A, Itri LM (Hoffman-La Roche Inc, Nutley, NJ)

Arch Dermatol 125:362–365, March 1989 7–5

The risk of major congenital malformations is increased in infants exposed to isotretinoin (13-cis-retinoic acid) during pregnancy. The safety of a subsequent pregnancy after discontinuation of isotretinoin is yet unknown. Pregnancy case reports of 88 patients in whom conception occurred after isotretinoin treatment had been discontinued were reviewed to determine the pregnancy outcome; of these pregnancies, 90% occurred within 2 months after discontinuation of the drug.

The incidence of both spontaneous and missed abortions in all pregnancies was 9% (8 pregnancies), and the incidence rate of congenital malformations among the live births was 5%. Both rates were not significantly different from those in women of reproductive age in the general population. Furthermore, the congenital malformations observed, such as a relatively small anterior fontanelle, congenital cataract, and hypospadias, were not characteristic of retinoic acid-induced congenital abnormalities.

There is no statistically significant risk of congenital malformation or spontaneous abortion in women who discontinue isotretinoin therapy before conception.

▶ This study reassures us that, as we would expect from animal studies and our knowledge of isotretinoin's metabolism, once this drug has been discontinued and sufficient time for complete clearance has elapsed, the risk of congenital malformations in subsequent pregnancies of former users is not increased.—R.S. Stern, M.D.

Acitretin Monotherapy in Darier's Disease

Van Dooren-Greebe RJ, Van de Kerkhof PCM, Happle R (Univ of Nijmegen, The Netherlands)

Br J Dermatol 121:375–379, September 1989 7–6

The dose-response relationship to the oral retinoid acitretin was investigated in 5 patients with Darier's disease.

Acitretin treatment was started at an initial dosage of 35 mg/day for the first 3 months, after which the daily dose was adjusted according to clinical response. Two patients had complete clearance of the eruption (Fig 7–1), 2 had marked improvement, and 1 had only moderate improvement. Isomorphic reactions resulting from a relative overdose occurred in 2 patients and improved with dose reduction. Maintenance therapy with 10–35 mg/day was effective in 4 patients. Acitretin was well tolerated by all patients.

Acitretin appears to be valuable in the treatment of Darier's disease. Acitretin treatment should be initiated at a dose of 10–25 mg/day with gradual adjustment of the dose. Its relatively short half-life and prompt response to dose reduction when side effects occur make it more practically advantageous than etretinate in the treatment of Darier's disease.

▶ I'm convinced that we need this drug—at least to try out—to see if we get the same results as investigators are reporting. As it appears to have less potential toxicity than etretinate (because of a shorter half-life), I wonder when our FDA is going to get around to approving it.—J.C. Alper, M.D.

Clinical and Ultrastructural Effects of Acitretin in Darier's Disease

Lauharanta J, Kanerya L, Turjanmaa K, Geiger JM (Univ Central Hosp, Helsinki; Inst of Occupational Health, Helsinki; Univ Central Hosp, Tampere, Finland; F. Hoffmann-LaRoche, Basle, Switzerland)

Acta Derm Venereol (Stockh) 68:492–498, 1988 7–7

Etretinate is an effective treatment for Darier's disease, especially its widespread and hyperkeratotic forms. A disadvantage of the drug, however, is its long elimination time from the body. Women of childbearing age must practice contraception for 2 years after stopping treatment with etretinate. The main metabolite of etretinate, acitretin, is rapidly eliminated from the body after oral administration.

The effect of acitretin on the faulty keratinization in Darier's disease was assessed in 13 patients aged 19–69. The duration of their disease varied from 11 to 41 years. Nine had previously taken etretinate with good or moderate results. For the current episode the patients were given 30 mg of acitretin daily for 8 weeks, followed by an individualized dosage to minimize side effects during the remainder of the 4-month course.

Of the 13 patients, 7 had good clearing of the lesions within 4–8 weeks. The involved area was increased in 1 patient and accompanied by intense pruritus, but a reduced dose almost completely cleared the lesions

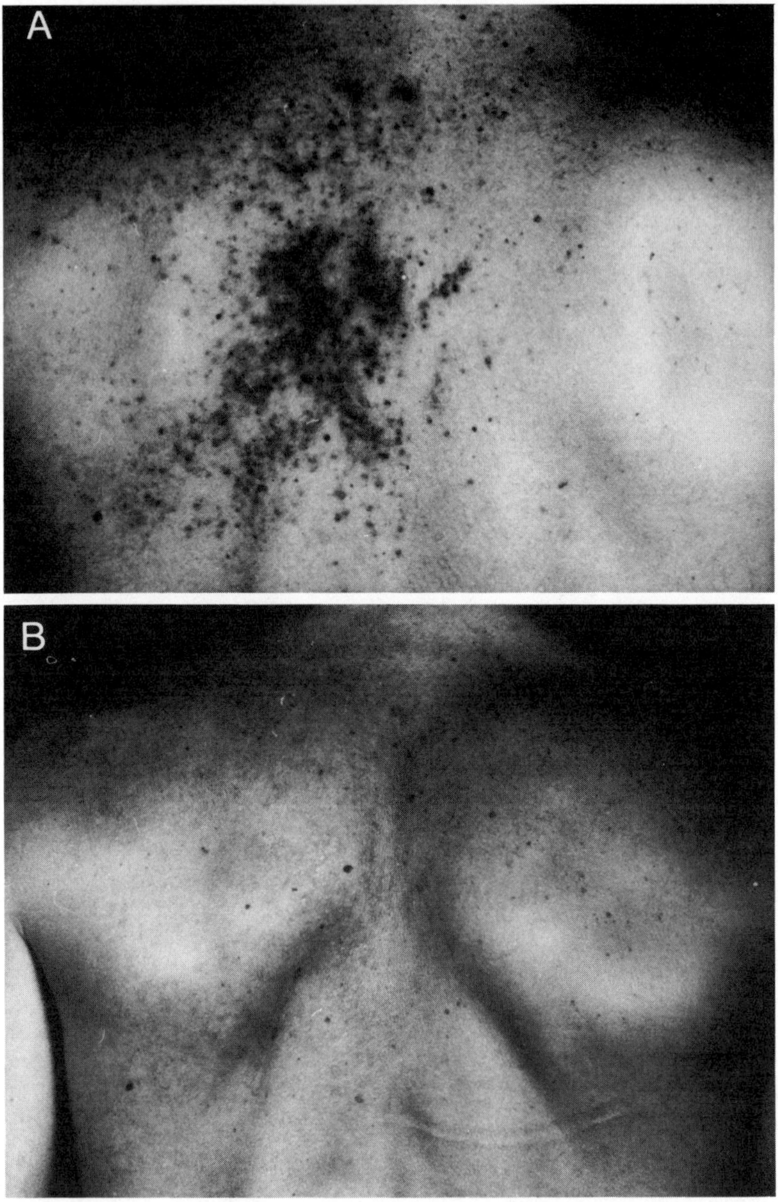

Fig 7–1.—Darier's disease. **A,** before treatment; **B,** after 5 months of treatment with acitretin. (Courtesy of Van Dooren-Greebe RJ, Van de Kerkhof PCM, Happle R: *Br J Dermatol* 121:375–379, September 1989.)

in 12 weeks. Three patients experienced only slight improvement with acitretin. Side effects included dry lips, pruritus, and moderate alopecia that was reversed after treatment stopped.

Most patients did well with 20 mg of acitretin daily, and none required more than 30 mg/day, a smaller dose than needed with etretinate. Darier's disease almost always recurs even when the skin appears completely cleared, because several pathologic features remain in the epidermis. Electron microscopy studies in 3 patients showed that normal stratification did not develop and the size and number of desmosomes remained reduced. Because maximum improvement was seen at about 12 weeks, acitretin should probably not be continued beyond this period.

▶ I expect to see a lot more of this type of investigation in many of the other chronic diseases such as the ichthyoses and psoriasis. It is hoped that more congeners of the retinoids with greater efficacy and less toxicity will be developed.—J.C. Alper, M.D.

Etretinate: Persistent Serum Levels After Long-Term Therapy

DiGiovanna JJ, Zech LA, Ruddel ME, Gantt G, Peck GL (Natl Cancer Inst, Bethesda, Md; Clinical Ctr, NIH, Bethesda)

Arch Dermatol 125:246–251, February 1989 7–8

Etretinate, a synthetic aromatic retinoid, is approved for use in the therapy of resistant psoriasis. It is also useful in a variety of uncommon, treatment-resistant dermatologic diseases. However, etretinate accumulates in subcutaneous fat and therefore might be stored to a greater extent in overweight patients. Whether overweight persons eliminate etretinate more slowly than persons of normal weight was investigated 1–244 weeks after therapy was discontinued in 47 patients who had received long-term etretinate treatment.

The earliest posttreatment, undetectable serum concentration of etretinate was noted 5 weeks after treatment. Serum concentrations were still detectable more than 2 years after treatment was stopped. Sequential samples of serum were obtained from 8 patients to determine half-lives for this late-phase elimination. The median half-life was 12.5 weeks. Each patient's deviation from ideal body weight as a measure of excess fat was then compared with various pharmacokinetic factors of etretinate elimination. Overweight patients tended to eliminate the drug more slowly, maintain higher serum concentrations, and clear the drug later (Fig 7–2).

▶ Because this drug binds so avidly to fat, longer half-lives in fat patients are not surprising.—R.S. Stern, M.D.

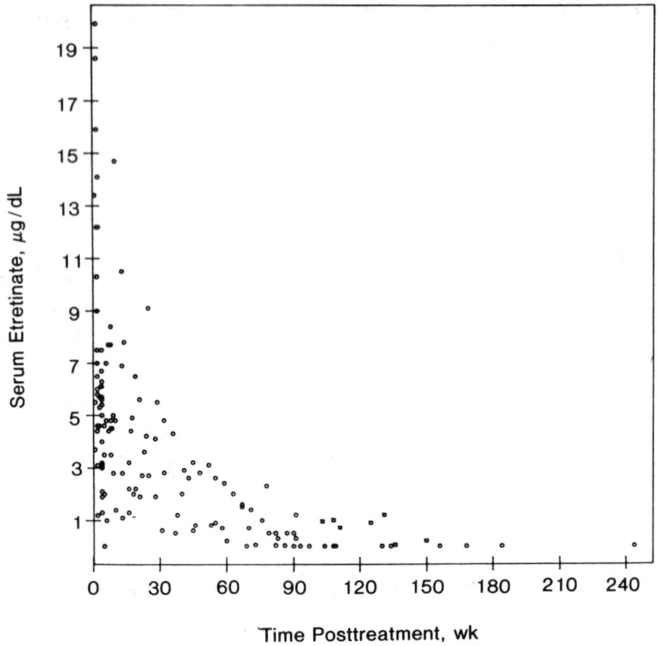

Fig 7–2.—Posttreatment serum etretinate concentrations. In 47 patients, serum etretinate concentrations were obtained 1 to 244 weeks after discontinuation of therapy. Detectable serum concentrations (0.05–1.2 µg/dL) were observed in 5 patients more than 2 years (108, 131, 136, and 150 weeks) after discontinuation of therapy. (Courtesy of DiGiovanna JJ, Zech LA, Ruddel ME, et al: *Arch Dermatol* 125:246–251, February 1989.)

Etretinate Treatment in Disseminated Porokeratosis

Danno K, Yamamoto M, Yokoo T, Ohta M, Ohno S (Tenri Hosp, Nara, Japan)

J Dermatol 15:440–444, October 1988 7–9

The treatment of porokeratosis of Mibelli is often disappointing, but systemic retinoid has proved beneficial in some cases.

Man, 77, with disseminated superficial porokeratosis of Mibelli over the entire body surface for 60 years, was treated orally with etretinate, 1 mg/kg/day, for 9 months after resection of 2 lesions of Bowen's disease. The hyperkeratotic edge of the annular plaques moderately regressed to a smooth, flat surface after 3 months of treatment (Fig 7–3). Histologic examination showed disappearance of parakeratosis and residual but less stacked cornoid lamella. Follow-up at 6 months showed gradual improvement of the lesions without relapse. Known side effects of retinoids were well tolerated.

Eight patients with porokeratosis of Mibelli have been treated successfully with oral etretinate (table, p 102), with all showing a remarkable response after an average 5 weeks of treatment. Etretinate may be the first choice of treatment in widespread porokeratosis of Mibelli.

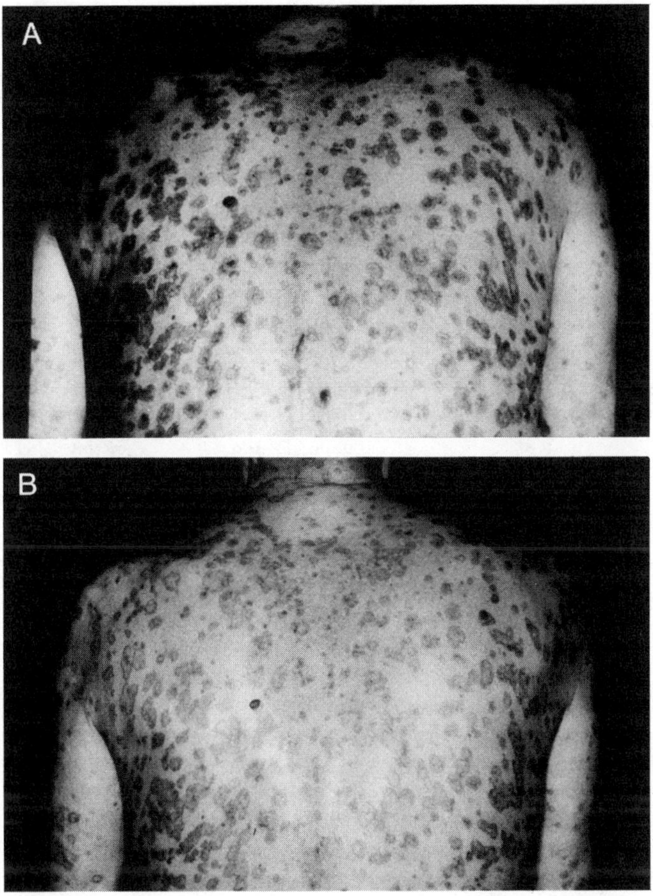

Fig 7–3.—Clinical features of upper back; **A,** before treatment, and **B,** after 3 months of treatment. (Courtesy of Danno K, Yamamoto M, Yokoo T, et al: *J Dermatol* 15:440–444, October 1988.)

▶ The efficacy of etretinate in both porokeratosis of Mibelli and disseminated superficial actinic parakeratosis raises questions as to whether its effect is on the basis of changes in keratinization, increased differentiation, or anticancer properties. Figure 7–3 clearly shows that some improvement is realized in these difficult conditions that are otherwise relatively refractory to therapy.—R.S. Stern, M.D.

Absorption of Minoxidil After Topical Application: Effect of Frequency and Site of Application
Eller MG, Szpunar GJ, Della-Coletta AA (Upjohn Company, Kalamazoo, Mich)
Clin Pharmacol Ther 45:396–402, April 1989 7–10

Summary of Successful Cases of Porokeratosis With Retinoid

Patient (Ref No)	Clinical form (duration)	Regimen and Tx period	Response and Comment
1/78/M (3)	Disseminated PM of head and thighs (15y)	75 mg/d × 10d 50 mg/d × 3wk 25 mg/d × mtn	remarkably regressed after 3–4wk
2/62/M (3)	Disseminated PM of forearm and legs, verrucous form (25y)	same as above	remarkably regressed after 3–4wk
3/15/M (4)	Linear PM of arm (6mo)	1 mg/kg/d × 7wk 0.5 mg/kg/d × 5wk	moderately regressed after 7wk and remarkably after 12wk
4/84/F (5)	DASP of trunk and extremities (4y)	100 mg/d × 10d 50 mg/d × 40d 25 mg/d × mtn	remarkably regressed after 6wk itching also ceased
5/46/F (6)	Linear PM of forearm, shoulder, and legs (10y)	1 mg/kg/d × 8wk 0.5 mg/kg/d × 1y	disappeared after 4wk
6/62/M (7)	Linear PM of buttocks and lower extremities (verrucous form)	75 mg/d × 3wk	remarkably regressed after 3wk associated with psoriasis
7/58/M (8)	Disseminated PM of whole body, palms and soles (40y)	50 mg/d × 4wk 25 mg/d × 1y	remarkably regressed after 3wk some of lesions disappeared
8/77/M (present case)	Disseminated PM of whole body (60y)	1 mg/kg/d × 9mo	slightly regressed after 2wk and moderately after 8–12wk

Abbreviations: mm, maintenance; *PM,* porokeratosis of Mibelli; *Tx,* treatment; *d,* day; *wk,* week; *mo,* month.
(Courtesy of Danno K, Yamamoto M, Yokoo T, et al: *J Dermatol* 15:440–444, October 1988.)

Minoxidil, a potent antihypertensive drug, lowers blood pressure by selectively relaxing the smooth muscle of peripheral arterioles. Most patients receiving maintenance treatment orally have hypertrichosis. Topically applied minoxidil has also been used for treatment of alopecias. To determine how the frequency and site of application influence the systemic absorption and accumulation of topically applied minoxidil, 52 nonobese, healthy men applied 1 mL of 3% minoxidil solution 4, 6, or 8 times daily to the scalp or 2, 4, 6, or 8 times daily to the chest for 14 days. Serum and urine were analyzed for minoxidil.

No minoxidil accumulated systemically from increasing frequency of application to the scalp. Data on chest application suggested that absorption may have been lower with the twice-daily application. Absorptions through the chest and scalp were similar after the lower-frequency regimens. Trends of the 8-times-daily regimen suggested that absorption from scalp application may have been greater.

It is unlikely that systemic minoxidil accumulation results from frequent application. Initial doses probably saturate the skin for a period longer than the dosing intervals examined.

▶ If, as this study suggests, minoxidil stays in the skin for a prolonged period, why do we use minoxidil twice a day rather than once a day? It would be interesting to see how absorption from once-a-day therapy compares to that with twice-a-day therapy. As the authors warn, absorption and biovailability may not be the same for an agent that is meant to affect the skin or its appendages. Not clear from this article is how much absorption of topical minoxidil is increased when this agent is used on inflamed skin or in conjunction with agents such as Retin-A.—R.S. Stern, M.D.

Topical Capsaicin Treatment of Chronic Postherpetic Neuralgia

Bernstein JE, Korman NJ, Bickers DR, Dahl MV, Millikan LE (GenDerm Corp, Northbrook, Ill; Case Western Reserve Univ; Univ of Minnesota; Tulane Univ)

J Am Acad Dermatol 21:265–270, August 1989 7–11

Uncontrolled studies have suggested that topically applied capsaicin may be a safe and effective treatment for postherpetic neuralgia. In a double-blind study, 32 elderly patients with chronic postherpetic neuralgia were treated with either capsaicin cream or its vehicle for 6 weeks. Treatment response was assessed by visual analogue scales of pain and pain relief along with changes in a categoric pain scale and in a physician's global evaluation. The patients given capsaicin had significantly greater relief on all efficacy variables than patients given the vehicle. Almost 80% of capsaicin-treated patients experienced some relief from pain after the 6 weeks of treatment.

This double-blind, vehicle-controlled study showed that topically applied capsaicin provides partial to complete relief from pain in almost 80% of patients with chronic intractable postherpetic neuralgia. Because problems with drug interactions and systemic toxicity are avoided with capsaicin, it should be considered in the initial management for postherpetic neuralgia.

Capsaicin in Dermatologic Disease

Bernstein JE (GenDerm Corp, Northbrook, Ill)

Semin Dermatol 7:304–309, December 1988 7–12

In consideration of its effects on substance P (SP) in cutaneous sensory neurons, topical capsaicin has been investigated in a variety of cutaneous disorders. The pain of postherpetic neuralgia is frequently so persistent and severe that neurosurgical procedures may be required to reduce it. Several studies evaluated the topical application of capsaicin in a cream base in patients with postherpetic neuralgia. In 1 study 75% of 12 patients reported relief from the chronic pain of postherpetic neuralgia. In another study of a larger group of patients, 78% reported some relief and in 56% results were good to excellent. Other studies reported similar results.

An apparent relationship between pain and itching prompted several studies on the use of capsaicin for pruritus. Although data on pruritus studies are sparse, a multicenter study has shown the application of topical capsaicin to be as effective in relieving itching as it is in relieving pain. Capsaicin has a very short action time, so it is necessary to apply the cream 3–4 times daily to obtain relief. About 20% of patients experience burning, stinging, or redness at the site of application. Reactions usually disappear within 72 hours of regular use. Pretreatment with xylocaine may reduce the severity of burning. Relief of symptoms is usually obtained within 2–4 weeks. Younger patients can usually stop treatment after 3–5 months of pain relief. Very elderly patients might continue to be treated for life.

Topically applied capsaicin cream appears to provide relief of pain and pruritus in patients with postherpetic neuralgia or other cutaneous disorders. The treatment is safer and more effective than other systemic therapies.

▶ Both papers on capsaicin (Abstracts 7–11 and 7–12) report that it relieves discomfort, at least partially, in about 80% of patients with post zoster neuralgia. Capsaicin is a phytochemical that both induces the release of substance P from a neuron and blocks its synthesis and transport within the neuron. Substance P is an undecapeptide neurotransmitter involved in the communication of pain, and possibly itch, from the peripheral to the central nervous system. Hence the rationale for the use of substance P in attempts to relieve the pain of post zoster neuralgia. Relief, according to the authors, may be achieved within 2–6 weeks of topical therapy. The effect of any given topical application is short lived, thus it must be applied 3–4 times a day. The duration of relief after 6 weeks of therapy is unclear—some patients, particularly older individuals, may have to continue treatment indefinitely. The topically applied drug may produce local irritation but seems to have no systemic side effects, in contrast to the anticonvulsants, antidepressants, and narcotics that currently may be used systemically.—R. Masters, M.D.

Clofazimine: Therapeutic Alternative in the Treatment of Necrobiosis Lipoidica and Granuloma Anulare

Mensing H (Universitäts-Hautklinik Hamburg-Eppendorf, West Germany)

Hautarzt 40:99–103, February 1989 7–13

Necrobiosis lipoidica (NL) and disseminated granuloma annulare (DGA) are noninfectious skin disorders of unknown etiology. The prognosis of both dermatoses is favorable, and spontaneous resolution can be expected. However, it may take months or even years before symptoms clear completely. Whereas DGA often has a benign course, NL usually follows a stubborn course and is often complicated by ulceration. Clinical trials of various anti-inflammatory agents such as aspirin have shown little effect. Corticosteroids, although effective, are not suitable for long-term use and cause numerous side effects. The efficacy of clofazimine, a phenothiazine drug used in the treatment of leprosy, was assessed because it has shown promise in the treatment of DGA and NL.

Ten patients aged 23–56 years with biopsy-confirmed NL and 10 patients aged 22–54 years with biopsy-proved DGA were treated with 100 mg of orally administered clofazimine taken twice daily. Drug therapy was stopped if no improvement was observed after 6 months of treatment. Patients underwent routine laboratory testing after 14 days of treatment and every 4 weeks thereafter. The dosage was reduced to 100 mg daily as soon as more than 50% improvement was observed.

Clofazimine therapy was discontinued in 4 patients with NL and in 4 patients with DGA because there was no change in the lesions after at least 6 months of therapy. Three patients in each group had complete resolution of their lesions, and 3 patients in each group improved by more than 50%. However, after clofazimine therapy was discontinued, 3 patients in the NL group and 2 in the DGA group had a recurrence that required reinstatement of drug therapy. Two patients with DGA were lost to follow-up.

All patients experienced a reddish-brown skin discoloration that was not resolved with a reduction in dosage but that disappeared completely within 2–3 months after clofazimine therapy was discontinued. Two patients experienced transient diarrhea. Results of all laboratory studies remained normal throughout the study, and the drug was generally well tolerated. Although the study population was too small for any definite conclusions to be drawn, the preliminary results obtained with oral clofazimine in the treatment of DGA and NL are encouraging and warrant further investigation.

▶ Clofazimine was originally developed for use in tuberculosis. It is currently an important drug in the management of nonreactive and reactive leprosy and has been used against infections caused by the *Mycobacterium avium-intracellulare* group. It has also been useful in conditions associated with a vasculitis such as erythema nodosum leprosum and in facial granuloma. Some neutrophilic dermatoses (e.g., pyoderma gangrenosum and pustular dermatoses of the palms and soles) reportedly respond to clofazimine therapy. The drug has also been used in patients with cheilitis granulomatosa (Melkersson-Rosenthal syndrome) and generalized granuloma annulare (1); the mechanism of action of this drug in these conditions has not been adequately defined or understood.—S.L. Moschella, M.D.

Reference

1. Djawari E, Felgner K: *Aktuel Dermatol* 14:15, 1988.

Colchicine Therapy in Behçet's Syndrome: A Report of Five Cases

Muzulu SI, Walton S, Keczkes K (Hull Royal Infirmary, Hull; General Infirmary, Leeds England)

Clin Exp Dermatol 14:298–299, July 1989 7–14

The treatment of Behçet's syndrome remains a challenge, because presently available drugs are only moderately effective. Colchicine was used with benefit in 5 patients with Behçet's syndrome when given in doses of 500 μg twice daily. The patients improved clinically; 1 has remained clear for 1 year after treatment. Paresthesias persisted in 1 patient with neurologic symptoms. All patients initially had orogenital ulceration, and 3 had ocular and joint involvement.

Four patients have required ongoing colchicine therapy for continued clinical improvement. Because colchicine is relatively free of side effects, it is most useful in a chronic, multisystemic disorder, such as Behçet's syndrome, as long-term immunosuppression could have serious side effects in these patients.

▶ There are potentially 7 cardinal features associated with Behçet's disease. Typically, the diagnosis is made in the presence of oral aphthosis ulcerations and at least 2 other features, most commonly arthritis and uveitis, after disorders mimicking them are excluded. Behçet's syndrome has responded not only to colchicine but also to dapsone and thalidomide. In the more severe and refractory cases, oral prednisone and chlorambucil have been used.—S.L. Moschella, M.D.

Treatment of Scabies With Permethrin Versus Lindane and Benzyl Benzoate

Haustein U-F, Hlawa B (Karl Marx Univ, Leipzig, East Germany)

Acta Derm Venereol [Stockh] 69:348–351, 1989 7–15

Lindane has long been used for treatment of scabies, but because of its neurotoxicity and percutaneous absorption, alternative treatments have been sought. The efficacy and side effects were compared after 2 applications of lindane hydrochloride ointment 1% (0.3% in children in a single or split application), 3 applications of benzyl benzoate liquid 20% (10% in children), and 1 application of permethrin emulsion 5% (2.5% in children) at bedtime. The patients included 114 adults and 80 children no older than 5 years of age.

Treatment failures, assessed at 22 days, occurred in 3 adults and 2 children treated with lindane but not with the other medications. The incidence of postscabies eczema at day 8 was much higher after 20% benzyl benzoate than after the other treatments, and burning, redness, and dryness were significantly more frequent after benzyl benzoate treatment.

Permethrin is an effective, reliable treatment for scabies. It is preferred to benzyl benzoate because of the latter's odor and irritating quality. Permethrin is especially suitable for infants and small children, patients with neurologic disorders, and those in whom lindane treatment has failed.

▶ This study and subsequent studies of synthetic permethrins provide evidence for the ease of use, apparent low toxicity, and high efficacy of these agents in scabies therapy.—R.S. Stern, M.D.

Creeping Eruption Stopped in Its Tracks by Albendazole

Williams HC, Monk B (Kings College Hosp, London; Bedford Gen Hosp, Bedford, England)

Clin Exp Dermatol 14:355–356, September 1989 7–16

Because more and more people are taking advantage of low air fares to exotic destinations, creeping eruption disease is becoming common in Britain. Treatment of 5 patients aged 19–44 with a new antihelminthic agent, albendazole, was carried out. Three patients had recently been to Barbados, 1 to Thailand, and 1 to Antigua.

The first patient had 5 independent serpiginous tracks and a secondary infection from excoriation. Albendazole, 400 mg twice a day orally for 3 days, produced dramatic relief of pruritus and cessation of worm movement within 24 hours without side effects. The second woman had a solitary lesion on the abdomen 3 weeks after returning from Thailand. The itching was so intense that she had been unable to sleep for several days. Albendazole orally for 3 days was curative; her symptoms resolved within 24 hours. The third patient had a typical creeping eruption on the foot that did not respond to topical 10% thiabendazole; she was cured, however, with oral albendazole. The fourth and fifth patients, traveling together, returned from Barbados with typical creeping eruption and distressing pruritus. Itching and movement resolved within 48 hours of oral albendazole therapy.

Creeping eruption is the distinctive serpiginous eruption caused by the accidental invasion of skin by parasites. The most common parasites are dog and cat hookworm larvae. The worms ultimately die, but in the meantime the patient experiences intense pruritus and the sensation of worms crawling through the skin. Albendazole in a dosage of 400 mg twice daily for 3 days is a rapid, safe treatment for this unpleasant condition.

▶ Creeping eruption (cutaneous larva migrans) is not uncommon in the Northeast and in the Florida Gulf coastal areas, and in Caribbean vacationers. Currently, isolated lesions and generalized lesions are treated with topical and oral thiabendazole, respectively. Unfortunately, oral thiabendazole causes side effects relatively frequently including nausea, vomiting, and vertigo; potentially severe side effects such as leukopenia, hallucinations, olfactory disturbances, tinnitus, Steven-Johnson syndrome, and shock also may develop. The benzimidazoles, oral albendazole and mebendazole, and intramuscular flubendazole are effective in various intestinal and extraintestinal parasitosis. Albendazole, in the therapeutic dose of 400 mg twice daily, is the best tolerated and least toxic, and apparently is very effective against creeping eruption.—S.L. Moschella, M.D.

8 Adverse Drug Reactions

Cutaneous Drug Reactions: Clinical Types and Causative Agents: A Five-Year Survey of In-Patients (1981–1985)

Alanko K, Stubb S, Kauppinen K (Univ Central Hosp Helsinki)

Acta Derm Venereol (Stockh) 69:223–226, 1989 8–1

The development of new therapeutic drugs increases the risk of drug eruptions. From 1981 to 1985, there were 225 cutaneous drug reactions reported in 219 patients; 128 of the reactions were confirmed by provocative testing.

Fixed drug eruptions, exanthematous eruptions, and urticaria/angioedema were the most common clinical reactions. Antimicrobial drugs and antipyretic/anti-inflammatory agents were the most frequent causative agents. A comparison of recent drug eruptions with those treated at the same hospital during the previous 25 years showed a decrease in the number of skin reactions (table, p 110). Although the drugs chiefly responsible for reactions have remained the same, the importance of sulfonamides as causative agents has decreased.

Drugs that cause the most common skin reactions appear to remain the same throughout the years. However, fewer skin reactions seem to have occurred in the early 1980s, perhaps because of purification of such drugs as penicillin, lack of use of the long-acting sulfonamides, and better diagnoses of drug eruptions. The only certain way of confirming that a skin reaction is caused by a particular drug is by provocative testing.

▶ An update of the elegant work of Kauppinen. Using provocation tests, this Finnish group was able to verify suspected drug reactions in more than half of the patients studied. Of interest is the large number of fixed drug eruptions in their series. The most frequent suspect agents for these reactions include the antimicrobial and anti-inflammatory drugs. These are similar to the causative agents suggested by other studies in other populations.—R.S. Stern, M.D.

Skeletal Toxicity With Isotretinoin Therapy: A Clinico-Radiological Evaluation

Carey BM, Parkin GJS, Cunliffe WJ, Pritlove, J (Gen Infirmary, Leeds, England)

Br J Dermatol 119:609–614, November 1988 8–2

Skeletal toxicity occurs with high doses of isotretinoin. The clinical significance and extent of musculoskeletal toxicity associated with lower

Skin Reactions to Drugs, Causative Agents, and Clinical Reactions

Drug	Exanthematous eruption	Fixed drug eruption	Urticaria angioedema	Other reaction types	Positive provoc./Total
Antimicrobial agents.					
Penicillin	–	–	15	1	0/16
Ampicillin/bacampicillin	8	–	1	–	3/9
Amoxicillin	7	–	–	–	1/7
Tetracyclines	–	5	2	–	4/7
(Doxycycline)	–	(3)	(1)	(–)	(2/4)
Erythromycin	2	–	–	–	2/2
Sulphonamides	17	8	–	1	24/26
(Sulphasalazine)	(5)	–	–	(–)	(5/5)
Trimethoprim	11	3	1	–	14/15
Sulpha-trimethoprim	5	1	2	2	1/10
Others*	3	–	–	–	3/3
Antipyretic analgesic drugs					
Phenazone derivatives	1	32	2	1	32/36
Acetylsalicylic acid	–	–	17	–	17/17
Chlormezanone	1	1	–	–	1/2
Oxyphenbutazone	–	–	–	2	0/2
Others †	2	–	1	1	3/4
Drugs acting on the central nervous system					
Barbiturates	–	6	1	–	5/7
Carbamazepine	4	3	–	2	6/9
Phenytoin	2	1	–	1	1/4
Others ‡	–	3	–	–	2/3
Gold sodium thiomalate	–	–	–	15	0/15
Other drugs§	5	1	3	4	9/13
Positive provocation/Total	47/68	51/64	26/45	4/30	128/207

*Metronidazole, nitrofurantoin, and methenamine hippurate.
†Indomethacin, sulindac, tolphenamic acid, and proquazone.
‡Chloralhydrate-phenazone, klopoxide, and tioridazine.
§Allopurinol (2), nifedipine (2), hydroxyzine, kinidine sulfate, methamizole, methoxsalen, tranexamic acid, amiloride-hydrochlorothiazide combination, Disofrol mite R, Toclase esp R, and Urografin R.
(Courtesy of Alanko K, Stubb S, Kauppinen K: *Acta Derm Venereol (Stockh)* 69:223–226, 1989.)

doses of isotretinoin used to treat severe acne were investigated in 120 patients. The received a 4-month course of isotretinoin in oral doses of 0.1–1 mg/kg/day. Radiographs were then obtained.

Twelve percent of the patients had minor changes. Four had spinal hyperostoses, and 10 had calcaneal hyperostoses, but none of these changes was clinically significant. Matched control radiographs showed that 8% of the control group had similar nonsignificant changes. The 11 patients with abnormal radiographic results were followed up: 1 patient had minor deterioration, 4 had no change, and 6 had improvement.

Doses of isotretinoin, 0.5 mg/kg/day, do not lead to any significant long-term musculoskeletal changes. Dermatologists should be aware of the possibility of skeletal toxicity when treating patients with this drug.

▶ The findings of this study are quite reassuring, showing that in acne patients isotretinoin administered orally for 4 months produced no major bony problems (12% incidence vs. 8% in nonacne controls). Moreover, when changes did occur, follow-up radiologic studies revealed either improvement or no further progression in virtually all cases.

It should be noted, however, that the dose of oral isotretinoin in 75% of the patients was 0.5 mg/kg/day or less. For individuals with body weights ranging from 50 to 80 kg (110–175 lb), a dosage of 0.5 mg/kg/day would translate to a dose range of 25–40 mg/day. These amounts are clinically effective in acne, but there is much published information indicating that the most significant factor in acne relapse after successful isotretinoin treatment is the dosage used. So, a question remains whether the probability of the need for more than 1 course of isotretinoin is more (or less) desirable, from the point of view of skeletal toxicity, than a higher dose in the initial course.—P.E. Pochi, M.D.

Skeletal Hyperostosis and Extraosseous Calcification in Patients Receiving Long-Term Etretinate (Tigason)

Wilson DJ, Kay V, Charig M, Hughes DG, Creasy TS (John Radcliffe Hosp, Oxford, England)

Br J Dermatol 119:597–607, November 1988 8–3

The synthetic analogues of vitamin A are widely used to treat skin disorders but are associated with various side effects, especially during long-term use. These effects include skeletal changes, with bone spurring and ossification of ligaments, mimicking diffuse idiopathic skeletal hyperostosis. However, there are conflicting reports on the relationship between total dose and skeletal effects, and the incidence of these effects is unclear.

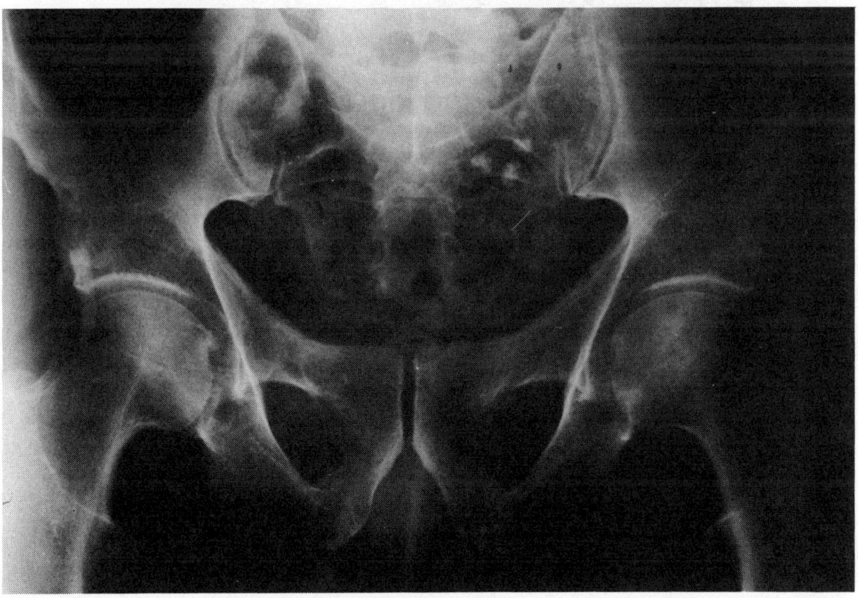

Fig 8–1.—Areas of new bone in the iliopsoas insertions at both lesser trochanters and at the anterior inferior iliac spines. (Courtesy of Wilson DJ, Kay V, Charig M, et al: *Br J Dermatol* 119:597–607, November 1988.)

Neither is there agreement on the best technique for monitoring patients given long-term therapy.

Thirteen patients with a congenital or inherited disorder of keratinization and 10 with psoriasis were receiving long-term etretinate therapy. Skeletal scintigraphy, plain radiographs, and hematologic and biochemical studies were done. Using all criteria, 7 patients in the first diagnostic group had evidence of hyperostosis. No single study was able to detect all of these cases. Results of skeletal scintigraphy were positive for only 9 of the 13 patients with hyperostosis. Eleven patients with hyperostosis had a history of musculoskeletal symptoms, compared with only 3 of the 10 patients without hyperostosis. No clear association with total dose or treatment duration could be found. Serum chemistry and hematologic

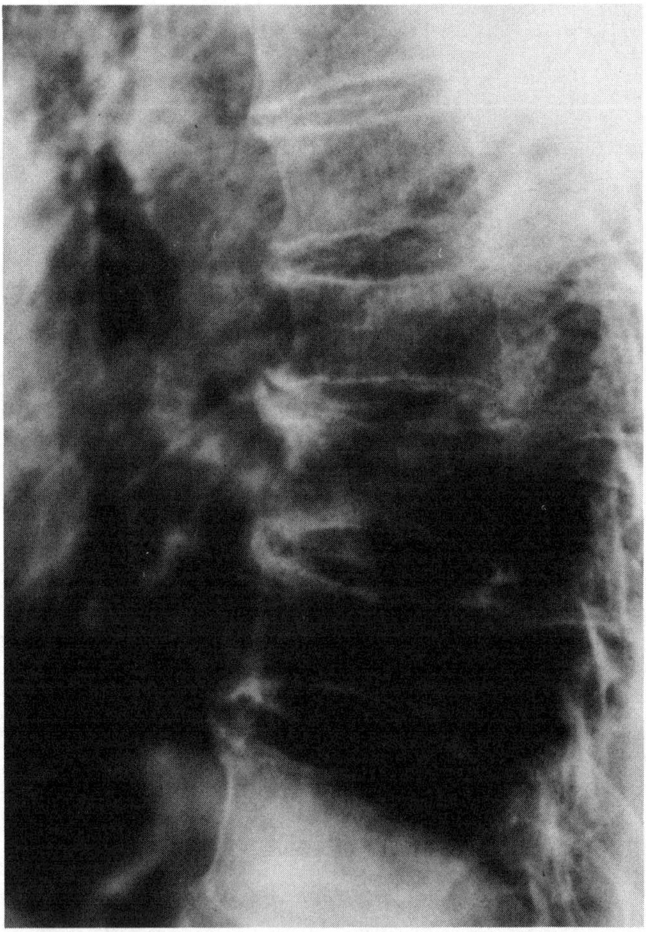

Fig 8–2.—Lateral radiograph of the thoracic spine showing early hyperostosis that might be considered normal in an older patient. (Courtesy of Wilson DJ, Kay V, Charig M, et al: *Br J Dermatol* 119:597–607, November 1988.)

evaluations yielded normal results. In 2 patients the 24-hour urinary calcium excretion was significantly increased, an abnormality not described previously. Annual lateral thoracic spine radiographs with additional views of symptomatic areas were recommended for patients receiving long-term etretinate therapy (Figs 8–1 and 8–2).

Detectable hyperostosis is fairly common among patients given long-term etretinate treatment. It is not known whether these patients will deteriorate, or whether withdrawal of the drug would lead to reversal of the hyperostosis.

▶ The incidence and type of osseous changes caused by etretinate therapy, and how often they are symptomatic, have not been well established despite a large number of published reports. From the results of this study by a group of radiologists in which patients with disorders of keratinization and psoriasis were evaluated retrospectively, the conclusion was reached that hyperostosis is common but that the dose and duration of drug are not causative factors; the latter findings are rather surprising and as likely a reflection of the small numbers of patients studied. The authors could show, however, that scintigraphy was not superior to plain x-ray examination, and their recommendation that annual x-ray studies be performed of the lateral thoracic spine and of other areas where pain is experienced seems reasonable.— P.E. Pochi, M.D.

Beta-Adrenoceptor Antagonist-Induced Psoriasiform Eruption: Clinical and Pathogenetic Aspects

Heng MCY, Heng MK (Univ of California, Los Angeles; VA Med Ctr, Sepulveda, Calif)

Int J Dermatol 27:619–627, November 1988 8–4

Reportedly, certain β-adrenoreceptor blocking drugs can induce a papulosquamous eruption resembling psoriasis. However, at present it is unknown whether the β-blocker-induced eruption is an entity unto itself, or whether these drugs aggravate an existing psoriatic tendency. It is also unclear whether it is β blockade or the drug itself that is responsible for the syndrome. A group of 16 patients given β-adrenoreceptor-blocking agents who had psoriasiform cutaneous eruptions were studied. Nine patients had no past or family history of psoriasis, and 6 had ongoing psoriasis aggravated by β blockers. All patients underwent punch biopsies of involved skin; punch biopsy specimens also were obtained from uninvolved skin in 4 patients in each group. Direct immunofluorescence of the skin was carried out.

Clinically, it appeared that the psoriasiform lesions induced by β blockers were thinner, less scaly, and less erythematous in the drug-induced group than in the drug-aggravated group. The trunk and limbs were usually involved symmetrically, but the face was spared in the group with drug-induced lesions. Palms, soles, and elbows were seldom involved (table). With treatment, the eruption typically subsided within 6 weeks of discontinuation of the β blocker. The group with drug-aggra-

β-Adrenoreceptor Blocker Induced Eruptions—Clinical Data

Patients	Age/Sex	Psoriasis		Beta Blocker	Duration on Drug	Type of Skin Eruption	Time Taken for Rash to Resolve
		P/H	F/H				
1	68/M	–	?	Atenolol*	6 months	Psoriasiform with pustules, generalized	6–8 weeks
2	52/M	–	–	Metoprolol*	4 months	Psoriasiform, generalized, pustules	4–6 weeks
				Atenolol*	2 weeks	Psoriasiform, generalized	4–6 weeks
3	60/M	–	–	Propranolol	33 months	Psoriasiform, generalized	12 weeks
4	69/M	–	–	Propranolol	12 months	Psoriasiform, generalized	6–8 weeks
5	53/M	+	–	Nadolol	12 months	Psoriasis—asymptomatic plaques	Partial resolution
6	66/M	+	+	Nadolol	18 months	Psoriasis—asymptomatic plaques	Partial resolution
7	62/M	+	–	Metoprolol*	6 months	Psoriasis, generalized	Partial resolution
				Atenolol*	4 weeks	Psoriasis—plaques	Partial resolution

8	68/M	–	–	Metoprolol*	12 months	Psoriasiform, with pustules, generalized	6–8 weeks
9	56/M	–	–	Propranolol	9 months	Psoriasiform, generalized	6–8 weeks
10	54/M	–	–	Atenolol*	12 months	Psoriasiform generalized	8–10 weeks
11	64/M	+	–	Propranolol	6 months	Psoriasis—plaques	Partial resolution
12	54/F	–	–	Metoprolol*	6 months	Psoriasiform, with pustules, generalized	12–14 weeks
13	74/M	–	–	Propranolol	12 months	Psoriasiform, generalized	6–8 weeks
14	58/M	+	–	Sotalol	3 months	Psoriasis—asymptomatic plaques	Partial resolution
15	63/M	–	–	Propranolol	9 months	Pustules, itch	4–6 weeks
16	61/M	–	–	Propranolol	9 months	Pustules, itch	4–6 weeks

*β_1-selective.
(Courtesy of Heng MCY, Heng MK: *Int J Dermatol* 27:619–627, November 1988.)

vated lesions had only partial remission after β blocker withdrawal. Skin immunofluorescence did not reveal the presence of antibody or complement deposits. The composition of biopsy specimens of eruptions caused by selective β blockers differed from that caused by nonselective β blockers.

β-Blocker-induced eruptions may result from increased proliferation, motility, and activity of lymphocytes, neutrophils, and cells of the macrophage-Langerhans cell series. This action may stem from depressed intracellular cyclic adenosine monophosphate levels caused by the β blockade.

Cutaneous Adverse Reactions Associated With Calcium Channel Blockers

Stern R, Khalsa JH (Beth Israel Hosp, Boston; Food and Drug Administration, Rockville, Md)

Arch Intern Med 149:829–832, April 1989 8–5

The calcium channel blockers nifedipine, verapamil, and diltiazem are widely used to treat patients with cardiovascular disease. However, there is little information on the frequency and spectrum of cutaneous reactions associated with these agents.

Between 1978 and 1985, the Food and Drug Administration (FDA) and the American Academy of Dermatology's Adverse Drug Reaction Reporting System (ADRRS) received 379 case reports of cutaneous adverse drug reactions associated with these 3 calcium channel blockers. Of these, 146 were associated with nifedipine, 153 with verapamil, and 72 with diltiazem (table). Thus, although the frequency of adverse cutaneous events associated with these drugs is low, severe reactions can occur on occasion. The more serious include toxic epidermal necrolysis associated with diltiazem, Stevens-Johnson syndrome and erythema multiforme with all 3 agents, and exfoliative dermatitis with all 3. Most of the serious reactions have occurred within 2 weeks of initiation of drug therapy. Physicians should be alert to the possibility of cutaneous reactions when calcium channel blockers are given.

Eczema-Like, Erythematous, Infiltrated Plaques: A Common Side Effect of Subcutaneous Heparin Therapy

Klein GF, Kofler H, Wolf H, Fritsch PO (Univ of Innsbruck, Austria)

J Am Acad Dermatol 21:703–707, October 1989 8–6

Studies suggest that erythematous, infiltrated plaques are a common but neglected reaction to heparin treatment. In 14 women and 1 man with heparin intolerance, erythematous, infiltrated plaques developed that resembled contact dermatitis clinically and histologically. The plaques developed within 3–21 days after initiation of subcutaneous heparin treatment. All had received 5,000–7,500 units of heparin 2 or 3 times a day after surgery or for the treatment of prophylaxis of thromboembolic disease.

Cutaneous Adverse Drug Reactions (ADRs) Associated With New Calcium Channel Blockers (Reactions Are Expressed as COSTART* Terms)

Adverse Reactions	Nifedipine	Verapamil	Diltiazem
Acne	0	1	20
Alopecia	21	24	2
Angioedema	3	4	0
Applicate site reaction	4	3	2
Contact dermatitis	0	2	0
Exfoliative dermatitis	11	1	7
Lichen dermatitis	0	1	0
Edema injection site	1	0	0
Eczema	2	0	0
Erythema multiforme	2	2	5
Erythema nodosum	3	0	0
Hair discolor	5	0	0
Hemorrhage injection site	2	0	0
Herpes zoster	0	0	1
Hirsutism	1	1	1
Hypertrophy skin	0	1	0
Hypersensitivity injection site	1	0	0
Inflammatory injection site	1	2	0
Injection site reaction	1	5	0
Nail dystrophy	4	3	1
Necropsy skin	0	0	1
Nodule skin	0	1	0
Pain injection site	0	2	1
Pruritus	27	25	8
Psoriasis	1	0	1
Rash	54	58	24
Lupuslike rash	0	0	1
Rash maculopapular	12	21	8
Rash petechia	0	1	0
Rash purpura	0	1	0
Rash pustular	0	0	1
Rash vesicular bullae	4	0	2
Skin discolor	4	1	0
Skin dry	3	1	0
Stevens-Johnson syndrome	4	6	3
Sweat	6	6	2
Urticaria	22	16	12
Ulcer skin	1	0	0
Total, all ADRs	**190**	**190**	**103**

*COSTART terms are assigned to each case report to facilitate retrieval from the FDA database. Numbers denote the times the event is reported in association with the drug regardless of causality. Case reports received under a generic name of the drug, e.g., nifedipine or its trade name (Procardia), are shown under its generic name.

(Courtesy of Stern R, Khalsa JH: *Arch Intern Med* 149:829–832, April 1989.)

The presence of a delayed hypersensitivity reaction was suggested by the clinical appearance, routine histopathologic and immunohistopathologic findings, and results of various skin tests. Subcutaneous provocation tests were superior to intracutaneous or epicutaneous tests in establishing the diagnosis of erythematous, infiltrated plaques. The plaques were caused by heparin constituents in all of the women; in the man, chlorocresol was implicated.

Erythematous, infiltrated plaques are not often diagnosed as a cutaneous reaction to heparin. However, they may occur in reaction to such treatment much more often than previously believed. Neither epicutaneous nor intracutaneous testing is suitable for the diagnosis of heparin sensitivity reaction underlying erythematous, infiltrated plaques. However, subcutaneous provocation is reliable. Low-molecular-weight heparin analogues cannot be universally recommended as a substitute; 3 of the 6 patients in the series tested had reactions to at least 1 low-molecular-weight heparin analogue.

Anaphlactic Symptoms Due to Chlorhexidine Gluconate

Okano M, Nomura M, Hata S, Okada N, Sato K, Kitano Y, Tashiro M, Yoshimoto Y, Hama R, Aoki T (Osaka Univ; Han-nanchuo Hosp; Habikino Hosp of Osaka, Japan)

Arch Dermatol 125:50–52, January 1989 8–7

Chlorhexidine gluconate, or Hibitane, has been widely used as a medical disinfectant. Although it is thought to be safe, there have been several previous reports of adverse reactions to the agent. Six patients had adverse, life-threatening anaphylactic reactions to this disinfectant.

Boy, 15 years, was seen with a forehead wound. The injury was disinfected with 0.5% chlorhexidine gluconate, injected with 1% lidocaine, and stitched. Just after treatment, coughing, dyspnea, wheezing, cyanosis, facial urticaria, and edema of the palpebral conjunctiva developed in the patient. The dyspnea vanished 1 hour after emergency treatment, which included an intramuscular injection of epinephrine and an intravenous injection of hydrocortisone. However, the urticaria persisted for several hours. The next day, scratch tests with 0.02% chlorhexidine gluconate and 0.05% lidocaine were done. Only chlorhexidine gluconate produced a positive reaction in 15 minutes.

In all 6 cases, chlorhexidine gluconate was confirmed as the causative agent of type I hypersensitivity by intradermal, scratch, and epicutaneous tests. It is important to use chlorhexidine gluconate on wound surfaces in a concentration of 0.05%, as recommended by the manufacturer, to prevent life-threatening adverse reactions. Chlorhexidine gluconate may not be suitable for use on mucous membranes.

▶ An important but, we hope, rare hypersensitivity reaction to Hibiclens, an agent that we use so often.—R.S. Stern, M.D.

Protracted Systemic Illness and Interstitial Nephritis Due to Minocycline
Wilkinson SP, Stewart WK, Spiers EM, Pears J (Ninewells Hosp and Med School, Dundee, Scotland)
Postgrad Med J 65:53–56, January 1989 8–8

Tetracycline therapy can aggravate azotemic renal failure through an antianabolic action, but acute interstitial nephritis with this class of antibiotics is unusual. A prolonged hypersensitivity-like illness occurred after minocycline therapy in 1 patient.

Boy, 16 years, was given minocycline, 50 mg twice weekly, for sycosis barbae and acne vulgaris. Malaise and rigors developed 2 weeks later. A morbilliform rash developed on his face, neck, and upper trunk, and he vomited twice. After 3 days the boy was hospitalized with suspected glandular fever. Acute renal failure was diagnosed, and hemodialysis and steroid therapy were begun. His illness remitted but recurred after steroid withdrawal. After further steroid treatment, the patient recovered completely. Lymphocyte function tests, done in an attempt to positively incriminate minocycline, were inconclusive because of a general suppression of the patient's lymphocytes to in vitro stimulation.

Hypersensitivity reactions previously attributed to minocycline include skin rashes, lymphadenopathy, and, in 1 case, acute interstitial nephritis.

▶ Another case of a peculiar hypersensitivity syndrome apparently seen with minocycline but not to my knowledge observed with tetracycline. In this case, in addition to the usual fever, malaise, rash, and lymphadenopathy that usually occur in this syndrome, the patient also had acute nephritis.—R.S. Stern, M.D.

Camphor Ingestion
Gibson DE, Moore GP, Pfaff JA (Madigan Army Med Ctr, Tacoma, Wash; Darnall Army Community Hosp, Fort Hood, Tex; Womack Army Community Hosp, Fort Bragg, NC)
Am J Emerg Med 7:41–43, January 1989 8–9

Camphor is an ingredient in many widely available, over-the-counter products. It is rated as a class 4 (very toxic) agent but is usually not distributed in child-proof packaging. Often used as a liniment, camphor is noted for its characteristic odor.

Boy, 2 years, with canker sores, accidentally swallowed about 9.5 mL of Camphophenique (10.8% camphor). He was taken immediately to the emergency department but experienced a tonic-clonic seizure en route. At admission, he had the odor of mothballs on his breath. Treatment with orogastric lavage followed by instillation of activated charcoal was given; phenobarbital was given intravenously for 24 hours and then orally after apparently full recovery and discharge.

In 1985, 1,173 patients (mostly young children) with camphor poisoning were treated in the United States. Toxicity manifests rapidly, within 5–90 minutes after ingestion, and causes feelings of warmth followed by nausea, epigastric burning, and often vomiting. These symptoms are followed by muscular excitability with twitching and can lead to confusion and seizures, with delirium, coma, apnea, and asystole possible. Quick treatment is crucial to successful management, but induced emesis should be avoided; no antidote is known. The most effective management of camphor poisoning would be removal of the substance from over-the-counter medications.

▶ A nice review of the toxicity of camphor after oral ingestion. The authors point out that phenobarbital is the treatment of choice because it not only helps to prevent seizures but also has been shown to decrease neural damage in experimental animals. It also induces enzymes that metabolize camphor. As camphor is of very questionable, if any, therapeutic value, we should think seriously of supporting its removal from over-the-counter preparations.—R. Masters, M.D.

9 Fungal Infections

Sulconazole Nitrate 1% Cream in the Treatment of Chronic Moccasin-Type Tinea Pedis Caused by *Trichophyton rubrum*

Akers WA, Lane A, Lynfield Y, Greenberg J, Hall J, Mangan C, Tinker A (Syntex Research, Palo Alto; Univ of Rochester, NY; Veterans Hosp, Brooklyn; San Rafael, Calif; Greensboro, NC)

J Am Acad Dermatol 21:686–689, October 1989 9–1

Sulconazole nitrate is a synthetic imidazole derivative that is effective in treating patients with tinea pedis and other dermatomycoses. One percent sulconazole nitrate cream was compared with its vehicle in the treatment of chronic moccasin-type tinea pedis caused by *Trichophyton rubrum*. The series included 229 patients, in all of whom chronic moccasin-type tinea pedis was confirmed by positive results of a potassium hydroxide preparation. Of the 131 patients with positive dermatophyte cultures, *T. rubrum* was identified in 121. By random assignment 119 of the patients were given sulconazole and 110 were given the vehicle. Patients were treated twice daily for 4 weeks and then for 2 more weeks if needed.

Sulconazole cream was significantly more effective than the vehicle in patients with chronic *T. rubrum* tinea pedis. Overall, 57% of sulconazole-treated patients, but only 13% of vehicle-treated patients, were cured. Two-week relapse rates were also significantly lower in patients given active treatment. The 103 patients with moccasin-type tinea pedis but with cultures negative for *T. rubrum* had comparable results.

One percent sulconazole nitrate cream applied twice a day is significantly more effective than its vehicle in producing clinical and mycologic clearing in patients with and without culture-proved *T. rubrum* infection. Some patients may need more than 4 weeks of therapy for optimal results.

▶ This comparison study of twice-daily applied 1% sulconazole nitrate cream vs. the vehicle cream in treatment of moccasin-type tinea pedis reports that sulconazole is more effective. Results of future studies comparing sulconazole cream with other topical antifungals such naftifine, which is effective when applied only once daily, will be of interest.—R.A. Johnson, M.D.

Double-Blind Randomized Comparative Study of Naftifine Cream and Clotrimazole Cream in the Treatment of Dermatophytosis

El Darouti MA, Al Raubaie S, Shandrashekhar CR, Al Sawaf MH, Movahadi GA (Rashid Hosp; Sief Hosp, Ras al Khaimah, United Arab Emirates)

Int J Dermatol 28:345–346, June 1989 9–2

Naftifine is a new antifungal allylamine-derivative intended for use against dermatophytes, yeasts, and molds. The efficacy of naftifine in the treatment of dermatophytosis was compared with clotrimazole in a double-blind trial. Seventy-six patients with dermatophytosis were randomly assigned to apply 1% naftifine cream once daily or 1% clotrimazole twice daily. Clinical and mycologic healing and tolerability were monitored 1, 2, and 4 weeks after treatment began.

Overall, naftifine proved superior to clotrimazole. After 4 weeks, cultures were negative in 92% of the naftifine-treated group compared with 78% of the clotrimazole-treated group. Clinical symptoms disappeared in 90% of those given naftifine and in 74% of those given clotrimazole. Side effects were minimal. In addition to the superiority of naftifine cream in treating dermatophytosis, the compliance factor with once-daily application favors this drug.

▶ Naftifine, along with terbinafine, are fungistatic allylamine derivatives that inhibit squalene epoxidase, resulting in decreased ergosterol production. Previous clinical studies found naftifine to be as effective against yeast as clotrimazole, effective in a gel preparation against onychomycosis, and as effective as gentamycin in bacterial pyodermas. Compared with clotrimazole, the higher cure rates, both clinical and mycologic, as well as the once-daily application rate vs. twice daily, of naftifine make this new topical antifungal very attractive.—R.A. Johnson, M.D.

Dermatophyte Onychomycosis in Children

Philpot CM, Shuttleworth D (Univ Hosp of Wales, Cardiff)

Clin Exp Dermatol 14:203–205, May 1989 9–3

Unlike in adults, fungal infections of the nail plate are uncommon in children. The prevalence of dermatophyte onychomycosis was determined in 494 children aged 5–10 years and 200 children aged 3–12 years attending a pediatric medical outpatient clinic. In addition, data on fungal nail infections diagnosed from 1984 to 1987 in children younger than 12 years were reviewed.

Only 1 fungal infection of the nail plate was found, and culture grew *Trichophyton rubrum*. The prevalence of fungal nail infection was 0.2%. A parent of the affected child also had *T. rubrum* infection of the toe nails. Seven fungal infections of the toe nails were reported in a 3-year period in children younger than 12 years. Culture of the nail was positive in 6 and grew *T. rubrum*. At least 1 parent of 4 of these children had dermatophyte onychomycosis, and all specimen cultures grew *T. rubrum.*

Dermatophyte onychomycosis is uncommon in children and, when present, a parental source should be suspected and sought. The low infectivity of dermatophyte onychomycosis in children may result from differences in nail plate structure or lack of cumulative trauma and increased growth rate of nails, thus preventing colonization by a "washout" effect.

▶ A prevalence of only 0.2% of onychomycosis in children is certainly consistent with our experience as dermatologists. When onychomycosis is present in children, a parental source of infection is likely. The low prevalence of onychomycosis in children is in contrast with predilection of tinea capitis for children. The reason for the low prevalence is unclear.—R.A. Johnson, M.D.

Tinea Nigra Palmaris and Plantaris: A Black Fungus Producing Black Spots on the Palms and Soles

Palmer SR, Bass JW, Mandojana R, Wittler RR (Tripler Army Med Ctr, Honolulu)

Pediatr Infect Dis J 8:48–50, January 1989 9–4

The relationship between sun exposure and skin cancer has been widely publicized. Tinea nigra palmaris and plantaris is a rare, benign

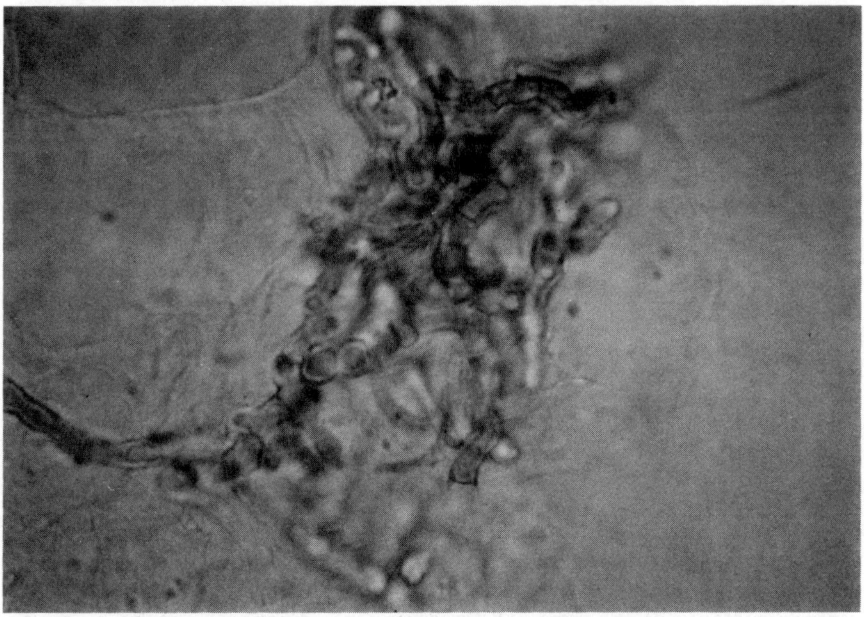

Fig 9–1.—Photomicrograph of skin scrapings from palmar lesion showing pigmented branching septate hyphae. Potassium hydroxide preparation; original magnification, ×1,000. (Courtesy of Palmer SR, Bass JW, Mandojana R, et al: *Pediatr Infect Dis J* 8:48–50, January 1989.)

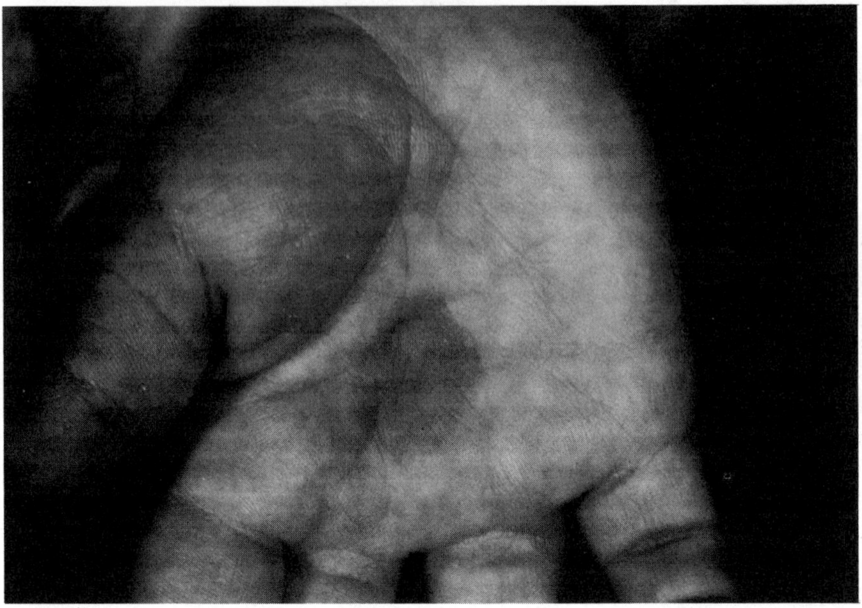

Fig 9–2.—Pigmented skin lesion on palm of the right hand. (Courtesy of Palmer SR, Bass JW, Mandojana R, et al: *Pediatr Infect Dis J* 8:48–50, January 1989.)

fungal infection that could be confused with cancers such as malignant melanoma or pigmented junctional nevi. Such confusions could lead to unnecessary and expensive invasive diagnostic procedures.

Boy, 9 years, had a slowly enlarging dark spot on the skin of the instep of his right foot. The lesion was flat with an irregular border and uneven pigmentation ranging from dark brown to black. It measured 2 × 2.5 cm. No vesicles, erythema, scales, or desquamation at the outer edge or central clearing were noted. The lesion was neither tender nor pruritic. It tended to clear when superficial layers of skin were scraped off. Microscopic evaluation of scrapings revealed numerous light brown to dark green branching septate hyphae (Fig 9–1). Laboratory testing identified the organism as *Phaeoannellomyces werneckii*. The lesion disappeared after several days of treatment with half-strength Whitfield's ointment 4 times daily.

Findings were similar in 2 other patients with palmar lesions. One had an oval-shaped lesion 2.5 × 3.0 cm having a sharply defined border but no erythema, vesicles, scaling, or central clearing (Fig 9–2). Treatment with clotrimazole or ketoconazole resulted in cure of both patients.

Tinea nigra usually is found on the palmar surfaces of the hand or the plantar surfaces of the foot. The presumptive diagnosis can be made by direct microscopic examination of skin scrapings prepared with 10% potassium hydroxide. Clinicians should consider tinea nigra in children with any enlarging hyperpigmented macular lesion, especially when lesions are found on the hand or foot.

▶ Tinea nigra is of interest because of possible confusion with a pigmented melanocytic lesion occurring on the palm or sole. It is unlikely than many pediatricians, internists, or surgeons are cognizant of this superficial mycosis. If a unfortunate patient with tinea nigra encounters an aggressive surgeon, the consequence might be an unnecessary biopsy or excision.—R.A. Johnson, M.D.

Sporotrichoid Pyogenic Bacterial Infection

Tanaka S, Mochizuki T, Watanabe S (Shiga Univ of Med Science, Otsu, Japan)
Dermatologica 178:228–230, 1989 9–5

Various organisms can cause lymphocutaneous sporotrichoid infection; similarly, various etiologic agents have induced sporotrichosis-like lesions. Pyogenic bacterial infection, which at first resembled lymphocutaneous sporotrichosis, was diagnosed in 2 patients.

Case 1.—Man, 43, injured his right thumb. Wound healing was slow, and new lesions having a sporotrichoid pattern developed along his forearm. Four nodules in linear distribution with erosion and ulcers were noted 75 days after the injury (Fig 9–3). No subjective or systemic symptoms were present. Cultured biopsy specimens from a nonulcerated lesion of the wrist were positive for *Staphylococcus aureus* and *Streptococcus* group A. The nodules disappeared after 10 days of treatment with orally administered cefaclor, 1,000 mg daily.

Case 2.—Man, 68, had a similar linear distribution of nodules on the hand and forearm. This patient had previously had diffuse normolipidemic plane xanthoma. Histologic examination of a biopsy specimen revealed gram-positive

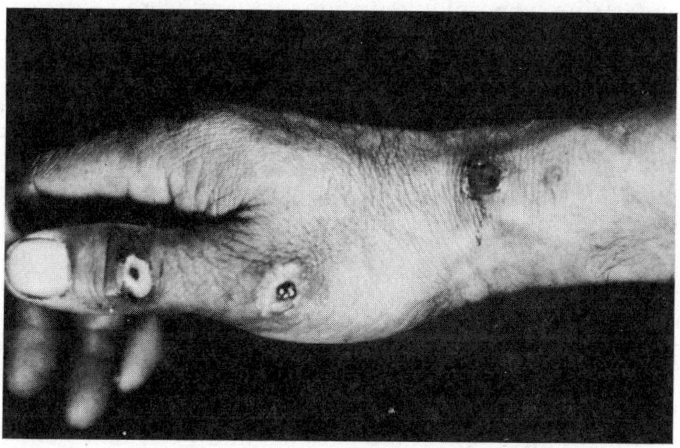

Fig 9–3.—Right hand of patient showing sporotrichoid pattern of lesions. (Courtesy of Tanaka S, Mochizuki T, Watanabe S: *Dermatologica* 178:228–230, 1989.)

cocci, and *S. aureus* was grown in culture. Cefaclor also brought dramatic improvement in this case.

This clinical picture rarely results from pyogenic bacteria. But when patients have cutaneous lesions resembling lymphocutaneous sporotrichosis but negative results of standard sporotrichin skin tests, the possibility of common pyogenic bacteria should be explored.

▶ Sporotrichoid infections are characterized by nodular lesions of the cutaneous and subcutaneous tissues and adjacent lymphatics that suppurate, ulcerate, and drain, and are acquired by traumatic inoculation into the skin. The infectious agents that we associate with this clinical syndrome are *Sporotrix schenkii, Mycobacterium marinum, Francisella tularensis, Nocardia brasiliensis, Bacillus anthracis, Pseudoallescheria boydii,* and *Leishmania tropica.* In that *S. aureus* was cultured from biopsy specimens in both cases, as well as group A β-hemolytic. *Streptococcus pyogenes* in 1 case, that neither mycobacterium nor fungus was isolated on culture, and that the lesions cleared within 10 days of treatment with cefaclor, makes it hard to refute that *S. aureus* should be added to this list of infectious agents causing sporotrichoid lesions.—R.A. Johnson, M.D.

Cutaneous *Rhizopus* and *Aspergillus* Infections in Five Patients With Cancer

Khardori N, Hayat S, Rolston K, Bodey GP (Univ of Texas MD Anderson Cancer Ctr, Houston)

Arch Dermatol 125:952–956, July 1989 9–6

Primary skin infection can produce localized or disseminated disease in immunocompromised patients. Primary cutaneous infection with *Aspergillus* species and *Rhizopus* species occurred in 5 patients, all of whom had an underlying hematologic malignancy and were neutropenic (table). All were receiving broad-spectrum antibiotics at the time of appearance of the skin lesions, and 3 were receiving corticosteroids.

In all 5 patients characteristic skin lesions developed as a result of skin trauma caused by intravenous catheter insertion in 4 and maceration after a sweat rash in the lower back in the fifth patient. The lesions started as erythematous macules that became purpuric and eventually developed into hemorrhagic ulcers with eschar formation (Fig 9–4). The diagnosis was confirmed in each case with histopathologic studies and culture of skin biopsy specimens. Cultures grew *Aspergillus* species in 3 and *Rhizopus* species in 2.

All patients were treated with amphotericin B. Three responded to antifungal therapy and local care without surgical débridement; in 2 of these patients granulocyte recovery was noted. Two patients died of disseminated fungal infection; these patients had persistent neutropenia.

Patients with hematologic malignancies are at risk of contracting opportunistic fungal infections in areas of skin trauma that can disseminate

Clinical Characteristics of Patients With Primary Opportunistic Cutaneous Fungal Infections

Patient/ Age, y/Sex	Underlying Malignancy	Signs and Symptoms	Site	Organism	Therapy	Neutropenic/ Recovery	Dissemination	Outcome
1/30/F	Chronic myelogenous leukemia in blast crisis	Fever, eschar on anterior part of L forearm	IV site	*Aspergillus* species	Amphotericin B, 1.5 g; WBC transfusion	Yes/yes	No	Improved
2/52/F	Acute myelogenous leukemia	Fever, eschar on R forearm	IV site	*Rhizopus* species	Amphotericin B, 1.2 g; rifampin	Yes/no	No	Improved
3/20/F	Aplastic anemia	Fever, nodular lesion on R forearm	IV site	*Rhizopus* species	Amphotericin B, 0.5 g	Yes/no	Probable	Died
4/52/M	Multiple myeloma	Fever, erythematous skin lesion with ulceration and eschar	IV site	*Aspergillus* species	Amphotericin B, 1 g	Yes/yes	No	Improved
5/58/M	Acute myelogenous leukemia	Fever, erythematous papular lesion with central necrosis and eschar formation	Lower part of back	*Aspergillus* species	Amphotericin B, 1.8 g	Yes/no	Yes	Died

Abbreviations: IV, intravenous; *WBC,* white blood cell.
(Courtesy of Khardori N, Hayat S, Rolston K, et al: *Arch Dermatol* 125:952–956, July 1989.)

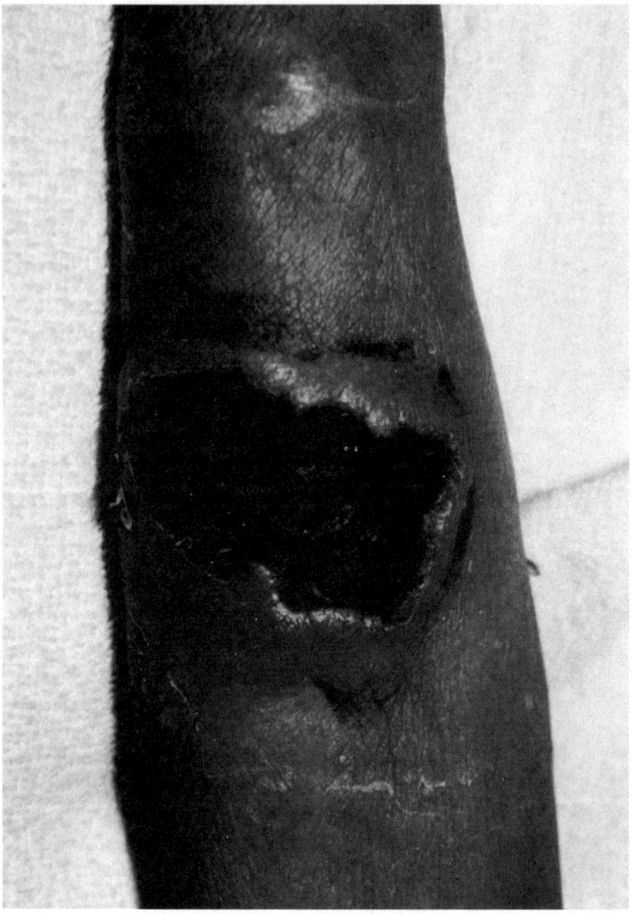

Fig 9–4.—Anterior part of right forearm shows large hemorrhagic, necrotic ulcer around insertion site of intravenous catheter. (Courtesy of Khardori N, Hayat S, Rolston K, et al: *Arch Dermatol* 125:952–956, July 1989.)

in the presence of persistent neutropenia. The development of these fungal infections may be associated with the moist and humid conditions created by occlusive dressings or excessive perspiration.

▶ *Aspergillus* and *Rhizopus* are molds present ubiquitously in our environment. As with the majority of other deep fungal infections, the most common clinical presentation of infection in the immunocompromised host is a primary pulmonary site, with secondary hematogenous dissemination to distant sites. These 5 cases of primary cutaneous infection by *Aspergillus* and *Rhizopus* are distinctly unusual in that the primary infection occurred at the site of an intravenous line in 4 patients and in macerated skin in the other. Two patients in this series died, 1 without autopsy and the other of documented disseminated angioinvasive aspergillosis.

Of interest during the past few years are the reports of *Malassezia furfur*

(Pityrosporum orbiculare) fungemia in neonates and adults as a complication of hyperalimentation (1–3). Major risk factors for these patients were prolonged hospitalization, presence of central venous catheters, and the use of fat emulsions. Given the right circumstances, even our resident follicular fungus can be invasive.—R.A. Johnson, M.D.

References

1. Danker WM, et al: *Rev Infect Dis* 9:743, 1987.
2. Mickelsen PA, et al: *J Infect Dis* 157:1163, 1988.
3. Wurtz RM, Knospe WN: *Ann Intern Med* 109:432, 1988.

Secondary Cutaneous Cryptococcosis: Case Report and Review of 22 Cases

Barfield L, Iacobelli D, Hashimoto K (Wayne State Univ, Detroit)
J Cutan Pathol 15:385–392, December 1988 9–7

Secondary cutaneous cryptococcosis has a multitude of presentations. Because these lesions can mimic a variety of other diseases, a high index of suspicion and histologic confirmation are needed for accurate diagnosis. Secondary cutaneous cryptococcosis presenting as abdominal wall ulcerations occurred in an immunosuppressed patient.

Man, 51, had a 2-day history of dizziness and blurred vision. Adenocarcinoma in both lungs had been treated palliatively with radiotherapy 3 years later. After

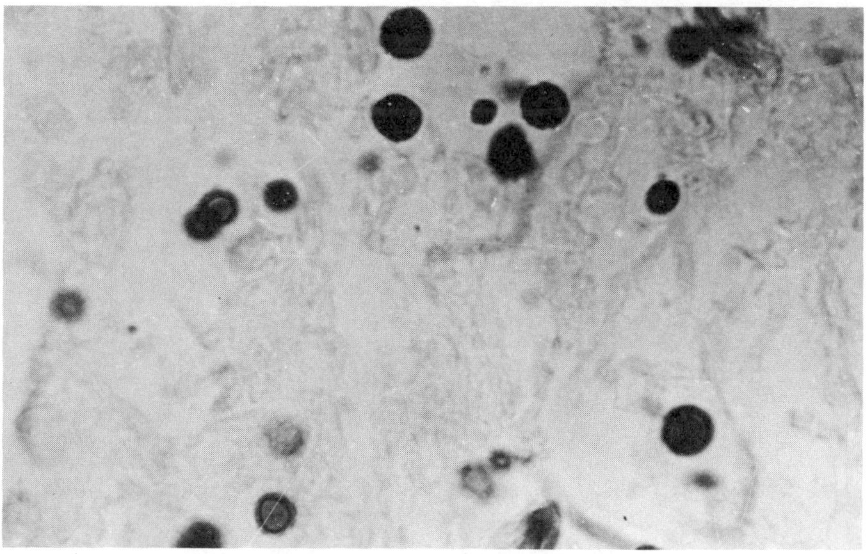

Fig 9–5.—Methenamine silver stain identifies organisms in the lesion as black dots; however, it masks details except for occasional cells, which were sectioned and oriented properly. It also stains small fragments and shadows of degenerated cell wall (×700). (Courtesy of Barfield L, Iacobelli D, Hashimoto K: *J Cutan Pathol* 15:385–392, December 1988.)

Summary of 23 Patients With Secondary Cutaneous Cryptococcosis

	Age	Sex	Race	Underlying Disease	Immunosup. Therapy	Additional Organ Involvement	Location of Skin Involvement	Type of Skin Involvement	Therapy	Outcome	Confirmation of Diagnosis	Reference
1	51	M	W	CA lung	steroids	CNS	abdomen	ulcers	ampho B 5–FC	died	biopsy ulcer	
2	31	M	W	AIDS	none	CNS	lip	herpetiform vesicles	ampho B 5–FC	survive	tzanck & culture	2
3	29	M	B	AIDS	none	CNS, liver bone marrow, lungs, kidneys	face & neck	white papules	ampho B 5–FC	died	biopsy & culture	6
4	33	M	W	ulcerative colitis	steroids		legs, arms, abdomen, shoulder, chest	pyoderma gangrenosum-like ulcers	ampho B 5–FC	died	biopsy & culture	8
5	31	F	W	nephrotic syndrome	steroids azathioprine	CNS	legs, thighs, wrist, forearm	ulcers, abscesses subcutaneous nodules, cellulitis	IV miconazole ampho B 5–FC	survive	biopsy & culture	4
6	40	M		renal transplant	steroids azathioprine cyclophosphamide	CNS	thigh	cellulitis	ampho B 5–FC	survive	culture aspirate, India ink of aspirate	9

7	62	F	W	chronic active hepatitis	steroids azathioprine	lungs CNS	thigh	cellu-litis	ampho B 5–FC	died	biopsy & culture	10
8	46	M		renal transplant	steroids azathioprine cyclophos-phamide	CNS	ankle abdominal wall	cellu-litis	ampho B 5-FC	survive	culture aspirate	9
9		M		lymphoma	chemo-therapy radiation	CNS lungs, renal	neck, anterior chest	palpable purpura	ampho B	died	biopsy	11
10	38	M	W	lymphoma	steroids	none mentioned	back, face	ulcer	ampho B	died	biopsy	12
11	31	M	W	none	none	liver	chest, forehead	subcu-taneous nodule	sulfadiazine hydroxystil-bomide, ise-thionate, ampho B	survive	biopsy & culture	12
12	59	M	W	not mentioned	none	bone marrow prostate, CNS, lung	pinna of ear	ulcer	ampho B	died	biopsy & culture	12
13	49	F	W	not mentioned	not mentioned	lung, CNS	forehead	subcuta-neous nodule	ampho B	survive	biopsy & culture	12

(Continued)

Table (*continued*)

	Age	Sex	Race	Underlying Disease	Immunosup. Therapy	Additional Organ Involvement	Location of Skin Involvement	Type of Skin Involvement	Therapy	Outcome	Confirmation of Diagnosis	Reference
14	35	M	W	cervical medullary tumor	radiation steroids	lung	thigh	cellulitis	ampho B 5–FC	survive	biopsy	13
15	74	M		chronic lymphocytic leukemia	radiation steroids	none	calves	vesiculobullous	topical ampho B	died	biopsy, tzanck, culture, India ink of culture	3
16	48	F		SLE renal failure	steroids azathioprine cyclophosphamide	lung, pleura cecum	arm, foot, vulva	vesiculobullous	ampho B 5–FC	died	India ink of vesicular fluid, tzanck	3
17	65	F		multiple myeloma	steroids, melphalan	inconclusive	finger	ulcer, vesicles	ampho B	survive	bioposy, culture vesicle	3
18	35	F		SLE	steroids cyclophosphamide	CNS bone marrow	antecubital fossa	cellulitis	ampho B	died	culture of aspirate	3

19	17	M		SLE, auto-immune hemo-lytic anemia	steroids azathioprine cyclophos-phamide	CNS	thigh	cellu-litis	ampho B 5–FC	survive	biopsy, India ink of needle aspirate	3
20	33	M		sarcoid	steroids	CNS	scalp, chest wall	ulcer	ampho B 5–FC	survive	culture	1
21	44	M		renal transplant	steroids azathioprine	none	thigh, groin	cellu-litis	ampho B	died	culture aspirate India ink of aspirate	14
22	33	M	W	renal transplant	steroids	blood, renal	thigh	cellu-litis	ampho B	died	culture	5
23	21	F	B	SLE	steroids	blood, CNS	abdominal wall	ulceration of striae	5–FC ampho B	survive	biopsy	5

(Courtesy of Barfield L, Iacobelli D, Hashimoto K: *J Cutan Pathol* 15:385–392, December 1988.)

2 masses in the cerebellar hemispheres were discovered, the patient was given whole brain irradiation and dexamethasone; maintenance treatment was with steroids. Physical examination at the patient's latest admission showed a distended abdomen with marked striae distensae. Cryptococcal meningitis, suspected because of the clinical symptoms, was confirmed by high titered CSF cryptococcal antigen. Amphotericin B and 5-fluorocytosine treatment was begun. However, abdominal wall ulcers developed that were unresponsive to 2 weeks of conservative treatment. These multiple ulcerations were 1–10 cm in diameter, with discrete margins; sanguinous and purulent material exuded from the margins and center of the lesions. The ulcerations extended to the subcutaneous fat and were nontender. Deep underlying vessels of medium sizes were uninvolved. A culture grew mucoid colonies identified as *Cryptococcus neoformans*. Light microscopy studies were done (Fig 9–5). The patient died without any improvement in the cutaneous lesions.

In this case, biopsy of the ulcer margin was needed for the diagnosis of cutaneous cryptococcosis. Because many opportunistic organisms can present with nonspecific cutaneous lesions, these infections must be ruled out by tissue diagnosis in all immunosuppressed patients. An additional 22 cases have been reported (table, pp 130–133).

▶ The patient reported above was immunosuppressed as a result of 3 years of oral corticosteroid therapy and secondary cutaneous cryptococcosis. Other disease states altering the immune status and predisposing to disseminated infection include lymphoreticular malignancies, diabetes mellitus, connective tissue disease, hepatitis, alveolar proteinosis, sarcoidosis, renal transplantation, renal failure, and HIV infection. During the past decade the incidence of secondary cutaneous cryptococcosis has markedly increased, associated with the immunodeficiency of HIV disease. Cryptococcal disease accounts for approximately 5% to 8% of all opportunistic infection in HIV-infected individuals; 10% of patients with cryptococcal disease experience hematogenous dissemination to the skin. The most common presentation of secondary cutaneous cryptococcosis in patients with AIDS is multiple molluscum contagiosum-like lesions, erupting on the face, scalp, and neck. These papules and nodules may become crusted or ulcerate; they are usually 3 mm to 6 mm in size, but may reach 1 cm in diameter. Patients may appear to be in relatively little distress, or may be obtunded with meningitis.

Fluconazole has just been released for treatment of cryptococcal meningitis and is given at a daily dose of 200–400 mg. In that cryptococcosis is never regarded as cured in the HIV-infected patient, fluconazole may be administered as chronic prophylaxis as well as for treatment of meningitis.—R.A. Johnson, M.D.

Infantile Seborrhoeic Dermatitis and *Pityrosporum ovale*

Broberg A, Faergemann J (Univ of Gothenburg; Sahlgren's Hosp, Gothenburg, Sweden)

Br J Dermatol 120:359–362, March 1989 9–8

The cause of infantile seborrheic dermatitis (ISD) is unknown, but an allergic reaction to *Candida albicans* antigen has been suggested. *Pityrosporum ovale* is a saprophytic organism commonly found in healthy adults but not in healthy children. However, *P. ovale* has been implicated in various skin diseases. Its role in the cause of ISD was investigated in 20 infants aged 4–16 weeks with clinical evidence of ISD and 20 healthy infants aged 3–12 weeks. Samples were taken from the skin of the forehead or temporal area. All specimens were studied directly under the microscope. Cultures for bacteria, *P. ovale*, and other fungi were also obtained.

Pityrosporum ovale was cultured from 18 infants with ISD but from only 4 control infants. *Staphylococcus aureus* was cultured from 14 infants with ISD but from only 1 control infant. These findings suggest that *P. ovale* is the etiologic agent of ISD. However, the sample was small, and further studies are needed to clarify the role of *P. ovale* in ISD. The role of *S. aureus* in ISD is also not known, but it could be a secondary invader.

▶ Do you remember when we used to take college exams to test whether we knew how to prove cause and effect scientifically? If 2 statements were true concerning an occurrence, it was left to us to decide if causality was proven. If not, the answer was true-true, unrelated. I think that is where the results of this paper are. Whether the organisms cause the seborrhea or are just commensals on scaly skin has not been proved.—J.C. Alper, M.D.

Association of *Pityrosporum orbiculare (Malassezia furfur)* With Seborrheic Dermatitis in Patients With Acquired Immunodeficiency Syndrome (AIDS)

Groisser D, Bottone EJ, Lebwohl M (Mt Sinai Hosp and Med Ctr, New York)
J Am Acad Dermatol 20:770–773, May 1989 9–9

The possible causative role of the yeastlike fungus *Pityrosporum orbiculare* in the pathogenesis of seborrheic dermatitis in patients with and without AIDS is still debated. The association of *P. orbiculare* with seborrheic dermatitis was investigated in 10 patients with AIDS by analyzing the patients' skin scrapings.

In each of the 9 men and 1 woman a correlation was established between severity of the clinical presentation and number of *Pityrosporum* organisms observed on Giemsa-stained smears. Yeast cells ranged from 3 to 10 per keratinocyte and were numerous throughout the smear. Small numbers often were seen in areas of slight scaling. Skin scrapings from uninvolved areas had 0–1 yeast cell per keratinocyte. *Pityrosporum* organisms were cultured readily from the skin scrapings. Microscopic assessment of colonies rarely demonstrated budding yeast cells with rudimentary hyphae. Two patients with overt seborrheic dermatitis were treated for 2 weeks with 2% topical ketoconazole, with rapid clearing and a drastic decrease resulting in the number of *Pityrosporum* cells per keratinocyte.

On the basis of a quantitative correlation between the numbers of yeast cells adherent to and extruded from keratinocytes and the clinical severity of seborrheic dermatitis, an association, if not a causative role, between *Pityrosporum* and seborrheic dermatitis in HIV-infected patients was strongly suggested. The marked clinical response of 2 patients to ketoconazole, with a concomitant reduction in the number of *Pityrosporum* cells per keratinocyte, further strengthens the evidence for this association.

▶ *Pityrosporum orbiculare* and *Pityrosporum ovale* appear to be 2 morphologically distinct species of lipophilic yeast; there is evidence, however, that the spherical and the ovoid types are only different morphological forms of the same yeast. Normally, *Pityrosporum* colonizes the skin, in greatest density on the scalp, upper trunk, and flexures. *Pityrosporum* is known to cause tinea versicolor and *Pityrosporum* folliculitis. Its role in the pathogenesis of seborrheic dermatitis occurring in normal hosts and HIV-infected individuals is less clear, however. In 1 study (1) comparing HIV-seropositive and HIV-seronegative homosexual men, the mean number of *P. ovale* per cm^2, the mean serum antibody titers against this yeast, and the occurrence of cutaneous disorders did not differ significantly between the 2 study groups. It does seem clear, however, that some patients with seborrheic dermatitis do respond to ketoconazole, administered either orally or topically.—R.A. Johnson, M.D.

Reference

1. Håkansson C, et al: *Acta Derm Venereol (Stockh)* 68:422, 1988.

Seborrhoeic Dermatitis and *Pityrosporum ovale:* A Cultural and Immunological Study

Bergbrant I-M, Faergemann J (Univ of Gothenburg; Sahlgren's Hosp, Gothenburg, Sweden)

Acta Derm Venereol [Stockh] 69:332–335, 1989 9–10

The role of *Pityrosporum ovale* in seborrheic dermatitis is not clear, although a connection between the organism and the disease is recognized. This association was explored in 30 patients with seborrheic dermatitis through quantitative culture for *P. ovale* from skin and scalp lesions and normal skin, serum IgG antibody titers against the organism, and lipid measurements. Results were compared with those from 60 healthy controls.

No significant difference was noted between numbers of organisms in clear skin and numbers in skin or scalp lesions in the patients. Fewer organisms were found in the normal skin of patients than in the skin from controls. Skin lesions in patients and skin in controls had similar numbers of *P. ovale*. No significant difference in serum antibody titers was found between patients and controls. The amount of lipid, however, was significantly higher in the patients. Neither the antibody titers nor the amount of lipid was correlated with the number of organisms on the skin.

The number of *P. ovale* on the skin has little importance in seborrheic dermatitis. The inflammation is theorized to be caused by an abnormal reaction in the skin against the organism, possibly because of a weakness of cell-mediated immunity.

▶ I'm pretty sure that the issue of *P. ovale* and seborrheic dermatitis has been debated since I was a first-year resident (and I'm rather old). And you know what? The controversy hasn't changed one bit. I think that the only way it will ever be solved (if it's really worth solving) is to develop an animal model of seborrhea in which both the organism and the host response to it can be manipulated at will. Otherwise, the current first-year dermatology residents will be saying the same things that I'm saying about this topic when they are my age.—J.C. Alper, M.D.

A Double-Blind Trial of Treatment of Seborrhoeic Dermatitis with 2% Ketoconazole Cream Compared With 1% Hydrocortisone Cream

Katsambas A, Antoniou Ch, Frangouli E, Avgerinou G, Michailidis D, Stratigos J (Univ of Athens; Janssen Research Found, Athens, Greece)

Br J Dermatol 121:353–357, September 1989 9–11

Pityrosporum ovale plays a role in the pathogenesis of seborrheic dermatitis. Of 50 patients with seborrheic dermatitis, 24 were treated with 2% ketoconazole cream and 26 with 1% hydrocortisone cream applied twice daily for 4 weeks.

Symptomatic improvement was observed in 81.6% of patients treated with ketoconazole cream and 87.2% of patients treated with hydrocortisone cream. The number of *P. ovale* yeasts was reduced significantly after application of ketoconazole compared with hydrocortisone cream. The incidence of adverse effects was low in both groups.

In the treatment of seborrheic dermatitis, 2% ketoconazole cream is almost as effective as 1% hydrocortisone cream. That a role exists for *P. ovale* in the pathogenesis of seborrheic dermatitis was supported.

▶ Isn't it interesting how 2 different people can look at the same data and come to 2 antithetical conclusions? In this study, the levels of *P. ovale* were decreased with the use of ketoconazole cream, and the conclusion is that a role for *P. ovale* in the pathogenesis of seborrhea is supported. The levels of *P. ovale* were slightly decreased by the hydrocortisone also, however. The latter cream was just as, or more, effective than ketoconazole. I would interpret these findings as showing that both creams somehow increase the integrity of the skin barrier, and that levels of *P. ovale* decrease because of this. More research is needed!—J.C. Alper, M.D.

10 Genodermatoses

X-Linked Ichthyosis and Ichthyosis Vulgaris: Comparison of Their Clinical Features Based on Biochemical Analysis

Okano M, Kitano Y, Yoshikawa K, Nakamura T, Matsuzawa Y, Yuasa T (Osaka Univ School of Medicine, Osaka, Japan)

Br J Dermatol 119:777–783, December 1988 10–1

The clinical distinction between X-linked ichthyosis and ichthyosis vulgaris is in many cases difficult because the cutaneous manifestations of the disorders are similar. Polyacryalamide gel disc electrophoresis is useful in detection of the electrophoretic mobility of low-density lipoprotein (LDL). Also, other researchers have found that in X-linked ichthyosis there is a deficiency in steroid sulfatase activity, and that the electrophoretic mobility of LDL is elevated because of accumulated plasma cholesterol sulfate in X-linked ichthyosis. In a study of 30 patients with X-linked ichthyosis and 32 patients with ichthyosis vulgaris the diagnoses based on clinical features were compared with diagnoses based on determination of the steroid sulfatase activity of peripheral lymphocytes or the electrophoretic mobility of serum LDL, or both.

In both diseases a family history of the condition was evident in 63% to 66% of patients. Ichthyosis appeared in infancy in 68% of patients with ichthyosis vulgaris, whereas ichthyosis was noted at birth or immediately afterward in 59% of those with X-linked ichthyosis. Most patients with ichthyosis vulgaris had small brown or light-brown scales, whereas those with X-linked ichthyosis had mostly large brown or dark-brown scales. In 44% of those with ichthyosis vulgaris the back was more scaly than the abdomen; however, in X-linked ichthyosis the abdomen was more severely involved than the back in 63% of the patients. In both types the extensor surface of the extremities was more severely affected than the flexor surface. Ninety-three percent of the patients with X-linked ichthyosis had scales in the preauricular area, whereas preauricular involvement was seen in only 17% of those with ichthyosis vulgaris.

In more than 80% of the patients with X-linked ichthyosis who had relatives with ichthyosis the diagnosis was confirmed by biochemical analyses. However, a clinical diagnosis of ichthyosis vulgaris was made in most sporadic cases of X-linked ichthyosis. In half of the sporadic ichthyosis vulgaris cases the clinical diagnosis was correct. Clinically, X-linked ichthyosis seems to be characterized by preauricular involvement, which could be an important feature for distinguishing that form from ichthyosis vulgaris.

▶ None of the material is really new in this paper, but the correlation of the clinical appearance with the biochemical findings is interesting. I would recommend reading this paper, especially to all dermatology residents. The finding of scales in the preauricular area (also on top of the pinna, in my experience) deserves emphasis. I have found it to be the most helpful differentiating clinical sign.—J.C. Alper, M.D.

The Expression of Congenital Ichthyosiform Erythroderma in Second Trimester Features of the Same Family: Morphologic and Biochemical Studies

Holbrook KA, Dale BA, Williams ML, Perry TB, Hoff MS, Hamilton EF, Fisher C, Senikas V (Univ of Washington; Univ of California, San Francisco; VA Med Ctr, San Francisco; McGill Univ)

J Invest Dermatol 91:521–531, December 1988 10–2

Biopsy specimens of skin and amniotic fluid cells from 3 fetuses of the same family at risk for congenital icthyosiform erythroderma were examined using microscopy, immunohistochemistry, and protein and lipid biochemistry. Specimens obtained from the skin of the first fetus at both 21 weeks and 25 weeks appeared normal. A healthy infant was born at term. Examination of the skin samples from the second infant yielded conflicting results. In 1 sample the epidermis appeared normal, but the second had 5–15 layers of incompletely keratinized cells superficial to the basal and intermediate layers. Hair canals in both infants were hyperkeratotic. Pelleted amniotic fluid cells contained incompletely keratinized epidermal cells surrounded by keratinized cells. The pregnancy was terminated, and regional variability in epidermal thickness and keratinization was noted in the fetus. The follicles were hyperkeratinized. Epidermal lipids were abnormal. All 4 biopsy samples obtained from the third fetus appeared normal; however, a male infant was born with severe congenital ichthyosiform erythroderma. The biopsy scars were identified, all in less affected regions of the body.

The onset of congenital ichthyosiform erythroderma in utero appears to coincide with keratinization; therefore, biopsies performed after 24 weeks provide more accurate diagnoses. Several biopsy specimens from different body regions should be examined because of the regional variation in disease expression; also, several methods of analysis should be used. Morphological examination of the follicular epidermis may be the most useful test. However, with present methods, false negative results remain common in prenatal testing for congenital ichthyosiform erythroderma.

▶ This is an extremely important paper concerning the prenatal identification of one of the ichthyoses. The most important point for clinicians is that false negatives can occur. We hope that research based on this study will continue and will identify more definite indicators of the disorder in utero.—J.C. Alper, M.D.

Progress of a Harlequin Fetus to Nonbullous Ichthyosiform Erythroderma
Lawlor F (Coventry and Warwickshire Hosp, Coventry, England)
Pediatrics 82:870–873, December 1988 10–3

The term *harlequin fetus* refers to the most severe form of congenital ichthyosis, in which the infant is deformed by the contraction and thickness of its skin, resulting in strangulation of the ears, lips, nose, and digits. Most such infants die within weeks of birth. The development of 1 harlequin fetus, still living at age 2 years 6 months was monitored.

Girl, 2 years 6 months, twelfth child of unrelated parents, was the fifth harlequin fetus born in her family. At birth her body was covered with large, thick, rigid scales that separated to reveal moist fissures. Severe ectropion and eclabium were noted. The nose was absent, but nostrils were visible (Fig 10–1). Rudimentary ears were covered in thick keratin, and scalp keratin was fissured, but hair was present. The hands and feet were deformed and clenched in flexion; large

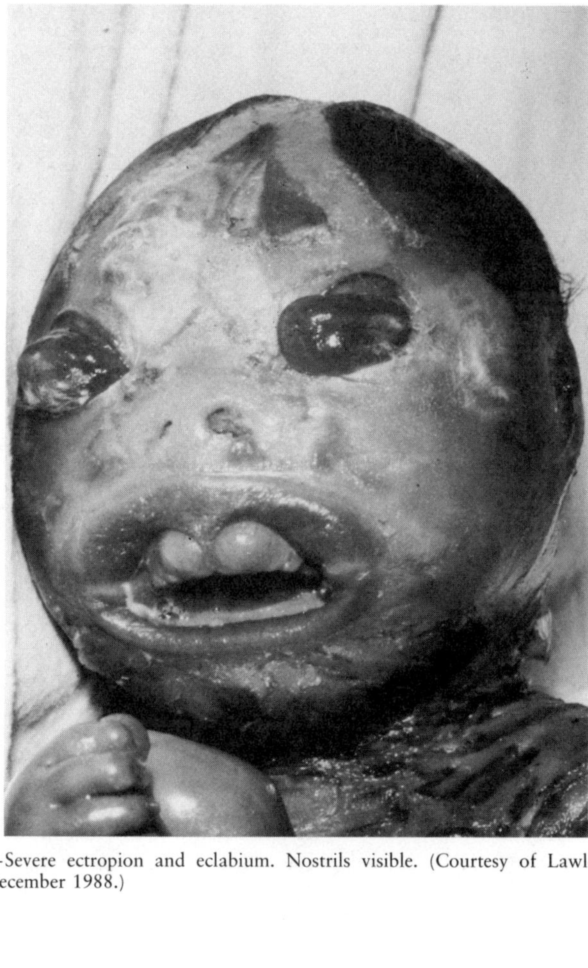

Fig 10–1.—Severe ectropion and eclabium. Nostrils visible. (Courtesy of Lawlor F: *Pediatrics* 82:870–873, December 1988.)

joints also were held in fixed flexion. The infant could neither move nor suck, and she had an offensive odor. She was placed in a humidified incubator and given baths containing oil twice daily. Liquid paraffin with soft white paraffin was applied every 2 hours. Tube feeding was initiated. Systemically, she was treated with etretinate; ectropion was covered with a strip of Geliperm and saline-soaked eye pads. The infant was removed from the incubator at 9 weeks; bottle feeding was begun at 8 weeks. She received an early blood transfusion for anemia. Skin scales gradually thinned, features began to develop, and she began to move. At 11 months she underwent plastic surgery on her eyelids, and at 1 year she had normal features, some ectropion, and erythematous skin with fine scaling. At 2.5 years of age, her weight is less than the third percentile and motor development is retarded, but the child is otherwise normal. Ectropion persists, the ears appear crumpled (Fig 10–2), and background erythema with fine scaling is present.

The fine scaling with a diffuse background erythema in this patient is

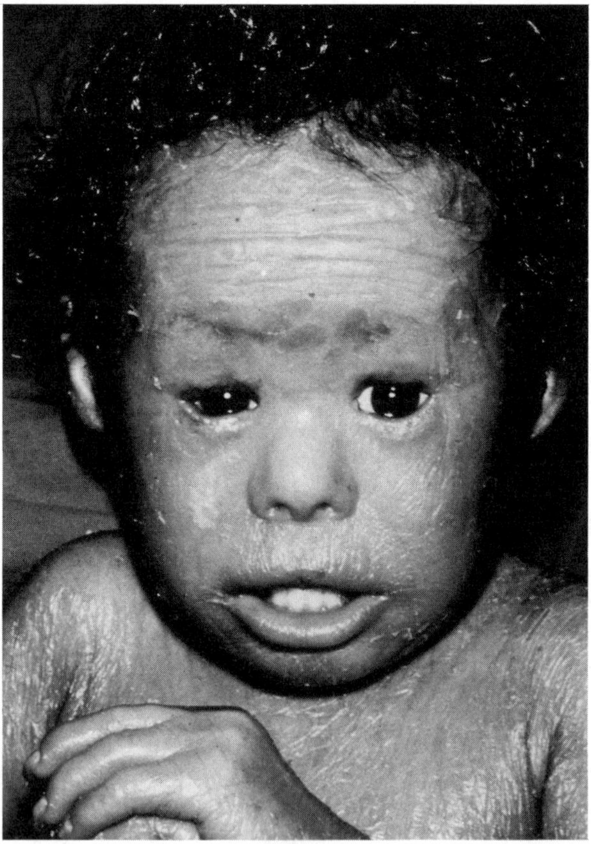

Fig 10–2.—At 24 months of age ectropion persists. (Courtesy of Lawlor F: *Pediatrics* 82:870–873 December 1988.)

compatible with a diagnosis of nonbullous ichthyosiform erythroderma. The specific genetic abnormality that causes harlequin fetus could not be determined.

▶ This very interesting paper shows that the harlequin fetus condition is not uniformly fatal if early, aggressive therapy is begun. The child at 2 years of age, however, was far from normal. Perhaps more effective and less toxic derivatives of etretinate will be derived so that these children can lead productive lives.—J.C. Alper, M.D.

Genetic Aspects of Tuberous Sclerosis in the West of Scotland

Sampson JR, Scahill SJ, Stephenson JBP, Mann L, Connor JM (Duncan Guthrie Inst of Med Genetics, Glasgow; Royal Hosp for Sick Children, Glasgow)

J Med Genet 26:28–31, January 1989 10–4

Failure to find signs of tuberous sclerosis in obligate carriers of the tuberous sclerosis gene has previously suggested gonadal mosaicism or nonpenetrance. The chief genetic aspects of tuberous sclerosis in western Scotland as well as its prevalence were studied.

In a population of 2,763,000, slightly more than 100 patients were identified. The minimum prevalence overall was 1/27,000, but in children younger than 10 years it was 1/12,000. Of 84 cases analyzed, the parents in 51 instances had no signs of tuberous sclerosis, thus the mutation rate was about 60%. As estimated elsewhere in Great Britain the mutation rate per gene per generation was at least 2.5×10^{-5}. Thirty-five patients came from families having more than 1 affected person and autosomal dominance prevailed, but no evidence of heterogeneity was found. Assessment of parents of apparently sporadic cases revealed a new mutation in 1 (involving monozygotic twins), nonpaternity in another, and nonpenetrance or gonadal mosaicism in a third. When parental ages for new mutations were analyzed, no significant age effect was found.

The proportion of new mutations may have been overestimated. Genetic counseling of normal parents of what seem to be children with sporadic cases remains difficult, but at present the recurrence risk appears to be 1%.

▶ This excellent study provides helpful information. The overall prevalence of tuberous sclerosis in this population in Western Scotland was determined to be 1/27,000 overall, and 1/12,000 in persons younger than age 10 years. This prevalence is similar to previous estimates. Of the 84 natural parents evaluated clinically using Wood's light and funduscopic examination but no other laboratory tests, there was no evidence of tuberous sclerosis in 51 sets of parents (i.e., a sporadic rate of 61%). It is possible that the true spontaneous mutation rate is lower if ascertainment of disease in parents is biased on the low side. More detailed examinations may sometimes be required to determine tuberous sclerosis in parents of bona fide cases. There were 4 generations affected in 1 family and 3 generations in 4 families. Great variation of expression is reported within and among the familial cases of tuberous sclerosis in this study with no skipped generations seen.—A.R. Rhodes, M.D., M.P.H.

Von Recklinghausen Neurofibromatosis: A Clinical and Population Study in South-East Wales

Huson SM, Harper PS, Compston AS (Univ of Wales, Cardiff)

Brain 111:1355–1381, December 1988 10–5

With the development of recombinant DNA techniques there has been renewed interest in the clinical problems of diagnosis and management of neurofibromatosis. Von Recklinghausen, or type 1, neurofibromatosis (NF-1), a relatively common autosomal dominant disorder, was studied to complement genetic linkage investigations. An attempt was made to determine the prevalence of NF-1 in a British population and the age of appearance of the major definitive features.

Index cases with NF-1 were located by survey of general practitioners and consultants and review of hospital records. Cooperating index cases were evaluated clinically along with all first-degree relatives. Within the study area 135 cases of NF-1 were identified, for a prevalence of $20:10^5$. Sixty patients were male and 75 female. The age range at evaluation was 11 months to 83 years. In addition to dermal neurofibromas and/or café-au-lait spots (Fig 10–3), 67% of the patients had freckling in the axilla and 44% had freckling in the groin; 29% of the females had freckling in the submammary areas (table). Most patients had Lisch nodules in the iris.

Plexiform neurofibroma was the most common complication. There were 6 patients each with epilepsy, scoliosis requiring surgery, and visceral and endocrine tumors; 3 had pseudarthrosis; 2 each had optic

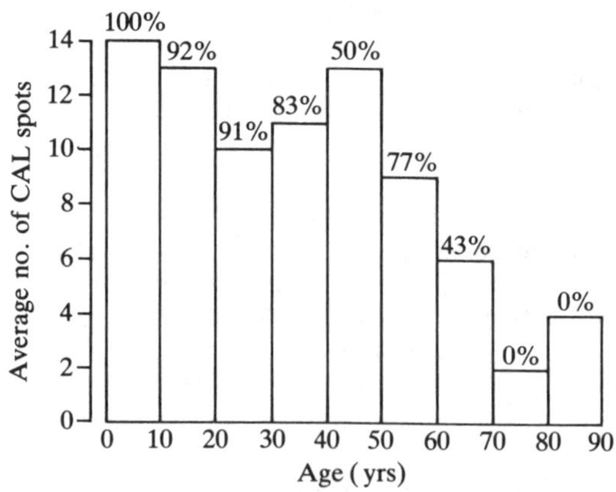

Fig 10–3.—Average number of café-au-lait (CAL) spots per person in 122 cases of NF-1 with a diameter of >0.5 cm for those aged less than 10 years and >1.5 cm for the remainder. The percentage of patients with more than 6 spots is shown for each group. (Courtesy of Huson SM, Harper PS, Compston DAS: *Brain* 111:1355–1381, December 1988.)

Age-Related Frequency of Freckling

Age (yrs)	*No. of cases*	*Axillary freckling* (%)	*Inguinal freckling* (%)	*Submammary freckling in females* (%)
0–5	5	0	0	0
6–10	12	42	8	0
11–20	29	72	41	8
21–30	23	70	43	16
31–40	18	89	56	58
41–50	10	80	50	38
51–60	13	69	23	20
61–70	7	57	14	0
71–85	5	60	20	0

(Courtesy of Huson SM, Harper PS, Compston AS: *Brain* 111:1355–1381, December 1988.)

glioma, spinal neurofibroma, aqueduct stenosis, and delayed puberty; and 1 each had severe mental retardation, meningioangiomatosis, and congenital glaucoma. No patient had acoustic neuroma. The frequency of CNS or malignant tumors related to the disease was 4.4% to 5.2%.

Uncomplicated NF-1 is disfiguring, but the disease is not a major cause of morbidity. Management is complication related and can be divided into 3 categories: childhood complications that may cause lifelong morbidity, treatable complications that can occur at any time, and malignancies. In this survey the combined frequency of these complications was 12%, 16%, and 4.4% to 5.2%, respectively.

▶ Neurofibromatosis (NF) is now divided into 4 types: (1) von Recklinghausen's neurofibromatosis, termed NF-1; (2) bilateral acoustic or central neurofibromatosis, NF-2; (3) segmental neurofibromatosis, with features of NF-1 confined to one region of the body (very rare)—this may represent a somatic mutation of the NF-1 gene (1); and (4) familial café-au-lait macules (very rare). In this new study from Wales the importance of pigmentary hamartomas of the iris, Lisch nodules, is emphasized as a marker of NF-1. Lisch nodules are present in the iris in the majority of NF-1 patients (in this reported series the incidence was 96%), and this eye finding is a highly important criterion for diagnosis of NF-1; *they are not present in NF-2.*

Lisch nodules of the iris are dome shaped and can be seen only on slit-lamp examination; they appear as "glassy," transparent, dome-shaped, yellow-to-brown papules up to 2.0 mm in size. They do not correlate with disease severity. Although Lisch nodules are usually brown in color, in this, as in other series, the nodules were pale or almost white; they are easily distinguished from iris nevi.

Lisch nodules "were not seen in any of the at-risk relatives who were otherwise normal, nor in parents of new mutations." However, a study done in Holland (2) reported that Lisch nodules were present in a sister and a daughter of a man with NF-1, and neither of the "normal" persons had any signs of NF-1.

If a child presents with a number of café-au-lait macules but neurofibromata have not yet appeared, it is impossible to make a diagnosis of NF-1 because the Lisch nodules are not detectable before age 16. This situation poses a problem in doing genetic counseling.

The criteria for the diagnosis of NF-1 have been stated previously following multidisciplinary discussions at national NF meetings held in the United States (3): Two or more of the following criteria are necessary for diagnosis of NF-1: (1) multiple café-au-lait macules, more than 6 with a diameter of 15 mm in adults and more than 5 with a diameter of 5 mm or more in children younger than 5 years; (2) multiple freckles in the axillary and/or inguinal regions; (3) based on clinical and histologic grounds, 2 or more neurofibromas of any type, or 1 plexiform neurofibroma; (4) sphenoid wing dysplasia or congenital bowing or thinning of long bone cortex, with or without pseudarthrosis; (5) optic nerve gliomas (usually unilateral in NF-1) (6) 2 or more Lisch nodules (iris hamartomas); and (7) a first-degree relative (parent, sibling, or child) with NF-1 by the above criteria.—T.B. Fitzpatrick, M.D., Ph.D.

References

1. Miller RM, Sparkes RS: *Arch Dermatol* 100:1635, 1977.
2. Toonstra J, et al: *Dermatologica* 174:232, 1987.
3. *Neurofibromatosis* 1:172, 1988.

Dyskeratosis Congenita

Davidson HR, Connor JM (Duncan Guthrie Inst of Med Genetics, Glasgow)
J Med Genet 25:843–846, December 1988 10–6

Frequencies of Clinical Features of Dyskeratosis Congenita

	At time of reporting (%)	*At onset of disease (%)*
Skin manifestations		
Hyperpigmentation	99	53
Nail dystrophy	92	59
Leucoplakia	82	10
Epiphora	79	5
Hyperhidrosis	87	—
Hyperkeratinisation (palms and soles)	69	—
Bullae on minimal trauma	23	7
Alopecia	34	—
Extensive caries/dental loss	12	—
Other manifestations		
Haematological abnormalities	51	5
Neoplasia	12	—
Mild mental retardation	10	—
Hepatomegaly	7	—
Splenomegaly	15	—
Growth retardation	13	—
Bone involvement	8	—

(Courtesy of Davidson HR, Connor JM: *J Med Genet* 25:843–846, December 1988.)

Dyskeratosis congenita is an uncommon condition characterized by prominent dermatologic features. Serious manifestations include bone marrow involvement with pancytopenia and a predisposition to malignancy. The nature of the disease, based on 104 patients' courses, was reviewed.

Dermatologic features of dyskeratosis congenita include reticulate skin pigmentation (Fig 10–4), nail dystrophy, and leukoplakia, which appears later than the other features. Other late-appearing features are epiphora, conjunctivitis, and blepharitis resulting from hyperplasia of the epithelial lining of the lacrimal punctum (table). When they occur, hematologic abnormalities usually are serious. Anemia and thrombocytopenia are early signs, but progression to pancytopenia is usual. Bone marrow aspirates could be either hypocellular or hyperplastic. There is a high incidence of solid tumors. Malignancies include squamous carcinomas of

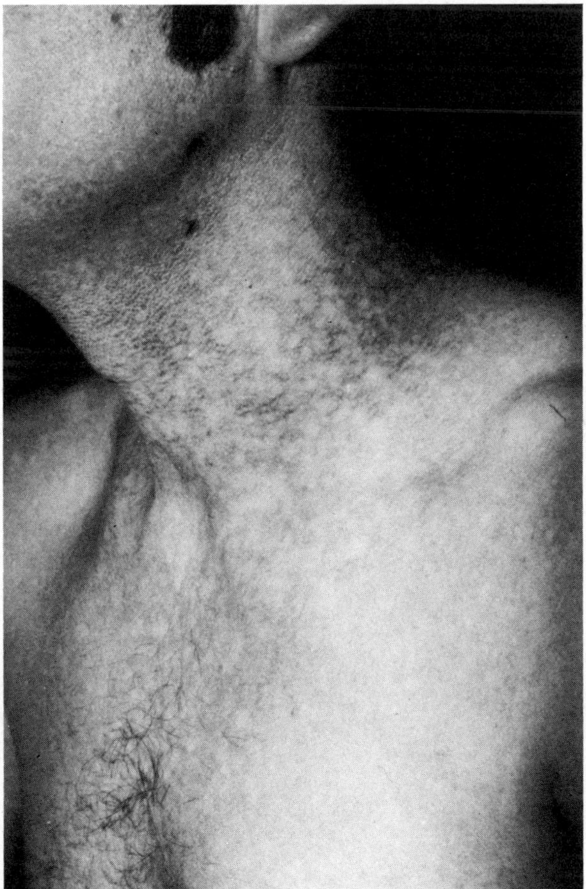

Fig 10–4.—Typical reticulate hyperpigmentation of skin. (Courtesy of Davidson HR, Connor JM: *J Med Genet* 25:843–846, December 1988.)

the mucosa or skin, esophageal and pancreatic tumors, and Hodgkin's lymphoma. Unaffected family members also seem to have an increased incidence of malignancy.

Features usually appear in childhood, and the mean age of onset is 7 years. In 92% of the patients at least 1 characteristic of the disease is present by age 10 years. Serious complications begin to develop by the midteens. Bone marrow transplantation for the pancytopenia and retinoids is the only known treatment. However, etretinate has been useful in controlling keratinizing disorders and may cause regression of lesions in leukoplakia oris, thus reducing the incidence of malignancy.

Of the 104 reported patients, 24% had died by the time of reporting. The mean age at death was 24 years. Half of the deaths were caused by infection, 20% by bleeding, and 30% by malignancies. The primary defect has not been identified, but typical disease in males usually follows X-linked recessive inheritance. If females are affected or mild atypical features are seen in males, autosomal dominant inheritance should be considered.

▶ This is an excellent, complete, but succinct summary of the syndrome. The bibliography is relatively complete and makes this paper a good place to start for review of the topic.—J.C. Alper, M.D.

Proteus Syndrome

Samlaska CP, Levin SW, James WD, Bendon PM, Walker JC, Perlik PC (Walter Reed Army Med Ctr, Washington, DC)

Arch Dermatol 125:1109–1114, August 1989 10–7

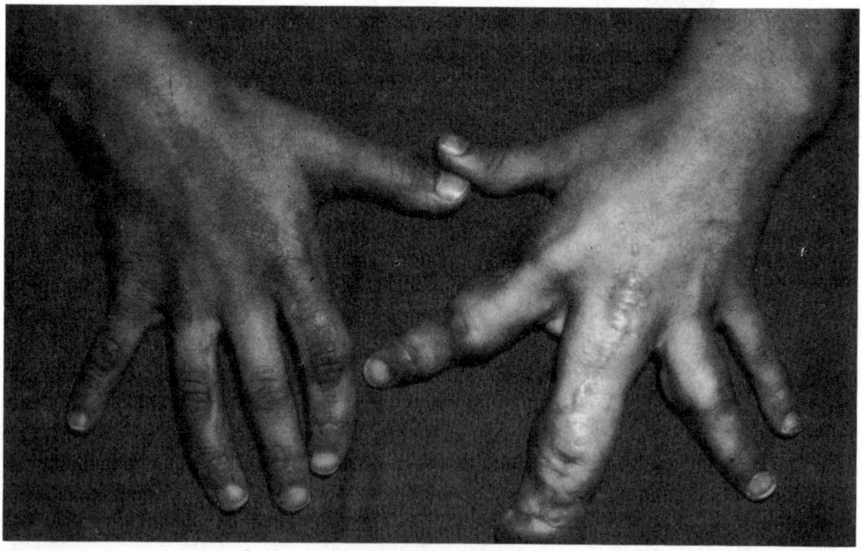

Fig 10–5.—Macrodactyly involving the left middle and index fingers (patient's age, 5 years). (Courtesy of Samlaska CP, Levin SW, James WD, et al: *Arch Dermatol* 128:1109–1114, August 1989.)

Major Clinical Findings in 34 Patients With Proteus Syndrome

Finding	**No. of Cases**
Hemihypertrophy (partial or complete)	31
Macrodactyly	30
Subcutaneous masses	26
Lipomatosis (including pelvic)	12
Pelvic lipomatosis	2
"Hamartomas"	5
Cavernous hemangiomas	4
Lymphangiohemangioma	1
Lymphohemangioma	1
Lipohemangioma	1
Lipolymphohemangioma	1
Hemolymphangiomatous hamartoma	1
Plantar or palmar masses	22
Connective tissue nevus	3
Lipomatosis	3
Exostoses	21
Cranial	9
Distal extremities	17
Epidermal nevus	17
Linear	16
Whorled	1
Scoliosis	17

Major clinical findings are defined as those identified in more than half of all 34 reported cases.

(Courtesy of Samlaska CP, Levin SW, James WD, et al: *Arch Dermatol* 128:1109–1114, August 1989.)

Proteus syndrome is a newly described congenital disorder of mesodermal malformations seen as partial gigantism of the hands or feet, or both, hemihypertrophy, macrocephaly, a variety of subcutaneous tumors, and other malformations. The cause of Proteus syndrome is unknown. There is no male or female predominance, and all occurrences appear to be sporadic. No abnormal chromosomes have been identified; a new dominant gene mutation has been suggested.

In the literature before 1983, 8 patients were identified as having manifestations suggestive of Proteus syndrome. Subsequent reports and clinical series have shown that patients with this syndrome have a wide variability in clinical findings. In all, 34 patients with Proteus syndrome have been identified (table).

The main confirmed clinical features of Proteus syndrome include hemihypertrophy, macrodactyly (Fig 10–5), subcutaneous tumors, plantar or palmar masses (or both), exostoses, epidermal nevi, and scoliosis. Most patients have had at least 4 of these findings.

▶ If you want to read about the syndrome, this is the place to do it because the entire literature is reviewed. The authors attempt to structure a clinical classification of this syndrome in order to differentiate it from others that share morphological features such as Klippel-Trenaunay-Weber or neurofibromatosis.

I caution against adhering to such a classification, however, no matter how well developed. In the past, many syndromes that were thought to be different based on clinical findings eventually were found to be attributable to the same gene defect when it was identified. We must wait for genetic or biochemical elucidation of this syndrome before rigidly adhering to exclusionary clinical definitions.—J.C. Alper, M.D.

Incidence, Severity, and Prevention of Infections in Chronic Granulomatous Disease

Mouy R, Fischer A, Vilmer E, Seger R, Griscelli C (Hôp des Enfants-Malades, Paris; Kinderspital, Zurich)
J Pediatr 114:555–560, April 1989 10–8

Chronic granulomatous disease is an inherited disorder of bacterial and fungal killing by phagocytic cells. Affected patients contract recurrent infections from the first year of life, usually involving skin, lymph nodes, lungs, liver, and gastrointestinal tract. The clinical features of 48 patients with chronic granulomatous disease were reviewed retrospectively to delineate the relative frequency, types, and sites of infections and their consequences. The long-term use of trimethoprim-sulfamethoxazole and ketoconazole as a preventive therapy for infections also was assessed.

The most frequently occurring infections were lymphadenitis, lung in-

Microorganisms Cultured From 169 Infection Sites in Patients With Chronic Granulomatous Disease

	Patients		Infections	
Microorganisms	**No.**	**%**	**No.**	**%**
Staphylococcus aureus	25	52	53	31
Aspergillus	19	40	24	16
Salmonella	16	33	22	14
Serratia	8	17	11	7
Escherichia coli	8	17	11	7
Mycobacteria	8	17	8	5
Staphylococcus epidermidis	7	15	10	6
Proteus	6	12.5	7	4
Candida albicans	5	10	5	3
Klebsiella pneumoniae	4	8	4	2
Pseudomonas	3	6	4	2
Enterobacter cloacae	2		5	3
Haemophilus influenzae	2		2	
Cephalosporium	1		1	
Pneumocystis carinii	1		1	
Campylobacter	1		1	

(Courtesy of Mouy R, Fischer A, Vilmer E, et al: *J Pediatr* 114:555–560, April 1989.)

fections, dermatitis, enteral infections, and hepatic abscesses. The main microorganisms found were *Staphylococcus aureus, Salmonella,* and *Aspergillus* (table). Twelve patients died, 5 of lung aspergillosis, 3 of hepatic abscesses, 2 of pneumonopathy of unknown origin, 1 of salmonellosis, and 1 of another probable infection that could not be proved. The actuarial survival rate at 10 years of age was 50%, followed by a prolonged plateau. Analysis of the occurrence of bacterial and fungal infections in patients receiving trimethoprim-sulfamethoxazole and ketoconazole as infection prophylaxis revealed that the former was effective against bacterial infections and the latter provided no protection against *Aspergillus.*

Chronic granulomatous disease is associated with repeated and life-threatening bacterial and fungal infections. Far more deaths occur in the first decade of life. There has been significant improvement in survival rates, probably because of better diagnostic procedures and the use of more efficient antibacterial and antifungal agents.

▶ The authors describe 2 types of inheritance of chronic granulomatous disease—X-linked recessive, associated with a lack of cytochrome 559, and autosomal recessive, associated with abnormal flavoproteins, low-affinity NADPH oxidase, or extreme glucose-6-phosphate dehydrogenase deficiency. The X-linked recessive type is the most common. Recurrent infections are the rule. Skin infections affected 73% of the 48 children studied. Ten children had neonatal pustulosis, with *Staphylococcus epidermidis* the proven agent in 3 cases. Ketoconazole, as noted, did not prevent pulmonary aspergillosis, but it did prevent *Candida* infections in those patients.—R. Masters, M.D.

11 Hair and Nails

Androgens in Hirsute Women Referred for Electroepilation

Fogh H, Worm A-M, Forkert B, Bennett P (Bispebjerg Hosp; Statens Seruminstitut, Copenhagen)

Acta Derm Venereol (Stockh) 69:179–182, April 1989 11–1

Studies were made in 105 hirsute women referred for electroepilation to define those in whom endocrinologic evaluation was indicated. The level of androgens was correlated with a hirsutism score and menstrual disturbances. The effect of epilation, as performed by an experienced person, also was evaluated.

Increased values of at least 1 androgen were found in 58 women, most often free testosterone, dehydroepiandrosterone sulfate, and delta-4-androstendione. The level of androgen did not correlate significantly with the hirsutism score or with the frequency of menstrual irregularities other than amenorrhea. Fifty-three women were followed for at least 6 months after epilation. There was a significant decrease in the frequency of self-treatment and in the hirsutism score in these women, and scarring was not noted.

It is not possible to identify hirsute women with abnormal androgens by applying clinical parameters such as a hirsutism score or menstrual disturbances other than amenorrhea. The Danish recommendation that endocrinologic investigation should be restricted to women with moderate to severe hirsutism and hirsute women with menstrual irregularities, infertility, or virilization still applies. Epilation should be recommended as an excellent alternative treatment for hirsutism.

▶ The stated purpose of this study was to "identify those hirsute women in whom endocrinological evaluation should always be done." The authors then proceeded to measure blood androgen levels in 105 hirsute women undergoing electrolysis and found at least 1 androgen abnormality in 55% of them. One would have presumed that the authors would conclude that those hirsute women with elevated androgens were (or should have been) investigated further, but no such statement was proffered.—P.E. Pochi, M.D.

Reduction in Undesired Sexual Hair Growth With Anandron in Male-to-Female Transsexuals: Experiences With a Novel Androgen Receptor Blocker

Asscheman H, Gooren LJG, Peereboom-Wynia JDR (Free Univ Hosp, Amsterdam; Erasmus Univ, Rotterdam)

Clin Exp Dermatol 14:361–363, September 1989 11–2

Male sexual hair growth is undesirable in male-to-female transsexuals who wish to adapt to the female gender. A total of 14 male-to-female transsexuals aged 19–33 years began treatment with Anandron, a pure nonsteroidal androgen receptor antagonist. For the first 8 weeks, Anandron, 150 mg, was taken orally twice a day; in weeks 9–20, ethinyl estradiol, 100 μg/day, was added to the Anandron regimen.

In the first 8 weeks the mean serum testosterone level increased significantly from 19.2 mmol/L to 44.9 mmol/L, and the mean serum estradiol level increased significantly from 0.08 mmol/L to 0.24 mmol/L. Hair growth, as scored by the Ferriman and Gallwey system, hair weight, and number of terminal hairs in the trunk and limbs (the areas assessed) decreased significantly in the first 8 weeks and in weeks 9–20. Less hair growth was experienced subjectively by all patients on the trunk and limbs after 5 months' treatment, but beard growth decreased only little.

Treatment with Anandron alone initially, and thereafter with Anandron plus estrogen, effectively reduces undesired sexual hair growth on the trunk and limbs but not beard growth. The discrepant results in facial and body hair may be because of differences in the life cycle and density of hair in these areas.

▶ A modest diminution in hairiness on the trunk and extremities, but none on the face, was observed in men (male-to-female transsexual subjects) treated for 20 weeks with nilutamide (Anandron). This oral antiandrogen, a product of Roussel-UCLAF but not as yet available in the United States, differs from the older antiandrogen, cyproterone acetate, in being "pure," i.e., having no gonadotropin-inhibition property. It is difficult to conclude, however, how much of the overall reduction in hairiness can be attributable to the drug, because a high dose of estrogen (100 μg of ethinyl estradiol daily) was added to the regimen after 2 months.—P.E. Pochi, M.D.

Acquired Progressive Kinking of the Hair
Cullen SI, Fulghum DD (Univ of Florida)
Arch Dermatol 125:252–255, February 1989 11–3

Acquired progressive kinking of the hair (APKH) is a rare disturbance of scalp hair growth. Three additional patients, females aged 8–22 years, were seen.

Woman, 22, was seen initially at 14 years of age with the primary complaint of excessively curly hair developing on the dome of her scalp. It spread slowly to the mid and central parts of the scalp. The patient's general health was good, and her history was unremarkable. Physical examination revealed a marked difference in the texture and curliness of the hair on the dome and central part of the scalp compared with the hair on the lateral or posterior portions of her scalp. Her scalp showed no erythema, scaliness, or other abnormalities. A punch biopsy specimen of the involved central scalp revealed slight hyperkeratosis of the follicular infundibula but no other abnormalities. Treatment consisted of regular washing with a nonmedicated shampoo and benign neglect. The abnormality slowly regressed during an 8-year period, with the lateral and frontal borders of involved hair the first to regain their usual configuration. Complete restoration of the patient's usual hair appearance occurred recently during the first trimester of pregnancy.

Acquired progressive kinking of the hair is an acquired disorder of hair formation in which patches of hair become tightly curled, resembling pubic hair. It appears to be more common in males and is associated with darkening of the involved hair in approximately two thirds of the affected individuals. The differential diagnosis includes inherited forms of kinky hair and kinky hair secondary to mechanical, chemical, or traumatic manipulation. Drugs are rarely implicated in the etiology of this disorder.

▶ Some people pay big bucks to have their hair look like this. Too bad the etiology hasn't been determined so that it could be marketed. The good news is that it regresses, even if it takes 8 years to do so.—J.C. Alper, M.D.

Loose Anagen Syndrome

Price VH, Gummer CL (Kaiser Permanente Med Ctr, San Francisco; Univ of Calif, San Francisco)

J Am Acad Dermatol 20:249–256, February 1989 11–4

The loose anagen syndrome is a distinct new hair condition characterized by anagen hairs that are loosely anchored and easily pulled from the scalp. Observations were made in 22 children and 5 adults from 24 families with this syndrome.

Characteristic Features of Loose Anagen Syndrome

In childhood	
History	*Hair "does not grow," "grows very slowly"
	*Seldom requires cutting
	*Often blond
Clinical findings	*Hair sparse, short but adequately covers scalp
	*Pulls out easily, painlessly
	*No fragility, no breakage
	Occipital hair often matted, sticky
	*No associated abnormalities
Light microscopy (pulled hairs)	*Distorted anagen bulbs, ruffled cuticle, absent outer root sheath
In adolescence and adulthood	
History	*Hair thicker, longer
Clinical findings	*Hair density, length increased
	Pigmentation increased
	*Pulls out easily, painlessly
	*No fragility, no breakage
	*No associated abnormalities
Light microscopy (pulled hairs)	*Distorted anagen bulbs, ruffled cuticle, absent outer root sheath

*Essential features.
(Courtesy of Price VH, Gummer CL: *J Am Acad Dermatol* 20:249–256, February 1989.)

Most of the patients were blond girls, aged 2–5 years, but both sexes and those with dark hair also were affected. The children had sparse hair that was relatively short and fine in texture, having a slightly matted appearance over the occiput. The hair could be pulled easily from the scalp but was not fragile and did not break. The easily pulled hairs were misshapen anagen hairs without an outer root sheath (table).

The children were observed for 2–18 years. The length and density of the hair gradually increased with age, but even in adulthood the anagen hairs remained loosely anchored. Analysis of the folliculogram showed that the size of the follicles was small and most were the size of vellus follicles. Twenty-seven percent of the follicles were in the telogen phase and 73% in the anagen phase. Histologic examination of the hair showed abnormally premature keratinization of Huxley's and Henle's layers of the inner root sheath in some samples.

There is no treatment for loose anagen syndrome, but the appearance improves with time. Apart from the hair characteristics, there are no associated abnormalities.

▶ There is an interesting report. I had the distinct feeling while reading this paper that some toxic substance was at fault. I think that a detailed exposure history should be taken, paying attention to the area where these people live or have lived.—J.C. Alper, M.D.

Quantitative Assessment of 2% Topical Minoxidil in the Treatment of Male Pattern Baldness

Rushton DH, Unger WP, Cotterill PC, Kingsley P, James KC (Philip Kingsley Trichological Clinic, London; Univ of Wales College Cardiff; Toronto)

Clin Exp Dermatol 14:40–46, January 1989 11–5

Reports on the efficacy of topical minoxidil in the treatment of male pattern baldness have been contradictory. A recent review of the published literature concluded that topical minoxidil can be expected to produce cosmetically satisfactory results in no more than 10% of the patients treated. In a double-blind clinical trial of topical 2% minoxidil solution, quantitative hair measurement was carried out by visual counting of hairs and the use of the unit area trichogram.

The study population consisted of 47 men aged 18–49 years with male pattern baldness who were randomly assigned to treatment with topical 2% minoxidil solution or a placebo solution. Twelve men were selected at random for quantitative hair evaluation with the objective unit area trichogram and by visual hair counting performed at the initial sites at 6-month intervals.

After 6 or 12 months of treatment with 2% minoxidil solution, there was no significant difference in total hair density, meaningful hair density, percent of hair in the anagen growth phase, or percent of meaningful hair in the anagen growth phase. Significantly fewer hairs were recorded with the visual hair counting method than with the unit area trichogram. Also, there was a significant difference between experienced and inexperienced observers with respect to hair counts, with inexperienced observers recording fewer hairs within the 1-in. diameter sample area. However, there was no significant deterioration in total hair density or in meaningful hair density, perhaps suggesting a prophylactic effect of topical minoxidil.

The findings indicate that topical minoxidil solution is unlikely to affect the long-term course of male pattern baldness. The continued use of topical minoxidil for this indication should be reviewed.

▶ This paper elegantly indicates the problems of qualification of hair growth in studies of alopecia. Its conclusion about the lack of efficacy of minoxidil is marred by the high probability of type 2 error, given the small number of subjects studied and the relatively modest efficacy documented in far larger studies of this agent.—R.S. Stern, M.D.

Psoriasis of the Nails Treated With Grenz Rays: A Double-Blind Bilateral Trial

Lindelöf B (Karolinska Hosp, Stockholm)

Acta Derm Venereol [Stockh] 69:80–82, March 1989 11–6

There are various treatments for psoriatic nails, but the results are unpredictable and not always satisfactory. Studies were made in 22 patients to learn how grenz rays affect the nail changes of psoriasis. Patients had been untreated for at least 6 months before the study. Each patient received 5 Gy of grenz rays on 10 occasions. Nails on 1 hand received active treatment; irradiation was simulated for the nails of the other hand. The hands were evaluated clinically before and after treatment. After a 10-week evaluation, the nails of the placebo-treated hand also received active treatment. Patients were followed for 6 months.

Only 1 patient had almost complete recovery of the treated hands, 7 had slight improvement, and 14 had no improvement at all. In 1 patient the placebo-treated nails improved slightly. All nails that responded were of normal thickness. Treatment was unsuccessful in hyperkeratotic nails. After 6 months the grenz-ray-treated nails had improved moderately in 2 patients and worsened slightly in another 2. The remaining patients were unchanged. The only side effect noted was slight pigmentation of the treated nailfold in 5 patients.

Grenz-ray treatment appears to be useful only in psoriatic nails of normal thickness. The treatment is safe, and side effects are minimal.

▶ There is a need for an effective topical therapy for psoriasis of the nails. It is apparent that the only acceptable form of radiotherapy is grenz, and it has at best only moderate and limited usefulness. An intralesional steroid may be helpful, but it is painful, not predictable, and is not readily accepted by patients. Systemic methotrexate and PUVA and RePUVA, when given for generalized disease, do have a favorable effect, not only on the skin but also on the nails.—S.L. Moschella, M.D.

Red Lunulae Revisited: A Clinical and Histopathologic Examination

Wilkerson MG, Wilkin JK (Med College of Virginia, Richmond; McGuire VA Med Ctr, Richmond)

J Am Acad Dermatol 20:453–457, March 1989 11–7

Red lunulae are associated with alopecia areata, systemic lupus erythematosus, dermatomyositis, rheumatoid arthritis, congestive heart failure,

Reports of Patients With Red Lunulae

Investigator	Diagnosis	Corticosteroids	Other conditions
Leider[2]	AA	Yes	None
Ringrose and Bahcall[3]	AA	No	Eosinophilia, lymphadenopathy
Misch[4]	AA	No	None
Jorizzo et al.[5]	Rheumatoid arthritis	Yes	None
	SLE	No	None
	Dermatomyositis	Yes	None
Terry[6]	Heart failure	—	—
DeNicola et al.[8]	Lymphogranuloma venereum	—	—
	Reticulosarcoma	—	—
	Hepatic cirrhosis	—	—
Runne[9]	Twenty-nail dystrophy	—	—
Daniel[7]	Carbon monoxide poisoning	—	—
	Psoriasis	—	—
Present report	COPD	No	Diabetes mellitus, alcohol abuse, cirrhosis
	COPD	Yes	Anemia of chronic disease, alcohol abuse
	Drug-induced SLE	Yes	Diabetes mellitus, hypertension, psoriasis
	COPD	No	Hypertension, chronic urticaria, proteinuria

Abbreviations: AA, alopecia areata; — not given; *COPD,* chronic obstructive pulmonary disease; *SLE,* systemic lupus erythematosus.
(Courtesy of Wilkerson MG, Wilkin JK: *J Am Acad Dermatol* 20:453–457, March 1989.)

hepatic cirrhosis, reticulosarcoma, psoriasis, carbon monoxide poisoning, 20-nail dystrophy, and lymphogranuloma venereum (table). Four patients with red lunulae were examined. Three had chronic obstructive pulmonary disease, 2 were alcohol abusers, 2 had no evidence of any conditions previously associated with red lunulae, and another 2 had histories of chronic corticosteroid therapy. None of the patients was aware of lesions. Half had palmar erythema. Histopathologic examination of the red lunulae in 1 patient found no signs of capillary proliferation or dilation. Screens for antinuclear antibody and rheumatoid factor were negative in all patients.

In the absence of evidence of neovascularization, it is postulated that red lunulae result from increased arteriolar blood flow, a vasodilatory capacitance phenomenon, or changes in the optical properties of the overlying nail so that normal blood vessels become more apparent.

▶ The number of diseases reported previously to be associated with red lunulae, plus the findings in this paper, suggest that it is a relatively nonspecific phenomenon. The presence of red lunulae does not appear to be a reliable bedside pearl.—R. Masters, M.D.

12 Leprosy and Other Mycobacterial Diseases

Genetic Susceptibility to Leprosy on a Caribbean Island: Linkage Analysis With Five Markers

Abel L, Demenais F, Baule M-S, Blanc M, Muller A, Raffoux C, Millan J, Bois E, Babron M-C, Feingold N (Unite de Recherches de Genetique Epidemiologique, Bois de Boulogne; Centre d'Hemotypologie, Toulouse; Centre Natl de Transfusion Sanguine, Paris; Hôp Saint-Louis, Paris; Institut Pasteur, Guadeloupe)
Int J Lepr 57:465–471, June 1989 12–1

The nature of genetic susceptibility to leprosy remains to be defined. A recent complex segregation analysis of 27 multigenerational pedigrees from a Caribbean island (Desirade) resulted in detection of a recessive major gene or genes controlling susceptibility to leprosy per se and to nonlepromatous leprosy. Analysis of linkage was performed subsequently between each of these 2 traits and any of the 5 markers typed in this Desirade population: HLA, Gm, and Km immunoglobulin genotypes, ABO, and Rhesus.

There were 82 patients with leprosy—54 nonlepromatous and 28 lepromatous. Linkage analyses showed no significant linkage between either of the 2 susceptibility genes and the 5 markers typed in this population. However, for leprosy per se, close linkage was excluded with Rhesus and Gm, and also for ABO and HLA considering a lower value for the frequency of the gene controlling susceptibility to leprosy per se. The highest lod score, although not significant, was observed between the gene for nonlepromatous leprosy and ABO.

These data suggest a 2-locus model of genetic susceptibility to leprosy. The gene controlling susceptibility to leprosy per se and that controlling for nonlepromatous leprosy may be different, acting at successive stages of the immune response to infection with *Mycobacterium leprae.*

► There has been accumulating inconclusive evidence of the role of genetics in the host response to *M. leprae,* including twin studies (1) and HLA studies (2). A genetic model that determines susceptibility could have important practical implications for the prevention and treatment of leprosy, i.e., clarifying the role of vaccine for prophylaxis or immunotherapy in leprosy.—S.L. Moschella, M.D.

References

1. Smith DG: *Hum Genet* 50:163, 1979.
2. van Eden W, de Vries RRP: *Lepr Rev* 89, 1984.

Leprosy in Infants: Report of Two Cases

Girdhar A, Mishra B, Lavania RK, Bagga AK, Malaviya GN, Girdhar BK (Central JALMA Inst for Leprosy, Agra, India)

Int J Lepr 57:472–475, June 1989 12–2

Leprosy during infancy is uncommon, but 2 infants were seen with the disease at ages 2 months and 4 months, respectively. Both had histologically confirmed indeterminate leprosy with nerve infiltration. The 2-month-old infant had specific anti-phenolic glycolipid IgM antibodies in both serum and urine. The mother of the 4-month-old did not have leprosy, but a relative staying in the same house had active borderline tuberculoid (BT) leprosy. The mother of the 2-month-old infant had smear-negative BT leprosy. The lesions in both infants responded to dapsone, with or without rifampin.

The incubation period in these 2 infants could not have been more than a few months, which could result from a more rapid multiplication of *Mycobacterium leprae* than usual in such highly susceptible hosts. It appears that clinical leprosy can become manifest at a very young age. When there is an index case in the family, infants and children should be examined for suspicious-looking lesions and a biopsy specimen should be taken, when necessary, to rule out leprosy.

▶ There have been about 50 recorded cases of leprosy in infants and 20 of them have been proven (1). In mothers with active lepromatous leprosy, a 5% prevalence in children under 2 years of age has been suggested, and transplacental transmission is possible (2). The occurrence of leprosy in the above reported cases raises important issues such as the source of infection, the route or mode of infection, and the incubation period of this disease.—S.L. Moschella, M.D.

References

1. Ganapti RR, et al: *Lepr India* 48:645, 1976.
2. Duncan ME, et al: *Int J Lepr* 51:7, 1983.

Improved Staining of Leprosy Bacilli in Tissues

Harada K, Suzuki K (Natl Tamazenseiyen Sanatorium, Tokyo)

Lepr Rev 60:124–128, June 1989 12–3

A technique was developed that can reliably demonstrate the leprosy bacilli, the tubercle bacilli, and certain fungi. It is based on oxidation of cell wall lipid substances by chromic or periodic acid and the release of free aldehydes, which are then capable of reducing ammoniacal silver salt solutions to metallic silver.

Human skin lesions of various forms of leprosy, pulmonary lesions of tuberculosis, and fungal lesions were examined. *Mycobacterium leprae,*

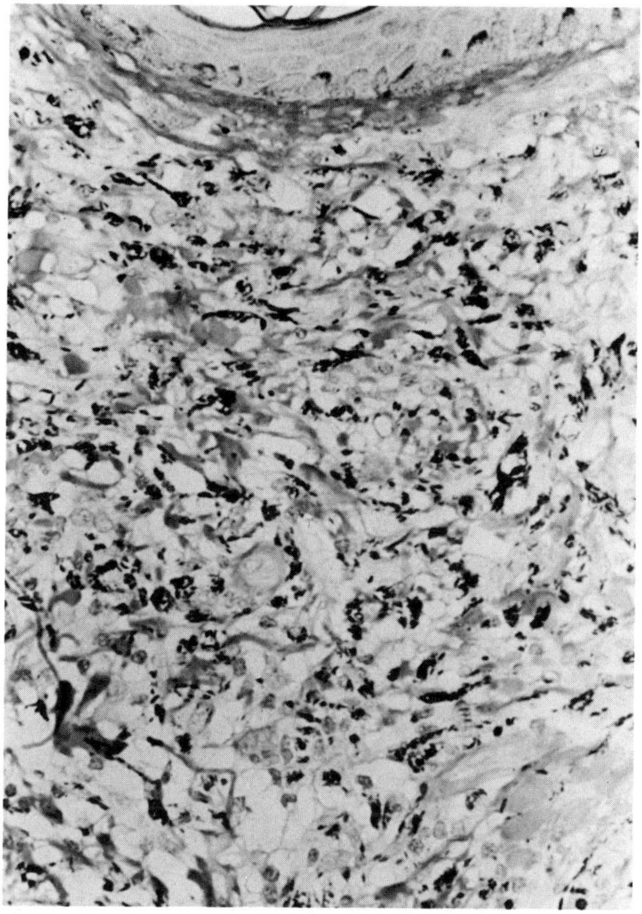

Fig 12–1.—Leprosy bacilli in lepromatous lesion of skin. Periodic acid-ammoniacal silver hydroxide stain. (Courtesy of Harada K, Suzuki K: *Lepr Rev* 60:124–128, June 1989.)

Mycobacterium tuberculosis, and fungi were stained black and appeared uniformly solid (Figs 12–1 and 12–2). Because of the sensitivity and ease of examination and recognition of bacilli and their products, this method is recommended in diagnosis and research, disregarding morphological appearances.

▶ The periodic acid-ammoniacal silver hydroxide stain described here can be helpful diagnostically when it is or may be difficult to demonstrate the *M. leprae,* such as in paucibacillary disease, in material that has been fixed for long periods of time, or when organisms are in an advanced state of decay or are resistant to modified Ziehl-Neelsen staining. Because nonsolid bacilli appear to be intact and rod-shaped with this stain, it is not useful for determination of the

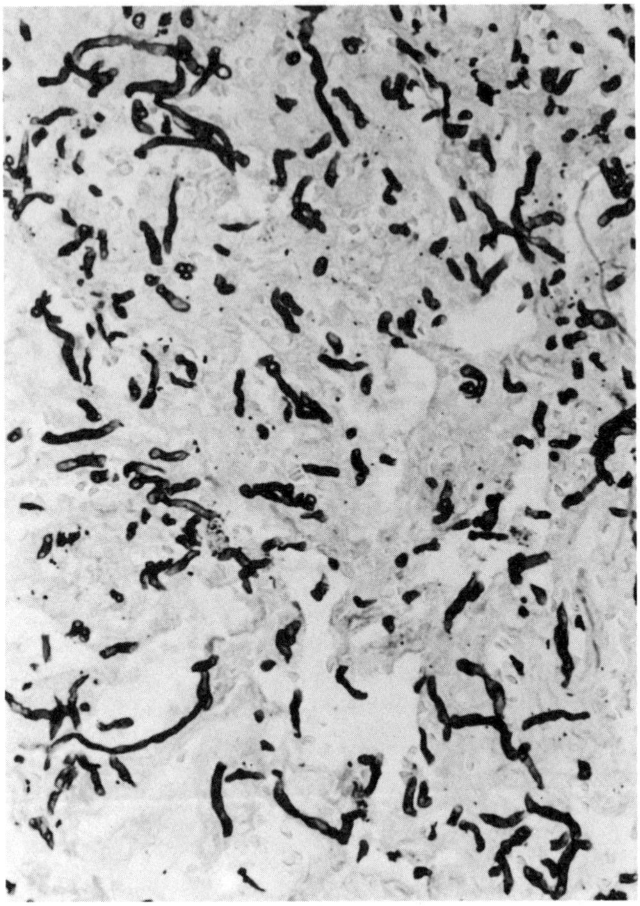

Fig 12–2.—Fungi in pulmonary tuberculosis. Periodic acid-ammoniacal silver hydroxide stain. (Courtesy of Harada K, Suzuki K: *Lepr Rev* 60:124–128, June 1989.)

morphological index or the directly related viability of the organisms.—S.L. Moschella, M.D.

Combined Regimens of One Year Duration in the Treatment of Multibacillary Leprosy: I. Combined Regimens With Rifampicin Administered During One Year

Pattyn SR, Bourland J, Grillone S, Groenen G, Ghys P (Univ of Antwerp; Service Natl de la lèpre au Burundi; Service Natl de la lèpre, République Fédérale Islamique des Comores; Damien Found, Brussels, Belgium, Kisangani, Zaire)
Lepr Rev 60:109–117, June 1989 12–4

A combined therapy regimen has been advocated by the World Health Organization for the treatment of leprosy. In a prospective therapeutic trial, a triple-drug regimen of 1 year's duration was evaluated in Burundi and on the island of Anjouan for the treatment of multibacillary (MB) leprosy. In all, 216 patients were treated daily with 600 mg of rifampicin, 500 mg of ethionamide, and 100 mg of dapsone or 100 mg of clofazimine for 8 weeks followed once weekly by 600 mg of rifampicin and daily by 500 mg of ethionamide and 100 mg of dapsone or 100 mg of clofazimine for 44 weeks. The results in patient cohorts of 1981, 1982, and 1983 who were followed for a mean of 4.24 years were reviewed. There were 109 previously untreated patients and 107 who had received dapsone monotherapy, including 16 who were infected with proven dapsone-resistant *Mycobacterium leprae.*

Clinical and bacteriologic results were excellent. The mean annual decrease in the bacteriologic index was 1.12 units per year. No relapses were observed during the 919 person-years of follow-up. Hepatotoxicity was the most serious complication; it occurred in 5.1% of patients, including 2 who died. Upgrading reactions were observed in 16.1% of patients, particularly among those previously untreated. Erythema nodosum leprosum reactions occurred in 16.8% of patients.

Multibacillary leprosy can be treated successfully with a regimen of 1 year's duration. However, hepatotoxicity remains a serious drawback to the applicability of this protocol. The search for less toxic, easily applicable regimens is warranted.

▶ This paper gives added support to the concept that multibacillary leprosy can be treated effectively by multiple drug therapy delivered for at least 1 year, but it also points out the need for closer surveillance of these patients. The problem with this therapeutic program is the potential hepatotoxicity, which is more than 5% and may even be fatal because of the administration of the combination of rifampin and etionamide. Thus there is a pressing need for alternative drugs that are effective, less toxic, and less expensive. Among the drugs currently being looked at are analogues of rifampin, minocycline, and the quinolines. Immunotherapy, such as vaccines and interferon, are being investigated as either solitary or adjunctive therapies.—S.L. Moschella, M.D.

Combined Regimens of One Year Duration in the Treatment of Multibacillary Leprosy: II. Combined Regimens With Rifampicin Administered During 6 Months

Pattyn SR, Groenen G, Janssens L, Deverchin J, Ghys P, and the Collaborative Study Group for the Treatment of Leprosy (Univ of Antwerp; Damien Found, Kisangani, Zaire; Musienene Hosp, Zaire; Head Foperda Hosp, Pawa, Zaire)
Lepr Rev 60:118–123, June 1989 12–5

Use of a combined regimen of 1 year's duration, with rifampicin (RMP) administered for 1 year, is efficacious in the treatment of multibacillary (MB) leprosy. However, there is a need for close supervision of patients so treated. The applicability of this regimen would be simplified if the supervised phase could be shortened to 6 months. In a prospective

peutic trial, 289 patients with MB leprosy in Zaire and Rwanda received treatment with 1 of the following regimens: a 6-month supervised daily regimen of 600 mg of RMP, 500 mg of ethionamide (ETH), and 100 mg of dapsone (DDS) or 100 mg of clofazimine (CLO), followed by a 6-month unsupervised daily regimen of 100 mg of DDS or 100 mg of CLO with or without 500 mg of ETH. The mean duration of follow-up was 3.88 years.

Clinical and bactericidal results were excellent. The mean annual decrease in the bacteriologic index was 1.01 units per year. No relapses occurred during the 1,121 person-years of follow-up. The addition of ETH during the second 6 months of therapy did not improve any of the results. The incidences of hepatotoxicity, reversal, and erythema nodosum leprosum reactions were similar to those previously reported in the combined regimen of 1 year's duration.

It is possible to treat MB leprosy successfully with a 1-year combined regimen with RMP administered for the first 6 months. However, because the incidence of hepatotoxicity remains unacceptable, other alternative short-course therapies need to be tested.

▶ Again, the authors demonstrate that a short course of therapy with multidrugs may be effective. In an attempt to reduce the hepatic toxicity, and thus the necessity for closer supervision, rifampin was administered for only 6 months; even so, hepatotoxicity remained an unacceptable complication. This again reinforces the need for alternative regimens that are less toxic and more applicable in difficult field situations, among which are the lack of adequate laboratory facilities.—S.L. Moschella, M.D.

Erythema Induratum (Bazin's Disease)

Rademaker M, Lowe DG, Munro DD (St Bartholomew's Hosp, London)
J Am Acad Dermatol 21:740–745, October 1989 12–6

Erythema induratum is a chronic nodular eruption on women's legs. Its cause is still disputed. Many researchers believe the disease has a tuberculous origin. Clinical and pathologic findings in 26 patients with erythema induratum were reviewed to determine whether tuberculosis was a likely cause.

The cutaneous lesions were characteristically violaceous, indurated, 1–2 cm in diameter, and painful (Fig 12–3). They were sometimes ulcerated and could heal with scarring. A strongly positive Mantoux test result and clearing of lesions after antituberculosis therapy confirmed the diagnosis in all cases. The histologic features varied, but they were mostly those of a vasculitis with a paraseptal and lobular panniculitis. The criteria to fulfill the diagnosis of tuberculosis in the lesions could not be met. However, sufficient circumstantial evidence supported the hypothesis that erythema induratum is a true tuberculid.

Erythema induratum is not rare and is often misdiagnosed. The initial Mantoux test must be done with a 1:10,000 dilution because ulcerative

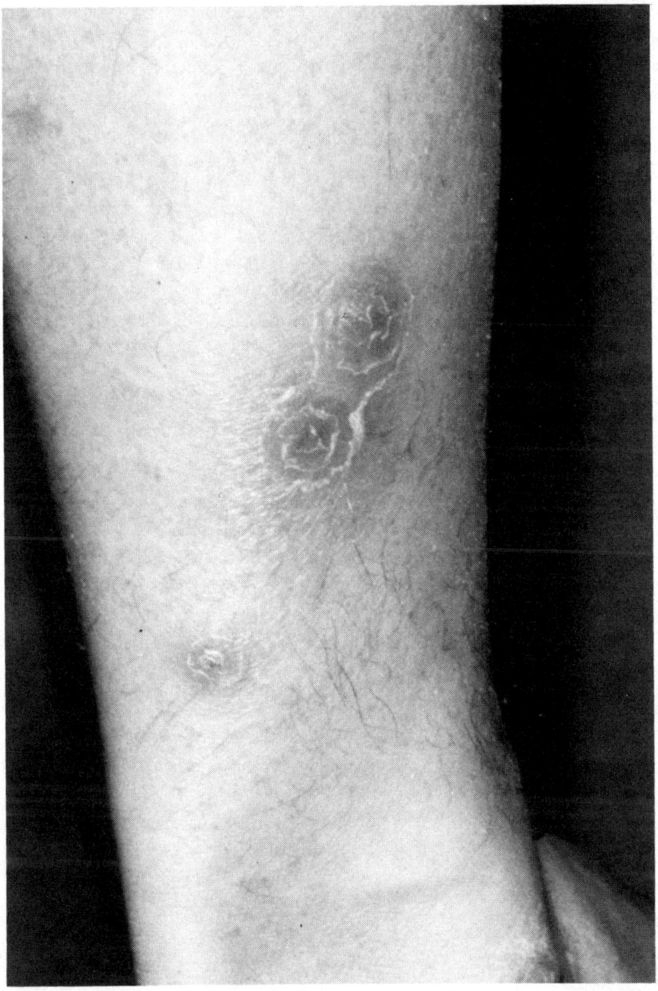

Fig 12–3.—Classic ulcerating erythematous nodules, 1–2 cm in diameter, of erythema induratum. (Courtesy of Rademaker M, Lowe DG, Munro DD: *J Am Acad Dermatol* 21:740–745, October 1989.)

reactions may result with a dilution of 1:1,000. Clinicians must be careful to inject the Mantoux test material into the dermis and not into the subcutis or false negative results may be obtained. Patients with erythema induratum require a full course of antituberculosis therapy: 9 months of triple-agent treatment.

▶ It appears that patients with the erythema induratum-nodular vasculitis complex can be divided into 2 groups: 1 rarely associated with tuberculosis (Bazin's disease) and the other unassociated. Erythema induratum (Bazin's disease) is rare in the United States and is seen occasionally in immigrants from areas having a relatively high incidence of tuberculosis. It is more easily suspected in the patient with active tuberculosis (1) than in a patient with a temporal association manifested by a positive skin test. No acid-fast bacilli are demonstrable in the skin biopsy specimen or its culture. Some of these patients may have an accompanying more superficial, symmetrical, papular necrotic eruption, the so-called papulonecrotic tuberculid (2).—S.L. Moschella, M.D.

References

1. Hassou PM, et al: *Am J Med* 84:784, 1988.
2. Chen AMK, Graham-Brown RAC: *Clin Exp Dermatol* 15:21, 1990.

13 Melanocytic Nevi and Melanoma

Racial Differences in Mole Proneness

Rampen FHJ, de Wit PEJ (Sint Ana Hosp, Oss; Univ of Nijmegen, The Netherlands)

Acta Derm Venereol (Stockh) 69:234–271, 1989 13–1

Hereditary factors, such as skin complexion, may be related to the frequency of pigmented nevi. Racial differences in the number of nevocytic nevi were studied in 14 nonwhite children aged 7–13 years, 31 nonwhite adults aged 18–30, and 2 age- and sex-matched white controls for each group.

Total mole counts were significantly higher in the white groups than in the nonwhite groups. In children, the median total number of nevocytic nevi was 17 in whites and 2.5 in nonwhites. Similarly, in young adults the total mole count was 61 and 16 in whites and nonwhites, respectively. In a subgroup of students with moles 2 mm in diameter, whites again had a higher median count than nonwhites. The median number of moles steadily declined from "fair" to "dark" skin complexion. The highest number were found in individuals of white complexion, followed by those of mixed or Oriental ancestry. The lowest number were found in blacks.

There is a strong racial background predisposing to the development of nevocytic nevi. This is the first study to indicate a relationship between nevocytic nevi and phenotypic factors.

▶ This study suggests that racial differences in melanoma risk may be related to mole proneness rather than skin color per se. It is important to remember that the prevalence of darkly pigmented lesions on acral surfaces has been associated with melanoma in blacks. Dysplastic nevi have not been described in blacks. Lentigo maligna is a disease of whites, not blacks. Congenital nevi occur in 1% of all races. Still, after all is said and done, the mole factor needs to be reconciled with the sun factor in melanoma causation. This study goes a long way in correlating mole proneness with race.—A.R. Rhodes, M.D., M.P.H.

Frequency of Acquired Melanonevocytic Nevi and Their Relationship to Skin Complexion in 939 Schoolchildren

Sigg C, Pelloni F (Univ Hosp of Zurich)

Dermatologica 179:123–128, 1989 13–2

The increased frequency of cutaneous malignant melanoma (CMM) appears to be related to the increased number of common melanonevocytic nevi (MNN); MNN occurrence is closely associated with skin complexion. However, this phenomenon in children is not well understood. The number of moles in prepubertal and pubertal white children related to skin complexion was determined on the basis of a differentiated classification of skin pigment content in 939 schoolchildren, aged 8–16 years.

Skin complexions were categorized into 1 of 7 types. Anamnestic data on tanning ability and history of sunburns were not considered. The mean nevus count was 17.97. This count was significantly higher in boys than in girls and increased with age. The mean nevus number was clearly related to skin complexion. Nevi were most frequent in children with fair skin types and decreased in number as pigment content increased. Children with freckles had higher mean nevus counts in every category of skin complexion. Complexion type and freckles appear to be risk factors for mole proneness.

▶ The relationship among skin type, freckling, and nevus counts has been investigated numerous times. This is yet another study that investigates the same issue, with the null hypothesis that skin type has nothing to do with nevi. In fact, the null hypothesis is rejected based on the data presented. However, this study will be difficult to reproduce. Macular and raised nevi and freckles were counted but the distinguishing characteristics of these lesins were not well defined. One might expect increased numbers of nevi in frecklers if one lesion is not clearly distinguished from the other.—A.R. Rhodes, M.D., M.P.H.

Excess Benign Melanocytic Naevi After Chemotherapy for Malignancy in Childhood

Hughes BR, Cunliffe WJ, Bailey CC (Gen Infirmary, Leeds; Seacroft Hosp, Leeds, England)

Br Med J 299:88–91, July 8, 1989 13–3

Patients who survive immunosuppressive therapy are at an increased risk of cutaneous infection and tumor. Effective chemotherapy for leukemia or lymphoma in some children appears to be followed by the development of an excess number of moles. A blind comparison of treated patients with age- and sex-matched control patients was carried out. The study group included 32 patients who received chemotherapy for acute lymphatic leukemia, lymphoma, or rhabdomyosarcoma.

Patients who completed chemotherapy had the most moles, which occurred chiefly on the trunk but also on the extremities. Macular, papular, and pigmented moles all were seen. More treated patients than controls had acral moles. The findings were independent of acute ultraviolet light exposure and skin type.

Children with an increased number of moles after receiving chemotherapy for malignancy may have an increased risk of melanoma. They, therefore, should be closely observed and cautioned about excessive exposure to ultraviolet light.

▶ Hughes et al. demonstrate a greater number of "moles" (clinically defined) in children who had completed chemotherapy for malignancy than in children who were actively receiving chemotherapy or in sex- and age-matched children in a dermatology outpatient clinic. This finding is consistent with observations of oncologists and parents of affected children. Assuming that the observation is real, the possible mechanisms are interesting to contemplate. It will be important to repeat this study using treated patients as their own controls (during and after chemotherapy).—A.R. Rhodes, M.D., M.P.H.

Dysplastic Melanocytic Nevi: A Reproducible Histologic Definition Emphasizing Cellular Morphology

Rhodes AR, Mihm MC Jr, Weinstock MA (Massachusetts Gen Hosp, Boston; Harvard Med School; Va Med Ctr, Providence, RI)

Mod Pathol 2:306–319, July 1989 13–4

Various diagnostic histologic criteria have been proposed for dysplastic melanocytic nevi (DMN), but none has been adequately correlated with biology or subjected to rigorous reproducibility studies. To address these failings, histologic criteria emphasizing cellular morphology were developed. The histologic definitions were based on the appearance of typical melanocytes in sun-protected buttock skin, fully evolved atypia in the vertical component of metastasizing primary cutaneous melanomas, and slight or moderate degrees of atypia defined within these limits in selected varieties of DMN (table). The minimum definition of DMN was hyperplasia of intraepidermal melanocytes manifesting variable and discontinuous cellular atypia in a lentiginous epidermal pattern.

Single routine tissue sections of 19 melanocytic lesions were studied by 2 pathologists on 2 occasions at least 6 months apart to assess the reproducibility of histologic criteria. The lesions included 5 previously diagnosed primary invasive cutaneous melanomas, 7 lesions selected for gross morphological features characteristic of DMN, 4 solar lentigines, and 3 common acquired nevomelanocytic nevi preselected for typical appearance and stable growth history.

For the primary pathologist, agreement rates between first and second readings were 84% for final diagnosis and 79% for the highest degree of cellular atypia. For the secondary pathologist, agreement rates for the first and second readings were 84% for both parameters. Agreement rates for the second reading by both pathologists were 89% for the final diagnosis and 79% for the highest degree of cellular atypia. Agreement rates for most architectural and host response features commonly associated with DMN were less reproducible for both pathologists.

These data suggest the potential for good reproducibility of histologic definitions used to differentiate the intraepidermal component of DMN from that of melanoma and benign melanocytic and nevomelanocytic hy-

Definitions of Cellular Morphology for Intraepidermal Melanocytes as Seen in Routinely Prepared Paraffin-Embedded Tissue Sections*

Feature	Normal†	Degree of cellular atypia in intraepidermal melanocytes: Slight	Moderate	Fully evolved ‡
Nucleus				
Area	Normal (N)§	1.5–2N	>2N	>2N
Variability in shape and size	Minimal	Marked	Marked	Marked
Chromatin	Small, regular aggregates in finely granular homogenous background	Condensed, with loss of all detail	Attenuated, widely spaced aggregates in pale background with condensation on nucleolar membranes	Few, large, irregular aggregates with pale, almost empty background, and condensation on nuclear membranes
Nucleolus	Not visible	Not visible	Large, pale, often multiple	Lavender, often multiple
Cytoplasm				
Quantity	Rarely visible	Small rim, eccentric around nucleus	Increased, eccentric around nucleus	Fully expanded around nucleus
Quality		Densely pink	Pink, pale, finely granular	Pink and finely granular, often bipolar streaming

*Routine sections embedded in paraffin, cut at 4 μm, and stained with hematoxylin-eosin.
†Defined as similar in appearance to single intraepidermal melanocytes in sun-protected buttock skin.
‡Defined as similar in appearance to the vertical component of invasive cutaneous melanomas that have metastasized to lymph nodes, viscera, or distant cutaneous sites.
§Normal size of intraepidermal melanocyte nucleus defined as about one half to two thirds the area of a basal keratinocyte nucleus.
(Courtesy of Rhodes AR, Mihm MC Jr, Weinstock MA: *Mod Pathol* 2:306–319, July 1989.)

perplasias based on a biologic correlation emphasizing cellular morphology.

▶ There is a spectrum of abnormalities in dysplastic nevi, and there are subtle differences at either end of this spectrum in the differentiation of slightly atypical dysplastic nevi from typical nevomelanocytic nevi on the one hand and markedly atypical dysplastic nevi from intraepidermal melanoma on the other. This study is a demonstration of a reproducible scheme for assessing the histology of melanocytic tumors. The concept of such a grading scheme is relevant to epidemiologic and experimental studies of melanoma and melanoma precursors, as well as communication among clinicians and pathologists. With recent papers by Klein (1) and Black and Hunt (2) demonstrating that many architectural features of dysplastic nevi are present in clinically benign appearing nevi, the absence of degrees of atypia greater than slight gives further importance to the need of reproducible grading systems.—A.J. Sober, M.D.

References

1. Klein LJ: *J Am Acad Dermatol* 22:275, 1990.
2. Black WC, Hunt WC: *Am J Surg Pathol* 14:44, 1990.

The Dysplastic Melanocytic Nevus: A Prevalent Lesion That Correlates Poorly With Clinical Phenotype

Piepkorn M, Meyer LJ, Goldgar D, Seuchter SA, Cannon-Albright LA, Skolnick MH, Zone JJ (Univ of Utah; VA Med Ctr, Salt Lake City)
J Am Acad Dermatol 20:407–415, March 1989 13–5

The diagnostic criteria for dysplastic nevus syndrome have not been defined. A review of the literature suggests that melanoma-prone families are at increased risk for dysplastic nevi. However, genetic modeling has not conclusively identified the dysplastic nevus syndrome phenotype as a genetic trait. Furthermore, recent reports have suggested that the prevalence of dysplastic nevi in the general population may be significantly higher than estimated previously. The prevalence of dysplastic nevi and the relationship between histopathologic features and clinical phenotype were investigated in 521 Caucasians with dysplastic nevi, representing 34 kindreds.

Biopsies were performed on the lesions of more than 80% of the participants. The rate of dysplastic nevi in the general population was estimated by examining spouses as controls. Two lesions, thought most likely to harbor histologic dysplasia, were selected for biopsy. All histologic findings were recorded without knowledge of clinical status. On the basis of the findings in the biopsy specimens, a grading scheme of histologic dysplasia was developed.

The prevalence of white persons who had histologic dysplasia in at least 1 of the 2 nevi selected for biopsy was 53%. This high prevalence was unexpected and indicated that such lesions may represent a normal variant of melanocytic nevi, perhaps those in the process of active proliferation. Comparison of histologic and clinical findings revealed that dysplasia was not related to lesion size, as lesions 3 mm in diameter or smaller were as likely to be dysplastic as the much larger ones. However, there was a statistically significant relationship between histologic dysplasia of a nevus and a patient's total number of melanocytic lesions.

The unexpected findings suggest that histologic dysplasia may occur as a normal phase of all melanocytic nevi, perhaps reflecting an active phase of radial growth. The data bring into question the clinical significance of a dysplastic nevus as an isolated finding, even though other studies have suggested that dysplastic nevi are histogenetic precursors for melanoma.

▶ The authors conclude that 53% of adult whites in Utah have at least 1 nevus displaying histologic dysplasia. However, their definition of dysplasia is based on architectural changes only, not requiring cellular atypia; cellular atypia is reserved for the definition of melanoma in situ. In other words, the definition for dysplastic nevus is not the same as that described in the classic studies of dysplastic moles and familial melanoma. One can only conclude from these studies that certain architectural changes are quite common in "typical nevi."—A.R. Rhodes, M.D., M.P.H.

Dysplastic Naevi in a Population-Based Survey

Cooke KR, Spears GFS, Elder DE, Greene MH (Univ of Otago, Dunedin, New Zealand; Hosp of the Univ of Pennsylvania; Natl Cancer Inst, Bethesda)
Cancer 63:1240–1244, Apr 15, 1989 13–6

The prevalence of dysplastic nevi was studied in a population-based survey of 380 non-Maoris aged 30–39 and 50–59, in Milton, a small town in the south of New Zealand. Photographs of pigmented nevi of ≥4 mm in diameter were evaluated by 2 experienced reviewers.

At least 1 dysplastic nevus was noted in 9% of the natives. The percentage was higher in men and younger individuals. There was a strong association between the total number of moles ≥2 mm in diameter and the presence of dysplastic nevi. Persons with 3 or more dysplastic nevi were 40 times more likely to have 50 or more moles ≥2 mm in diameter. Furthermore, the association between numbers of nevi and numbers of dysplastic nevi also was evident when independent judgments on individual nevi were collated.

These findings suggest that, in the general population, dysplastic nevi may be markers of an expended nevus cell system. Interobserver agreement on the diagnosis of dysplastic nevi was 85%. Dysplastic nevi are more common than previously estimated and are associated with an increased number of common moles.

▶ This study documents a high prevalence of dysplastic melanocytic nevi (DMN) in a population aged 30–39 and one aged 50–59, about 9% overall having at least 1 DMN and 4% having 3 or more, based on photographic assessment. Biopsies were not obtained, and criteria were not clearly stated. The high prevalence rate of DMN in this population in a small New Zealand town may be real (and relate to a unique high-risk group) or be biased by methods of ascertainment or selection. The true prevalence of DMN in the general population is central to estimating the relative risk for melanoma. This risk may be assessed using case/control methodology based on numbers of nevi over a certain diameter, numbers of atypical-appearing nevi, or the degree of cellular atypia in nevi. This paper begins to address one method of assessment.—A.R. Rhodes, M.D., M.P.H.

An Assessment of the Value of Ag NOR Staining in the Identification of Dysplastic and Other Borderline Melanocytic Naevi

MacKie RM, White SI, Seywright MM, Young H (Univ of Glasgow)

Br J Dermatol 120:511–516, 1989 13–7

Nucleolar organizer regions (NORs) are loops of ribosomal DNA in nuclei that direct formation of both ribosome and protein. In humans, NORs are found on the 5 acrocentric chromosomes 13–15, 21, and 22. The Ag NOR technique identifies argyrophilic NOR-associated proteins in a highly specific manner. Studies were made in 106 melanocytic lesions to assess the Ag NOR technique. Counts were possible in 79 instances.

The Ag NOR counts in banal melanocytic nevi were low. Malignant melanocytic lesions, in contrast, had high Ag NOR counts. No significant differences existed among lentigo maligna melanoma, superficial spreading melanoma, and secondary melanoma. Dysplastic nevi, Spitz nevi, and spindle nevi of Reed all had low Ag NOR counts in the range of banal nevi. The Ag NOR counts were similar in primary and secondary melanomas, and were not clearly related to tumor thickness. The Ag NOR method may have value in distinguishing difficult or borderline nevi from frank malignant melanomas.

▶ The authors attempted to determine whether the mean number of NORs may be a way of distinguishing intermediate lesions from banal nevi and melanoma. Although there was a suggestion that a greater proportion of cells in the intermediate lesions had a higher number of NORs than in the banal lesions, the mean number of NORs per specimen was not significantly different. Of note, the authors relate that about 25% of specimens were not evaluable because of excessive melanin. This may be an important limiting factor in implementing such a test. The histologic criteria used to separate intermediate lesions from banal and malignant lesions were not stated.—A.R. Rhodes, M.D., M.P.H.

Silver Staining of Nucleolar Organizer Regions in Malignant Melanoma and Melanotic Nevi

Leong AS-Y, Gilham P (Inst of Medical and Veterinary Science, Adelaide, South Australia)

Hum Pathol 20:257–262, March 1989 13–8

Nucleolar organizer regions (NORs) are chromosomal regions that can be detected in the nuclei of cells actively transcribe ribosomal RNA genes. A simplified silver staining technique was developed that allows NORs to be stained in paraffin sections. This staining technique was applied to 5 junctional nevi, 13 compound nevi, 7 Spitz nevi, 9 cellular blue nevi, 11 dysplastic nevi, 7 malignant lentigines, 12 superficial spreading melanomas, and 14 secondary melanomas to determine whether it could be used to distinguish between benign and malignant lesions.

Among the 45 benign lesions examined the mean number of NORs detected was 1.22. Among the 33 melanomas examined the mean number of NORs detected was 9.18. This difference was both significant and easily recognized on microscopic examination of silver-stained paraffin sections. The silver staining technique for NORs in paraffin sections may be useful in distinguishing malignant from benign lesions. It may reflect tumor cell proliferation and indicate prognosis.

▶ The numbers of AgNORs appear to be higher in the malignant lesions compared with the benign ones. The dysplastic nevi could not be differentiated from the other benign nevi in this study. The cases of lentigo maligna were not distinguishable from the primary and metastatic melanomas. Cytoplasmic melanin is also stained by the silver colloidal solution used in this technique, so there may be difficulty in evaluating heavily melanized tumors. This technique is worthy of further study.—A.R. Rhodes, M.D., M.P.H.

Cyanoacrylate Skin Surface Stripping: An Improved Approach for Distinguishing Dysplastic Nevi From Malignant Melanomas

Piérard GE, Piérard-Franchimont C, Arrese Estrada J, Delvoye P, Henry C, Damseaux M, Lê T, Hermans JF, Letot B, Mélotte P, Van Cauwenberge D, Ben Mosbah T, Gharbi R (Univ of Liège; Centre Hospitalier Hutois, Huy; Hôp Sainte Ode, Baconfoy; Centre de Diagnostic, Verviers; Hôp Miliaire Saint Laurent, Lieġe, Belgium; et al)

J Cutan Pathol 16:180–182, August 1989 13–9

The clinical distinction between dysplastic nevi and early evolving superficial spreading melanomas has been difficult. Conventional histologic study of an excised lesion is still considered the best way to reach the correct diagnosis of atypical melanocytic lesions, but there is a practical limit to the number of lesions that can be removed. A new technique, cyanoacrylate skin surface stripping (CSSS), was used to search for atypical melanocytes. The technique is based on the transepidermal migration of neoplastic cells being an early feature of superficial spreading melanomas, whereas atypical melanocytes of dysplastic nevi are confined to the deeper epidermis. The sensitivity and specificity of the CSSS method were evaluated over a 10-year period.

The study material consisted of 117 CSSS samples obtained from superficial spreading malignant melanomas from all regions of the body except the palms, soles, and genitalia and 98 CSSS samples obtained from

from pigmented neoplasms in 9 patients with the dysplastic nevus syndrome. Of the 117 superficial spreading malignant melanomas, 114 contained atypical melanocytes that appeared as oval or irregular cells containing nuclei and variable amounts of melanin. These cells were easily distinguished from other cell types. Three malignant melanomas had no atypical melanocytes in the stratum corneum. None of the 94 CSSS samples taken from dysplastic nevi contained melanocytes.

The CSSS method is an additional noninvasive procedure that is useful in the differential diagnosis of dysplastic nevi and malignant melanomas. The method is specific and sensitive and it is technically easy.

▶ This cytologic technique is an imaginative approach to an increasingly difficult management problem. Some caution should be exercised, however. The technique may take experience to master, particularly the interpretation of cytology. Also, of the 117 melanomas diagnosed, only 114 showed atypical melanocytes in the stratum corneum. Conceivably, there are evolving melanomas or melanomas on noncutaneous surfaces that may not show upward migration of atypical melanocytes. Note that melanomas on the acral and genital surfaces were excluded in this study. This method requires further investigation.—A.R. Rhodes, M.D., M.P.H.

Effect of Oral Isotretinoin on Dysplastic Nevi

Edwards L, Meyskens F, Levine N (Univ of Arizona; Tucson VA Med Ctr)

J Am Acad Dermatol 20:257–260, February 1989 13–10

Dysplastic nevi are direct melanoma precursors and markers for the risk of development of cutaneous melanoma. Surgical removal is impractical, and there are no known behavior adaptations to decrease the risk. Because favorable histologic responses have been noted in cutaneous melanoma metastases after application of topical retinoic acid, the effects of orally administered isotretinoin (Accutane) on dysplastic nevi were investigated.

Dysplastic nevi from 10 men and 1 woman were photographed and biopsy specimens were obtained. Dysplastic nevi were confirmed histologically before treatment. All patients were given Accutane orally, 40 mg twice daily for 4 months. Complete blood cell counts, blood chemistry studies, and urinalysis were performed at baseline and monthly thereafter. Studied dysplastic nevi were rephotographed and biopsy was again performed at cessation of treatment.

Eight patients completed the treatment. No clinical changes in the dysplastic nevi were observed. Analysis of biopsy specimens from the remaining lesions in 6 volunteers revealed that most lesions were dysplastic nevi. In 2 patients most of the lesions studied were normal benign nevi. This rate (28%) of normal benign nevi corresponds to that in other reports. With the treatment schedule used, oral administration of isotretinoin apparently has no significant biologic or clinical effect on the histologic appearance of dysplastic nevi. The recommended management continues to be regular follow-up, photographic documentation, and early biopsy to determine potentially curable cutaneous melanomas.

▶ Isotretinoin at an oral dosage of 40 mg twice daily for 4 months had no clinical or histologic effect on dysplastic nevi. This study was undertaken because of the observation of regression of metastatic cutaneous melanoma in 2 patients and "a more normal" histologic appearance of dysplastic nevi in 2 of 3 patients when lesions were treated topically with retinoic acid solution 0.05% under tape occlusion for 4 months. This sort of therapy should still be regarded as experimental.—A.R. Rhodes, M.D., M.P.H.

Histopathology of Congenital Pigmented Nevi

Everett MA (Univ of Oklahoma, Oklahoma City)

Am J Dermatopathol 11:11–12, February 1989 13–11

Histologic criteria are often used to distinguish between congenital and acquired pigmented nevi. Deep dermal involvement, aggregation in appendageal structures, and infiltration of single nevus cells between collagen bundles are considered very suggestive of congenital pigmented nevi. When these histologic features are observed in nevi associated with melanoma, it is presumed that the melanoma originated in a congenital pigmented nevi. The diagnostic features of this lesion and that assumption were investigated in 39 congenital pigmented nevi removed from children younger than 10 years. Multiple sections from each of the removed lesions were examined. Photographs taken at birth or neonatal data had confirmed the congenital status of the removed nevi.

Most of the smaller nevi did not have the features supposedly diagnostic of congenital pigmented nevi, whereas nearly all of the larger ones did have such features (table). The histologic features traditionally associated with these lesions apparently pertain primarily to the size of the nevus, rather than to the time of its appearance. Because small congenital pig-

Congenital Pigmented Nevi by Size and by Histologic Pattern

	Pattern			
Size (cm)	Superficial	Intermediate	Deep	Total
<1.5	9[a]	0	0	9
1.5–3	4	2	1	7
3–10	5	4	5	14
>10	1	2	6	9
Total	19	8	12	39

Pearson chi-square = 17.851 (P = .007) and linear trend analysis = 13.288 (P = .0003).

[a]Two of the small nevi were pedunculated, and nevus cells extended to the fat within the pedicle.

(Courtesy of Everett MA: *Am J Dermatopathol* 11:11–12, February 1989.)

mented nevi are much more common than large ones, histologic examination is not a reliable method for identifying this lesion.

▶ The author documents what has been demonstrated before in at least 3 other studies, namely, that small nevi present at birth (according to family documentation) may not have the histologic features classically associated with large varieties of congenital nevi. This study investigated the sensitivity of the classic histologic features in 39 congenital pigmented nevi. The specificity of the classic features was not investigated in a group of well-documented acquired nevi. Based on this study, no additional statements can be made about the usefulness of the "classic congenital features" of nevi in contiguity with melanoma.—A.R. Rhodes, M.D., M.P.H.

Congenital Giant Hairy Nevus: Implications for Treatment

Llaneras MR, Morgan RF, Pham ST, Paley RJ, Kaulbach HC, Clapp CG, Edlich RF (Univ of Virginia, Charlottesville)

J Emerg Med 7:25–28, January–February 1989 13–12

Congenital giant hairy nevi are predisposed to become malignant melanomas. The history of a patient with such a lesion and new data on the diagnosis and treatment of these dermatologic lesions were reviewed.

Man, 24, was seen for treatment of an unrelated illness. Physical examination of the medial aspect of the right arm revealed a brown skin lesion 25 × 20 cm with irregular margins and multiple satellite lesions around the periphery of the nevus. The lesion contained numerous papillomatous projections and long hairs. The patient said he had the lesion since birth, and that he had been advised that the only indications for removal were cosmetic. The lesion was diagnosed as a giant hairy nevus that had a significant risk of converting to malignant melanoma. It was excised with a 1-cm margin of uninvolved skin. The excision extended to the fascia, and all underlying subcutaneous tissue was removed. The defect was covered with a split-thickness skin graft.

Congenital giant hairy nevi always are discernible because of their size. These lesions can be distinguished histologically and clinically from acquired nevi and have a potential for progressing to malignancy. Prompt, complete excision of all congenital giant hairy nevi is recommended.

▶ The authors describe a 24-year-old man who visited their medical facility several times before his large congenital nevus was noticed. The lesion was eventually excised, and the histology was benign. The authors provide their interpretation of available information about the malignant potential and management of congenital nevi.—A.R. Rhodes, M.D., M.P.H.

An Approach to Excision of Congenital Giant Pigmented Nevi in Infancy and Early Childhood

Bauer BS, Vicari FA (Children's Mem Hosp, Chicago)
Plast Reconstr Surg 82:1012–1021, December 1988 13–13

Complete prophylactic excision of congenital giant pigmented nevi in infancy and early childhood has been recommended, but the multiple procedures required to achieve this purpose frustrate many surgeons. A timely coordinated approach to complete excision of congenital giant pigmented nevi is based on the coordinated use of early grafting, tissue expansion, and combined graft/flap coverage. Complete excision of giant nevi of the head and neck, trunk, or an extremity based on this approach was undertaken in 78 patients aged 3 months to 12 years at the time of initial nevus excision. The nevi covered a minimum of 2% to 45% of the total body surface area.

Giant nevi of the scalp were treated most effectively with tissue expansion, beginning as early as 3 months of age. For giant nevi of the face, tissue expansion of the forehead, neck, and cheek facilitated early complete excision. Large expanded full-thickness skin grafts proved invaluable in obtaining single-unit, color-compatible skin coverage of the periorbital/nasal area. Giant nevi of the trunk were treated using a combination of abdominoplasty technique, tissue expansion, and split-thickness skin graft. Extensive nevi of the posterior trunk and buttocks were best treated with early "large segment" excision and immediate sheet grafting. Excision and grafting was the best treatment modality for extensive lesions of the extremity, and expanded full-thickness skin grafts gave excellent coverage on the hands and feet. Most circumferential lesions in the extremities could be excised in 2 stages, the extensor and flexor surfaces.

Timely use of combined modalities of tissue expansion, early excision, and reconstruction beginning in infancy for congenital giant pigmented nevi may minimize the risk of malignant transformation as well as the late psychological sequelae caused by the appearance of the lesion. In addition, this combined approach may significantly improve the final cosmetic result.

▶ *Complete* excision of many giant congenital nevi is not possible because of size, location, multifocality of associated smaller congenital nevi, and the tendency of nevus cells in these lesions to penetrate deeply within the skin, sometimes into underlying muscle or within the covering membranes of the brain and/or spinal cord. The greatest concern for malignant degeneration has been noted during the first 5 years of life. In contrast, the risk of small congenital nevi progressing to melanoma seems greatest after puberty. Given the above information, surgical intervention, if to be effective, would have to occur early in life for patients with giant congenital nevi, but the prophylactic removal of normal-appearing "small" congenital nevi can be deferred until around the time of puberty. This article outlines one approach to the removal of giant congenital nevi. Another approach involves use of the patient's own cultured keratinocytes for coverage of the defect.—A.J. Sober, M.D.

Typical, Dysplastic, Congenital, and Spitz Nevi: A Comparative Immunohistochemical Study

Palazzo J, Duray PH (Yale Univ)

Hum Pathol 20:341–346, April 1989 13–14

The antigenic profile of malignant melanoma has been well characterized. To further delineate benign nevi, formalin-fixed paraffin sections of 44 cutaneous nevi were examined immunohistochemically with melanocyte-specific HMB.45, S-100 protein, RAP-5, epithelial membrane antigen, and neuron-specific enolase (NSE) antibodies.

Of the 44 tumors, 13 were typical; 7, congenital; 12, dysplastic; and 12, Spitz nevi. Epithelial membrane antigen and RAP-5 were negative in all 44 tumors. The antibody HMB.45 reacted strongly with the epidermal component and weakly with the dermal component in the typical nevi (Table 1). There was a heterogeneous reaction in the junctional component of dysplastic, congenital, and Spitz nevi with this antibody (Tables 2 and 3). All nevomelanocytes were labeled with S-100 protein. In some of the dysplastic nevi the reaction to this antibody was heterogeneous. Neuron-specific enolase stained the central component in some Spitz nevi more than the lateral component.

Because S-100 protein and NSE stained fairly uniformly, they were not very useful in distinguishing between the subsets of these benign nevi. The monoclonal antibody HMB.45 demonstrated heterogeneous staining

TABLE 1.—Immunohistochemical Staining of Typical Nevi

Case No.	Histology	S-100 Protein	HMB.45	NSE
1 (738)	Intradermal nevus	5+	1+*	5+
2 (7116)	Intradermal nevus	5+	1+	5+
3 (11278)	Intradermal nevus	5+	1+	5+
4 (4636)	Intradermal nevus	5+	4+	5+
5 (11979)	Intradermal nevus	5+	0	4+
6 (7116)	Junctional nevus (1)	0	4+	5+
7 (8588)	Junctional nevus	2+	4+	4+
8 (4874)	Junctional nevus	4+	5+	4+
9 (7116)	Junctional nevus (2)	3+	1+	5+
10 (11278)	Junctional nevus	4+	2+	5+
11 (2337)	Blue nevus	4+	Not interpreted	
12 (8450)	Junctional nevus	4+	2+	5+
13 (8248B)	Compound nevus	4+	2+	4+

Note: Percentage of cells staining: 0, negative; 1+, 0 to 25%; 2+, 25% to 50%; 3+, 50% to 75%; 4+, 75% to 90%; 5+, 90% to 100%.

*Scattered B-45 reactivity in papillary dermal nevomelanocytes.

(Courtesy of Palazzo J, Duray PH: *Hum Pathol* 20:341–346, April 1989.)

TABLE 2.—Immunohistochemical Staining of Spitz Nevi

Case No.	Histology	S-100 Protein	HMB.45	NSE
1 (12133)	Atypical Spitz nevus	5+	2+	4+
2 (4617)	Junctional Spitz nevus	4+	2+	3+
3 (7516)	Atypical Spitz nevus	4+	3+	3+
4 (7894)	Desmoplastic Spitz nevus	4+	0	4+
5 (13691)	Classic Spitz nevus	3+	2+	2+
6 (4617)	Classic Spitz nevus	4+	2+	3+
7 (12591)	Classic Spitz nevus	5+	2+	4+
8 (13691)	Compound Spitz nevus	4+	1+	3+
9 (3056)	Pigmented staining of Spitz nevus	4+	5+	2+
10 (8058)	Desmoplastic Spitz nevus	3+	3+	4+
11 (3700)	Classic Spitz nevus	4+	2+	5+
12 (11479)	Classic Spitz nevus	4+	0	3+

Note: Percentage of cells stained: 0, negative; 1+, 0 to25%; 2+, 25% to 50%; 3+, 50% to 75%; 4+, 75% to 90%; 5+, 90% to 100%.
(Courtesy of Palazzo J, Duray PH: *Hum Pathol* 20:341–346, April 1989.)

TABLE 3.—Immunohistochemical Staining of Dysplastic and Congenital Nevi

Case No.	Histology	S-100 Protein	HMB.45	NSE
1 (8311)	Dysplastic nevus	4+	0	4+
2 (6990B)	Dysplastic nevus	4+	1+	5+
3 (8337)	Dysplastic nevus	5+	2+	4+
4 (1690C)	Dysplastic nevus	4+	2+	4+
5 (2323C)	Dysplastic nevus	4+	2+	4+
6 (8232)	Dysplastic nevus	3+	2+	5+
7 (8365B)	Dysplastic nevus	4+	0	4+
8 (1691B)	Dysplastic nevus	3+	1+	3+
9 (8245)	Dysplastic nevus	4+	1+	4+
10 (8528B)	Dysplastic nevus	4+	2+	5+
11 (15195)	Dysplastic nevus	5+	2+	4+
12 (1490)	Dysplastic nevus	4+	5+	4+
13 (11673)	Congenital nevus	4+	4+	5+
14 (5619)	Congenital nevus	4+	2+	5+
15 (10563)	Congenital nevus	4+	0	5+
16 (10563-B2)	Congenital nevus	5+	1+	5+
17 (8745-A2)	Congenital nevus	4+	0	4+
18 (6366)	Congenital nevus	4+	0	4+
19 (11673)	Congenital nevus	3+	2+	5+

Note: Percentage of staining: 0, negative; 1+, 0 to25%; 2+, 25% to 50%; 3+, 50% to 75%; 4+, 75% to 90%; 5+, 90% to 100%.
(Courtesy of Palazzo J, Duray PH: *Hum Pathol* 20:341–346, April 1989.)

in all nevus subtypes, particularly in the junctional zones. Dysplastic nevi were the most likely to have HMB.45 staining, although with weak reactivity. At times, HMB.45 and S-100 demonstrated an inverse expression. The significance of this relationship is not yet known.

▶ This paper emphasizes the heterogeneity of immunohistochemical studies on a variety of nevi. The biological significance of these differences is not clear. This study is an interesting counterpoint to some of the articles on immunohistochemical studies of malignant melanoma.—T.J. Flotte, M.D.

Deep Penetrating Nevus

Seab JA Jr, Graham JH, Helwig EB (Armed Forces Inst of Pathology, Washington, DC)

Am J Surg Pathol 13:39–44, January 1989 13–15

Because of their characteristic cellular pleomorphism and deep infiltration of the reticular dermis, lesions of the deep penetrating nevus (DPN) are frequently misinterpreted as malignant melanoma by pathologists. Findings in a series of 70 patients were reviewed to define and document the diagnostic histologic features and clinical behavior of this cutaneous pigmented lesion.

Each patient had a single melanocytic lesion termed a DPN. Lesions occurred most often on the face, upper trunk, or proximal extremities of patients aged 10–30 years. Typically, the lesions were darkly pigmented. Histologically, they were characterized by loosely organized nests of pleomorphic pigmented cells penetrating deep into the reticular dermis and frequently to the subcutaneous fat. Of the patients, 48 were followed from 1 to 23 years. There were no local recurrences nor distant metastases despite an initial histologic diagnosis of malignant melanoma in 29% of the patients.

The characteristic histologic features of DPN allow it to be differentiated from malignant melanoma, as well as from spindle cell and epithelioid cell nevi and blue nevi.

▶ This paper attempts to describe a new entity that appears to have certain atypical features yet has a good prognosis. The relationship of this lesion to minimal deviation malignant melanoma and congenital nevi needs to be established. It will be interesting to learn of other investigators' experience with similar lesions.—T.J. Flotte, M.D.

Effects of a Health Education Campaign for the Earlier Diagnosis of Melanoma

Whitehead SM, Wroughton MA, Elwood JM, Davison J, Stewart M (Univ of Nottingham; Queen's Med Centre, Nottingham; City Hosp, Nottingham, England)

Br J Cancer 60:421–425, September 1989 13–16

The incidence of and rate of death from cutaneous malignant melanoma have been steadily increasing in the white population. According to the Breslow classification of tumor thickness, tumors with depths of less than 0.76 mm are associated with a virtual 100% 5-year survival rate, whereas tumors with depths of more than 3.5 mm are associated with a 5-year survival rate of less than 40%. Because delay by patients in consulting physicians about pigmented lesions greatly contributes to delayed diagnosis, a 6-month health education campaign was carried out in Nottingham, England. The number of referrals for evaluation of pigmented lesions before and after the campaign were analyzed.

During the 6 months before the public education campaign, general practitioners referred patients to dermatologists at an average of 10 per week. During the first week after the launch of the campaign, there were 120 referrals. The referral rate was almost 55 per week for the first 3 months immediately after launch of the campaign, and remained at about 23 referrals per week during the next 3 months. Of the referred patients, only about 40% had 3 or more of the 7 suggested danger signs of melanoma, but 6% of these patients actually had melanomas, compared with only 0.4% of those who had fewer than 3 of the 7 suggested danger signs. The effect on the work loads of general practitioners was less dramatic, as the weekly number of consultations for pigmented lesions rose from 0.5 to 3. Of the melanomas diagnosed during the first 6 months after the campaign, 64% had Breslow thicknesses of less than 1.5 mm, whereas only 16% had thicknesses of more than 3.5 mm. However, this distribution did not differ significantly from that during the 3.5 years before the campaign.

Attempts to improve early diagnosis of melanoma with health education campaigns are justified, but referral criteria need to be more precisely defined and further evaluation of the long-term effects of such campaigns is still needed.

▶ The changes in referral rate from 10 per week to about 55 per week for 3 months immediately after the public education campaign is clear evidence that physicians can be alerted to detecting suspicious pigmented lesions; consequently, melanomas are discovered in earlier stages and survival is improved. The general practitioners were sent a letter announcing the availability of a new pigmented lesion clinic and also received a copy of a booklet on the early diagnosis of melanoma written by Dr. Rona Mackie (1).

Two decades earlier, in 1966, the first group effort in the study of pigmented lesions, known as the Pigmented Lesion Clinic, was established at the Massachusetts General Hospital (MGH) in Boston by Drs. Wallace H. Clark, Jr. (dermatopathologist,) John Raker (general surgeon), and Thomas B. Fitzpatrick, (dermatologist.) It was in this MGH clinic that the now widely accepted classification of primary melanomas was first proposed by Clark; also the 2 important clinical characteristics of early melanoma—irregular border and variegation of color—were first proposed by Fitzpatrick (2).

Before 1965 most melanomas were recognized by the presence of ulceration, bleeding, and nodularity—these lesions were all late in the stage of development and consequently had a poor prognosis. Clark emphasized in 1969, 3 years after the beginning of the Pigmented Lesion Clinic of the MGH, that melanomas appeared to have a biphasic growth, spreading laterally for months to years (*radial* growth) and then spreading vertically (*vertical* growth). Clark introduced the term "superficial spreading melanoma," emphasizing that certain melanomas had a time period of radial growth, and that not all melanomas were exclusively nodular but had a lateral spread indicated by the "surround" portion of the nodule.

The evolution of these concepts by Clark's group and others in the past 2 decades has led to a complete reorientation of the beliefs regarding malignant melanoma of the skin and has changed the whole approach to pathogenesis, diagnosis, and treatment. Clark's classic paper, recently published in the *Journal of the National Cancer Institute* (3), should be read in the original and the tables carefully studied by all dermatologists, surgeons, and pathologists who are confronted with the problems of patients with malignant melanoma of the skin.—T.B. Fitzpatrick, M.D., Ph.D.

References

1. Mackie RM: *An Illustrated Guide to the Recognition of Early Malignant Melanoma.* Glasgow, University of Glasgow, 1986.
2. Fitzpatrick TB, Clark WH Jr: *Tumors of the Skin.* Chicago, Year Book Medical Publishers, 1963.
3. Clark WH Jr, et al: *J Natl Cancer Inst* 81:1893, 1989.

Nonfamilial Cutaneous Melanoma Incidence in Women Associated With Sun Exposure Before 20 Years of Age

Weinstock MA, Colditz GA, Willett WC, Stampfer MJ, Bronstein BR, Mihm MC Jr, Speizer FE (Brigham and Women's Hosp, Boston; Harvard School of Public Health; Massachusetts Gen Hosp, Boston)

Pediatrics 84:199–204, August 1989 13–17

There has been a rapid increase in the incidence and mortality attributable to malignant melanoma. The details of the relationship between sun exposure and malignant melanoma remain unclear despite strong evidence that sun exposure causes malignant melanoma. A nested case-control analysis was conducted within the Nurses' Health Study cohort to examine the relationship between timing of severe sun exposure and the incidence of melanoma.

The series included 130 white women aged 38–65 years with confirmed cutaneous melanoma whose first-degree relatives had no history of melanoma. Controls included 300 women matched by race, data of birth, and cycle of questionnaire who also reported no melanoma in first-degree relatives. Conditional logistic regression was used to evaluate the relationship of sun damage after 30 years of age and sun damage from 15 to 20 years of age with the incidence of melanoma.

There was a significant association between blistering sunburns at 15–20 years of age and risk of melanoma, with a relative risk of 2.2 for 5 or more burns vs. none. The association persisted after controlling for blistering burns after 30 years of age and latitude of residence at 15–20 years of age. No statistically significant association was found between sunburns after age 30 years and melanoma. A more equatorial latitude of residence between ages 15 and 20 years was more strongly associated with melanoma than was residence after 30 years of age.

Preventive efforts to reduce the incidence of melanoma attributable to sun exposure should be focused on children and adolescents. Measures that should be taken by white persons, particularly those younger than 20 years of age, include minimizing exposure to direct summer sunlight from 10 AM to 3 PM and covering the skin with clothing or sunscreen lotions when the skin is exposed to sun. Sunbathing should be considered a potentially hazardous behavior.

▶ The impetus for this study originated from the findings of a case-control study by Lew et al. from the Massachusetts General Hospital Melanoma Group (1), which indicated that blistering sunburns during adolescence were associated with a twofold increased risk for the development of melanoma later in life. The Lew et al. study had employed a rather unorthodox control group in that it was comprised of same-sex friends of the cases whose ages were within 5 years of the matched cases. The present study, which used a much more orthodox type of control group with more than 2:1 matching of controls with cases, confirms the findings of Lew et al. These papers do not prove causality of traumatic solar exposures during adolescence and melanoma but certainly suggest a relationship. These studies have important public health implications. Further exploration of this complex issue is warranted.—A.J. Sober, M.D.

Reference

1. Lew R, et al: *J Dermatol Surg Oncol* 4:891, 1983.

Accuracy in Clinically Evaluating Pigmented Lesions

Curley RK, Cook MG, Fallowfield ME, Marsden RA (St George's Hosp, London)
Br Med J 299:16–18, July 1, 1989 13–18

Previous studies have suggested that benign melanocytic nevi can be distinguished clinically from other banal pigmented lesions. In all, 120 pigmented lesions from 86 patients who were first seen mainly at a pigmented lesion clinic were evaluated clinically by 3 physicians experienced in managing melanocytic lesions to evaluate their ability to correctly diagnose melanoma, dysplastic nevi, and various pigmented lesions. The clinical diagnosis was compared with the histopathologic diagnosis for each lesion.

Histopathologic diagnoses included melanoma (3), dysplastic nevus (39), compound nevus (22), intradermal nevus (30), lentigo (6), seborrheic warts (8), and miscellaneous (12). Overall, the sensitivity accuracy for the 3 physicians for all types of lesion was 50%. Of the 39 dysplastic nevi only 19 were correctly identified by all observers. Another 24 banal lesions were incorrectly diagnosed as dysplastic by at least 1 observer. It was particularly difficult to identify small (<5 mm), flat lesions, which could be either banal or potentially malignant. The overall sensitivity for lentigines was only 27%.

Critical decisions concerning diagnosis and management of pigmented lesions should always be based on both clinical and histopathologic assessments as well as history of the patient.

▶ The authors stated how inaccurate they were in diagnosing pigmented lesions using histologic assessment as the gold standard. Whereas the histologic criteria for various diagnoses were stated, the gross morphological criteria used by the 3 clinicians were not. In fact, there was no attempt to standardize gross morphological assessment. Other clinicians may perform better or worse, but there seems to be a need for developing simple, reproducible methods for gross morphological assessment of melanocytic tumors.—A.R. Rhodes, M.D., M.P.H.

Dysplastic Nevi: Markers for Increased Risk for Melanoma

Rigel DS, Rivers JK, Kopf AW, Friedman RJ, Vinokur AF, Heilman ER, Levenstein M (New York Univ)

Cancer 63:386–389, Jan 15, 1989 13–19

The degree of risk of malignant melanoma developing in patients with dysplastic nevi remains uncertain. A review was made of 452 consecutive white patients having a clinical and histologic diagnosis of dysplastic nevi.

Cutaneous malignant melanoma developed in 16 patients (3.5%) after an average follow-up of 27 months. Of the 18 melanomas, 12 were in situ lesions. All 6 primary invasive melanomas were less than 0.9 mm in Breslow thickness. No patient has had a recurrent lesion or metastasis. Eight of the 18 melanomas were associated with contiguous dysplastic nevi.

In about 2 years these patients with dysplastic nevi exceeded the lifetime risk for malignant melanoma in the general U.S. population—for whites, about 1%. Malignant melanoma likely to develop in patients who have a personal or family history of the lesion. It may well be appropriate to increase surveillance of persons with dysplastic nevi.

▶ Rigel et al. demonstrate in a "prospective" study that patients who have dysplastic melanocytic nevi (DMN), regardless of a personal or family history of melanoma, have a significantly increased risk for the development of melanoma. (Most of the melanomas identified in this cohort of patients were preinvasive or very thin lesions associated with a very high cure rate.) If one logically presumes that preinvasive (in situ) melanoma eventually progresses over time to invasive melanoma, the results reported have even greater implications. The message for physicians is that patients who have any DMN, regardless of a personal or family history of melanoma, require periodic lifetime follow-up.—A.R. Rhodes, M.D., M.P.H.

Association of Early Malignant Melanoma With Nevocytic Nevi

Stolz W. Schmoeckel C, Landthaler M, Braun-Falso O (Univ of Munich, West Germany)

Cancer 63:550–555, Feb 1, 1989 13–20

It has been suggested that nevocytic nevi can act as precursors of malignant melanoma. Recent reports indicate that the histologic association of malignant melanoma and nevocytic nevi varies between 8.3% and 54%, with a maximum frequency between 20% and 30%. The difference could be explained partially by the fact that tumors in more advanced stages may have overgrown preexisting nevocytic cells. This association was investigated in 150 patients with early stage malignant melanoma (tumor thickness ≤1.5 mm; level of invasion ≤III).

A total of 33 patients (22%) had malignant melanoma associated with nevocytic nevi. An additional 6% had a possible, but doubtful, association with nevocytic nevi. Nevus cells could be detected below the tumor in 45.4% of the patients, at the laterally adjacent sides in 18.2%, and at both sides in 36.4%. When nevus cells were located to the side of the melanoma, junctional activity was noted in 50% of them.

Some nevocytic nevi can potentially develop into malignant neoplasms. Other studies have found that 9% to 45% of nevocytic nevi associated with malignant melanoma having junctional activity could be indications that at least some malignant melanomas develop within or next to a preexisting and still-proliferating nevocytic nevus.

▶ This report documents an in-contiguity histologic association between nevomelanocytic nevi and cutaneous melanoma in at least 22% of early melanomas (level III or less, 1.5 mm or thinner). The type of nevi in contiguity (dysplastic, acquired, congenital, spindle cell/epithelioid cell) was not investigated. A detailed review of similar studies is provided. This study does not address the central question: What kind of melanocytic lesions are at highest risk of progressing to melanoma?—A.R. Rhodes, M.D., M.P.H.

Mapping the Gene for Hereditary Cutaneous Malignant Melanoma–Dysplastic Nevus to Chromosome 1p

Bale SJ, Dracopoli NC, Tucker MA, Clark WH Jr, Fraser MC, Stanger BZ, Green P, Donis-Keller H, Housman DE, Greene MH (Natl Cancer Inst, Bethesda, Md; Massachusetts Inst of Technology, Cambridge; Univ of Pennsylvania; Collaborative Research Inc, Bedford, Mass)

N Engl J Med 320:1367–1372, May 25, 1989 13–21

Approximately 10% of cutaneous malignant melanomas occur in persons with a familial predisposition, usually in association with dysplastic nevi. Early studies indicated that the gene of hereditary melanoma is on the short arm of chromosome 1 (chromosome 1p) near the rhesus blood group locus. Twenty-six polymorphic loci on 1p in 6 families with melanoma, including 99 relatives and 26 spouses, were analyzed. Linkage analysis was used to detect the cosegregation of any of the loci with the disease trait.

A total of 34 family members had cutaneous malignant melanoma, 31 of whom also had dysplastic nevi. An additional 24 relatives had dysplastic nevi alone. Linkage analysis indicated the presence of a gene for susceptibility to melanoma between an anonymous DNA marker and the locus for pronatrodilatin, a common reference gene, in chromosome band 1p36.

Further knowledge of the function of this susceptibility gene may help to explain the role of ultraviolet radiation and other environmental factors in the pathogenesis of melanoma. The findings may be especially important in relation to the 30% to 50% of sporadic melanomas associated with dysplastic nevi.

▶ Based on the studies of 6 melanoma-prone kindreds, Bale et al. demonstrate the gene responsible for melanoma/dysplastic nevus trait to be in chromosome band 1p36, with odds greater than 260,000:1 in favor. There are at least 2 other groups studying melanoma-prone kindreds that dispute these data. A Dutch study of large melanoma-prone families excluded a region up to 25 centiMorgans on either side of band 1p34 (1). A Utah study of melanoma-prone families refuted linkage of either melanoma alone or a combined melanoma/clinical dysplastic nevus trait to markers for the short arm of chromosome 1 (2). We await further studies that clarify the molecular basis of the melanoma/dysplastic nevus trait.—A.R. Rhodes, M.D., M.P.H.

References

1. van Haeringen A, et al: *Genomics* 5:61, 1989.
2. Piepkorn M, et al: Unpublished data.

Nevomelanocytic Proliferations in Association With Cutaneous Malignant Melanoma: A Multivariate Analysis

Gruber SB, Barnhill RL, Stenn KS, Roush GC (Yale Univ)

J Am Acad Dermatol 21:773–780, October 1989 13–22

Nevi are thought to be precursors of melanoma and markers of increased melanoma risk. A nevus in histologic contiguity has been associated with several features of melanoma. Separate independent studies have linked a contiguous nevus with the level and depth of invasion of a melanoma and with an increased likelihood of superficial spreading melanoma. For this study, 248 new cases of melanoma accessioned from 1984 through 1985 were subjected to multivariate analysis. The 248 pigmented lesions were reviewed independently by 2 dermatopathologists for the presence of benign or dysplastic nevi.

After 51 cases were excluded from analysis for a variety of reasons, the study sample comprised 197 primary cutaneous malignant melanomas in 197 patients. The level of invasion and anatomical distribution in this population were consistent with the distribution in larger studies of melanoma.

Statistical analysis revealed that 32.5% of the melanomas were associated with a benign or dysplastic nevus in histologic contiguity. Sex, age, number of slides, and number of histologic sections were not significantly related to the presence of a contiguous nevus. Melanoma type and location were significant predictors of contiguous nevomelanocytic proliferations when considered alone. However, after adjustment for confounding variables, melanoma type only was significantly predictive of a contiguous nevus, whereas anatomical location was no longer significantly associated with a contiguous nevus. Superficial spreading melanomas were approximately 11 times more likely to contain histologic evidence of a precursor nevus than were nodular melanomas, and were almost 22 times more likely to be associated with a nevus than were lentigo maligna melanomas. Thus melanoma type remains a significant predictor of nevi in contiguity after adjustment for anatomical location.

► In this series of melanomas, which appeared to include lentigo maligna and varieties of in situ melanoma, about a third of cases were in histologic contiguity with a benign (48%) or a dysplastic (52%) nevus. Melanoma subtype was the most important predictor of association with a nevus. This study highlights the heterogeneity of the origin of melanoma, particularly the association of dysplastic nevi with certain subtypes of melanoma.—A.R. Rhodes, M.D., M.P.H.

Malignant Melanoma of the Skin in Children (0 to 14 Years of Age) in Denmark, 1943–1982

Partoft S, Østerlind A, Hou-Jensen K, Drzewiecki KT (Rigshospitalet: Danish Cancer Registry, Copenhagen)

Scand J Plast Reconstr Surg 23:55–58, 1989 13–23

Sixty-three cutaneous malignant melanomas in children aged from less than 1 to 14 years were reported to the Danish Cancer Registry from 1943 to 1982. Because malignant melanoma in prepubescent children is extremely rare, the possibility of overdiagnosis was entertained. Clinical and pathologic evaluations of the reported cases were undertaken to define the true incidence of childhood melanoma in Denmark.

Nine childhood melanomas were identified among the 23 slides available for study. Seven of the 9 patients (78%) were aged 10–14 years. Malignant melanoma developed in congenital giant nevi in 2 cases. The crude incidence rate of childhood melanoma for the 40-year period was estimated to be between 0.24×10^{-6} and 0.32×10^{-6}. This corresponds to 1 new case of childhood melanoma every 3–4 years in Denmark. The remaining 14 lesions were classified as Spitz nevi in 7 patients, blue nevi in 4, and nevocytic nevi in 3.

Childhood melanoma in Denmark was seriously overdiagnosed between 1943 and 1982. This overdiagnosis could result from the histologic resemblance of malignant melanoma to the more commonly occurring Spitz nevus, which was not defined as an entity until 1948.

▶ Of the 9 cases of verified melanomas (7 definite, 2 suspected), 2 that resulted in death were associated with congenital nevi (dimensions, 10 × 8 cm and 15 × 17 cm, ages 13 years and 6 years, respectively). These congenital nevi would qualify as large but not giant according to definitions proposed by Kopf. This study confirms the rarity of melanoma in children, the frequent problem of misdiagnosis of melanoma in children, and the malignant potential of congenital nevi in children.—A.R. Rhodes, M.D., M.P.H.

Juvenile Malignant Melanoma

Reintgen DS, Vollmer R, Seigler HF (H Lee Muffitt Cancer Ctr, Tampa, Fla; Duke Univ)

Surg Gynecol Obstet 168:249–253, March 1989 13–24

Because published reports involving the incidence, differential diagnosis, and outcome of malignant melanoma in children and adolescents are confusing or contradictory, a computer-assisted review of charts was conducted at the melanoma clinic of Duke University. Among 4,246 patients with melanoma, 78 were younger than age 20 years (1.8%). Clinical characteristics such as sex, race, and primary site, and pathologic features such as histologic type, Clark level, ulceration, and Breslow thickness, were similar in adult and juvenile patients.

The 5-year actuarial survival rates were 76% in both groups, and the median survival time was similar—12.9 years in adults and 11.9 years in juveniles. A trend toward less time to recurrence was observed in the juvenile group. In children and adolescents the thicker lesions tended to be associated with a decreased disease-free survival time.

This is the largest series of melanomas in children and adolescents reported thus far. Physicians with patients younger than age 20 years need to be aware of the differentiation between malignant melanoma and benign nevus and must watch for irregular borders, ulceration, bleeding, regressive areas, and varied colors. Changes in a pigmented mole should be approached aggressively and studied by excisional biopsy, as in adults.

▶ Based on a stepwise logistic regression and Cox proportional hazard model, age younger than 20 years was not determined to be an independent prognostic variable for the development of metastasis. Of the 78 childhood cases, 46% had a relapse 6 months to 20 years after the original diagnosis. There was no investigation of melanoma risk factors in childhood melanoma.—A.R. Rhodes, M.D., M.P.H.

Clinical and Histopathologic Characteristics of Early Lesions of Subungual Malignant Melanoma

Saida T, Oshima Y (Shinshu Univ, Matsumoto, Japan)

Cancer 63:556–560, February 1989 13–25

Malignant melanoma rarely affects the subungual region in white persons, but approximately 10% of Japanese patients with these cancers

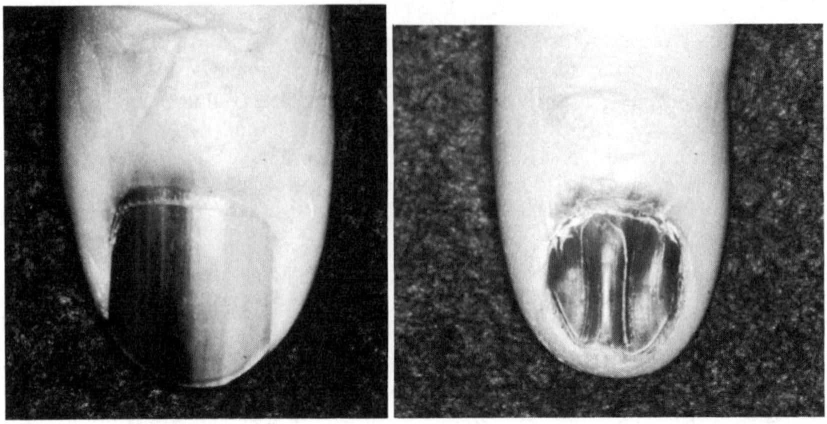

Fig 13–1.—Early subungual melanomas. **A,** patient 1. **E,** patient 5. (Courtesy of Saida T, Oshima Y: *Cancer* 63:556–560, February 1989.)

have subungual melanomas. The lesions are often diagnosed during the late clinical period when the prognosis is poor. A better understanding of the clinical characteristics of early lesions of subungual melanoma might lead to earlier diagnosis and better prognosis.

Within a 16-year period at 1 institution, 67 Japanese patients were first seen with malignant melanomas. Twenty-one of the melanomas were in the subungual region. Researchers reviewed photographs and records of these patients and elicited further information by questionnaire. Early lesions, i.e., Clark's level I or the early phase of level II, were studied in detail.

Almost 86% of the subungual melanomas occurred on the hand; 14% occurred on the foot. Usually, the initial sign of disease was confirmed to be melanonychia striata. In all 5 Clark's level I melanomas, melanonychia striata was the initial sign of disease. The risk of early subungual melanoma developing was increased when melanonychia striata was observed during adulthood, when it was broader than 6 mm, when it was either black or variegated shades of brown, and when it was accompanied by Hutchinson's sign (Fig 13–1).

Prompt detection of early lesions of subungual melanoma can improve the prognosis. The prospects for preserving the affected phalanx also are enhanced.

▶ The diagnosis of subungual melanoma is problematic because the populations at greatest risk (blacks and Orientals) are also the same populations having the greatest frequency of benign pigmented streaks from nevi of the nailfold. Thin longitudinal streaks present for a long duration, without involvement of the posterior nailfold, are less ominous than wider, newer streaks or those involving the posterior nailfold (Hutchinson's sign). When in doubt, biopsy of the nailfold region, including the matrix, is necessary for diagnosis. With early lesions amputation may be avoided. Wide excision and graft coverage are usually sufficient for the early lesions. With late lesions, aggressive surgery often fails secondary to systemic disease.—A.J. Sober, M.D.

Desmoplastic Malignant Melanoma and Its Variants: A Study of 45 Cases
Jain S, Allen PW (Queen Elizabeth Hosp, Woodville, South Australia; Woden Valley Hosp, Woden, Australia)
Am J Surg Pathol 13:358–373, May 1989 13–26

To examine neurotropism or neuroid differentiation in desmoplastic malignant melanomas, data on 45 tumors that satisfied the criteria for desmoplastic malignant melanoma were reviewed. The 31 male and 14 female patients were white and were aged 42–91 years.

The tumors were subdivided into 3 groups: 12 were desmoplastic melanomas with an atypical intraepidermal melanocytic component (the classic desmoplastic melanoma); 21 were desmoplastic melanomas without an atypical intraepidermal melanocytic component (de novo desmoplastic melanoma); and 12 were predominantly nerve-centered superficial malignant tumors with or without an atypical intraepidermal melanocytic component. Three of the nerve-centered tumors were associated with pigmentary abnormalities in the overlying skin. Most tumors were found in sun-exposed areas. The tumors were located in the head and neck in 35 patients. Three tumors arose in irradiated areas and 1 occurred on the face of a radiotherapist.

Microscopically, tumors involved the dermis, subcutis, or nerves. The histologic features varied considerably, but certain growth patterns were common. The appearance of the individual neoplastic spindle cells in the dermis and subcutis was similar. A continuous histologic pattern was noted. Melanin was found in 4 tumors, but the S-100 protein stain was positive in 19 tumors and negative in 3.

Follow-up data were available for 42 patients. The mean follow-up period was 4.6 years (range, 4 months to 15 years). Fifteen patients (36%) died or were terminally ill, 24 (57%) were alive with no apparent residual tumor, and 3 (7%) died of other causes. Local recurrences developed in 23 patients, distant spread including extension into the cranial cavity along nerves in 17, and both local and distant recurrences in 14. Nine of 11 patients with nerve-centered tumors died or were terminally ill. Surgery was the usual treatment. Most uncontrolled recurrences were resistant to chemotherapy and radiotherapy, but 2 patients responded well.

▶ Desmoplastic melanoma is frequently a difficult diagnosis to make. I personally believe that it is always worth looking at more series and examples of desmoplastic melanoma. The authors' definition, however, of desmoplastic melanoma would appear to differ considerably with those of other authors. In particular, they define a nerve-centered desmoplastic tumor that most authors, I think, would classify as neurofiber sarcoma. It is interesting that this category of lesion has a dramatically different course than the more traditional desmoplastic melanoma. Therefore, this paper should be read with some caution.—T.J. Flotte, M.D.

Trends in Cutaneous Malignant Melanoma in Denmark 1943–1982 by Anatomic Site

Østerlind A, Engholm G, Møller Jensen O (Danish Cancer Society; Danish Cancer Registry; Inst of Cancer Epidemiology, Copenhagen)

Acta Pathol Microbiol Immunol Scand 96:953–963, November 1988 13–27

The incidence of cutaneous malignant melanoma (CMM) has increased significantly among many white populations in all parts of the world, but the incidence of CMM in Denmark has been low. The dramatic increase, coupled with the marked geographical variations in incidence, suggests that exogenous factors play a role in the etiology of CMM. Time trends in the incidence of CMM in Denmark were assessed by analyzing data from the Danish Cancer Registry recorded between 1943 and 1982.

During the 40-year study period, 3,509 men and 5,305 women with CMM were reported to the Registry. The average annual number of cases increased from 59 (27 men, 32 women) reported in 1943–1947, to 476 (189 men, 287 women) reported in 1978–1982. During the study period the age-standardized incidence rate for CMM in Denmark increased by fivefold to sixfold. However, changes in the age-standardized incidence rates over calendar-time differed for anatomical sites and between the sexes. The increases were particularly marked for CMM of the trunk in both sexes and of the arms and legs in women. Steep increases in risk were observed in progressively younger birth cohorts (table). This association was particulary pronounced for sites other than the face, scalp, and neck. With regard to the latter sites, the increase among younger cohorts was much smaller.

The dramatic increase in the incidence of CMM reflects a substantial increase in exposure to 1 or more important generation-specific risk factors. Although the risk for CMM in Denmark increases in relation to intermittent sun exposure, particularly during childhood, it is not known to what degree the difference in melanoma risk between cohorts can be explained by differences in sunburn experience. However, preventive action based on current knowledge of risk factors for CMM (e.g., sun exposure) is highly warranted.

Risk for Malignant Melanoma at Various Sites in 1 Generation Relative to a Generation Born 25 Years Earlier

Anatomic site	Males	Females
Face, scalp, and neck	2.2 (1.9-2.6)	2.1 (1.8-2.4)
Trunk	6.1 (5.3-7.1)	4.9 (4.2-5.7)
Arms	4.1 (3.1-5.4)	4.2 (3.5-5.1)
Legs	2.8 (2.4-3.4)	4.5 (4.0-5.0)

Note: relative risk = 1.0.

(Courtesy of Østerlind A, Engholm G, Møller Jensen O: *Acta Pathol Microbiol Immunol Scand* 96:953–963, November 1988.)

▶ Cancer registries in small countries such as Denmark have always been exemplary because of complete reporting by the physicians. This very large number of melanomas identified over a 40-year period further underscores an important new trend in melanoma around the world in the white populations, excluding acrolentiginous melanoma. This trend is an increase in melanomas on sites not necessarily the most sun exposed such as the face, scalp, and neck, the traditional sites of nonmelanoma skin cancer. Furthermore, there has been a dramatic increase in the number of melanomas in younger cohorts, whereas nonmelanoma is a disease of persons in the older age groups. This is the same pattern reported from Norway by Magnus (1), which also shows an increased incidence, compared with earlier data, on the trunk in both sexes and of the arms and legs in women. The incidence has been rising in cohorts in a manner consistent with changes in patterns of exposure, particularly with respect to increasing intermittent, intense, sun exposure of certain anatomical sites, i.e., the backs of males and females and the lower legs of females. Consistent with this fact is a higher incidence in higher social classes (professional) and in indoor workers.

The type and site of origin of malignant melanoma are related to age and sex. Everyone agrees that one form of melanoma is clearly related to prolonged exposure to sunlight: lentigo maligna melanoma (LMM), which occurs almost invariably on sites in which there is marked dermatoheliosis (sun-damaged skin). Also, the incidence of LMM increases progressively with age except for an early peak at ages 60–69, but superficial spreading melanoma (SSM) reaches a peak at 50–59 years and then declines. More than 80% of LMM occurs on the head and neck; SMM, which occurs on the trunk and lower limbs (in females), increases in incidence from age 20–29 (females) and 30–39 (males.) Lentigo maligna melanoma is the least common melanoma, and its incidence has not changed over time in a number of series.—T.B. Fitzpatrick, M.D. Ph.D.

Reference

1. Magnus K: *Cancer* 48:2329, 1981.

Additional Reading

1. National Academy of Sciences (NAS): *Halocarbons: Effects on Stratospheric Ozone*. Washington DC, National Academy Press, 1976.
2. National Academy of Sciences (NAS): *Protection Against Depletion of Stratospheric Ozone by Chlorofluorocarbons*. Washington DC, National Academy Press, 1979.
3. National Academy of Sciences (NAS): *Causes and Effects of Stratospheric Ozone Reduction: An Update*. Washington DC, National Academy Press, 1982.
4. Fitzpatrick TB, Sober AJ: Sunlight and skin cancer *N Engl J Med* 313:818–820, 1985.
5. Hoffman JS, Longstreth JD (eds): *Ultraviolet Radiation and Melanoma with a Special Focus on Assessing the Risks of Stratospheric Ozone Depletion*. Washington DC, EPA 400/1–87/001D, December, 1987. (This is the best summary so far.)
6. Ley RD, et al: Ultraviolet radiation-induced malignant melanoma in *Monodelphis domestica. Photochem Photobiol* 50:1–5, 1989. (This is the first report of melanoma induction in a mammal with UV-B alone.)

Change of Epidemiological Characteristics of Malignant Melanoma During the Years 1962–1972 and 1983–1986 in the Federal Republic of Germany

Garbe C, Wiebelt H, Orfanos CE (Univ Med Ctr Steglitz, The Free Univ of Berlin; German Cancer Research Ctr, Heidelberg, West Germany)

Dermatologica 178:131–135, 1989 13–28

Two long-term, multicenter, prospective studies of malignant melanoma (MM) have been performed in West Germany. The basic characteristics of these 2 data collections were compared to detect any changes in the clinical epidemiology of MM diagnosed in the past 20 years.

The age distribution of patients at the time of first diagnosis did not appear to change over time. From 1962 to 1972 and from 1983 to 1986 similar proportions of patients were younger than 50 years (44% of men and 45% of women in the first period, and 44% of men and 47% of women in the second). In 1 study the percentage of men with MM rose, and the portion of tumors localized on the trunk increased markedly in both sexes. Comparison of the tumor thickness suggested a significant advance in early recognition of MM. The percentage of thick tumors decreased between periods, with a corresponding increase in thinner tumors. During both periods the first diagnosis was metastasizing melanoma in approximately 10% of all patients. The proportion of prognostically unfavorable, nodular malignant melanomas remained almost constant at about 30%.

Population-based data in West Germany reveal a continuous rise in mortality for MM beginning in the 1950s. The average annual increase in death rates was approximately 4%. Increased efforts are needed in improving the earliest possible recognition of MM and insuring its early surgical removal.

▶ There were some surprising findings in this study:

1. The age distribution of patients did not change in 2 decades; most countries have reported a trend to younger ages in the melanoma population.

2. The proportion (30%) of "prognostically unfavorable" nodular melanomas remained constant. There is a distinct trend in most reports from other countries of more "thin" melanomas being reported. This would suggest some type of different etiology or the need for an educational program of physicians and the general public in recognition of early melanoma, and the establishment of pigmented lesion clinics in Germany. (See Abstract 13–16.) Prof. L. Illig in Germany, during his tenure, created a very successful pigmented lesion clinic in the small town of Giessen.—T.B. Fitzpatrick, M.D. Ph.D.

Trends in Survival From Malignant Melanoma: Remarkable Improvement in 23 Years

Thörn M, Adami H-O, Bergström R, Ringborg U, Krusemo UB (Univ Hosp, Uppsala, Sweden; Natl Board of Health and Welfare, Karolinska Hosp, Stockholm)

J Natl Cancer Inst 81:611–617, Apr 19, 1989 13–29

Apparent discrepancies between trends in the incidence of and mortality from malignant melanoma suggest that death rates have changed over time. Temporal trends and relative survival (RS) from malignant melanoma in Sweden from 1960 to 1982 were analyzed.

The incidence rates of malignant melanoma rose annually by 5.4% in women and 5.8% in men, whereas death rates rose annually by 2.7% in women and 3.3% in men. Before 1970 the 5-year RS rates in women rose by about 15%; in men RS rates improved by 4.6% to 8.2% for each 5-year period of diagnosis. Multivariate analyses showed that the malignant melanoma-specific hazard decreased by 71% in women and 64% in men in the first 5 years of follow-up.

Improvement has been found in short- and long-term survival for both sexes in all age groups, except for men more than 70 years old. The average reduction in the expected life span decreased from 35% to 19% in women and from 46% to 27% in men.

▶ The increase in survival of patients with primary malignant melanoma of the skin in the time period covered by this study from Sweden (1960–1982) is truly remarkable. Although the incidence increased steadily each year by more than 5% in both males and females, the specific hazard decreased by 71% in women and 64% in men. This is a remarkable achievement in public education, and the increased survival is not related to a change in histologic criteria in which there are more lesions called malignant melanoma because, in fact, there was an increase in mortality in Sweden between 1960 and 1982, as there has been in England, Wales, Canada, and in the white population of the United States.

The increase in survival is because of patients with early disease being treated with surgery. The prognosis of primary melanoma of the skin is related to the stage of development of the tumor at the time of surgical removal. Wallace Clark and his group of the University of Pennsylvania recently presented an 8-year follow-up study of a large series (264) of primary melanomas of the skin in stage I (localized disease with no palpable regional lymph nodes) (1). Clark and his group carefully defined 2 types of growth pattern of malignant melanoma arising in the skin: *radial growth phase* and *vertical growth phase.* The 8-year survival for patients with radial growth tumors was 100%! Survival of patients with vertical growth tumors was 84%. Determination of the survival for the vertical growth phase was based on a logistic regression model possessing 6 independent prognostic attributes: (1) mitotic rate, (2) tumor infiltrating lymphocytes, (3) thickness, (4) site, (5) sex, and (6) histologic regression.

With increased awareness of pigmented lesions and skin cancers in general by the general public, and especially as a result of the recent intensive education of physicians in recognition of early melanoma, more tumors are being discovered *incidentally* on physical examination; these are melanomas in the radial growth phase of development, and the survival rate of affected patients is 100%.—T.B. Fitzpatrick, M.D., Ph.D.

Reference

1. Clark WH Jr, et al: *J Natl Cancer Inst* 81:1893, 1989.

Pathologic Prognostic Factors for Cutaneous Malignant Melanoma: The Western Canada Melanoma Study

Worth AJ, Gallagher RP, Elwood JM, Yang PC, Lamb C, Spinelli JJ, Wood WS, Threlfall WJ, Hill GB (Cancer Control Agency of British Columbia; Vancouver Gen Hosp; Univ of Otago, New Zealand)

Int J Cancer 43:370–375, March 15, 1989 13–30

The recent increase in the incidence of cutaneous malignant melanoma has prompted a number of investigations into prognostic factors. Data on 798 patients from a defined geographic region were reviewed to elucidate the course of cutaneous melanoma.

Depth of penetration was the chief overall predictor of survival. Also, women had a better prognosis. These factors were important only in lesions <4 mm deep; for lesions >4 mm deep, no factors were predictive. The prognoses of patients with primary tumors >4 mm deep, without further evidence of disease, was similar to that of patients with deep tumors and in-transit metastases or lymph node involvement. The improved survival of women is of special interest because of the increased attention to estrogen receptors in melanoma research.

Patients with lesions >4 mm deep are more likely to have hidden metastases at diagnosis. The value of elective lymph node dissection in such patients must be questioned.

▶ This study of a large series of patients will have to be reconsidered in light of the recently published "bench-mark" study of Clark and his group (1) in which a multivariate analysis was performed.—T.B. Fitzpatrick, M.D., Ph.D.

Reference

1. Clark WH Jr, et al: *J Natl Cancer Inst* 81:1893, 1989.

Objective Histopathologic Grading of Cutaneous Malignant Melanomas by Stereologic Estimation of Nuclear Volume: Prediction of Survival and Disease-Free Period

Sørensen FB (Univ of Aarhus, Denmark)

Cancer 63:1784–1798, May 1, 1989 13–31

Many prognostic indicators for malignant melanomas are without value or are not objective or reproducible. Determination of the nuclear volume by stereology is a useful prognosticator for bladder cancer and may have prognostic significance in stereologic estimates of the 3-dimensional nuclear volume of malignant melanomas. After 10 years of follow-up 47 patients with malignant melanoma were investigated retrospectively. The value of 3-dimensional nuclear volume was compared with that of traditional clinicopathologic prognostic parameters and 2-dimensional, shape-dependent morphometric estimates.

Stage I tumors had significantly smaller nuclear volume (226 μm^3) than stage II tumors (457 μm^3). High nuclear volumes were associated with ulceration, nodular melanoma, and Clark's levels IV and V. Nuclear volume and tumor ulceration were excellent prognostic parameters, but patient sex, age, anatomical site of tumor, histologic type, tumor thickness, and Clark's level of invasion were not significantly associated with prognosis. All ulcerated melanomas had metastatic recurrences.

Stereologic estimates of nuclear volume provided a powerful prognostic parameter in cutaneous melanomas. A cutoff point of 200 μm^3 was a sensitive indicator of metastatic recurrences and survival. Combined with tumor ulceration, the 2 parameters are powerful forecasters of the outcome of stage I malignant melanomas. Because nuclear volume is relatively fast and easy to determine, and is unbiased and objective, a prospective trial is planned on a large series of patients to confirm these results.

▶ This study of 47 patients with stage I and stage II melanoma followed for at least 10 years (or until death from melanoma) revealed important prognostic information from estimation of 3-dimensional nuclear volume using a complex analysis and a simple counting method. Surprisingly, Cox regression analysis indicated that 3-dimensional nuclear volume provides excellent prognostic information, rivaled only by tumor ulceration. The method does not have the simplicity of microscopic tumor thickness, but it may be more accurate in predicting recurrence/death from melanoma. This study needs to be confirmed.—A.R. Rhodes, M.D., M.P.H.

Local Recurrences and Metastasis With Thin Malignant Melanoma (≤1 mm): The Importance of Wide Safety Margins in Primary Surgical Management

Garbe C, Stadler R, Orfanos CE (Freie Universität, Berlin)

Hautarzt 40:337–343, June 1989 13–32

The prognosis for thin malignant melanoma (MM) lesions is considered extremely favorable. A study from the United States reported a 99% 7.5-year survival rate for patients with tumor thicknesses of 0.85 mm or less. Yet, larger European studies have reported a distinct mortality risk for patients with tumor thicknesses of less than 0.76 mm. The size of the safety margins for primary excision of MM lesions varies between studies.

Tumor thickness, size of safety margins, and mortality of 704 patients treated for MM at 1 institution between 1969 and 1987 were reviewed; 631 had stage I disease at the time of first diagnosis. Complete histologic data were available for 516 patients, 191 of whom had MM lesions with a thickness of 1 mm or less; 325 had thicker lesions. Of the 191 patients, 151 underwent total excision with safety margins of 3–5 cm; 37 others had excision with safety margins of 0.5–2 cm. The mean follow-up for both groups was 54 months.

None of the 151 patients who had wide surgical total excision of thin MM lesions had a local recurrence, but primary lymphogenous or other hematogenous metastases developed in 12 patients (8%). Six of the 37 patients with thin MM who had narrow excision of the lesion had a local recurrence; hematologic metastases later developed in 2. One of the 6 patients died of MM 13 years after the first diagnosis was made.

The 5-year survival rates were 90% for men with MM of 1 mm or less thickness, 59% for men with MM of more than 1 mm, 97% for women with thin MM lesions, and 80% for women with thicker MM lesions. A statistically signficant difference existed between the 10-year survival rates associated with thin and thicker MM lesions, particularly among men. The 10-year survival rate for men with thin lesions was 71%, compared with 52% for those with thicker lesions. For women, the 10-year mortalities were 87% for those with thin lesions and 76% for those with thicker lesions. The highest risk of death occurred an average of 48 months after primary excision for all cases but an average of 72 months after excision of MM lesions less than 0.76 mm thick.

Local recurrences and distant metastasis do occur, even if the excised MM lesions are 1 mm thick or less. Wide surgical total excision with safety margins of at least 3 cm is the safest form of treatment for MM.

▶ The "thin" melanoma is a mixture and not a pure lesion. Thickness or level alone can no longer be used to predict survival or recurrence. All studies on the treatment of melanoma with surgical excision of the primary, or the effect of regional node dissection, or of adjuvant therapy will have to consider more attributes of the tumor than level and thickness.

In a recent report of a large series of primary melanomas followed for 8 years, Clark et al. (1) analyzed 386 patients using multivariable logistic regression to develop a prognostic model for primary clinical stage I cutaneous melanoma. In this series, 23 attributes were tested but only 6 had "independently predictive prognostic information."—T.B. Fitzpatrick, M.D., Ph.D.

Reference

1. Clark WH Jr, et al: *J Natl Cancer Inst* 81:1893, 1989.

Effect of BANS Location on the Prognosis of Clinical Stage I Melanoma: New Data and Meta-Analysis

Weinstock MA, Morris BT, Lederman JS, Bleicher P, Fitzpatrick TB, Sober AJ (Harvard Med School; Massachusetts Gen Hosp, Boston)

Br J Dermatol 119:559–565, November 1988 13–33

Intermediate-thickness clinical stage I melanomas on the upper *b*ack, posterior *a*rm, posterior *n*eck, and posterior *s*calp (BANS) were initially said to have a worse prognosis than lesions of similar thickness at other subsites. The effect of BANS location on prognosis of clinical stage I melanoma was reinvestigated in 156 consecutive patients with melanomas 0.76–1.69 mm in thickness.

Patients with BANS lesions had recurrences at twice the rate of those with non-BANS lesions, although this difference was not statistically significant. A meta-analysis of the effect of BANS location on mortality was done using data from this investigation and 5 comparable published reports. To avoid bias, the original data set that led to the BANS hypothesis was excluded. The location of melanomas at BANS sites was associated with a 60% increase in risk of death. This difference remained significant after any 2 of the 6 studies analyzed were excluded.

▶ This new analysis of data on primary melanomas of intermediate thickness confirms the importance of site in the prognosis of melanoma, as originally reported by Day et al. (1). Clark et al., in their recent report (2), also include site as an important attribute in predicting prognosis of stage I melanoma; they divided the sites into 2 categories: extremities and axial, and there was a favorable prognosis for the melanomas of the extremities. They also stated that, "Primary melanomas located on the site group designated BANS (upper back, posterior arm, posterior scalp, posterior neck) by Day and associates, had a decreased 8-year survival when compared with primary melanomas not located in BANS areas."—T.B. Fitzpatrick, M.D., Ph.D.

References

1. Day CL, et al: *Ann Surg* 195:30, 1982.
2. Clark WH Jr, et al: *J Natl Cancer Inst* 81:1893, 1989.

The Incidence of Late Recurrence (Greater Than 10 Years); An Analysis of 536 Consecutive Cases of Cutaneous Melanoma

Callaway MP, Briggs JC (Frenchay Hosp, Bristol, England)
Br J Plast Surg 42:46–49, January 1989 13–34

Using a computerized database, the records of 536 patients with cutaneous melanoma diagnosed and treated during a 10-year period were studied in an attempt to establish possible prognostic factors. Five of these patients (all women, aged 38–76) had a late recurrence, for an incidence of 0.93%. The mean disease-free interval was 12.85 years. Two women were premenopausal and 3 were postmenopausal at the time of initial diagnosis. The primary site of the lesion was the extremities in 4 patients. The mean thickness of the initial tumor was 1.8 mm (range, 0.81–3.1 mm). There was no correlation between tumor thickness and length of disease-free interval. Histologically, only 1 melanoma had ulceration, a poor prognostic indicator.

Between 1% and 7% of patients treated for cutaneous melanoma will have a late recurrence, and women with tumors of intermediate thickness on their extremities appear to be at higher risk for this event. Patient education is necessary for early recognition and treatment of a late recurrence.

▶ This study should be redone using the risk attributes established by Clark et al. (1).—T.B. Fitzpatrick, M.D., Ph.D.

Reference

1. Clark WH Jr, et al: *J Natl Cancer Inst* 81:1893, 1989.

Ten Years' Experience of Treating Lentigo Maligna With Topical Azelaic Acid

Nazzaro-Porro M, Passi S, Zina G, Breathnach AS (Istituto Dermatologico San Gallicano, Rome; Clinica Dermatologica Università, Turin; St Mary's Hosp Med School, London)

Acta Derm Venereol Suppl (Stockh) 143:49–57, 1989 13–35

Since 1979, azelaic acid has been used to treat lentigo maligna (melanotic freckle of Hutchinson), with satisfactory results occurring in more than 50 patients. Twenty-seven remained free of disease 5–10 years later. In 11 patients relapse occurred, but renewed treatment brought resolution.

Woman, 70, had typical lentigo maligna of 10 years' duration. In the basal epidermal layer, normal interkeratocyte relationships were disrupted by an excessive number of abnormal melanocytes. After 1 year's treatment with topically applied azelaic acid, clinical and histologic resolution was complete. Five years after treatment the skin was still normal clinically. Electron microscopic sections of the basal layer of the epidermis had normal interkeratinocytic organization and no abnormal melanocytes. No lymphocytic infiltration of the epidermis or dermis was evident, and the epidermal-dermal junction was intact. Sebaceous and sweat glands and hair follicles in the area of the former lesion were normal.

The progression of lentigo maligna can be arrested and reversed by treatment with azelaic acid. The beneficial results usually are lasting.

▶ The management of lentigo maligna in nonfacial skin is surgical excision. Large lesions on the face and lesions around the eyes or on the bridge of the nose are a problem in management; because the very large size of some lesions considerable disfigurement can result from surgical removal. Radiation therapy has been used successfully, but the recurrence rate is high, and this treatment has been largely abandoned in recent years. The use of topical azelaic acid for the treatment of lentigo maligna has been proposed as an alternative (1–3). There has been 1 report of melanoma developing in a patient with lentigo maligna while undergoing treatment with azelaic acid. (4).

The development of azelaic acid is an interesting story in itself. Dr. Nazzaro-Porro and her colleagues, investigating the mechanism of depigmentation in tinea versicolor, isolated azelaic acid as the chemical structure produced in the skin after the action of lipases present in the organism causing tinea versicolor, *Pityrosporum orbiculare.* Azelaic acid, which is also present in rancid butter, has a selective melanocytotoxic effect on *pathologic* melanocytes, not on *normal* melanocytes. It has been reported to be effective in the treatment of melasma.—T.B. Fitzpatrick, M.D., Ph.D.

References

1. Nazzaro-Porro N, et al: *J Invest Dermatol* 78:331, 1983.
2. Leibl H, et al: *J Invest Dermatol* 85:417, 1985.
3. Nazzaro-Porro M, et al: *J Invest Dermatol* 87:438, 1986.
4. McLean D, Peter KK: *Br J Dermatol* 114:685, 1986.

Isolated Regional Perfusion for Treatment of Limb Melanoma in the American Black

Muchmore JH, Krementz ET, Carter RD, Sutherland CM, Cieutat EG (Tulane Univ; Univ of Texas, Dallas)

Am Surg 55:232–237, April 1989 13–36

Malignant melanoma is rare in the American black population; however, the overall survival rate in this population is low, which suggests that the disease may be more aggressive in blacks. Survival rates of patients with limb melanoma were analyzed to determine whether survival in blacks is equivalent to that in other patients with same-stage disease.

Of 961 patients treated for invasive malignant melanoma of the limbs, 48 (5%) were black. Of the black patients, 21 had stage I lesions, 63% of which showed level IV or greater invasion. The average depth of invasion was 3.7 mm. Of 21 black patients, 15 with stage III disease had an intact primary lesion in addition to regional disease at the time of diagnosis. Most lesions arose on a plantar site with level V invasion. Acral lentiginous melanoma was found in 80% of the black patients. All melanoma patients were treated by isolated regional perfusion with wide excision of the primary site. Regional lymph node dissection was performed for biopsy-proven regional disease.

At 10 years, patients with stage I disease had a 71% survival rate, whereas those with stage III disease had a 12.5% survival rate. Black patients had survival rates equivalent to those of whites in a similar stage of disease.

Black and white patients have equivalent prognoses if they are compared in the same stage of disease. Apparently, more aggressive disease in blacks may be explained partially by the fact that blacks often have more advanced disease at diagnosis.

▶ This report is from a pioneer group doing regional perfusion in a large number of patients over a period of many years. Regional perfusion is a very good method of control of melanoma of the extremities and should be more widely used.

This new study from the New Orleans group, however, presents some important observations that underscore the need for public education regarding malignant melanoma among the American black population. The poor prognosis of malignant melanoma in blacks, especially black males with melanoma on the plantar surface, is related to the advanced stage of the tumor at the time of presentation to the physician. The prognosis of malignant melanoma of the foot in black males is the same if the stage of the disease is taken into consideration. There had been a belief that melanoma in the black population had a worse prognosis. As in the white population, it was found that black men have a worse prognosis than black women. However, both black men and black women with distal lower extremity melanomas have a poor prognosis, ". . . the poorest survival rate of all the melanoma subgroups . . . when compared with SSM and LMM." The black population should be alerted to look for changes in pigmented lesions on the sole and around the nail.—T.B. Fitzpatrick, M.D., Ph.D.

14 Nonmelanoma Skin Cancer

▶ ↓ With each passing year the association between DNA viruses of the human papillomavirus (HPV) group and malignancy of squamous epithelia strengthens. From the earliest reports of epidermodysplasia verruciformis to association of viral particles with squamous cell carcinoma in transplant patients to the recent reports of increased cervical intraepithelial dysplasias in women with genital warts or in women whose consorts have genital warts, a convincing case has been proposed for an oncogenic role for wart viruses of certain serotypes. The present studies add to this growing study. Abstract 14–1 reaffirms the premalignant nature of wart-induced giant condyloma accuminata and suggests the need to biopsy large anogenital warts that are poorly responsive to therapy or appear to behave in an aggressive manner. Abstract 14–2 documents the presence of HPV-16 in periungual squamous cell carcinomas in healthy nonimmunocompromised patients, and indicates that the same serotype associated with tumors of mucous membranes is associated with the digital sites. Abstract 14–3 extends the sites of association between HPV-16 and dysplasia/malignancy to ocular tissues. The application from molecular biology of the polymerase chain reaction, which can greatly amplify the presence of low levels of viral DNA sequences to detectable levels, has been a major breakthrough in this area of research. Abstract 14–4 attempts to incorporate oncogenes in the interaction of viruses of more than 1 type in the etiology of human genital tumors. None of the samples was positive for all 3 agents simultaneously, but several had 2 agents present. At this point, the effect of interaction between 2 factors is highly speculative but raises the concern that the presence of more than 1 of these factors in the same lesion may be even more problematic than the presence of 1 alone.—A.J. Sober, M.D.

Malignant Transformation of Anorectal Giant Condyloma Acuminatum (Buschke-Loewenstein Tumor)

Creasman C, Haas PA, Fox TA Jr, Balazs M (Henry Ford Hosp, Detroit; St John's Hosp, Budapest)

Dis Colon Rectum 32:481–487, June 1989 14–1

Giant condyloma acuminatum was originally described as a penile lesion, but it is seen more rarely in the anorectal region. Eight anorectal lesions were seen at 2 surgical centers in a 13-year period. Previously malignant transformation was described in 15 patients with "ordinary" condylomata acuminata. Six of 20 giant condylomatas reported earlier progressed to squamous cell carcinoma.

The mean age of the 3 women and 5 men in the present study was 41

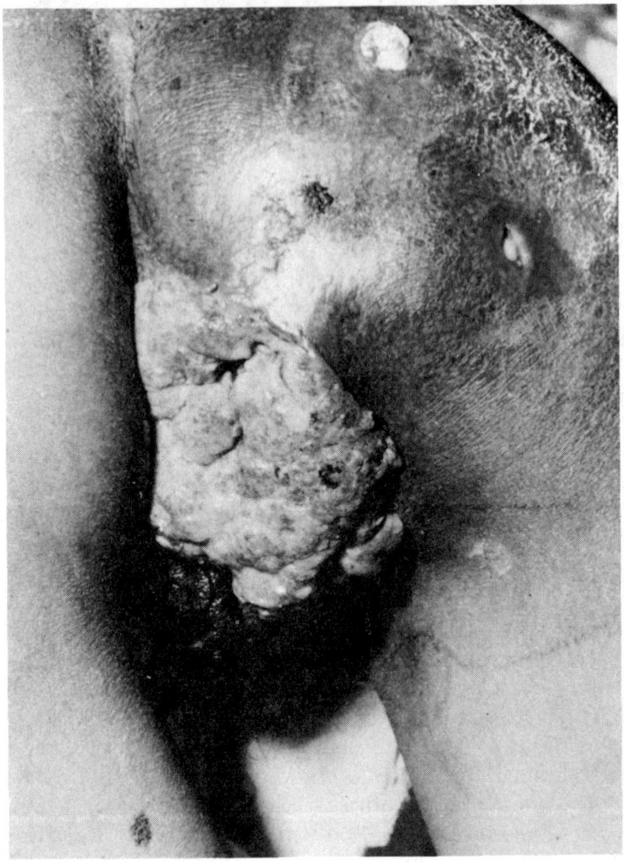

Fig 14–1.—Giant perianal condyloma acuminatum (gross photo) in woman aged 26 years. (Courtesy of Creasman C, Haas PA, Fox TA Jr, et al: *Dis Colon Rectum* 32:481–487, June 1989.)

years. Most lesions arose on the perianal skin (Fig 14–1). The patients underwent radical excision with fulguration; 3 also received radiation therapy. Three with advanced disease had abdominoperineal resection. Four of the 8 patients had histologic evidence of frank squamous cell cancer with local invasion, but none had detectable metastases. Two of the 8 patients died.

Malignant transformation of giant condylomata acuminata seems to have increased in the past 3 decades, but overall mortality has steadily declined.

The keys to ultimate survival are early control of local disease with radical excision and recognition of the potential for malignant transformation. Abdominoperineal resection is best in cases of recurrence, pelvic invasion, or malignant transformation. Human papillomavirus is known to induce these tumors, but the precise role of the virus itself in malignant transformation remains uncertain.

Human Papillomavirus Type 16 DNA in Periungual Squamous Cell Carcinomas

Moy RL, Eliezri YD, Nuovo GJ, Zitelli JA, Bennett RG, Silverstein S (Univ of California, Los Angeles; Columbia Univ; Montefiore Hosp, Pittsburgh)
JAMA 2669–2673, May 12, 1989 14–2

Periungual carcinomas may arise in preexisting verrucae, suggesting an etiologic role for human papillomavirus (HPV). Nine patients underwent microscopically controlled excision of periungual squamous cancers of the digits. Of 10 carcinomas analyzed, 8 were found to have DNA sequences homologous to HPV.

The 10 tumors were analyzed for DNA homology by dot blot hybridization. Most of the lesions, which were presented clinically as verrucae, resisted conventional treatment. Six of the 8 lesions containing HPV DNA sequences were related to HPV-16. The restriction endonuclease digestion pattern of DNA in 4 of these lesions was diagnostic of episomal HPV-16.

The frequent association of HPV-16 with periungual squamous cell carcinoma is similar to that described at other mucous membrane sites, such as the genital tract. Human papillomavirus type 16 may have a role in the transformation of warts into squamous cell carcinoma.

DNA of Human Papillomavirus Type 16 in Dysplastic and Malignant Lesions of the Conjunctiva and Cornea

McDonnell JM, Mayr AJ, Martin WJ (Univ of Southern California, Los Angeles)
N Engl J Med 320:1442–1446, June 1, 1989 14–3

Human papillomaviruses (HPVs) have been associated with anogenital malignancy and with benign lesions of the conjunctiva. To investigate their role in the pathogenesis of malignancy in the conjunctiva, the polymerase chain reaction (PCR) was used to detect HPV types 16 and 18 DNA in paraffin-embedded specimens or mucosal scrapings from 6 neoplastic lesions of the conjunctiva.

The PCR technique detected DNA sequences related to HPV-16 in all embedded and swab specimens. These sequences were not detected in 6 control specimens from patients with conjunctival melanoma, papilloma, nevus, or pterygium.

These results indicate that sufficient DNA for the PCR assay can be obtained from paraffin-embedded conjunctiva specimens and from mucosal swabs. It appears from this limited sample that DNA from HPV-16 is present in many conjunctival malignancies and may be involved in the pathogenesis of these lesions.

Search for Human Papillomavirus, Herpes Simplex Virus, and c-*myc* Oncogene in Human Genital Tumors

Di Luca D, Costa S, Monini P, Rotola A, Terzano P, Savioli A, Grigioni W, Cassai E (Istituto di Microbiologia, Ferrara; Il Dipartimento di Ostetricia e Ginecoligia, Bologna; Istituto di Anatomia Patologica, Bologna, Italy)

Int J Cancer 43:570–577, Apr 15, 1989 14–4

Previous findings have demonstrated the simultaneous presence of DNA sequences homologous to herpes simplex virus type 2 (HSV-2) and human papillomavirus (HPV) in the same genital neoplastic lesions. An investigation was made of the possible interaction of HSV-2 and HPV as well as of oncogenes in cervical carcinogenesis. Using molecular probes, the concomitant presence and expression of HSV-2, HPV DNA, and the c-*myc* oncogene were investigated in 63 genital samples, including grade III cervical intraepithelial neoplasms (CIN), genital invasive carcinomas, and healthy genital tissues.

Homologies to HSV-2 DNA fragments were identified in about 30% of genital tumors by Southern blot analysis, and HPV-16 DNA was identified in nearly half of the tumor samples by dot-blot hybridization. Of 8 tumors with HSV-2 DNA, 6 also contained HPV-16 DNA. Immunoreactivity to the HSV-2 specific protein ICP 10 was found in 29 of 55 genital tumors but was absent from all healthy genital tissue or nongenital tumors tested. No tumors positive for HPV DNA were immunoreactive for HPV capsid protein or HPV-16 E6 protein. Four tumors were positive for c-*myc* expression but none showed amplification of c-*myc* DNA. No tumor was positive for every factor tested.

These results provide evidence that HSV-2, HPV-16, and c-*myc* expression are independent risk factors for cervical carcinogenesis. Because some tumors contained evidence of several of these factors simultaneously, it is possible that different carcinogenic factors act independently or synergistically at different steps of tumor development. This may explain why HPV-16 DNA is found in many tissue samples from healthy women.

Dermatologic Lesions in a Transplant Population

Brown JH, Hutchison T, Kelly AMT, McGeown MG (Belfast City Hosp, Northern Ireland)

Transplantation 46:530–532, October 1988 14–5

Increases in renal transplantation have resulted in larger numbers of persons receiving long-term immunosuppression. An increased incidence of skin infections and neoplasms in such patients has been reported. The 223 Celtic Caucasian patients who underwent renal transplantation between 1965 and 1984 were examined for the presence of skin lesions. All had received routine immunosuppression therapy.

Nine patients had malignant skin lesions, including 7 squamous cell carcinomas and 2 basal cell carcinomas; none of these 9 patients reported excessive exposure to sunlight. Two patients with squamous cell carcinoma previously had recurrent viral warts. In 42 patients hyperkeratoses developed and in 51, simple warts, often multiple and resistant to treatment. Four patients had keratoacanthomas. Acne and purpura were common among these patients. All 3 surviving patients who received transplants between 1965 and 1969 had skin malignancies.

These data confirm the evidence of other investigators that in renal transplant patients receiving long-term immunosuppression, an increase in skin neoplasia occurs. The incidence of frank malignancy in the population studied was 4 times that expected for the general population in Northern Ireland. It seems likely that prolonged immunosuppression has a cumulative effect, because the risk of neoplasia seems to increase with increasing graft survival times.

▶ The most impressive cutaneous manifestation of long-term immunosuppression is the increased incidence of skin cancer, particularly squamous cell carcinoma. This survey covered patients who are not normally exposed to the excessive doses of ultraviolet whose effects we are accustomed to see. All the more should we be on guard for skin cancer in renal transplant patients who have had much actinic damage.—R. Master, M.D.

The Incidence of Immunosuppression-Related Skin Disease in Long-Term Transplant Patients

McLelland J, Rees A, Williams G, Chu T (Hammersmith Hosp, London)

Transplantation 46:871–874, December 1988 14–6

Concerns have been expressed regarding the risk of skin lesions developing after an immunosuppression regimen that includes cyclosporine compared with conventional immunosuppression after organ transplantation. The incidence of immunosuppression-related skin disease in long-term allograft recipients on different immunosuppression regimens was studied in 121 patients who had received a renal allograft at a mean of 71 months previously (range, 4 months to 21 years). of these, 72 received conventional immunosuppression with azathioprine and prednisolone and 36 received the current treatment regimen of cyclosporine, azathioprine, and prednisolone.

Fungal skin infections occurred in 10 patients (7%). The prevalence was greater in patients with skin types that tanned easily than in those who burn. Viral warts were present in 45 patients, 20 of whom had more than 10 warts. The presence of warts was significantly associated with excess sun exposure, skin types 1 and 2, and longer duration of transplant. Warts were significantly more common in those receiving conventional immunosuppression, but this could result from differences in duration of immunosuppression. Dysplastic or neoplastic skin lesions developed after transplantation in 12 patients. The incidence of dysplasia increased with age and was significantly associated with skin types 1 and 2, excess sun exposure, and with duration of allograft. Despite the shorter duration of treatment with the new regimen, there was no difference between the groups in the proportion of patients with dysplastic skin lesions.

Immunosuppression-related skin disease can cause significant problems in allograft recipients. Patients receiving cyclosporine will have skin problems similar to those in patients given conventional immunosuppression. All immunosuppressed patients should be advised to avoid sun exposure, use sunscreens, and be regularly examined for the development of dysplastic lesions.

▶ The cutaneous complications of long-term immunosuppression in transplant patients include warts, tumors, and fungal infections. The authors emphasize the importance of protection from sunlight in patients with type 1072 skin, because sun-induced tumors may be very aggressive in this situation.—R. Master, M.D.

Non Melanoma Skin Cancer of the Scalp: On the Etiology

Frentz G, Sørensen JL, Flod K (The Finsen Inst, Rigshospitalet, Copenhagen)

Acta Derm Venereol (Stockh) 69:142–146, April 1989 14–7

The role of previous exposure to grenz rays was evaluated in 82 patients treated for nonmelanoma skin cancer of the scalp from 1976 to 1985. Twelve patients had previously been treated with grenz rays on the scalp. Eight patients were treated for psoriasis. Ten had been exposed to at least 1 additional skin carcinogen, whereas no skin carcinogen other than exposure to grenz ray was found in 2. Characteristically, 11 scalp cancers associated with previous grenz ray treatments were basal cell cancers. They developed more commonly in females than in males (male: female ratio, <0.1), and two thirds occurred in patients with multiple skin cancers.

A very small subgroup of the human population may be abnormally sensitive to the carcinogenic effect of grenz rays. Additional grenz ray therapy should be administered with caution in patients exposed to other skin carcinogens. Screening for skin cancer should be performed in previously multifactorially exposed patients with dermatologic conditions.

▶ Although this study lacks an appropriate control group, it would be hard to imagine that in a cohort of randomly selected age- and sex-matched Danes one would find that 15% had previous grenz ray exposure to the scalp. Basal cell carcinoma caused, or co-caused, primarily by grenz rays appears to be proven. It would seem prudent to add grenz ray exposure to the list of possible exposures in the history taken for patients being evaluated for skin cancer, along with chronic ultraviolet light, other forms of ionizing irradiation, arsenicals, and tars. Also noteworthy is the observation that 1 in 10 nonmelanoma skin cancers arising on the scalp does so from a precursor sebaceous or verrucous nevus. (See also Abstract 14–8.)—A.J. Sober, M.D.

Grenz Ray-Induced Nonmelanoma Skin Cancer
Frentz G (Rigshospitalet, Copenhagen)
J Am Acad Dermatol 21:475–478, September 1989 14–8

Grenz ray irradiation is used in the treatment of benign skin disorders. Only 22 occurrences of nonmelanoma skin cancer in areas previously exposed to grenz rays have been reported. However, 10 of these 22 patients also had been exposed to at least 1 additional carcinogen, and 10 patients had been treated for psoriasis. The effects of age at onset, latency period, and total grenz ray exposure were compared in 11 patients with psoriasis and 17 without psoriasis. All were questioned about exposure to carcinogens such as ionizing and ultraviolet irradiation and sun exposure. Exposure to tar preparations, thorium, radium, and arsenic also was recorded.

Nonmelanoma skin cancers developed in grenz-ray-exposed skin areas in 8 women and 3 men who had received grenz ray treatment for psoriasis. The tumors appeared on the scalp in 9 patients and on the legs in 2. Ten of the 11 patients also had been exposed to large amounts of ultraviolet irradiation, coal tar, thorium, radium, and oral arsenic.

In 15 women and 2 men who had undergone treatment for pityriasis, seborrheic dermatitis, acne, rosacea, and neurodermatitis, the nonmelanoma skin cancers also developed within the grenz-ray-exposed areas. The involved sites included the scalp in 10 patients, the face in 5, the neck in 1, and the lower part of the abdomen in 1. Only 2 of the 17 patients had undergone occasional ultraviolet radiation treatments.

Development of nonmelanoma skin tumors after grenz ray therapy occurred most frequently in women. No statistically significant difference was found between psoriasis and nonpsoriasis patients with regard to average age at first exposure to grenz rays. No threshold dose of grenz rays could be established for the development of nonmelanoma skin tumors. Whereas the latency time was significantly lower for nonpsoriatic patients, the distribution of their latency times was normal. Most of the tumors were basal cell cancers, and most patients had multiple tumors.

Common therapeutic doses of grenz rays, when used as a single treatment modality, can cause nonmelanoma skin cancer but apparently only in a few predisposed individuals. Whether such patients can be identified beforehand by testing their cellular sensitivity to irradiation has not been determined.

▶ This study describes the patients with basal cell carcinoma of the scalp previously reported in Abstract 14–7. Noteworthy is the predominance of women and patients with psoriasis. Without epidemiologic controls, a predisposition cannot be established from the present series because the cases reported may reflect exposure opportunities rather than an inherent predisposition.—A.J. Sober, M.D.

Long-Term Follow-Up of Skin Cancer in the PUVA-48 Cooperative Study

Forman AB, Roenigk HH Jr, Caro WA, Magid ML (Northwestern Univ)
Arch Dermatol 125:515–519, April 1989 14–9

Worldwide experience with psoralen plus ultraviolet A light (PUVA) therapy in patients with psoriasis is now sufficient to draw some conclusions about the associated risk of epidermal tumors. One report demonstrated a substantial dose-related increase in squamous cell carcinomas. Evaluation was made of the results of a long-term follow-up study of skin cancer in 551 PUVA-treated patients with psoriasis seen at 7 medical centers in a 10-year period.

Basal cell carcinoma developed in 13 patients (2.4%) and squamous cell carcinoma in 9 (1.6%), an incidence significantly higher than that in the general population. The increase in basal cell carcinoma occurred only in patients exposed to other carcinogenic agents, whereas the increase in squamous cell carcinoma occurred in patients without such exposures. The cumulative UVA dosage did not correlate with the development of basal cell carcinoma, but there was a trend of increasing numbers of squamous cell carcinomas in patients who received higher doses. Five of 9 patients had squamous cell carcinomas at sites not exposed to the sun. All of the patients with tumors underwent surgery, and none of the tumors recurred.

The incidence of squamous cell carcinoma is increased in patients with psoriasis who are treated with PUVA. To limit the risk, patients with a history of therapeutic ionizing radiation, arsenic exposure, or previous skin cancer should be excluded from PUVA therapy. Patients with type I skin who are receiving PUVA therapy should be watched closely. Minimum phototoxic dosage testing should also be done, because minimum dosages appear to be associated with a reduced risk. Sites that are not involved with psoriasis, especially scrotal skin, should be carefully shielded.

▶ Although this cohort is smaller and has received far less treatment than the PUVA Follow-Up Study cohort (1), after correction for differences in dose these findings are comparable. There is an increased risk of squamous cell carcinoma. Squamous cell carcinoma occurs in sites not usually exposed to the sun, and a disproportionate number of genital squamous cell carcinomas were observed.—R.S. Stern, M.D.

Reference

1. Stern RS, Lange R: Nonmelanoma skin cancer occurring in patients treated with PUVA five to ten years after first treatment. *J Invest Dermatol* 91:120, 1988.

Frequency of Occurrence of Diagnostic Cytologic Parameters in Basal Cell Carcinoma: A Retrospective Review of 25 Cases

Youngberg GA, Laucirica R, Leicht SS (VA Med Ctr; East Tennessee State Univ, Johnson City)
Am J Clin Pathol 91:24–30, January 1989 14–10

The utility and accuracy of cytology in the diagnosis of basal cell carcinoma have been reported by several investigators. Useful cytologic features include strong cellular coherence, small tumor cell size, hyperchromatic nuclei with absent or inconspicuous nucleoli, peripheral palisading of tumor cells, and uniformity of tumor cells. However, some features, such as prominent nucleoli, keratinization, and nuclear enlargement and pleomorphism, can be misleading. The frequency of occurrence of several microscopic findings that could be diagnostically helpful or misleading was tabulated.

Twenty-five cytologic preparations from basal cell carcinomas documented by subsequent tissue material were studied. A major criterion for the histologic diagnosis of basal cell carcinoma—peripheral palisading—was seldom evident in the cytologic preparations. Large clusters of cells with crowded nuclei were observed in each case, and that finding is therefore a useful cytologic parameter. Because of the frequent absence of peripheral palisading, there could be diagnostic confusion with lesions of small cell squamous carcinoma. The absence of large clusters of cells with contiguous nuclei should raise doubt about a diagnosis of basal cell carcinoma. Clinicians should be careful not to confuse the clusters with hair follicles.

▶ Clearly, the diagnosis of basal cell carcinoma is much more easily established with biopsy specimens as small as those obtained by a 2-mm punch in comparison to cytologic preparations, which may be problematic even to skilled cytopathologists. It appears that important architectural features such as "peripheral palisading," which help to establish the diagnosis in biopsy specimens, are often lacking in cytologic preparations. This situation appears similar to that occurring with dysplastic nevi in which appreciation of both architectural abnormalities as well as the cytologic features are required for accurate diagnosis.—A.J. Sober, M.D.

Analysis of Morpheaform Basal Cell Carcinoma

Richman T, Penneys NS (Univ of Miami)
J Cutan Pathol 15:359–362, December 1988 14–11

Morpheaform basal cell carcinoma (MBCC) is a relatively uncommon subtype of basal cell carcinoma (BCC) having poorly defined histologic and clinical borders. It frequently occurs on the face. When specimens of MBCC were analyzed, 2 histologic subtypes were identified. Of 11,187 specimens identified as BCC, 87 (0.1%) were classified as MBCC. This entity was considered pure if it was composed solely of thin strands of basaloid epithelium and complex if the neoplasm was composed of thin strands of basaloid epithelium and some other pattern, such as nodular aggregates.

Both pure and complex subtypes are more often found on the face, especially the midface, than is pigmented BCC. Pure MBCC is more common in women, in whom these lesions are more likely to occur on the midface. Men are less likely to have midface lesions, pure or complex. Although MBCC histologically resembles some eccrine tumors, immunohistochemical evidence for eccrine differentiation is lacking. The frequency of both subtypes on the midface and their infiltrative margins justify their inclusion among the potentially recurrent cancers often needing aggressive therapy.

▶ Perhaps the reason that a greater number of "pure" subtypes occurred in women (76%) is that this is an earlier presentation of MBCC. As more nodular areas "grow," an event probably correlated with more clinically evident tumors, a more typical proportion of men and women are seen (49% and 5%, respectively). There is no doubt that women are more conscientious about noting subtle changes in their faces, and early MBCCs can indeed be very subtle. No data on the duration of the lesions are given in the article, but this information would be very interesting.—J.L. Fewkes, M.D.

Long-Term Recurrence Rates in Previously Untreated (Primary) Basal Cell Carcinoma: Implications for Patient Follow-Up

Rowe DE, Carroll RJ, Day CL Jr (Univ of Texas, San Antonio; Texas A & M Univ, College Station)

J Dermatol Surg Oncol 15:315–328, March 1989 14–12

No uniform method exists for reporting recurrence rates among patients with previously untreated (primary) basal cell carcinoma. To address this problem, all studies since 1947 reporting recurrence rates after treatment of primary basal carcinomas using surgical excision, radiotherapy, cryotherapy, curettage and electrodesiccation, and Mohs' micrographic surgery were reviewed.

Thirty percent of all recurrences appeared during the first year after treatment, 50% appeared within the first 2 years, and 66% appeared within the first 3 years. Generally, the 10-year recurrence rate was twice that of the 2-year recurrence rate. Furthermore, 18% of recurrences appeared between 5 and 10 years after treatment. Basal cell carcinomas tended to recur at the same cumulative rate through time regardless of treatment modality.

The weighted average recurrence rate among the 72 short-term studies with follow-up of less than 5 years was 4.2%, whereas the rate was 8.7% among the 34 long-term studies with follow-up of 5 or more years. The mean 5-year recurrence rate associated with Mohs' micrographic study of 1.0% was 8.7 times less than the weighted average of all 4 non-Mohs' modalities combined (table). Furthermore, the average 5-year recurrence

Summary of Short-Term Versus Long-Term Recurrence Rates: All Modalities

Treatment Modality	Recurrence Rates Short-Term (< 5 years)	Long-Term (5 years)
Surgical excision	2.8% (157/5560)	10.1% (264/2606)
Curettage and electrodesiccation	4.7% (173/3664)	7.7% (274/3573)
Radiation therapy	5.3% (318/6072)	8.7% (410/4695)
Cryotherapy	3.7% (90/2462)	7.5% (20/269)
All non-Mohs modalities	4.2% (738/17,758)	8.7% (968/11,143)
Mohs micrographic surgery	1.4% (5/367)	1.0% (73/7670)

(Courtesy of Rowe DE, Carroll RJ, Day CL Jr: *J Dermatol Surg Oncol* 15:315–328, March 1989.)

rate of 8.7% for non-Mohs' modalities combined was more than twice the 4.2% average recurrence rate of short-term studies.

Reporting of recurrence rate data after treatment of primary basal cell carcinoma should be standardized using 5-year life-table analysis. Recurrences after treatment of primary basal cell carcinoma appear later than is generally acknowledged in the literature. Lifetime follow-up is necessary for detection of recurrences and new primaries.

▶ The authors put tremendous effort and thought into this article in an attempt to evaluate the recurrence rates found in the literature. With sophisticated number crunching, they come up with some very interesting figures (table). The bottom line is that patient with BCC must be followed routinely for the rest of their lives; and recurrences *do* occur, even 10–20 years after the original procedure. Any change in a scar is suspect and must be biopsied.—J.L. Fewkes, M.D.

Factors Predictive of Recurrence of Basal Cell Carcinoma

Dixon AY, Lee SH, McGregor DH (Univ of Kansas, Kansas City; VA Med Ctr, Kansas City)

Am J Dermatopathol 11:222–232, June 1989 14–13

Basal cell carcinoma (BCC) commonly occurs on the head and neck area of elderly persons with light complexions. Most BCCs are slow-growing, relatively nonaggressive tumors that are readily cured by local treatment. However, a some BCCs behave aggressively, causing extensive tissue destruction, and some keep recurring, causing patients to undergo repeated operations. Whether any clinical and histologic parameters are predictive of recurring BCC was investigated in 30 patients (mean age 68 years) with recurrent BCC and 74 patients (mean age, 64 years) with nonrecurrent BCC.

Of the former group, 23 had 1 recurrence, 5 had 2 recurrences, and 2 had 3 recurrences. The mean interval between original BCC excision and first recurrence was 36.9 months. All recurrent BCCs had developed on the head only, whereas nonrecurrent BCCs had occurred on the head, neck, trunk, and extremities. The mean duration of BCC was 1.1 years in the group with recurrence and 2.2 years in the group with nonrecurrence. Statistical analysis of the clinical parameters showed that a location other than on the head was significantly associated with nonrecurrence and could therefore serve as a prognostic indicator. Age and tumor location had no prognostic validity.

Assessment of the histologic data revealed statistically significant differences between recurrent and nonrecurrent BCCs. Prognostic indicators included the measured distance to resection margins, the shape of cell groups, growth pattern, contour of the invading edge, degree of peripheral palisading, and nuclear pleomorphism. Parameters of possible prognostic significance included degree of fibrosis, cystic change, and atypical squamous change. Thus the histologic findings of excised BCCs may be prognostic of which BCCs are more likely to recur. The clinical findings are not particularly helpful as prognostic indicators of recurrence.

▶ Perhaps it is now time to make up a set of histopathologic parameters for the diagnosis of BCC (much as is done for melanoma) to aid the surgeon in his treatment of a particular lesion. For example, when should incompletely excised tumors or "close to margin" specimens be reexcised? Which need close follow-up? This article takes a step toward addressing such questions. Mohs' surgeons have for years been using the criteria mentioned here to direct their treatment of tumors. One of the most important and unique aspects to Mohs is that the surgeon and pathologist are one and the same person. There is no doubt this is integral to its high cure rate.—J.L. Fewkes, M.D.

Periocular Basal Cell Carcinoma in Adults 35 Years of Age and Younger

Nerad JA, Whitaker DC (Univ of Iowa)

Am J Ophthalmol 106:723–729, December 1988 14–14

The most common malignancy in human beings, basal cell carcinoma, usually occurs in the sixth or seventh decade of life. Little attention has been given to periocular basal cell carcinoma in the younger adult population. Of 409 patients of all ages with basal cell carcinoma, 13 individuals (6 men) aged 21–35 years were identified. Factors related to patient traits, tumor characteristics, and reconstructive technique were analyzed.

Eight patients had light pigmentation, including fair complexion, blue or green eyes, and blond hair; the other 5, including 3 with basal cell nevus syndrome, had normal or dark pigmentation. None of the patients had a history of excessive sun exposure. Two patients had other skin tumors previously and had basal cell nevus syndrome. In these 2 patients tumor was present bilaterally with several accompanying tumors of the face.

Clinically, the tumors were small (average size, 0.77 cm^2). The appearance was not that of a typical nodular basal cell carcinoma. Most lesions were erythematous and flat or slightly raised, often with scaling. Telangiectasia was common. The cell subtype at biopsy was most often morpheaform. The area of excision averaged 5.4 times times larger than the average size of the lesion based on clinical appearance Mohs' micrographic surgery was used to remove tumors, which insured a tumor-free surgical margin before reconstruction. Reconstruction was performed most commonly with the use of myocutaneous advancement flaps.

Features related to the characteristics of the patient and tumor may be helpful in identifying young persons with basal cell carcinoma. The first group includes those with no personal or family history of basal cell carcinoma and generally a light-colored complexion and hair, suggesting susceptibility to ultraviolet light injury. The second group includes those with multiple skin tumors, a family history of many relatives with basal cell carcinoma, and basal cell nevus syndrome.

▶ This is an excellent reminder that (1) young people (21–35 years) do have skin cancer, and (2) periorbital tumors are often diagnosed relatively late, leading to greater than necessary morbidity.—J.L. Fewkes, M.D.

Malignant Lesions of the Eyelid

Mamalis N, White GL Jr, Pedersen DM, Holds J, Anderson RL (Univ of Utah)
Am Family Physician 39:95–102, January 1989 14–15

Malignant tumors of the eyelid pose a great risk to the eye and have a significant potential for metastasis and mortality. Early diagnosis is important, and any chronic eyelid lesion or chronic unilateral keratoconjunctivitis should be biopsied for histopathologic examination.

Basal cell carcinoma accounts for 80% to 95% of all malignant lesions of the eyelid. The lesion often begins as a small, raised nodule with poorly defined edges. Of the 4 basic morphological patterns the nodular is most common. The ulcerative pattern may be associated with chronic inflammation. The morphea or sclerosing form is potentially aggressive, extending deep into the dermis. Least common is the multicentric pattern. Basal cell carcinoma of the eyelid seldom metastasizes and is rarely fatal.

Squamous cell carcinoma accounts for 5% to 10% of malignant eyelid lesions. It may appear as a scaly, crusting patch, especially at the margin of the lower lid. Inadequate treatment may result in invasion of the orbit and metastasis to regional lymph nodes. From 1% to 6% of malignant tumors of the eyelid are sebaceous gland carcinomas. They appear most often in patients aged 50–70 years. The most common sites of origin are the meibomian glands in the tarsus of the eyelid. Because the lesions may have a broad spectrum of clinical features and mimic other eyelid disorders, a biopsy is mandatory. These tumors are aggressive and have potential for multicentric origin. Further, 1% to 5% of malignant lesions are melanomas. A newly acquired pigmented lesion of the eyelid, particularly one that changes in color, size, shape, or consistency, should undergo excisional biopsy.

Malignant lesions of the eyelid occur most frequently in fair-skinned adults and are related to prolonged exposure to sunlight. Complete surgical excision is the preferred treatment, with Mohs' micrographic surgery recommended for recurrent or difficult tumors. Biopsy should be performed promptly when any questionable mass is observed on the eyelid.

▶ This is a good basic review of eyelid tumors, an area that dermatologists often overlook. Because 80% to 95% of all eyelid tumors are basal cell carcinomas, dermatologists should be finding them. Eyelids need to be carefully examined, usually by stretching the periorbital skin, especially in elderly patients.—J.L. Fewkes, M.D.

The Incidence of Non-Melanocytic Skin Cancers in an Australian Population: Results of a Five-Year Prospective Study

Marks R, Jolley D, Dorevitch AP, Selwood TS (Anti-Cancer Council of Victoria, South Carlton; AP Dorevitch & Assoc, Camberwell; Monash Univ, Praham, Victoria, Australia)

Med J Aust 150:475–478, May 1989 14–16

Nonmelanocytic skin cancers are common in Australia, but their exact incidence is not known. A longitudinal study of a sample population in Victoria was done to determine the incidence of symptomatic and asymptomatic nonmelanocytic skin cancers in that community. The effects of age, sex, occupation, country of birth, and skin type on the incidence of these cancers also were assessed. Of the eligible population, 2,669 persons (81%) participated in the 5-year study. They were 1,187 men and 1,482 women whose mean age was 58.6 years. The light-exposed areas of the head and neck, forearms, and dorsa of the hands were examined.

At the first examination, 60 persons (2.25%) had at least 1 nonmelanocytic skin cancer: 12 had a squamous cell carcinoma and 48 had a total of 51 basal cell carcinomas. Of the study population, 74% was seen on more than 1 occasion, resulting in 6,288 person-years of follow-up for determination of the incidence of new cancers. The calculated minimal age-standardized incidence rate was 873 nonmelanocytic skin cancers per 100,000 population each year. The minimal incidence rate for basal cell carcinomas was 672/100,000 population each year, and for squamous cell carcinomas, 201/100,000 each year. Age, sex, skin reaction to sunlight, and occupation were significant factors in determining the risk for nonmelanocytic skin cancer developing.

The incidence for nonmelanocytic skin cancers is more than 3 times the combined rate of all other cancers in Australia. The cumulative risk of a nonmelanocytic skin cancer developing by age 70 years was estimated to be more than 2 in 3.

▶ There are no surprises in the data collected here. However, it does begin to give actual numbers to the magnitude of the problem. It is interesting that the last paragraph of the full-length article specifically addresses cost at a minimum of $100 million per year—an interesting figure that might cause us to seriously reconsider how we deal with skin cancer in the United States and the importance of public education.—J.L. Fewkes, M.D.

Skin Cancer in a Queensland Population

Green A, Beardmore G, Hart V, Leslie D, Marks R, Staines D (Queensland Inst of Med Research, Brisbane; Royal Brisbane Hosp; Anti-Cancer Council of Victoria; Community Health Ctr, Nambour, Australia)

J Am Acad Dermatol 19:1045–1052, December 1988 14–17

Solar ultraviolet levels are high in tropical Australia, and the opportunity for outdoor recreation is available almost all year. Recently, greater numbers of young persons have been seen with signs of skin cancer and sun damage, but there have been few published studies of the prevalence of skin cancer in Queensland. A survey was made of a representative Queensland community to determine the current prevalence of actinic skin disease in young and middle-aged adults. In response to a letter of invitation, 2,095 people were interviewed by questionnaire and examined by a dermatologist. A random 10% received a full-body examination; in the remainder, examination was confined to the head, neck, backs of the hands, and forearms.

In 43 patients 54 invasive, histologically confirmed skin cancers were diagnosed. Eleven of these cancers occurred in patients receiving full-body examination. Overall, 4.6% of the patients aged 20–69 years had skin cancer, principally basal cell carcinoma; 40% had solar keratoses. Individuals younger than 40 exhibited substantial sun-related skin damage. In this sample a large proportion of actinic lesions occurred on sites other than the head, backs of hands, or forearms.

After adjustment for age and sex, the greatest risk factors for skin cancer and solar keratoses were fair skin and clinical signs of solar damage, such as solar lentigines, actinic elastosis of the neck, and facial telangiectasia. Self-reported tendencies toward sunburn, frequent painful sunburn, work-related sun exposure, and history of skin cancer correlated with findings.

▶ These large studies to assess the prevalence of sun-related skin damage are critical to our better understanding and treatment of all patients. Of note here was the highest correlation of *clinically* assessed actinic damage and skin cancer. This means that the dermatologist can easily, and at an early stage, make the diagnosis in patients at greatest risk. Also, there was actually a slightly greater risk for skin cancer in patients who "burn, then tan" than in those who "burn only." Therefore, our type III patients may need us more than fairer types who may self-select to avoid the sun. Also, eye color and hair color were not as significant as skin type.—J.L. Fewkes, M.D.

Treatment of Nonmelanoma Skin Cancer at a Large Australian Center

Ashby MA, Smith J, Ainslie J, McEwan L (Peter MacCallum Cancer Inst, Melbourne)

Cancer 63:1863–1871, May 1, 1989 14–18

Australia has the highest incidence of malignant melanoma and nonmelanoma skin cancer in the world. The case records of all 1,154 public patients seen in a cancer center in Melbourne during 1980 with primary or recurrent basal cell carcinoma, squamous cell carcinoma, or basosquamous cancer were reviewed. The median age was 68 years.

A final diagnosis of basal cell carcinoma was made in 901 patients (78%), of squamous cell carcinoma in 242 patients (21%), and of basosquamous carcinoma in 11 patients (1%); 62% of these diagnoses were biopsy proven. On the basis of histologic diagnoses, basal cell carcinoma was diagnosed correctly in 85% of cases, whereas squamous cell carcinoma was diagnosed correctly in only 53%. The predominant sites of lesions were the head and neck (75%), limbs (11%), and trunk (4%); 94% of the patients had primary lesions and 6% had recurrent lesions. Further, 55% of the patients were treated with surgery, 39% with superficial radiotherapy, 3% with other types of radiotherapy, 1% with cryotherapy, and 0.2% with 5-fluorouracil.

Increased treatment failures were associated with recurrent lesions or lesions on the eyelids, ears, or nose, and stage T_4 lesions. When other prognostic factors were taken into account, superficial radiotherapy resulted in a 2.3-fold higher failure rate than surgery, and nonsuperficial radiotherapy had an 11.5-fold higher failure rate than surgery.

Biopsy of suspected skin cancers before treatment is recommended in most cases. Radiotherapy is indicated as treatment in older patients or those unfit for or unwilling to have surgery, in those with multiple or large superficial lesions, for lesions with positive surgical margins or recurrence after surgery in elderly or infirm patients in whom further surgery would be extensive, and in those with advanced incurable disease. Surgery is recommended for young patients, for lesions involving underlying cartilage, bone, or tendon, or are deeply infiltrating or of uncertain depth, solitary lesions, lesions of clinically uncertain pathologic type, recurrent lesions after radiotherapy, and lesions subjected to constant trauma.

▶ This large study has several interesting aspects: (1) It is a rare study that splits nonmelanoma skin cancer patients between treatment with irradiation and plastic surgery; (2) cure rates are excellent; (3) the Australians have a male:female ratio of 1.5:1, whereas most of our large studies are 1:1; (4) 94% of the lesions were primary, which certainly accounts for the high cure rate; (5) a second lesion developed in 38%, which is similar to Robinson's findings (1); (6) only 14% of the lesions treated with irradiation were biopsied. Included in the latter group were unknown numbers of superficial basal or squamous cell carcinomas, hypertrophic actinic keratoses, and so on.—J.L. Fewkes, M.D.

Reference

1. Robinson JK: *Cancer* 60:118, 1987.

Basal Cell Carcinoma in a Patient With Acquired Immunodeficiency Syndrome: Treatment With Mohs Micrographic Surgery Fixed-Tissue Technique
Hruza GJ, Snow SN (Washington Univ; Univ of Wisconsin)
J Dermatol Surg Oncol 15:545–551, May 5, 1989 14–19

Patients with AIDS often have various malignant neoplasms involving the skin.

Man, 28, had a 2-year history of a right alar groove growth. The lesion had been treated with electrodesiccation and curettage after biopsy showed it to be basal cell carcinoma (BCC). However, the patient was referred for Mohs surgery because of lack of healing. The patient had been found to have *Pneumocystis carinii* and AIDS 14 months earlier. He had done well with dapsone and acyclovir prophylaxis for *P carinii* pneumonia and herpes simplex, respectively. Before biopsy of the BCC, 100% dichloroacetic acid and zinc chloride fixative paste were applied to the lesion. The specimen was obtained by shave excision. The lesion was extirpated after 4 stages of the Mohs surgery fixed-tissue technique. Specimens were handled with appropriate precautions for HIV. The defect was repaired with a split-thickness skin graft. Postoperatively, the patient experienced recurrent episodes of sinusitis, oral thrush, fevers, and severe anemia but no severe opportunistic infections.

Mohs micrographic mapping makes possible complete removal of a potentially life-threatening neoplasm in a patient with AIDS. If the tissue is fixed before excision and appropriate infectious disease precautions are followed, health-care personnel will minimize their exposure to the HIV virus.

► Appropriate precautions here include wearing double gloves, masks, gowns, caps, and eye protection, as well as taking extreme caution in handling any sharp instruments. Also, cleansing of all surfaces, the cryostat, and instruments was done after each procedure with one of several common agents known to inactivate HIV. With current restrictions on testing, shouldn't we be doing this for *all* patients?—J.L. Fewkes, M.D.

Metastases From Squamous Cell Carcinoma of the Skin and Lip: An Analysis of Twenty-Seven Cases
Dinehart SM, Pollack SV (Univ of Arkansas; Duke Univ)
J Am Acad Dermatol 21:241–248, August 1989 14–20

Squamous cell carcinoma accounts for 20% of all cutaneous malignancies. Clinical and histopathologic criteria have been suggested to identify tumors with an increased risk of metastasis, including size, location, histologic differentiation, tumor depth, age, etiologic findings, invasion, duration before treatment, and previous treatment. Data on 27 metastatic squamous cell carcinomas originating in the lip or in sun-damaged skin were compared with data on 338 nonmetastasizing squamous cell carcinomas. All had been treated by Mohs surgery.

Tumors of the temple, dorsa of the hands, and the lips were more likely to metastasize than those in other locations. Metastatic lesions did not develop in antecedent inflammatory or degenerative conditions. No single factor was helpful in predicting the likelihood of metastasis. However, metastatic lesions on average were significantly larger and deeper than nonmetastatic tumors. The primary lesions of patients with metastasis were much more difficult to control. Metastatic tumors caused death in 5 patients despite aggressive surgery and/or radiation therapy.

Metastatic behavior was difficult to predict on the basis of any single variable. Lesions that are large and deep appear to have a greater tendency to metastasize than small, shallow ones; tumors less than 1 cm long rarely metastasized. The primary lesion in half of the patients with metastatic disease was not controlled by Mohs surgery.

▶ It is difficult to get a true handle on which squamous cell carcinomas act aggressively. Because these are some of the most lethal lesions that we treat, and early adequate treatment can be curative, it is important to consider the important variables elucidated in thoughtful articles such as location and size when we encounter squamous cell carcinoma and plan treatment and follow-up intelligently.—J.L. Fewkes, M.D.

Carcinoma of the Skin of the Head and Neck With Perineural Invasion

Mendenhall WM, Parsons JT, Mendenhall NP, Brant TA, Stringer SP, Cassisi NJ, Million RR (Univ of Florida, Gainesville)

Head Neck 11:301–308, July–August 1989 14–21

Little information exists on carcinoma of the skin of the head and neck associated with perineural extension. Most reports involve a small number of patients with pathologic but not clinical evidence of perineural involvement who have been observed for only a short time. Clinical evidence of perineural invasion in 25 patients with carcinoma of the skin was evaluated.

Sixteen patients were managed by radiotherapy alone and 9 with surgery and radiotherapy. All patients had at least 5 years of follow-up. Local control after treatment was noted in 20% of patients treated with radiotherapy alone and in 38% of those treated with surgery and radiotherapy. Local control was diminished for recurrent lesions and tumors that also involved bone or cartilage. The 5-year absolute survival rate for patients treated with radiotherapy alone was 31%, and for patients treated with combined therapy, 33%. The incidence of significant complications was 25% with radiotherapy alone and 33% with surgery and radiotherapy.

The recommended treatment for patients with completely resectable disease is combined surgery and postoperative radiotherapy. Each patient's management is individualized regarding the use of pre- or postoperative radiotherapy. If preoperative radiotherapy is used, the dose must be high. Surgery is not recommended if all gross tumor cannot be resected, or if the functional or cosmetic consequences would be unacceptable. Patients who are not surgical candidates can be managed with radiotherapy alone.

▶ This paper emphasizes the clinical course of patients with squamous cell carcinoma with perineural invasion. It is worth emphasizing that the search for potential adverse factors in pathologic specimens is worthwhile.—T.J. Flotte, M.D.

Squamous Cell Carcinoma Arising in Previously Burned or Irradiated Skin

Edwards MJ, Hirsch RM, Broadwater JR, Netscher DT, Ames FC (Univ of Texas, Houston)

Arch Surg 124:115–117, January 1989 14–22

Squamous cell carcinoma (SCC) rarely arises in previously injured skin (Marjolin's ulcer). The natural history, patterns of recurrence, and survival of 66 patients treated from 1944 to 1986 for SCC arising from previously burned or irradiated skin were reviewed. Injured skin complicated by chronic ulcer was expected to undergo malignant transformation, and natural histories of the resulting carcinomas were expected to be similar and independent of the initial wound.

Initial injury healing was complicated in 70% of 66 patients. The mean interval from initial injury to diagnosis of SCC was 37 years. Most patients had a chronic intractable ulcer in previously injured skin. Regional relapse after surgical excision occurred in 58% of the patients. Of the recurrences, 93% were in local skin and regional lymph nodes. Overall survival rates at 5, 10, and 20 years were 52%, 34%, and 23%, respectively. The 5-year survival rates among burned and irradiated patients were comparable.

Squamous cell carcinoma arising in previously burned or irradiated skin appears to be a locally aggressive disease distinct from SCC arising in sunlight-damaged skin. More awareness of the significance of chronic ulceration in scar tissue may permit earlier diagnosis. Regional disease control and survival depend on surgical resection of all disease and possibly on radical lymph node dissection or amputation.

▶ The authors emphasize late diagnosis as a factor in these cases. Therefore, any change in a chronic scar, such as a fissure, especially in areas of repeated trauma, should be biopsied immediately. Of note also is that all SCC in radiation scars occurred in patients treated before 1959, and that, overall, SCC in both types of scars has been declining in recent years.—J.L. Fewkes, M.D.

Skin Cancer in Patients With Chronic Radiation Dermatitis

Davis MM, Hanke CW, Zollinger TW, Montebello JF, Hornback NB, Norins AL (Indiana Univ; Indiana Univ–Purdue Univ, Indianapolis)

J Am Acad Dermatol 20:608–616, April 1989 14–23

Reportedly, the most important risk factor in patients with radiation-induced skin cancer is the total accumulated dose. Facial skin apparently is more susceptible to x-ray damage than skin on the hands. It is often difficult to obtain information on the total accumulated dose in patients with chronic radiation dermatitis. Other risk factors might also be involved.

In all, 67 patients referred for skin cancer, who had chronic dermatitis resulting from radiation treatment for benign disease, were followed from 1979 to 1985. They were categorized according to clinical appearance and scarring. Hair color, eye color, skin reactive type, benign disease treated, area treated, age at treatment, and age at development of first skin cancer were determined.

Of these patients, 37% had sun-reactive skin type I, 27% had skin type II, and 36% had skin type III. No patients had skin types IV through VI. Types I and II appeared to be overrepresented, indicating that increased melanin pigmentation may be directly or indirectly protective against the development of skin cancer in patients receiving low-dose radiation for benign disease.

When the total dose of ionizing radiation is unknown, the sun-reactive skin type of patients with chronic radiation dermatitis may serve as a predictor of the risk of skin cancer. The history of excessive sunlight or ultraviolet radiation exposure is also important regardless of sun-reactive skin type.

▶ When you see a patient with multiple tiny basal cell carcinomas and no evidence of basal cell nevus syndrome, always determine whether previous radiation has been given. These patients need to be followed carefully with a high index of suspicion because, typically, lesions 1–2 mm in diameter will form.—J.L. Fewkes, M.D.

Signet-Ring Squamous Cell Carcinoma

Cramer SF, Heggeness LM (Univ of Rochester, NY)

Am J Clin Pathol 91:488–491, April 1989 14–24

Signet ring features have been considered pathognomonic of adenocarcinoma. A patient with a poorly differentiated cutaneous squamous cell carcinoma had a monodispersed, invasive signet ring component.

Man, 69, had a forehead lesion thought to be a keratoacanthoma. A year later, an ulcerated nodule classed as a well-differentiated squamous cell carcinoma arose in association with actinic keratosis. Skeletal muscle was involved. Thirteen operations were done in the next 5 years for multiple recurrent squamous cell cancers of the forehead and contiguous scalp; there were at least 4 separate primary tumors. Tumor cells continued to contain large amounts of eosinophilic cytoplasm; a clear-cell component was noted occasionally. An invasive signet ring carcinoma component was found 5 years after the first examination. The cells were negative for mucin by the Kreyberg stain, but some contained flocculent, periodic acid-Schiff-positive, diastase-sensitive material. Occasional signet ring cells were found on reviewing past specimens. Immunostaining of the signet ring carcinoma was strong for keratin in concentric rings at the periphery of the cells. A node aspirate contained metastatic squamous cell carcinoma, including the signet ring component. The tumor proved radioresistant and locally aggressive. The patient became hypercalcemic and septic and died 6 years after presentation.

This is the first known report of signet ring squamous cell carcinoma. The carcinoma arose in a field of actinic keratosis but led to the patient's death. This case may be an example of greater aberrations from normal differentiation reflecting greater solar carcinogenic action and therefore more aggressive neoplasms.

▸ This is 1 of 2 papers in this volume reporting signet cell tumors. This squamous carcinoma has a very rare variant. The differential diagnosis includes a variety of tumors; however, diagnostic features of squamous carcinoma are still present.—T.J. Flotte, M.D.

Signet Ring Cell Lymphoma of T Cell Type

Cross PA, Eyden BP, Harris M (Christie Hosp; Holt Radium Inst, Manchester, England)

J Clin Pathol 42:239–245, 1989 14–25

Signet ring lymphoma is a rare histologic variant of non-Hodgkin's lymphoma. The clear vacuole type of signet ring appearance is rare in T cell lymphoma.

Man, 75, with a 1-year history of a painless, slow-growing pimple on his chin, was otherwise in good general health. A biopsy was done on 2 pale, firm lesions 0.7 cm in diameter on the left side of the chin; later, a smaller pink papillomatous lesion medial to the previous biopsy scar was noted. The chin nodule grew somewhat in the next 3 months and was further excised. The patient was well 15 months after the first examination. Most cells were medium to large, with round or bean-shaped nuclei having finely granular chromatin. Smaller cells with hyperchromatic nuclei and scattered cells with a single clear cytoplasmic vacuole also were present. The signet ring cells comprised 15% to 20% of cells in the second biopsy specimen. Vascular proliferation was moderated. The tumor cells stained variably for T cell markers and were uniformly negative for B cell markers.

Because the ultrastructural appearance of the signet ring vacuoles was identical to that of the more common B cell signet ring lymphoma of the clear vacuole type, the vacuoles presumably are derived from multivesicular bodies. All 4 patients encountered to date with T cell signet ring lymphoma were first seen for cutaneous disease. The prognosis may be good; the 3 previous patients responded to radiotherapy and combination chemotherapy despite nodal and even widespread disease.

▶ This paper describes an unusual signet cell tumor that was a variant of non-Hodgkin's lymphoma, illustrating the light and electron microscopic findings. The differential diagnosis includes a variety of tumors including signet cell carcinoma (see Abstract 14–24).—T.J. Flotte, M.D.

Cutaneous Lymphoid Hyperplasia: Immunologic Characteristics and Assessment of Criteria Recently Proposed as Diagnostic of Malignant Lymphoma

Medeiros LJ, Picker LJ, Abel EA, Hu C-H, Hoppe RT, Warnke RA, Wood GS (Stanford Univ; VA Med Ctr, Palo Alto, Calif)

J Am Acad Dermatol 21:929–942, November 1989 14–26

Distinguishing benign from malignant lymphocytic infiltrates can be difficult. The clinical features of patients who do not have evidence of extracutaneous lymphoma are not distinctive. Data on 15 patients with cutaneous lymphoid hyperplasia were studied immunohistologically with a large panel of monoclonal antibodies to determine the immunoarchitectural composition and to learn whether immunologic criteria recently proposed to identify lymphoma can occur in benign skin lesions.

All lesions consisted of T cells, polytypic B cells, macrophages, and Langerhans cells. Only 6 lesions containing lymphoid follicles were identified in routinely stained sections, but 5 more were recognized in immunoperoxidase-stained sections. These follicles were both primary and secondary and contained dendritic reticulum cell networks. The immunophenotypic features of these follicles were comparable to those of reactive follicles in lymphoid organs and contrasted sharply with those reported previously for follicular lymphomas. Helper T cells were predominant in 11 patients. In assessing the proposed criteria for T cell lymphoma, loss of pan T cell antigens CD2, CD3, CD5, or BF-1 were not detected, nor were there populations of T cells with abnormal co-expression or loss of subset antigens such as $CD4^-8^-$ or $CD4^+8^+$. However, 2 patients in whom relatively sparse infiltrates were present were moderately deficient in CD7. In assessing proposed criteria for B cell lymphoma, populations of B cells that were immunoglobulin-negative were not detected, nor was preferential loss of 1 or more B lineage antigens, histocompatibility complex-associated antigens, or lymphocyte function-associated antigens. No $CD5^+$ B cells were identified. A comparison of these data with those of previous studies suggests that the general criteria for differentiating lymphoma from lymphoid hyperplasia are applicable to cutaneous lymphoid lesions.

▶ This paper is interesting because it provides an approach to understanding and using immunohistochemistry in differential diagnosis of lymphoid lesions. The authors emphasize that the utility of the commonly accepted hematopathology criteria are applicable to cutaneous lesions.—T.J. Flotte, M.D.

Follicular Mucinosis: Clinical and Histopathologic Study
Gibson LE, Muller SA, Leiferman KM, Peters MS (Mayo Clinc and Found, Rochester, Minn)
J Am Acad Dermatol 20:441–446, March 1989 14–27

Follicular mucinosis has a common histopathologic pattern of follicular mucinosis, but the clinical presentation may vary. A study was made

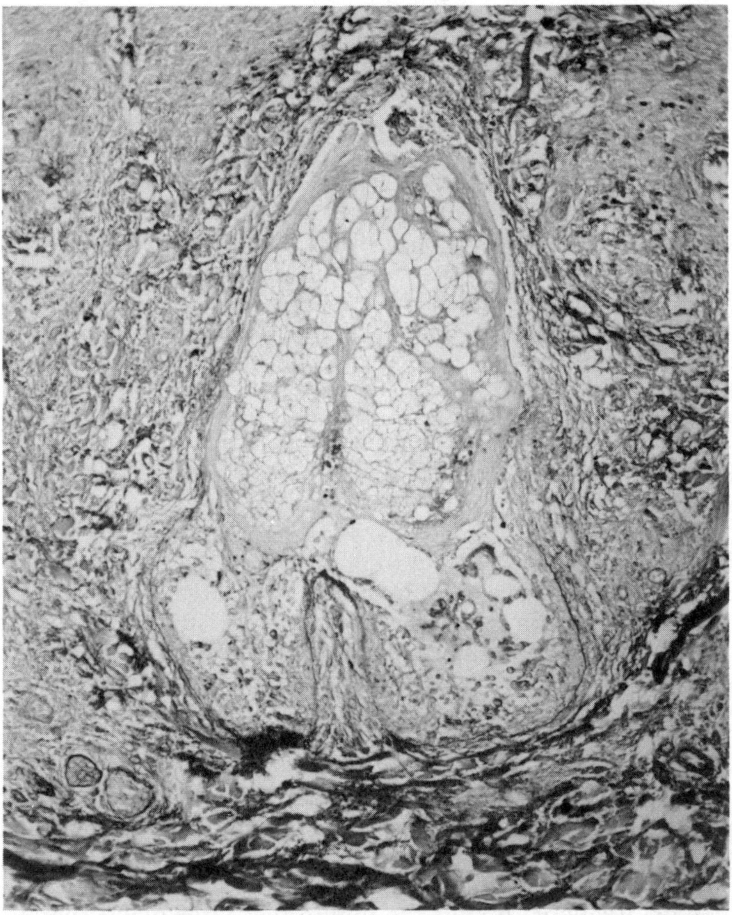

Fig 14–2.—Photomicrograph of biopsy specimen shows lymphocytic follicular inflammation and follicular mucin. Hematoxylin-eosin; original magnification, ×80. (Courtesy of Gibson LE, Muller SA, Leiferman KM, et al: *J Am Acad Dermatol* 20:441–446, March 1989.)

of 59 patients to determine whether any specific feature might provide pathophysiologic or prognostic clues to this disorder. All patients had undergone at least 1 biopsy, and for some, biopsy specimens were also obtained from lymph nodes or viscera. An additional 22 skin biopsy specimens from 15 patients with mycosis fungoides also were reviewed. The mean follow-up was 10 years.

Of 19 patients with mycosis fungoides, 16 had initial lesions of follicular mucinosis on the trunk or extremities. Of the group, 2 patients younger than 20 years had Hodgkin's disease and follicular mucinosis. Of 9 teenaged patients, 2 had persistent plaques of follicular mucinosis up to 18 years after diagnosis. Evaluation of biopsy specimens (Fig 14–2) revealed no significant features to differentiate patients with benign disease from those with mycosis fungoides.

No single clinical or histopathologic feature predicts which patients with follicular mucinosis will have benign disease and which will progress to malignancy. Evaluation of multiple clinical and histologic variables is necessary to determine the course of follicular mucinosis.

▶ This paper on follicular mucinosis confirms the current thoughts that follicular mucinosis may or may not be associated with lymphomas. However, that distinction cannot be based on evaluation of the follicular mucinosis itself. Careful evaluation and follow-up, both histologically and clinically, is important in the management of these patients.—T.J. Flotte, M.D.

Parapsoriasis and Mycosis Fungoides: The Northwestern University Experience, 1970 to 1985

Lazar AP, Caro WA, Roenigk HH Jr, Pinski KS (Northwestern Univ)

J Am Acad Dermatol 21:919–923, November 1989 14–28

Attempts have been made to subdivide parapsoriasis into papular and macular varieties. The macular type appears to be related to the eventual development of mycosis fungoides. To determine if certain common features would allow the physician to predict those patients in whom mycosis fungoides would develop, 89 patients with large plaque parapsoriasis and 106 patients with mycosis fungoides were studied. A total of 160 skin biopsy specimens from the patients with large plaque parapsoriasis and 240 specimens from the patients with mycosis fungoides were studied. Sex, age, history of eczema/atopy, and occupation were considered.

Mycosis fungoides developed in 30% of the patients with parapsoriasis. Of the patients with mycosis fungoides, 19% had worked in industry. An average of 4 biopsy specimens were needed to establish the diagnosis of mycosis fungoides. The average time from first visit to diagnosis of mycosis fungoides from biopsy specimens was 22 months.

These observations support the notion that large plaque parapsoriasis is an important precursor of mycosis fungoides. The designation premycosis fungoides is recommended to stress this relationship.

▶ In spite of the reported 30% development of mycosis fungoides in patients with large plaque parapsoriasis, to call all cases of large plaque parapsoriasis "premycosis fungoides" can be misleading to the uninformed physician and emotionally traumatic to the patient. It is hoped that definitive laboratory markers will become available to allow us to identify those cases of plaque type parapsoriasis that will become mycosis fungoides.—S.L. Moschella, M.D.

Long-Term Efficacy, Curative Potential, and Carcinogenicity of Topical Mechlorethamine Chemotherapy in Cutaneous T Cell Lymphoma

Vonderheid EC, Tan ET, Kantor AF, Shrager L, Micaily B, Van Scott EJ (Temple Univ; Natl Cancer Inst, Bethesda, Md; Hahnemann Med Ctr, Philadelphia)

J Am Acad Dermatol 20:416–428, March 1989 14–29

Topical applications of mechlorethamine hydrochloride (HN2) have long been used in the treatment of cutaneous T cell lymphoma. Patients with patch or plaque phase mycosis fungoides (MF) are more likely to respond completely to topical HN2 chemotherapy than those in later stages when tumors or generalized erythroderma, including Sézary syndrome, are present. The results and long-term outcome of cutaneous T cell lymphoma treated with topical HN2 chemotherapy were assessed during a 14-year period in 331 patients (mean age, 58 years). Of these, 244 had classic MF, 3 had MF *d'emblée,* 31 haderythrodermic MF, 29 had Sézary syndrome, 17 had lymphomatoid papulosis coexisting with MF, and 7 had lymphomatoid papulosis alone.

Topical HN2 chemotherapy resulted in a complete response in 191 (59%) of the 324 patients with MF or Sézary syndrome and in 4 of the 7 patients with lymphomatoid papulosis. Sixty-five of the 191 patients who had a complete response, or 20% of the total study population, have had remissions lasting 4 or more years. Most long-lasting remissions occurred in patients with patch or plaque phase MF without palpable lymphadenopathy.

Despite the long-lasting duration of complete responses in the 65 patients, 11 had a relapse between 8 and 88 months after discontinuation of maintenance topical HN2 chemotherapy. The remaining 54 patients had no signs of relapse from 4 to 168 months after discontinuation of maintenance therapy. None of the 35 patients in whom the duration of complete response has thus far lasted more than 8 years have experienced a relapse of cutaneous T cell lymphoma, for an overall cure rate of 11%.

The patients were at a significantly increased risk for the development of squamous and basal cell carcinoma of the skin, Hodgkin's disease, and colon cancer, but not for the development of systemic cancers, which are known to be induced by the systemic administration of alkylating drugs. Genetic factors and related pathogenic mechanisms other than the carcinogenic action of alkylating drugs appear to account for the association.

Topical HN2 chemotherapy should be administered aggressively to patients with potentially curable cutaneous T cell lymphoma. Maintenance therapy should be discontinued after 6 months in those in whom a sustained complete response is achieved.

▶ This is an excellent comprehensive and critical analysis of these authors' extensive experience with nitrogen mustard therapy for MF. The following conclusions can be drawn from their presentation: (1) A minority of so-treated patients are cured (11%). (2) Those cured were free of disease for at least 8 years. (3) Widely disseminated skin disease generally needs systemic drugs or radiation for effect or for the inapparent extracutaneous component of the disease, if the objective of treatment is curative. (4) One should reduce maintenance to 6 months after clearing in an attempt to minimize the occurrence of a complicating cutaneous malignancy, especially squamous cell carcinoma with its metastatic potential. (5) One should be aware of the increased incidence of complicating visceral cancer, especially Hodgkin's disease and colon cancer. (6) The patient should avoid or protect himself from ultraviolet light during and after therapy.—S.L. Moschella, M.D.

Interferon Alfa-2A in the Treatment of Cutaneous T Cell Lymphoma

Olsen EA, Rosen ST, Vollmer RT, Variakojis D, Roenigk HH Jr, Diab N, Zeffren J (Duke Univ-VA Hosp; Northwestern Univ-VA Lakeside Med Ctr; Hoffmann-La-Roche Inc., Nutley, NJ)

J Am Acad Dermatol 20:395–407, March 1989 14–30

Early-stage cutaneous T cell lymphoma is usually treated with topical therapy or electron beam radiation therapy; reportedly, however, early aggressive therapy may lead to more prolonged remissions and improved survival rates. Twenty-two patients were treated with recombinant human leukocyte interferon alfa-2a (Roferon-A) for cutaneous T-cell lymphoma, stages Ia to IVa.

The patients initially received either 3 million international units (IU) of Roferon-A or a dosage escalated to 36 million IU. Dosage was administered intramuscularly daily for a 10-week induction period. After 10 weeks, patients with complete remission received maintenance doses determined by the induction doses. Those with partial response continued with the same or a reduced dose of Roferon-A; the dose was escalated if patients relapsed or failed to improve during the next few months. Blood studies were taken at 1- to 2-month intervals during induction and monthly thereafter. Chest x-ray studies were made initially and at the end of the study.

Of 22 patients 14 had an objective antitumor response at the end of induction; 3 patients had a complete, 10 a partial, and 1 a minor response. Responders included patients with stages Ia to IVa disease. Remissions continued for at least 4–27 months. With further treatment 3 patients progressed from a partial to a complete response, for an overall complete response rate of 27%. Chronic dose-related side effects included malaise, depression, weight loss, and anorexia, and these were the most frequent reasons for dose reduction or termination of treatment.

The most common laboratory side effect was leukopenia, which was also dose related.

Roferon-A therapy is a well-tolerated, effective treatment for all stages of cutaneous T cell lymphoma. It is particularly helpful in patients with advanced stage disease who are refractory to other treatments.

▶ Like Bunn et al. (1), the above authors' data support the evidence that higher doses of recombinant interferon alfa-2A are more effective than low-dose therapy; as expected, however, the side effects are more numerous and greater in severity. Also interferon therapy has at best only an alternative temporary palliative role in the management of cutaneous T cell lymphoma.—S.L. Moschella, M.D.

Reference

1. Bunn PA, et al: *Ann Intern Med* 101:484, 1984.

Treatment of Cutaneous T Cell Lymphoma With Intermediate Doses of Interferon Alpha 2a

Nicolas JF, Balblanc JC, Frappaz A, Chouvet B, Delcombel M, Thivolet J (Hôp E. Herriot, Lyon, France)

Dermatologica 179:34–37, 1989 14–31

Epidermotropic cutaneous T cell lymphoma (CTCL), which includes mycosis fungoides and Sézary syndrome, cannot be cured by available chemotherapy. Intermediate dosages 10–50 × 10^6 international units per m^2/k of recombinant interferon-alpha (IFN-α)-2a were administered to 6 patients with histologically confirmed CTCL for 2–6 months.

One patient had a complete clinical remission; 3 had a partial remission. Two patients did not improve. The clinical and histologic responses were parallel. There were wide individual variations in tolerance to IFN. A flulike syndrome, partially prevented by paracetamol, was the most limiting side effect. One patient had reduced libido, and 1 had a transient increase in liver enzymes.

Interferon can effectively treat epidermotropic CTCL. Long-term treatment might be needed to induce remission. The efficacy of IFN-α in conjunction with other treatments, such as vinblastine, is being evaluated.

▶ Reports of the percentage of complete responses and overall therapeutic efficacy, of the best route of administration, and of the optimal dose of recombinant IFN-α in the treatment of cutaneous T cell lymphoma are contradictory and controversial. Interferon's best potential beneficial therapeutic role appears currently to be in combination with some other incompletely effective drugs such as etretinate (1), vinblastine or methotrexate (2).—S.L. Moschella, M.D.

References

1. Thestrup-Pedersen K, et al: *Br J Dermatol* 118:811, 1988.
2. Ohl S, et al: *J Leuk Biol* 42:577a, 1986.

Total Skin Electron Irradiation for Mycosis Fungoides

Le Bourgeois J-P, Levy E, Haddad E, Marinello G, Geara F, Pavlovitch J-M (Hôp Henri Mondor, Créteil, France)

Ann Dermatol Venereol 116:213–217, 1989 14–32

The results obtained with total cutaneous electron beam irradiation (TCI) in the treatment of mycosis fungoides (MF) are encouraging. Long-lasting remissions, some for more than 10 years, have been reported. However, TCI is costly and not without side effects. To better define which patients with MF might benefit from TCI therapy, during a 10-year period 17 males and 8 females aged 13–78 years were treated. The mean follow-up period for the entire study population was 34 months and ranged from 6 to 92 months.

A staging system, designed at Créteil, was used to classify the MF patients. Six patients had stage A disease, defined as superficial lesions covering less than 50% of the body surface; 9 had stage B disease, defined as superficial lesions covering more than 50% of the body surface; and 10 had stage C disease, that is, tumors of the skin, lymph nodes, or intestinal organs. Nineteen patients had received other forms of treatment, including psoralen ultraviolet (PUVA), systemic or topical chemotherapy, and corticosteroids.

All 6 patients with stage A disease had complete remissions. A mean follow-up of 40 months identified only 1 patient with a minor relapse 17 months after TCI. Six of 9 patients with stage B disease had complete remissions; the other 3 had partial remissions but have since died. Four of the patients with complete remissions subsequently had recurrences that were localized to the skin. Relapses were treated with local radiation therapy, local mechlorethamine chemotherapy, or PUVA. One of these 4 patients died of MF; the other 3 were alive after 14, 30, and 32 months. Five of the 10 patients with stage C disease initially had complete remissions but relapses occurred within 7 months, on average. Four of these 5 patients have since died of their disease. The only patient who was still alive 16 months after TCI had intestinal involvement.

Total cutaneous irradiation used in the treatment of MF is curative for patients with stage A disease and improves the quality of life for patients with stage B disease, but it does not benefit patients with stage C disease.

▶ This report, like others, demonstrates the relationship of the stage of disease to the anticipated response to the recommended amount of electron beam therapy of about 30 Gy. The fewer and more superficial the lesions in the absence of visceral lesions, the more complete and lasting the response, even "cure."—S.L. Moschella, M.D.

Risk of Second Malignancy After Cutaneous T-Cell Lymphoma

Kantor AF, Curtis RE, Vonderheid EC, Van Scott EJ, Fraumeni JF Jr (Natl Cancer Inst, Bethesda, Md; Temple Univ, Philadelphia)

Cancer 63:1612–1615, Apr 15, 1989 14–33

The findings of previous studies have suggested that patients with cutaneous T cell lymphoma (CTCL) may be at increased risk of a second primary malignancy. Because CTCL is uncommon, this risk has been difficult to evaluate. The incidence of second primary cancers was determined in a cohort of 544 patients with CTCL reported to the Surveillance, Epidemiology, and End Results (SEER) program of the National Cancer Institute. The mean age at diagnosis was 60 years. The cohort was followed for a total of 1,672 person-years, the average follow-up being 3.1 years.

During follow-up, a second primary malignancy developed in 35 patients (6%) whose first primary tumor was reported as CTCL. On the basis of age- and sex-specific incidence rates from the SEER program, 20.1 new cancers would have been expected. Thus the relative risk (1.7) for development of a second primary malignancy was significantly increased. There were significant excesses for colon cancer, which had a relative risk of 3.1; for lung cancer, with a relative risk of 2.8; and for non-Hodgkin's lymphoma, with a relative risk of 5.5. The elevated relative risk for colon cancer was seen for men and women, but the excess of lung cancer was limited to men. The risk of colon cancer increased with length of follow-up, whereas excesses of lung cancer and lymphoma were limited to the first 5 years of follow-up.

The increased risks for cancers of the lung and colon and for non-Hodgkin's lymphoma among patients with CTCL suggest the value of periodic screening for early detection of second primary malignancies. Further studies are needed to elucidate the host and environmental factors that may affect the risk of subsequent malignancies.

▶ Dermatologists have been aware of malignant epitheliomas occurring in patients with mycosis fungoides, especially during and after therapies, and have been concerned about the potential problems of increased melanoma risk. The authors have done us a service by alerting us to the potential and statistically significant malignant complications and by emphasizing necessary measures for the surveillance and management of patients with this chronic disease.—S.L. Moschella, M.D.

Cutaneous Diseases Preceding Diagnoses of Lymphoreticular Malignancies

Klapman MH (Kaiser Permanente Los Angeles Med Ctr)
J Am Acad Dermatol 20:583–586, April 1989 14–34

Dermatologic diseases observed before the diagnosis of lymphoreticular malignancies were considered in 258 patients. Data were compared with those in 258 age- and sex-matched controls. The charts of patients and controls were reviewed to determine the number of patients who visited the dermatology clinic and their dermatologic diagnoses during a 5-year period that ended 3 months before the diagnosis of lymphoreticular malignancy was made.

In all, 52 patients and 51 controls visited the dermatology clinic during the study period. Patients who later had lymphoreticular malignancies had 26 diagnoses, whereas controls had 111. Diagnoses found more often in patients included hemangiomas, fungus infections, and cutaneous malignancies. Six of 96 patients with leukemia, but no controls, initially were thought to have cutaneous malignancies, a significant incidence. The incidence of lymphoma in patients who initially had cutaneous malignancies did not differ from that in controls. There was an increased incidence of patients with lymphoreticular malignancies who had hemangiomas and fungal infections, but the increase was not significant.

The findings suggest that there may be a common factor predisposing to both cutaneous malignancy and leukemia. A defect in immunosurveillance might be responsible.

▶ The only meaningful association noted was the development of cutaneous malignancies in patients before the diagnosis of leukemia was made—3 basal cell cancers, 2 squamous cell cancers, and 1 Kaposi's sarcoma. Two theories were offered: (1) a defect in the immunosurveillance accounting for both malignancies, or (2) cutaneous malignancies causing persistent antigenic stimulation of lymphoreticular system, resulting in leukemia. The author is surprised and unable to explain the lack of increased specific and nonspecific cutaneous changes preceding the diagnosis of lymphoreticular malignancies.—S.L. Moschella, M.D.

Basal Cell Carcinomas and Lymphoma: Biologic Behavior and Associated Factors in Sixty-three Patients

Parnes R, Safai B, Myskowski PL (Mem Sloan-Kettering Cancer Ctr, New York; Cornell Univ)

J Am Acad Dermatol 19:1017–1023, December 1988 14–35

The role of the immune system in the development of basal cell carcinoma has been questioned. Studies of skin cancers in immunocompromised patients have lent credence to a suggestion that the behavior of basal cell carcinoma is more aggressive in patients with lymphoproliferative disorders. An analysis was made of the records of 63 patients who had both basal cell carcinoma and lymphoma. Patients were divided into 2 groups on the basis of the temporal relationship between onset of basal cell carcinoma and lymphoma.

Lymphoma developed in 50 patients before or concurrently with basal cell carcinoma; in 13 patients basal cell carcinoma was diagnosed at least 6 months before onset of lymphoma. Most patients had multiple basal cell carcinomas. The overall recurrence rate of the disease was 17%; 1 patient had metastatic disease.

These findings suggest that basal cell carcinoma behaves more aggressively in patients with lymphoma than in individuals who are otherwise healthy. Lymphoma patients who also have basal cell carcinoma should be treated aggresively and should be followed closely indefinitely.

▶ The authors call our attention to the immunosuppression created not only by lymphomas but also the contributory effects of radiation and chemotherapy on the incidence, type, clinical behavior, and therapeutic responses of the various potentially complicating or associated skin cancers, especially basal cell cancer. Similar effects can be seen in immunosuppressive diseases or states such as other malignant lymphoproliferative diseases, infections such as HIV, and chemotherapy for autoimmune diseases and organ transplantation.—S.L. Moschella, M.D.

Primary Cutaneous Follicular Centre-Cell Lymphoma: A Lymphoproliferative Disease With Favourable Prognosis

Pimpinelli N, Santucci M, Bosi A, Moretti S, Vallecchi C, Messori A, Giannotti B (Università degli Studi di Firenze, Italy)

Clin Exp Dermatol 14:12–19, January 1989 14–36

Patients with extranodal non-Hodgkin's lymphoma (NHL) appearing only in the skin seem to have a much better prognosis than those with extracutaneous involvement. The features, treatment, and outcome of NHL were reviewed in 11 patients with follicular center cell (B cell) NHL that was primarily observed in the skin.

All 11 patients had nodular, tumorous, and papulonodular skin lesions on the trunk (table). Eight patients had red to violaceous nodules or tumors, usually with a smooth, shiny surface and little scaling and ulceration, ranging from 2.5 to 15 cm in diameter and sometimes surrounded by slightly infiltrated plaques (Fig 14–3). The lesions had been present for 1–10 years before development of the rapidly growing skin tumors.

No clear correlation between age, clinical morphology of the lesions, and their histologic growth pattern was noted. Nine patients were treated initially with local orthovolt irradiation; the other 2 underwent surgical

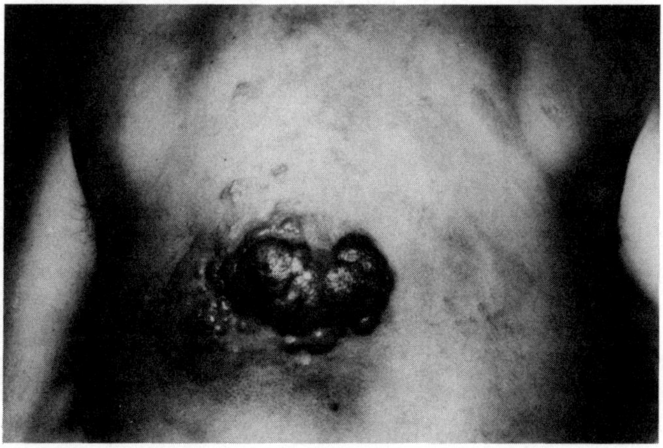

Fig 14–3.—Large tumor on the back. The lesion is surrounded by slightly infiltrated plaques. (Courtesy of Pimpinelli N, Santucci M, Bosi A, et al: *Clin Exp Dermatol* 14:12–19, January 1989.)

Clinical and Follow-Up Data

Patient	Age/sex	Clinical features at presentation	Past history	Initial therapy	Site of relapse	Therapy	Current status	Survival (months)
1	49/F	Large nodule surrounded by papules on the back	Papulonodular lesions for 17 months	RT	Skin after 6 months	RT+ COP (−Bleo)	CR	57
2	42/M	Large nodule on the left shoulder	Slowly progressing nodule for 11 months	Excision +RT	—	—	CR	55
3	58/M	Solitary tumour surrounded by slightly infiltrated plaques on the back	Slowly progressing plaque-like lesions for more than 14 years	RT	Skin and axillary lymh node after 9 months	RT+ COP	CR	52
4	51/M	Solitary ulcerated tumour on the left flank	Peripherally extending plaques for 7 months	RT	Skin after 23 months	RT	CR	45
5	69/M	Large tumour surrounded by many papules on the back	Slowly progressing papulonodular lesions for 10 years	RT	Skin after 10 months	RT+ COP (−Bleo)	CR	39
6	57/M	Multiple small papulonodular lesions on the back	Lesions present for more than 12 years	RT	Skin after 17 months	RT	CR	37

7	39/M	Multiple papulonodular and plaque-like lesions on the back	Lesions present for 5 months	RT	Skin after 9 months	RT	CR	35
8	34/M	Multiple small papulonodular lesions on the back	Lesions present for more than 3 years	RT	Skin after 11 months	RT	CR	19
9	66/M	Large nodule surrounded by annular erythema and plaques on the back	Small papular lesions for more than 2 years	Excision +RT	—	—	CR	16
10	69/F	Large plaque surrounded by papular lesions on the back	Small papular lesions for 8 years	RT	—	—	CR	14
11	61/M	Large tumour surrounded by annular erythema on the back	Small plaques for more than 6 years	RT	—	—	CR	13

Abbreviations: COP (—Bleo): cyclophosphamide, Oncovin, prednisone (—bleomycin); *CR*, complete remission; *RT*, radiotherapy.
(Courtesy of Pimpinelli N, Santucci M, Bosi A, et al: *Clin Exp Dermatol* 14:12–19, January 1989.)

excision before orthovolt therapy. All patients experienced complete remission. Only 1 patient later had extracutaneous disease, which was limited to a single drainage lymph node and appeared simultaneously with a cutaneous relapse. After a mean disease-free period of 15.5 months, 5 other patients had recurrences of skin tumors close to the initial site that were again treated with radiotherapy, with or without a short course of chemotherapy. All patients were alive and in good health at the time of this report. Immunohistochemical examinations confirmed the B cell nature of this typical cutaneous lymphoproliferative disorder.

The lack of extracutaneous spread in 10 of 11 patients strongly suggests a cutaneous origin for this NHL. The favorable outcome in these patients justifies a nonaggressive approach to treatment.

▶ Because cutaneous B cell lymphomas have been described as usually associated with nodal involvement early in the disease, we were very uncomfortable with the diagnosis and management of 4 elderly Lahey Clinic patients with only cutaneous lesions that were confined to the skin of the back and chest. These lesions, which had been present for more than 12 years, were clinically and cytomorphologically consistent with B cell lymphomas and were very responsive to electron beam therapy. Fortunately, European dermatologists (1–3) and the above authors have made the "Morbus Crosti" (a primary cutaneous follicular center cell lymphoma, a B cell lymphoma) more easily recognized and managed. Consequently, those of us who manage such diseases are more sanguine because of its more favorable prognosis.—S.L. Moschella, M.D.

References

1. Burg G, et al: *J Dermatol Surg Oncol* 10:256, 1984.
2. Willemze R, et al: *Am J Pathol* 126:325, 1987.
3. Giannotti R, et al: *J Invest Dermatol* 87:129, 1986.

Hodgkin's Disease of the Skin: A Case Report

Heyd J, Weissberg N, Gottschalk S (Shaare Zedek Med Ctr, Jerusalem)

Cancer 63:924–929, March 1, 1989 14–37

Hodgkin's disease seldom involves the skin, and the effect of skin involvement on the patient's outlook is not clear. In 26 cases reported since 1970, skin infiltration either was unrelated to nodal or visceral involvement and the prognosis was good, or skin infiltration was secondary to involvement of the lymph nodes. In the latter cases the prognoses depended on the course of the visceral disease.

Woman, 75, was first seen for axillary and inguinal lymphadenopathy and knee pain. Many large plaques and nodules 3 mm to 2 cm in diameter were seen in the lower right quadrant of the abdomen and in the vulvar, upper thigh, and inguinal areas (Fig 14–4). Biopsy of 1 inguinal lesion and a lymph node showed nodular sclerosing Hodgkin's disease. Combination chemotherapy achieved a

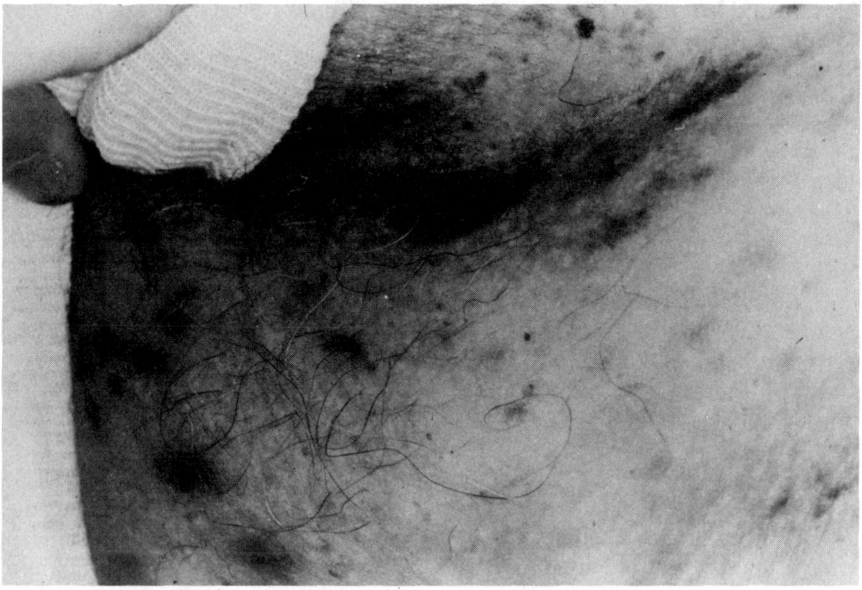

Fig 14–4.—Dark brown nodules and plaques over skin of right inguinal area. (Courtesy of Heyd J, Weissberg N, Gottschalk S: *Cancer* 63:924–929, March 1, 1989.)

temporary remission but, during more cycles of chemotherapy, the lesions reappeared, lymphadenopathy resumed, and a knee lesion progressed. The patient died 1 year later after refusing more treatment.

When skin infiltration is related to lymph node involvement, obstruction to lymph flow is involved in its pathogenesis. Skin "resistance" to chemotherapy probably is caused by mechanical factors resulting from obstruction of lymph flow through sclerosed lymph nodes. Assessment of prognosis should include the pattern of skin involvement and consideration of these mechanical factors.

▶ Hodgkin's disease of the skin is uncommon and reportedly occurs in only 0.5% patients with this disease (1). The patterns of cutaneous involvement of Hodgkin's disease are a primary type without visceral involvement, another type unrelated to existing nodal or visceral involvement, and a third type with skin infiltration from involved regional lymph nodes or bone. The primary type is very rare and was frequently misdiagnosed because of the absence in the past of appropriate cytologic markers. The authors have emphasized the impact of lymphatic obstruction by the disease process and/or local radiation on the clinical expression and therapeutic resistance of the disease.—S.L. Moschella, M.D.

Reference

1. Smith JL, Butler JJ: *Cancer* 45:354, 1980.

Classic and Immunodeficiency-Associated Kaposi's Sarcoma: Clinical, Histologic, and Immunologic Correlations

Santucci M, Pimpinelli N, Moretti S, Giannotti B (Università degli Studi di Firenze, Italy)

Arch Pathol Lab Med 112:1214–1220, December 1988 14–38

In its "classic" form, Kaposi's sarcoma (KS) is rare, but the disease has been seen with increasing frequency in patients receiving immunosuppressive treatment and in those with AIDS or AIDS-related complex. The clinical, histologic, and immunopathologic features of both classic and immunodeficiency-associated KS were compared with regard to the age of the lesions and the patient's immunologic status.

Multiple biopsy specimens were taken from skin lesions ranging in age from 1 month to 11 months in 10 patients with classic KS and 7 with immunodeficiency-associated KS. In all patients, peripheral blood mononuclear cells were separated from heparinized blood by centrifuge and incubated with CD2, CD3, CD4, and CD8 monoclonal antibodies. Fluorescence-activated cell-sorter analysis was used to determine the percentage of mononuclear cells that bound the monoclonal antibodies. The in vitro response to polyclonal activators phytohemagglutinin, concanavalin A, and pokeweed mitogen also was evaluated as was the response to allogeneic cells in the mixed cell lymphocyte reaction and the helper activity of the mononuclear cells.

Histologic findings were similar in patients with classic KS and in those with immunodeficiency-associated KS. A variably dense reactive infiltrate was present in classic KS; the amount was inversely related to the age of the lesions. In contrast, a scarce reactive infiltrate that lacked CD4+ cells was always found in immunodeficiency-associated KS lesions, even when the patient's immune status appeared normal.

A specific impairment of skin-associated lymphoid tissue may be key to the development of immunodeficiency-associated KS. The presence of normal absolute numbers of circulating lymphocytes, the CD4:CD8 ratio, and other immunologic findings has prognostic relevance in AIDS-associated KS. In these patients the disease is more stable and less aggressive; however, this status changes with time, and when frank immunodeficiency becomes detectable, a characteristic clinical evolution must be expected.

▶ Although it has been generally stated that the histopathologic features of KS are indistinguishable in the classic and AIDS-related form, this paper notes important differences in the local host response to the tumor that may well explain the lower biologic virulence of the classic form. Similar to the findings in melanoma, in which radial growth phase lesions have prominent mononuclear cell infiltrates that vertical growth phase lesions lack, the cellular infiltrate appears to diminish with time in classic KS lesions. In both tumor types, a sparse to absent infiltrate correlates negatively with prognosis. [See also the text by Gottlieb and Ackerman (1).]—A.J. Sober, M.D.

Reference

1. Gottlieb GJ, Ackerman AB (eds): *Kaposi's Sarcoma: A Text and Atlas.* Philadelphia, Lea & Febiger, 1988.

▶ ↓ The behavior of Kaposi's sarcoma (KS) in certain patients resembles a reactive process more than a neoplastic one in that shifts in immune function may lead to dramatic reversals of clinical activity. It is therefore noteworthy in the following 2 studies that biologic response modifiers [α interferon in the first paper and tumor necrosis factor (TNF) in the second] have shown activity in KS. The use of biologic response modifiers has a certain rational appeal in that their use does not result in further systemic immunosuppression associated with chemotherapeutic agents. As noted in the study by Lane et al. (Abstract 14–39), the interferon appears to be of benefit only in those patients who lack profound immunosuppression. The 94% response rate reported with TNF is promising; however, significant side effects limit the usefulness of both of these agents. The lack of distant antitumor effects in noninjected lesions is very reminiscent of that observed with intralesional BCG therapy of intracutaneous melanoma metastases.—A.J. Sober, M.D.

Anti-Retroviral Effects of Interferon-α in AIDS-Associated Kaposi's Sarcoma

Lane HC, Kovacs JA, Feinberg J, Herpin B, Davey V, Walker R, Deyton L, Metcalf JA, Baseler M, Salzman N, Manischewitz J, Quinnan G, Masur H, Fauci AS (Natl Inst of Allergy and Infectious Diseases, Bethesda, Md; Clinical Immunology Services, Frederick, Md; Georgetown Univ; Food and Drug Adm, Bethesda)

Lancet 2:1218–1222, Nov 26, 1988 14–39

Interferon-α (IFN-α) can reduce HIV replication in vitro by acting on viral assembly. It also has antitumor activity for AIDS-related Kaposi's sarcoma (KS), but is not of survival benefit in patients with late-stage AIDS. A prospective study was made of the antiviral effects of high doses of interferon-α_{2b} on 21 early-stage AIDS patients with KS.

Eight patients (38%) had complete or partial antitumor responses after 10–92 weeks of IFN-α treatment. Response was a function of immunologic competence. All 5 patients with CD4 cell counts of >400/μL had good responses, compared to 0 of 7 patients with CD4 counts of <150/μL; responders had a mean pretreatment CD4 count of 399/μL compared to 154/μL in nonresponders. Three patients had persistently reduced HIV activity in cultures and striking reductions in circulating levels of p24 antigen. Nearly all patients who had antitumor responses, but no nonresponders, had a reduction of >75% in circulating p24 levels after 12 weeks of IFN-α therapy. Side effects included leukopenia, hepatitis, asthenia, and reversible congestive cardiomyopathy. Discontinuation of therapy was necessary in 9 of 21 patients because of side effects.

Beneficial results of IFN-α therapy were found in some patients with early AIDS and KS, including both tumor reduction and reduced levels of circulating p24 antigen. Benefits occurred only to patients with good immune function only after long-term, high-dose treatment. Among some of these patients, improvement in quality of life was achieved.

Intralesional Recombinant Tumor Necrosis Factor-α for AIDS-Associated Kaposi's Sarcoma: A Randomized, Double-Blind Trial

Kahn JO, Kaplan LD, Volberding PA, Ziegler JL, Crowe S, Saks SR, Abrams DI (Univ of California, San Francisco; San Francisco Gen Hosp; VA Med Ctr, San Francisco; Genentech Inc, South San Francisco)

J AIDS 2:217–223, March 1989 14–40

Effective cosmetic treatment of lesions of Kaposi's sarcoma (KS) would substantially better the quality of life for many AIDS patients. Because production of tumor necrosis factor (TNF) is impaired in patients with AIDS, recombinant (r) TNF treatment was evaluated in 27 clinically stable patients who had AIDS and biopsy-proved Kaposi's sarcoma. In a preliminary toxicity trial the maximally tolerated intralesional dose was less than 100 $\mu g/m^2$, and a dose of 25 $\mu g/m^2$ was recommended.

A double-blind efficacy trial was carried out in 13 patients. Treatment decreased the cross-sectional area of all lesions except for 1; placebo-treated lesions did not change or progressed slightly. Three lesions disappeared after injection of rTNF, 25 $\mu g/m^2$. The total response rate of rTNF-treated lesions was 94%. Rigors occasionally occurred despite pretreatment with meperidine, alone or combined with acetaminophen. One patient had disseminated herpes zoster infection.

Intralesional rTNF injection is an effective approach to the management of KS. The cosmetic outcome is acceptable, but systemic toxicity and a lack of distant antitumor effect limit its usefulness.

Oral Etoposide for Kaposi's Mediterranean Sarcoma

Brambilla L, Boneschi V, Fossati S, Melotti E, Clerici M (Univ of Milan, Italy; S Carlo Borromeo Med Hosp, Milan)

Dermatologica 177:365–369, December 1988 14–41

Kaposi's Mediterranean sarcoma (KMS) is a rare variant of Kaposi's sarcoma (KS) that occurs predominantly in elderly patients. This rare sarcoma is only slightly symptomatic and has a slow course; the median survival ranges from 8 to 13 years. Mortality is directly attributable to KMS in 20% of the patients, but KMS is often associated with other neoplasms. Etoposide (VP16) has been used with good results in the treatment of AIDS-associated KS; it appears to have no cross-resistance with multidrug chemotherapeutic regimens.

The effects of orally administered VP16, used as monotherapy in the treatment of KMS, were assessed in 7 women and 15 men aged 47–87 years, 13 of whom had been pretreated with other chemotherapeutic regimens. Of the 17 evaluable patients, 10 had received previous treatment. Oral VP16 was administered at a dose of 100 mg daily for 3–5 days every 3 weeks 3 times during induction and every 4 weeks 10–12 times during maintenance. Follow-up was performed every 3 weeks during induction and every 4 weeks during maintenance.

Oral VP16 used as a single-drug therapy produced objective responses in 6 of the 7 non-pretreated patients (85.6%) and in 7 of the 10 pretreated patients (70%); 6 patients experienced hematologic toxicity, and 11 had gastrointestinal side effects. However, all drug-induced toxicities were mild and rapidly reversible.

Half of the patients who had already received other chemotherapeutic regimens in the treatment of KMS experienced an objective response. Monochemotherapy with orally administered VP16 insures better patient compliance, permits fewer outpatient follow-up visits, and causes fewer side effects than intravenously administered multiple-drug chemotherapeutic regimens.

▶ Classic KS is an indolent disease that responds to multiple forms of therapy including spot ionizing radiation and single- (vincristine) or multiple-drug chemotherapy. The attractiveness of VP16 is based on its ease of administration (oral), the relatively high response rate achievable in both untreated and previously treated patients, and its acceptable toxicity profile when administered to a group of largely elderly individuals, many of whom have baseline impairments in 1 or more organ systems. The surprising finding in this study was a higher complete remission rate in patients previously treated in comparison to those being treated for the first time (50% vs 14%). The number of patients in each group is too small, however, for meaningful statistical evaluation.—A.J. Sober, M.D.

Immunoreactivity for Laminin and Type IV Collagen in Malignant and Benign Fibrous Histiocytoma

Soini Y, Autio-Harmainen H, Miettinen M (Univ of Oulu, Finland)
J Pathol 158:223–228, July 1989 14–42

Malignant fibrous histiocytomas (MFHs) are soft tissue tumors that may be derived from mesenchymal cells. The distribution of 2 basement membrane proteins, laminin and type IV collagen, was investigated immunohistochemically in 16 samples of MFH; 13 were of the pleomorphic-storiform, 2 of the myxoid, and 1 of the giant cell subtype (table). Findings were compared with those in 10 benign fibrous histiocytomas of the skin. Specific antibody probes had been raised against proteins of human origin.

Intracytoplasmic immunoreactivity for laminin was found in 11 MFHs, 2 of which were also positive for type IV collagen. Staining was found in large neoplastic cells, including large pleomorphic giant cells. No staining was found in multinucleated osteoclast-like giant cells, and in only 2 cases was extracellular staining for laminin and type IV collagen seen.

Clinical Data and Results of Immunostaining on MFHs

Case	Age (years)	Sex	Location	Subtype	Laminin Ic	Laminin Ec	TIVC Ic	TIVC Ec
1	63	Male	Chest wall	G	+++	−	−	−
2	77	Male	Left thigh	PS	++	−	−	−
3	65	Female	Right calf	PS	−	−	−	−
4	62	Female	Right axilla	PS	+++	−	−	−
5	14	Female	Right scapular region	PS	++	−	−	−
6	68	Female	Left upper extremity	PS	+	+	+	+
7	60	Female	Left clavicular region	PS	+++	−	−	−
8	68	Female	Right upper extremity	PS	++	+	−	+
9	65	Female	Left upper extremity	PS	−	−	−	−
10	77	Female	Left lower extremity	PS	−	−	−	−
11	53	Male	Abdominal region	PS	+	−	−	−
12	81	Female	Left axilla	PS	+	−	−	−
13	81	Female	Back	PS	+++	−	++	−
14	65	Female	Left upper extremity	PS	−	−	−	−
15	66	Female	Left scapular region	M	++	−	−	−
16	57	Male	Back	M	−	−	−	−

Abbreviations: G, giant cell subtype of MFH; *PS,* pleomorphic-storiform subtype; *M,* myxoid subtype; *TIVC,* type IV collagen; *Ic,* intracellular immunoreactivity; *Ec,* extracellular immunoreactivity.

(Courtesy of Soini Y, Autio-Harmainin H, Miettinen M: *J Pathol* 158:223–228, July 1989.)

The benign tissues tested showed neither intracellular nor extracellular staining in tumor cells.

Laminin and sometimes type IV collagen present intracytoplasmically in tumor cells of MFH. Although these findings do not permit definitive conclusions on the histogenesis of MFH, they are consistent with the possibility that at least some MFHs are primitive, undifferentiated mesenchymal tumors. The benign fibrous histiocytomas, which were all negative for basement membrane proteins, may be unrelated to MFH.

▶ This study of the immunohistochemistry of benign and malignant fibrous histocytomas for laminin and type IV collagen is inconclusive in determining the histogenesis of these tumors. This has been a hotly debated topic since the first descriptions of these entities. It is interesting to note the presence of basement membrane proteins in some of the malignant variants. The importance of this observation has yet to be determined.—T.J. Flotte, M.D.

Cutaneous Neuroendocrine (Merkel Cell) Carcinoma: An Immunophenotypic, Clinicopathologic, and Flow Cytometric Study

Visscher D, Cooper PH, Zarbo RJ, Crissman JD (Henry Ford Hosp, Detroit; Univ of Virginia)

Mod Pathol 2:331–338, July 1989 14–43

Cutaneous neuroendocrine carcinoma (CNEC) is an uncommon neoplasm usually seen as 1 or more dermal nodules in the head-neck region or extremities in elderly patients. The biologic behavior of this carcinoma is unpredictable.

Twenty-one patients with a mean age of 76 years who had CNEC were studied by the immunoperoxidase method with the use of monoclonal antibodies. In addition, flow cytometric DNA analysis was obtained. Twelve patients had tumors in the head-neck region and 7 had tumors in a lower extremity. Two patients had node metastases at presentation. Nine of 19 patients had recurrent or metastatic disease, or both, during a mean follow-up of 26 months. Five patients with recurrent disease died.

Light microscopy study usually showed an admixture of diffuse and organoid growth patterns. Mitotic figures were numerous in all cases. All tumors stained positively for cytokeratin. Weak, focal staining for 1 or more neuroendocrine markers was present in 17 cases. Staining for peptide hormones was infrequent. The usual findings on flow cytometric analysis were DNA content in the normal range and an elevated S-phase fraction.

Cutaneous neuroendocrine carcinoma consistently stains for cytokeratin and often expresses neurofilament staining as well. Ploidy and growth fraction do not seem to be significant prognostic variables.

▶ This well-documented study of 21 Merkel cell tumors demonstrates findings similar to those reported previously and confirms the utility of keratin stains in particular and the neuroendocrine markers. In addition, they show that flow cytometric analysis is not useful. This is consistent with flow cytometric studies of other neuroendocrine tumors.—T.J. Flotte, M.D.

Primary Cutaneous Neuroendocrine (Merkel Cell or Trabecular Carcinoma) Tumour of the Skin: A Radioresponsive Tumour

Ashby MA, Jones DH, Tasker AD, Blackshaw AJ (Univ of Cambridge; Addenbrookes Hosp, Cambridge; Bedford Gen Hosp, Bedford, England)

Clin Radiol 40:85–87, January 1989 14–44

Primary neuroendocrine carcinoma of the skin is usually treated by surgical excision. The role of radiotherapy in management of this rare tumor has yet to be defined, but some reports have suggested that it is radio and chemotherapy sensitive. Four patients with the tumor were treated by radiotherapy.

Woman, 84, had a 6-month history of an increasing polypoid mass on the left elbow. The lesion was treated by excision and split-skin graft. Histologically, the tumor was a typical Merkel cell tumor. Nodal metastases developed in the left axilla and supraclavicular fossa within 7 months. Both areas were treated by radiation in fractional doses over 6 weeks. After a tumor dose of 12 Gy the tumor was markedly reduced in size, and after a dose of 21 Gy the disease disappeared completely. During treatment, contralateral supraclavicular nodes developed that were treated with a tumor dose of 20 Gy in 5 daily fractions over 1 week. This mass regressed rapidly and disappeared, but the patient died 2 months later of skeletal metastases.

The other 3 patients had a complete response with no local recurrence. One patient had postoperative irradiation after excision of an involved local node, which prevented the growth of further tumor in that nodal group; however, the tumor at the unirradiated primary site recurred.

Primary neuroendocrine tumor of the skin appears to be radioresponsive, but further data are needed to confirm this. A wider study of radiotherapy for the primary lesion after biopsy as well as prophylactic nodal irradiation is needed. Because these tumors occur principally in elderly persons, avoiding extensive surgery is particularly desirable.

▶ The primary treatment of Merkel cell carcinoma is surgical. Metastases to regional nodes is a frequent route of spread. If the radiosensitivity of this tumor is confirmed in a larger series with longer follow-up, this therapeutic approach may provide an option to surgery in older individuals. Large series will be difficult to acquire without multicenter trials because the Merkel cell tumor is rare. See Abstract 14–43 for a clinicopathologic description of Merkel cell carcinoma.—A.J. Sober, M.D.

Response of Eccrine Adenocarcinoma to Tamoxifen

Sridhar KS, Benedetto P, Otrakji CL, Charyulu KKN (Univ of Miami; Jackson Mem Hosp; VA Med Ctr, Miami)

Cancer 64:366–370, July 15, 1989 14–45

Adenocarcinomas of the skin adnexae are rare. Sweat gland carcinoma, commonly located on the scalp, is the least common of these tumors. About half of all sweat gland carcinomas are cured by surgical excision of the locoregional tumor, but the remainder give rise to potentially fatal metastases. Symptomatic metastases are difficult to palliate; they are often resistant to radiotherapy and chemotherapy. Two women aged 60 and 66 years with sweat gland carcinoma were tested for estradiol receptors and treated with tamoxifen.

The first woman had a hard scalp nodule, 2.5 cm in diameter, over the left occipital region; the second had a nodule behind her right ear. Both had systemic metastases. Poorly differentiated eccrine adenocarcinoma of the scalp was diagnosed. In 1 patient a tumor positive for estradiol receptors was found; after tamoxifen treatment, lymph node metastasis regressed completely. She had full relief of pain from osseous metastases for almost 3 years. Subsequently, progressive painful osseous metastases in her spine, skull, pelvis, and femur were palliated for shorter periods with sequential systemic treatment with megestrol acetate and fluoxymesterone. External radiation therapy was also used to palliate osseous metastases. The patient's brain metastases subsequently proved fatal. Tamoxifen was not effective in the patient who was estradiol receptor negative.

Determining the presence of estradiol receptor protein in eccrine carcinoma may be a valuable predictor of response to hormonal treatment.

▶ Unfortunately, this report must be viewed as anecdotal as only 1 of 2 patients treated with tamoxifen responded with tumor regression. It is noteworthy and biologically of interest that the patient with the positive response was estrogen receptor positive. Additional case reports on treatment of metastatic eccrine adenocarcinoma should be reported in order to develop a clearer view of this tumor's response to therapy.—A.J. Sober, M.D.

Acute Myelogenous Leukemia With Leukemia Cutis: Eighteen Cases Seen Between 1969 and 1986

Baer MR, Barcos M, Farrell H, Raza A, Preisler HD (Roswell Park Mem Inst, Buffalo)

Cancer 63:2192–2200, June 1, 1989 14–46

Relapse-free survival in patients with acute myelogenous leukemia (AML) has been prolonged by intensive consolidation chemotherapy; AML is potentially curable by intensive consolidation therapy and by bone marrow transplantation. Thus it is important to identify sites of extramedullary involvement and to insure that extramedullary leukemia is sufficiently treated to avoid local relapse and marrow relapse from marrow reseeding. Leukemia cutis can be recognized readily and documented by biopsy. The records of patients with AML with skin involvement were reviewed retrospectively to define optimal management of skin involvement at diagnoses of AML and at isolated relapse of AML in the skin.

Of 877 patients with AML seen between 1969 and 1986, 18 (2%) had leukemia cutis documented by biopsy. Five patients had a single large lesion at diagnosis (Fig 14–5), and 13 had multiple lesions. There were 4 French-American-British (FAB) types: four M2, one M3, ten M4, and three M5. Lysozyme was detected more consistently in skin sections than Leu-M1, α_1-antitrypsin, α_1-antichymotrypsin, or chloroacetate esterase activity. Sixteen patients had additional extramedullary sites of involvement, including meningeal leukemia in 6. Leukemia cutis preceded bone marrow leukemia in 2. In 11 patients the skin was the initial site of re-

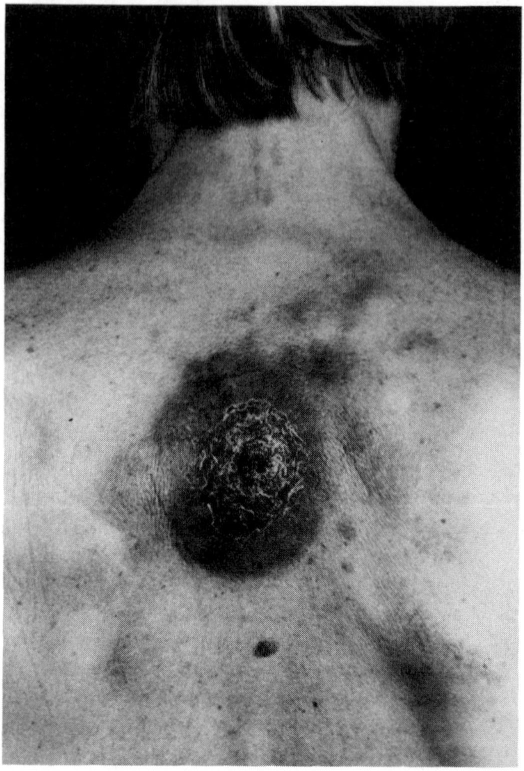

Fig 14–5.—Leukemia cutis appearing as a single large skin mass in a patient in bone marrow remission. (Courtesy of Baer MR, Barcos M, Farrell H, et al: *Cancer* 63:2192–2200, June 1, 1989.)

lapse without marrow relapse occurring as late as 5.5 years after diagnosis. Most of the patients were treated with radiation therapy or palliative chemotherapy, or both, and did poorly, with prompt marrow relapses and serial skin relapses. One patient, whose skin relapse was treated with whole-body electron-beam radiation therapy with reinduction and consolidation chemotherapy, achieved long-term, disease-free survival. In another patient severe skin toxicity was caused by doxorubicin 12 days after electron-beam irradiation, but this did not occur when cytosine arabinoside was given in doses of as much as 3 g/m^2 with radiation therapy.

The optimal management of AML involving skin may include whole-body electron-beam irradiation in conjunction with induction or reinduction chemotherapy without anthracyclines, followed by consolidation chemotherapy. Ongoing surveillance and treatment are needed for extramedullary disease at other sites including the meninges.

▶ Although skin involvement is a feature of monocytic leukemia, the above authors report skin involvement by myelomonocytic leukemia to be as frequent. Regardless of the type of leukemia, leukemia cutis appears frequently to be associated with extramedullary disease. The authors emphasize lysozyme to be a more consistent and readily detectable marker in skin sections than chloroacetate esterase activity (AE stain); however, this observation remains to be solidly established.

Systemic chemotherapy, which is adequate to induce and maintain bone marrow remission, appears to be insufficient to control leukemia cutis; conversely, electron beam therapy controls the skin disease but does not prevent bone marrow relapse.—S.L. Moschella, M.D.

15 Photobiology and Phototherapy

Skin Typing, Sun Exposure, and Sunscreen Use in a Population of Japanese

Kawada A, Hiruma M, Noda T, Kukita A (Natl Defense College, Saitama, Japan)

J Dermatol 16:187–190, June 1989 15–1

A skin typing system for the Japanese skin type (JST) has been proposed. The JST classification defines J-I when the skin burns easily and tan minimally, J-II when the skin burns moderately and tans moderately, and J-III when it burns slightly and tans markedly. To determine the distribution of JSTs and their relationship to sun exposure and sunscreen use, 379 new Japanese outpatients aged 15–68 years were studied.

Of the 379 patients, 65% had the J-II skin type, 24% had J-I, and 11% had J-III; 85% reported occasional sun exposure during summer and 24%, habitual exposure. Interestingly, 80% of those with occasional exposure and 62% of those with habitual exposure spent more than 3 hours per exposure day in the sun. More younger persons experienced occasional sun exposure than older persons, and more males had habitual sun exposure than females. Sunscreens were used by 41% of the patients, most often by J-I types and females. Of the sunscreen users only 23% knew the definition of the sun protector factor. Thus, although the

Comparison of Japanese Skin Type (JST) With Skin Phototype (SPT)

	Skin Phototype SPT no. = 1,139 (ages 30-69)	Japanese Skin Type JST no. = 379 (ages 15-68)
Burn easily, never tan	I (4%)	Not included
Burn easily, tan minimally	II (29%)	J-I (24%)
Burn and tan moderately	III (51%)	J-II (65%)
Burn slightly, tan markedly	IV (14%)	J-III (11%)

largest number of Japanese have JST J-I, there is a lack of knowledge about sun protection in this population.

▶ A new terminology was used for skin types by these authors. It is interesting to compare, in the table, the Japanese Skin Type system with the original skin type classification. Surprisingly, there were few differences in distribution of the different skin types in the 2 populations. A slightly greater percentage of Japanese populations had JST II (Skin Phototype III). Based on this study we could hardly call the Japanese population very different in their reactivity to sun exposure.

This raises the question of the classification of peoples into "races" based on their skin color. I recognize 3 skin colors: black, brown, and white. There are persons in South India who have "black" skin, for example. There are "blacks" in Africa with brown skin. There is, therefore, more to race than skin color. Although many Japanese may be brown skinned, it is likely that a greater number have, in fact, "white" skin and approximately the same sun reactivity as the white population.

A new program was undertaken to standardize skin prototypes by developing a reproducible set of questions. This has proved to be feasible and will be used in a worldwide survey of the various types.—T.B. Fitzpatrick, M.D., Ph.D.

UVA Sunbeds: Tanning, Photoprotection, Acute Adverse Effects, and Immunological Changes

Rivers JK, Norris PG, Murphy GM, Chu AC, Midgley G, Morris J, Morris RW, Young AR, Hawk JLM (Guy's and St Thomas' Hosps, London)
Br J Dermatol 120:767–777, June 1989 15–2

The use of ultraviolet irradiation skin tanning units, particularly ultraviolet A (UVA) sunbeds, has increased rapidly. It is generally believed that UVA sunbeds will tan the skin without burning or causing other significant adverse effects. However, many adverse reactions have been reported, even with the short-term use of sunbeds. Prolonged UVA exposure has been associated with premature skin aging in human beings and accelerated development of skin cancer in animal studies. The possible development of pityriasis versicolor, atypical lentigines, and malignant melanoma after sunbed use has rendered the safety of such use even more questionable. Because significant UVB radiation in sunlamps may be responsible for the adverse cutaneous changes, a double-blind controlled trial was done to assess the effects of a course of exposure to sunbeds containing the newer UVA lamps, which emit much smaller amounts of UVB radiation.

Forty untanned, white, normal persons aged 16–54 years, with variable burning and tanning skin types, were randomly assigned to exposure to sunbeds containing UVA lamps with minimal UVB emission 3 times weekly for 4 weeks, or to similar sunbeds emitting only visible light with insignificant UVA and UVB emissions. Thirty-one subjects received the active treatment and 9 the control treatment.

All 31 subjects given active treatment had mild to moderate tans with only moderate protection against later UV exposure; all controls had minimal or mild tans. Exposure to sunbeds containing the new UVA lamps emitting only minute amounts of UVB radiation appeared to have no obvious advantage over exposure to the older lamps with greater UVB output: The incidence of adverse effects was similar to that reported in previous studies. Pruritus was particularly frequent, and erythema, freckling, a burning sensation, skin dryness, and polymorphic light eruption also were common. Cutaneous Langerhans cell counts and blood CD_3^+ and CD_4^+ lymphocyte subsets were reduced in both active and control groups, as were $CD8^+$ cell counts. *Pityrosporon* yeast counts also were significantly reduced in both groups.

Previously issued warnings about the use of sunbeds were strongly supported.

▶ This well-documented, carefully designed study extends previous findings obtained using light sources containing a much greater proportion of UVB. As the authors state, it is especially interesting that the incidence of short-term adverse reactions was comparable with the newer light source. It seems certain, however, that the small carcinogenic risk, which we assume to be associated with original tanning, is greater with larger amounts of UVB.—R.W. Gange, M.D.

Possible Ultraviolet A-Induced Lentigines: A Side Effect of Chronic Tanning Salon Usage

Roth DE, Hodge SJ, Callen JP (Univ of Louisville)

J Am Acad Dermatol 20:950–954, May 1989 15–3

The role of ultraviolet B (UVB) in the formation of sunburn lentigines, as well as the causal role of psoralens plus ultraviolet A (PUVA) in the formation of so-called PUVA lentigines, have been well described. The effect on melanocytic cells of exposure to UVA alone was studied in a patient who had lentigines after prolonged exposure to UVA in a tanning booth.

Woman, 44, white, with blue eyes and brown hair, was first seen with multiple dark brown macules on her arms, neck, the dorsal aspect of her legs, and the anterior aspect of her chest. She had been exposing her whole body to UVA on a tanning bed twice a week for 1.5 years, having received a total dose of approximately 1,600 J/cm^2. The macules had started to appear after 1 year of tanning. The patient had no personal or family history of melanoma or other skin disorders and had not been exposed to psoralens or furocoumarins. Physical examination revealed multiple, irregular, dark-brown to black macules 2–5 mm in diameter, some of which were coalescent. Several of the heavily pigmented macules were removed. Histologic examination revealed 2 macules to be junctional nevi with moderate cell atypia and heavily pigmented melanophages in the dermis. Lamellar fibrosis and lymphocytes were seen in the papillary dermis. Biopsy of a smaller pigmented macule revealed marked melanocytic hyperplasia at the dermoepidermal junction. Four months after discontinuing UVA exposure another macule was excised. Histologic examination showed a lentigo without any atypia or actinic changes. A junctional nevus removed at the same time was not atypical.

The apparently UVA-induced pigmented macules in this patient support a previously suggested relationship between exposure to UVA in tanning beds and melanoma. Patients should be cautioned against the use of UVA tanning beds.

▶ This case report describes a patient in whom atypical pigmented lesions developed after approximately 1 year of tanning bed light therapy. The spectrum of the bulbs used was not described, but there is a presumption that the output was pure UVA or mostly UVA. (Even small amounts of UVB in the output could be additive or synergistic in the biologic effects produced.) Even if the melanocytic lesions did antedate therapy, the widespread use of UVA artificial radiation should be cause for concern. The long-term biologic hazards of recreational UVA are still unknown, including a potential promoter or initiator effect on melanocytic dysplasias. The UVA tanning salons are reminiscent of the widespread use of fluoroscopy for fitting shoes in the early 1950s.—A.R. Rhodes, M.D., M.P.H.

The Normal Range in Diagnostic Phototesting

Diffey BL, Farr PM (Dryburn Hosp, Durham; Royal Victoria Infirmary, Newcastle upon Tyne, England)

Br J Dermatol 120:517–524, April 1989 15–4

The purpose of phototesting is to determine the skin's response to a given ultraviolet (UV) radiation spectrum. Phototesting is commonly done in a geometric series of increasing exposure doses applied to normal-appearing skin. Response is usually assessed visually in terms of delayed erythema present at 24 hours after exposure. The minimal erythema dose (MED) is traditionally used as an index of cutaneous photosensitivity. Whether a correlation exists between the UVA and UVB MEDs in normal persons and, if so, whether such an association could be used to more accurately diagnose abnormal photosensitivity, were investigated in 254 normal subjects seen during a 7-year period. Phototesting consisted of up to 8 exposures of increasing radiation intensity (table).

Statistical analysis indicated a strong positive correlation between the UVA MED and the UVB MED in normal persons. By calculating the probability that a given combination of UVA and UVB MEDs is likely to occur in normal persons, it was shown that the UVA MED and the UVB MED may both be within normal range but that a particular combination of these values suggests abnormal photosensitivity. The implication is that normal findings on MED phototesting in a given subject do not always exclude a diagnosis of abnormal photosensitivity and abnormal findings do not always confirm such a diagnosis. Rather, the relationship

Number of Normal Subjects With a Given UVB (300 ± 5 nm) and UVA (350 ± 30 nm) Minimal Erythema Dose (MED)

UVA MED (J/cm²)	UVB MED (mJ/cm²) 10	14	20	28	40	56	80	112
10	0	0	0	0	0	0	0	0
14	0	2	5	3	1	0	0	0
20	0	1	24	31	20	11	0	0
28	0	1	12	28	33	29	0	0
40	0	0	5	14	15	10	5	1
56	0	0	0	0	0	1	0	2
80	0	0	0	0	0	0	0	0
112	0	0	0	0	0	0	0	0

(Courtesy of Diffey BL, Farr PM: *Br J Dermatol* 120:517–524, April 1989.)

between UVA MED and UVB MED values obtained in phototesting should be looked at to confirm the presence or absence of abnormal photosensitivity.

▶ This prolific pair of investigators, who have wide experience in phototesting, propose an interesting approach to the often difficult interpretation of results. This is based on disparity between UVA and UVB sensitivities, which they state may be significant even when the sensitivities to individual wave bands fall within the "normal" range.—R.W. Gange, M.D.

Photoallergy to Benzophenone

Knobler E, Almeida L, Ruzkowski AM, Held J, Harber L, DeLeo V (Columbia Univ)

Arch Dermatol 125:801–804, June 1989 15–5

Photosensitization to sunscreen products can present a unique problem. Ironically, sunscreen products intended to protect against such photosensitivity or a change to a sunscreen containing the same photoallergen may only exacerbate the condition.

Four patients were photoallergic to benzophenone 3 (oxybenzone) in sunscreens. Three had concomitant non-photocontact allergy to oxybenzone. The dermatitis occurred in sun-exposed areas, particularly the face. Half of the patients related their dermatitis to sunscreen usage, whereas the other 2 were unaware of this association.

Photoallergy to *p*-aminobenzoic acid and its esters in sunscreens has long been recognized, but benzophenone photoallergy is not so well known. It is likely that photoallergy to benzophenones will increase, because oxybenzone is the most frequently used component in modern, high-sun protection factor sunscreens (>8 sun protection factor). Benzophenones should be added to the list of antigens used for phototesting.

▶ This observation is important when photopatch testing is being considered.—R.W. Gange, M.D.

Adverse Effects of Sunscreens in Photosensitive Patients

Farr PM, Diffey BL (Royal Victoria Infirmary, Newcastle upon Tyne; Dryburn Hosp, Durham, England)

Lancet 1:429–431, Feb 25, 1989 15–6

Polymorphic light eruption, a common photosensitive skin disorder among indigenous northern European races, is caused by the ultraviolet A (UVA) component of terrestrial sunlight. Sunscreens afford little or no protection against the UVA component of sunlight, and the sun protection factor refers largely to ultraviolet B (UVB) wavelengths. An individual who uses a sunscreen to allow long-term exposure to the sun actually is exposed to greater amounts of UVA than would be possible without the sunscreen. Thus patients with polymorphic light eruption who use sunscreens can be exposed to excess UVA, which will aggravate the skin eruptions.

Because sunscreens distort the quality of sunlight reaching the skin, allowing much greater levels of UVA to be deposited than would otherwise be possible, patients with polymorphic light eruption should not use sunscreens; rather, they should sunbathe for a shorter time and move out of the sun before erythema develops.

▶ The title suggests the presence of data in this paper; in fact, the authors are presenting a hypothesis without even a single anecdote to support it; instead, they make liberal use of "we believe" and "we propose." The authors base their proposal on universal sensitivity to UVA among polymorphous light eruption patients, a debatable point. They ignore the unknown number of subjects who *do* benefit from UVB sunscreens and who consequently are not forced to make the pilgrimage to Durham, England.—R.W. Gange, M.D.

Photosensitizing Potential of Certain Nonsteroidal Anti-Inflammatory Agents

Kaidbey KH, Mitchell FN (Hosp of the Univ of Pennsylvania; Beecham Lab, Bristol, Tenn)

Arch Dermatol 125:783–786, June 1989 15–7

Nonsteroidal anti-inflammatory drugs (NSAIDs) have been associated with photosensitivity reactions. The underlying mechanism remains unknown, and the clinical features are not always consistent with either a phototoxic or photoallergic mechanism. To gain more insight into this, 4 NSAIDs were investigated for their phototoxicity potential in human volunteers using an oral dosing protocol. The volunteers were exposed to ultraviolet radiation on reaching the maximum plasma concentration of nabumetone, naproxen, ketoprofen, and piroxicam.

Phototoxicity was noted after administration of nabumetone and naproxen, but not piroxicam, a frequently cited NSAID causing photosensitivity reactions. All abnormal reactions were transient and of the immediate type, varying from erythema and flare to a wheal-and-flare reaction simulating solar urticaria. No abnormal delayed reactions were noted.

Although certain NSAIDs potentially can provoke phototoxicity reactions, others can presumably provoke clinical photosensitivity through other mechanisms. However, the incidence of this adverse reaction must be low, considering the widespread and long-term use of NSAIDs.

Phototoxic Potential of Thiazide Diuretics in Normal Subjects

Diffey BL, Langtry J (Dryburn Hosp, Durham, England)

Arch Dermatol 125:1355–1358, October 1989 15–8

To determine whether hydrochlorothiazide is more capable of inducing photosensitivity than bendroflumethiazide, 22 persons without a history of photosensitivity underwent monochromator phototesting just before and after 2 weeks of treatment with hydrochlorothiazide or bendroflumethiazide.

Several persons had increased erythemal sensitivity in wave bands of maximum absorption for each of the drugs. The phototoxic capabilities of the 2 drugs was similar. None of the subjects had clinical symptoms of photosensitivity. Although the clinical dose of bendroflumethiazide is 10 times less than that of hydrochlorothiazide, the extinction coefficients of both drugs were similar.

It could be hypothesized that the increased incidence of photosensitive reactions attributed to hydrochlorothiazide is simply related to the higher administered doses; however, it may be that the procedures used in phototesting were insufficient to detect a difference in weak phototoxic reactions. Also, the mechanism for photodamage in susceptible persons may not be the same as that causing increased photosensitivity in normal persons. Whatever the reason, clinical photosensitivity to thiazide diuretics is at present unpredictable.

▶ Both groups of investigators were able to provoke phototoxicity reactions in a significant proportion of normal individuals exposed orally to the drugs.—R.W. Gange, M.D.

Evaluating the UVA Protection of Sunscreens

Roelandts R, Sohrabvand N, Garmyn M (Univ of Leuven, Belgium)

J Am Acad Dermatol 21:56–62, July 1989 15–9

Because the protection factor of sunscreens concerns only ultraviolet B (UVB) protection, usually nothing is known about protection in the UVA range. Six commercially available sunscreens were compared to determine the UVA protection factors and thus select the most appropriate sunscreen. The effects of 2 clinical methods on human skin—inhibition of UVA-induced tanning with the use of a high-intensity UVA source and inhibition of methoxsalen plus UVA-induced phototoxicity—were compared with those of in vivo methods (inhibition of UVA-induced sunburn cell production in mice treated with methoxsalen) and 2 in vitro techniques (solution-dilution and sandwich spectrophotometry).

All 5 methods gave a quantitative estimate of UVA protection. However, different UVA protection factors were obtained, depending on the method used and the reading time.

It appears that none of the 5 methods can be accepted as a standard for quantifying UVA protection. It is probably more appropriate not to use numbers, i.e., protection factors, to classify sunscreens but, rather, to categorize them in terms of the UVA protection afforded.

Ultraviolet A Sunscreen Evaluations in Normal Subjects

Stanfield JW, Feldt PA, Csortan ES, Krochmal L (Bristol-Myers Pharmaceutical Research and Development, Buffalo; Johns Hopkins Univ)

J Am Acad Dermatol 20:744–748, May 1989 15–10

The ultraviolet A (UVA) portion of the solar spectrum, although less biologically active than the UVB range, can contribute to actinic damage and UV erythema. Over-the-counter sunscreens can provide all-day protection in the UVB region but may give incomplete protection against the UVA region. A specially modified xenon arc solar simulator was used to examine the UVA protection capability of a research sunscreen formula in 15 patients. The UVA doses were administered to sunscreen-protected and unprotected skin with the use of irradiance values of 50 mW/cm^2 and 100 mW/cm^2. Erythemal responses were determined approximately 5 hours later and again 24 hours later.

The overall mean unprotected UVA minimal erythema dose was 23.6 joules per cm^2. The mean UVA protection factor was 3.2 joules per cm^2. Neither irradiance nor evaluation time had a significant effect on minimal erythema dose or UVA protection factor.

These preliminary results suggest that the modified solar simulator allows convenient determination of sunscreen UVA protection factor. Similar minimal erythema dose and UVA protection factor values were noted for irradiance values of 100 mW/cm^2 and 50 mW/cm^2, indicating dose reciprocity.

▶ The difficulty of measuring topical protection against UVA is a currently discussed problem, and a perfect solution will not be found. Protection against UVA is sought to prevent a variety of undesirable responses (e.g., most photodermatoses, drug photosensitization, aging, and carcinogenesis), each of which may have different action spectra. Unlike the situation with UVB, protection against UVA erythema is important only if sunscreens are used to permit greatly prolonged solar exposure, that is to say, if our educational efforts fail. The results of measurements of screening efficiently will always depend on the action spectrum of the response used, the spectral irradiance of the source employed, and the absorption spectrum of the absorber. Because the responses against which protection is sought have varying action spectra, a single measurement made using a single response is not necessarily helpful. Providing this information to users may compare in value to knowing the riboflavin content of a breakfast cereal.—R.W. Gange, M.D.

Adolescent Use of Sun-Protection Measures

Cockburn J, Hennrikus D, Scott R, Sanson-Fisher R (Univ of Newcastle; Country Regions Skin Cancer Prevention Campaign, Tamworth, New South Wales, Australia)

Med J Aust 151:136–140, Aug 7, 1989 15–11

In Australia the most common form of cancer is skin cancer. In countries such as Australia that have substantial year-round exposure to ultraviolet light and a predominantly fair-skinned population, the incidence of skin cancer is higher than in similar countries with more temperate climates. Because adolescents represent an at-risk group, the prevalence of the use of sun-protection measures among adolescents and the variables that predicted use of and failure to use such measures were investigated. From 26 high schools in New South Wales (NSW) 3,002 students in years 9 and 10 were surveyed in the last term of 1986 and first term of 1987 as part of the NSW Department of Health's Country Regions Skin Cancer Prevention Campaign.

By standardized criteria, 1,412 (70%) students were classified as not using sun-protection measures. These included 636 (62%) male students and 776 (77%) female students. The association between sex and the use of sun protection was statistically significant. Significant predictors by stepwise regression analyses of whether a student used sun-protection measures included the number of opportunities for sun protection, sex, smoking status, skin type, and area of residence. Further regression analyses revealed that the attitudes and beliefs of students also were significant predictors of sun-protection use, independent of sociodemographic variables and the number of opportunities for sun protection. Students rated choice of sun protection as follows: Sunscreens were rated first by 44.5%, wearing a shirt by 35.3%, wearing a hat by 16.7%, and not going outdoors by 3.5%.

Interventions that are aimed at increasing the use of sunscreens may be more effective than other methods. However, increasing the use of sunscreens should be recommended as an adjunct to other sun-protection methods, such as wearing protective clothing and staying in the shade.

▶ The large percentage of non-sunscreen-using Australian adolescents is perhaps not surprising.—R.W. Gange, M.D.

Chronic Sunscreen Use Decreases Circulating Concentrations of 25-Hydroxyvitamin D: A Preliminary Study

Matsuoka LY, Wortsman J, Hanifan N, Holick MF (Jefferson Med College, Philadelphia; Southern Illinois Univ, Springfield; Boston Univ)
Arch Dermatol 124:1802–1804, December 1988 15–12

A single topical application of *p*-aminobenzoic acid (PABA) was found to prevent the increase of serum vitamin D levels in normal persons exposed to 1 minimal erythema dose of ultraviolet radiation. This metabolic change resulted from epidermal blockage in previtamin D_3 synthesis from 7-dehydrocholesterol, which requires the solar spectrum absorbed by PABA. Experiments with normal volunteers indicated suppression of cutaneous vitamin D formation during the short-term use of PABA. Thus vitamin D status was investigated in long-term users of this sunscreening agent.

The PABA-treated group consisted of 14 women and 6 men aged 35–89; 20 healthy white persons, aged 30–87, comprised a control group. After initial extraction in methyl alcohol:methylene chloride, lipid extracts of serum samples underwent preparative chromatography on silica cartridges for separation and purification of 25-hydroxyvitamin D (25-OH-D). The serum 25-OH-D concentration was determined by competitive protein-binding assay.

Overall, the mean serum concentration of 25-OH-D level was lower in sunscreen users than in controls. Two sunscreen users had levels compatible with vitamin D deficiency, indicated by serum 25-OH-D levels of less than 20 nmol/L. The normal range for this assay is from 20 to 137.3 nmol/L; the mean 25-OH-D level was not significantly lower than the population mean.

Long-term sunscreen users probably have lower circulating concentrations of 25-OH-D, suggesting lower vitamin D stores. The consequences of this phenomenon may be insignificant in young persons, whose vitamin D stores are derived from dietary intake as well as skin photosynthesis. However, the dietary contribution may be limited in elderly persons who are likely to ingest less vitamin D-fortified products. This population could be extremely dependent on cutaneous production to meet their requirements. These findings should not be taken as an indication to stop the continuous use of sunscreening agents in patients with skin cancer.

▶ This interesting study demonstrates a possible adverse effect of sunscreens, especially in elderly patients. Although the authors point out that defective mineralization of bone is a potential consequence of long-term usage of sunscreens, they do not advocate changing clinical practice with respect to their use, at least not in skin cancer patients.—R.W. Gange, M.D.

Actinic Reticuloid: A Clinical, Photobiologic, Histopathologic, and Follow-Up Study of 16 Patients

Toonstra J, Henquet CJM, van Weelden H, van der Putte SCJ, van Vloten WA
(Univ of Utrecht, The Netherlands)
J Am Acad Dermatol 21:205–214, August 1989 15–13

Actinic reticuloid, an infrequent photosensitive dermatosis usually seen in middle-aged and elderly men, was investigated in 16 Dutch patients seen in 1975–1987. All were middle-aged or older men who had prolonged or persistent erythroderma or, less often, extension of lesions to unexposed skin or persistent plaques on light-exposed skin only (Fig 15–1). The lesions were sensitive to ultraviolet B (UVB), UVA, and visible light (table). In most patients the dermal infiltrate consisted mainly of suppressor T cells. Many patients had a reversed helper-suppressor T cell

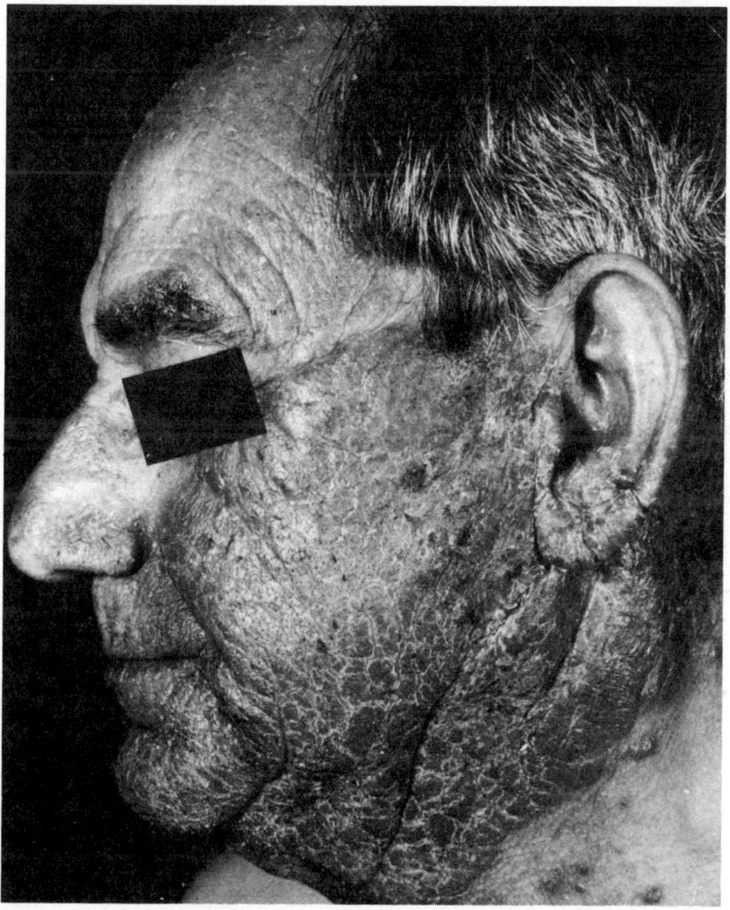

Fig 15–1—Diffusely infiltrated face of patient with actinic reticuloid. Note relative sparing of nose, forehead, and ears. (Courtesy of Toonstra J, Henquet CJM, van Weelden H, et al: *J Am Acad Dermatol* 21:205–214, August 1989.)

Clinical Data and Range of Photosensitivity in 16 Patients With Actinic Reticuloid

Patient No.	Sex	Age at time of diagnosis (yr)	Year phototested	Range of photosensitivity*					
							Visible light		
				UVC	UVB	UVA	Violet/blue†	Green	Orange/red
1	M	61	1975	ND	+				
2	M	68	1976	+	+				
3	M	66	1977	+	+	+	+		
4	M	63	1981	+	+	+	+		
5	M	49	1981	ND	+	+	+	+	+
6	M	69	1982	+	+	+	+	+	+
7	M	76	1982	+	+	+	+	+	
8	M	80	1983	ND	+	+			
9	M	65	1983	Normal	+	+	+		
10	M	53	1983	ND	+	+	+	+	
11	M	52	1984	ND	+	+	+		
12	M	63	1985	ND	+	+			
13	M	69	1985	+	+	+	+	+	
14	M	62	1985	+	+	+	+		
15	M	58	1986	+	+	+	+		
16	M	75	1987	Normal	+	+	+	+	

Abbreviation—*ND*, not done.
*Indicates sensitive to spectrum.
†For patients 1 and 2, sensitive for combination of UVA plus visible light. For patients 8 and 12, not possible to test wavelengths of the visible light spectrum separately.
(Courtesy of Toonstra J, Henquet CJM, van Weelden H, et al: *J Am Acad Dermatol* 21:205–214, August 1989.)

ratio. Active lesions exhibited focal or diffuse parakeratosis, often with marked acanthosis, and varying fibrosis and edema in the papillary dermis.

Thirteen of 15 patients had a good response when given slowly increasing doses of UVB radiation from an artificial sunlamp. The whole skin was treated, usually 5 times a week. The eruption recurred consistently when maintenance UVB therapy ceased.

Photosensitive eczema, persistent light reaction, and chronic photosensitivity dermatitis are closely related disorders than can precede actinic reticuloid. In actinic reticuloid the dermal infiltrate consists mainly of suppressor T cells. Contact allergy is of major importance. The condition is refractory to treatment, but tolerance induction with UVB is the best choice. Patients who respond are able to live a nearly normal life.

▶ This is an excellent and comprehensive review of the experience of this group in the diagnosis and management of actinic reticuloid. The authors emphasize the importance of allergic contact sensitivity in these patients, documented by patch testing in 12 of the 14 tested. The good results obtained using UVB phototherapy are impressive, although the authors point out that prolonged hospitalization was frequently necessary during such treatment.—R.W. Gange, M.D.

Treatment of Actinic Prurigo With PUVA: Mechanism of Action

Farr PM, Diffey BL (Royal Victoria Infirmary, Newcastle upon Tyne; Dryburn Hosp, Durham, England)

Br J Dermatol 120:411–418, March 1989 15–14

Actinic prurigo is an uncommon, chronic photosensitivity disorder that is difficult to treat. Action spectrum studies have shown that most patients with this disorder have increased erythemal sensitivity to ultraviolet radiation, particularly ultraviolet A (UVA). Psoralen plus UVA (PUVA) has been used to treat photosensitivity disorders such as polymorphic light eruption. Its effects in the treatment of actinic prurigo were investigated in 5 aged 30–39 years who were treated twice weekly with PUVA for 15 weeks.

The patients had been photosensitive since early childhood, with areas of erythema developing within hours of minimal sun exposure. All had abnormal augmentation of UVB erythema by topically applied indomethacin. None of the 5 patients had increasing tolerance to sunlight during the later months of summer, and symptoms continued throughout the year. One area on the back of each patient was protected from UVA exposure throughout the treatment period. Psoralen was administered orally 2 hours before UVA exposure.

Moderate pigmentation of the UVA-exposed skin occurred in 4 patients; 1 had only minimal pigmentation. After 4 weeks of treatment all patients had increased tolerance to sun exposure. After 15 weeks all 5 remained free of any photosensitive symptoms and rash despite long periods of summer sun exposure. However, the skin areas on the back that had been protected from exposure to UVA showed erythemal response that were unchanged from before PUVA therapy. Augmentation of UVB erythema by topically applied indomethacin also persisted after PUVA therapy. Whereas PUVA is effective in the treatment of actinic prurigo, it apparently does not modify the underlying mechanism of photosensitivity in these patients.

► This interesting study documenting the efficacy of PUVA therapy for actinic prurigo demonstrates a local rather than a systemic effect. The mechanism is still obscure despite the complacent title.—R.W. Gange, M.D.

Polymorphous Light Eruption: Results of a Prospective Survey and Study in 302 Patients

Diepgan ThL, Häberle M, Fartasch M, Stüben O, Hornstein OP (Univ of Erlangen, West Germany)

Z Hautkr 64:279–285, 1989 15–15

Polymorphous light eruption, a common photodermatosis, often is not recognized because standard diagnostic parameters have not been established. The diagnosis is based on clinical signs and symptoms, combined with a history of exposure to sunlight. Six types of polymorphous light eruption have been described; papular and plaque-forming are the most common. It is generally seen in women and usually develops within a few hours to several days after exposure to sunlight. Its prevalence is highest from March to June. The findings from a prospective study were compared with those from earlier Swedish, Finnish, and American studies.

All 500 Erlangen residents with suspected polymorphous light eruption were asked to complete a questionnaire. From these, data on 302 individuals, 87% of whom were women, were analyzed by statistical methods.

The median age was 34 years. The mean age at onset of disease was 24 years, and the average duration was 10 years. Of the group, 77% had polymorphous light eruption for more than 5 years; 40% of these reported that the intensity had increased yearly. Only 1% reported improvement over time. About 39% had consulted a dermatologist, and 6% had undergone skin biopsy. About 29% had a positive family history of allergy to sunlight. Eighty percent had polymorphous light eruption every summer; 67% reported a decrease in intensity toward the end of summer. Most had evidence of the disease in exposed skin areas only; less than 10% had polymorphous light eruption in nonexposed areas. Only 15% reported that symptoms usually appeared in less than half an hour after exposure to sunlight; generally, there was a latency of several hours. Itching was the most commonly cited symptom. Other symptoms were headache (14%), fever (6%), dizziness (9%), and nausea (9%).

► This study seems to be seriously flawed because of the sampling method used and the poor (302 of 500) response rate to the questionnaire.—R.W. Gange, M.D.

Polymorphic Light Eruption: An Immunopathological Study of Evolving Lesions

Norris PG, Morris J, McGibbon DM, Chu AC, Hawk JLM (St Thomas' Hosp; Hammersmith Hosp, London)
Br J Dermatol 120:173–183, February 1989 15–16

Polymorphus light eruption is a persistent acquired abnormal reaction to sunlight that probably affects 10% to 21% of the population in temperate regions. Its cause is unknown, but delayed type hypersensitivity is suspected by several researchers. The evolution of lesions was examined in 14 patients, 9 women and 5 men aged 20–67 years. A fully resolving, nonscarring papular eruption occurred within 48 hours of solar exposure. Three normal volunteers also were studied.

Papules were induced on previously affected sites in 11 of the 14 patients. Lesions appeared within 4–20 hours after single exposures to suberythemogenic doses of simulated solar radiation (table). Onset occurred within 5 hours of the appearance of perivascular cellular infiltration, with lymphocytes predominating. There was no epidermal pathology. Immunohistochemical studies showed a predominance of CD4+ cells in earlier lesions and of CD8+ cells in later infiltrates. Dermal macrophages and CD1b+ cells were increased shortly after irradiation.

The immunopathologic findings in evolving polymorphous light eruption lesions are consistent with a delayed type hypersensitivity response. The predominance of CD8+ cells in resolving lesions probably contributes to cessation of inflammation.

▶ In a careful study the investigators have expanded on previous reports characterizing the inflammatory infiltrate in polymorphous light eruption.— R.W. Gange, M.D.

Response to irradiation

Patient no.	Test site	35% MED	50% MED	70% MED	Time of onset of lesions (hours post irradiation)
1	Thigh	–	++	++	4
2	Upper arm	–	+	–	6–8
3	Forearm	+	+	–	8
4	Upper arm	+	+	–	10
5	Forearm	–	+	+	10
6	Thigh	–	++	–	12–20
7	Upper back	–	–	+	12–20
8	Upper arm	–	+	++	10
9	Upper back	–	+	+	12–20
10	Forearm	–	++	++	12–20
11	Upper back	++	++	++	6–8

+: sparse, scattered polymorphous light eruption (PLE) papules; ++: moderate/dense PLE papules.

(Courtesy of Norris PG, Morris J, McGibbon DM, et al: *Br J Dermatol* 120:173–183, February 1989.)

Preventive Effect of an *E. Coli*-Filtrate (Colibiogen) in Polymorphous Light Eruption

Przybilla B, Heppeler M, Ruzicka T (Ludwig-Maximilians-Universität, Munich, West Germany)

Br J Dermatol 121:229–233, August 1989 15–17

Colibiogen, a protein-free filtrate derived from *Escherichia coli* cultures, is manufactured in West German, where it has been used for many years in the treatment of gastrointestinal and allergic conditions. Because a woman with long-standing polymorphous light eruption reported that her photodermatosis disappeared while she was taking Colibiogen for an unrelated condition, its efficacy in other patients with polymorphous light eruption was investigated.

Three men and 6 women aged 21–47 years with papular-type polymorphous light eruption of 3–19 years' duration were studied. All patients underwent phototesting with ultraviolet A irradiation on 3 consecutive days during which incremental ultraviolet A doses were given to distinct test areas. In 2 patients test areas were also exposed to low-dose ultraviolet B irradiation. The administration of Colibiogen was started on day 7. Phototesting was repeated on 3 consecutive days, starting on day 21 of the study period. Colibiogen was discontinued after the second phototesting sequence. Control testing was carried out in 4 patients who had not taken the trial preparation for at least 8 months before the study.

After Colibiogen administration, the test dose of ultraviolet A required to cause skin papules was significantly increased in all 9 patients when in comparison with the baseline doses that elicited skin lesions. Controls, who did not receive Colibiogen, showed significantly less change after the second series of phototesting sessions.

How Colibiogen reduces skin reactivity to ultraviolet light is not known, but the agent seems to have a protective effect on mammalian cells and as such may be considered a biologic response modifier. Although the results of this small pilot study suggest that Colibiogen may be useful in the prophylactic treatment of patients with polymorphous light eruption, its clinical efficacy needs to be confirmed in controlled studies. A double-blind clinical trial of Colibiogen was in progress when this preliminary report was releated for publication.

▶ Colibiogen contains amino acids, peptides, polysaccharides, and fatty acids. It is to be hoped that the results of the ongoing double-blind study support this preliminary observation.—R.W. Gange, M.D.

Measurement of Plasma Uroporphyrin During Treatment and Long-Term Follow-Up of Patients With Porphyria Cutanea Tarda

Adjarov DG, Kerimova MA (Med Academy, Sofia, Bulgaria)

Clin Chim Acta 181:143–150, May 15, 1989 15–18

The amount of uroporphyrin in plasma reflects adequately the condition of patients with Porphyria cutanea tarda (PCT). A simple and reliable method was developed for assaying plasma highly carboxylated porphyrins during the treatment and follow-up of 91 patients with PCT. The controls included 33 nonporphyric persons.

With the precipitating and extracting properties of trichloroacetic acid (0.61 mol/L), the determined parameter consisted of a mixture of chiefly highly carboxylated porphyrins. The coefficient of variation in 10 determinations in a patient with remission was 4%, and no quenching of the fluorescence was established in higher plasma porphyrin concentrations. The recoveries of coproporphyrin and protoporphyrin were 14% and 8%, respectively.

The range of plasma uroporphyrin in the controls was 0–1.4 nmol/L. Among 17 patients with PCT requiring treatment, the range was 17.9–448 nmol/L. The correlation coefficient between the plasma and the urinary uroporphyrin levels in these patients was exceptionally high at 0.97. Among the 28 patients with remission, the values ranged from 0 to 12.8 nmol/L, which was correlated satisfactorily with urinary porphyrin levels.

This method is technically simple and rapid in monitoring the effects of treatment in patients with PCT, as well as the course during long-term follow-up.

▶ It was not stated whether this method would be useful in measuring plasma (serum) porphyrins in patients with variegate porphyria (tetracarboxylated coproporphyrins) or in patients with erythropoietic protoporphyria (dicarboxylated protoporphyrins.) The method proposed is simple, and it is recommended for patients with porphyria cutanea tarda undergoing multiple phelbotomy treatments.—T.B. Fitzpatrick, M.D., Ph.D.

Sunbed-Induced Pseudoporphyria

Murphy GM, Wright J, Nicholls DSH, McKee PH, Messenger AG, Hawk JLM, Levene GM (St John's Hosp for Diseases of the Skin; Guy's & St Thomas' Hosps, London; Royal Hallamshire Hosp, Sheffield, England)

Br J Dermatol 120:555–562, April 1989 15–19

The reported acute effects of sunbed exposure to date include erythema, intense itching, burning sensations, dryness of skin, freckling, and polymorphic light eruption. Photodermatoses may be aggravated or precipitated. Photosensitizing drugs or chemicals may also cause acute adverse effects. Sunbed exposure has been implicated as an etiologic factor in the development of melanoma. Four fair-skinned patients had striking skin fragility and blistering suggestive of porphyria after prolonged sunbed exposure.

Woman, 28, had a 3-year history of atopic eczema and recurrent blistering and erosions on the limbs after minor injured. She was not taking any medications.

The patient had used sunbeds regularly during the previous 3 years. Her total exposure to ultraviolet A (UVA) radiation was estimated in excess of 10 kJ/cm^2. Physical examination revealed an unusual orange/brown tan with many freckles. Her skin was dry, with loss of elasticity, and looked old for her chronologic age. There were striking linear purple streaks and excoriations on the legs, arms, and abdomen, and groups of blisters on the limbs (Fig 15–2). She also had eczema on both sides of her neck. Quantitative porphyrin studies of urine, blood, and stool were normal. Histopathologic examination of a blister from the arm showed a subepidermal split without associated inflammation. The suction-blister time test was normal. A toxicology screen for drugs known to cause pseudoporphyria also was negative.

The other 3 patients had similar, although somewhat less dramatic, findings. In all patients, porphyrin analysis excluded porphyria. Porphyrin found in normal amounts in blood and skin may cause porphyria-like tissue damage after excessive exposure to UVA over a prolonged period.

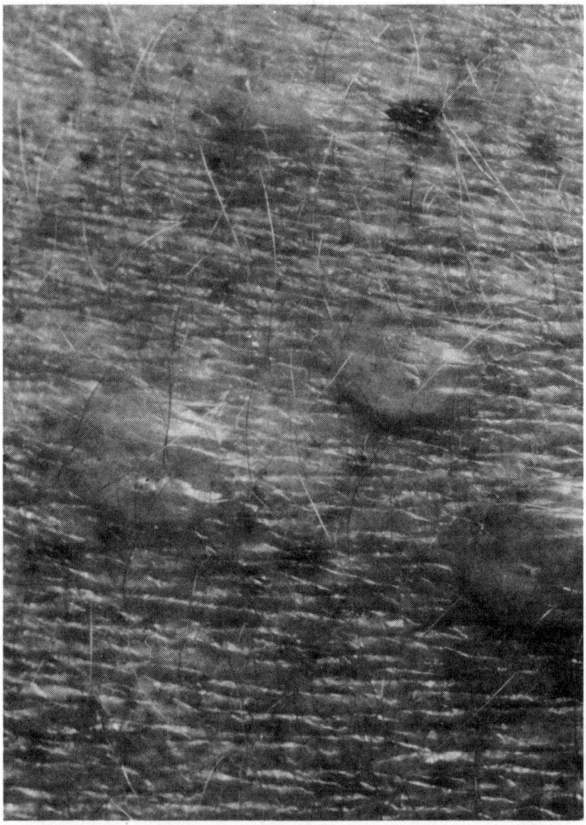

Fig 15–2.—Grouped blisters arising on noninflamed skin on the arm. (Courtesy of Murphy GM, Wright J, Nicholls DSH, et al: *Br J Dermatol* 120:555–562, April 1989.)

The use of sunbeds, particularly by fair-skinned individuals, should be strongly discouraged.

▶ Pseudoporphyria can mimic PCT so truly that it is only the chemical findings in the urine and stool that clinch the diagnosis; even the histologic findings in pseudoporphyria are typical for PCT. And it is essential that porphyrins be searched for in addition to the urine; stool porphyrins needed to be sought in order not to miss porphyria variegata (South African porphyria); in this disease the urine level of porphyrins may be normal, and the diagnosis is made based on the high levels of protoporphyrins in the stool. The list of agents and conditions that cause pseudoporphyria is long: furosemide, dapsone, tetracycline, naproxen, nalidixic acid, sulfonamides, hemodialysis, and epidermolysis bullosa acquisita.

The interesting aspect of this careful and thorough study from England is that the pseudoporphyria did not appear immediately but only after months or years of exposure to the sunbed. We noted previously that patients with PCT may present with a deep tan and bullae, the latter appearing only in late summer and not immediately on exposure to the sun. We learned at the time an interesting fact: Sunlight can photocatalyze the conversions of a nonsensitizing uroporphyrinogen to photosensitizing uroporphyrin. Apparently, the levels of uroporphyrin were high enough that bullae appeared, and this took some weeks (1).—T.B. Fitzpatrick, M.D., Ph.D.

Reference

1. Burnett JW, Pathak MA: *N Engl J Med* 268:1203, 1963.

Photodynamic Therapy for Cutaneous and Subcutaneous Malignant Neoplasms

McCaughan JS Jr, Guy JT, Hicks W, Laufman L, Nims TA, Walker J (Laser Med Research Found, Columbus, Ohio)
Arch Surg 124:211–216, February 1989 15–20

Photodynamic therapy was administered to 27 patients with cutaneous and subcutaneous malignant neoplasms. In all, 248 areas were treated during 72 sessions after 45 injections of sensitizer. A tunable dye argon laser system was used for the light source. Treatment was given either by surface radiation or interstitially. Seven patients had basal cell carcinoma, 3 had squamous cell carcinoma, 3 had malignant melanoma, 1 had liposarcoma, 12 had breast cancers, and 1 had Bowen's disease.

After 1 month of treatment, a complete response (no clinical evidence of tumor) was achieved in 48 (67%) of the 72 treatment sessions and a partial response >50% reduction in the number or size of tumors) in 19 (26%). Fifteen patients could be examined 12 months after treatment. In this subgroup sessions resulted in complete responses at 1-month after treatment and 15 (48%) retained this status at 1 year after treatment. In some patients, such as the patient with squamous cell cancer, no evidence of disease was evident even 5 years after photodynamic therapy. Adjuvant photodynamic therapy for tumor areas that showed a tumor in a resected margin led to pathologically complete responses that lasted for up to 24 months.

In comparing the ability of different light-delivery instrumentation, the Yellow Springs radiometer provided the most reliable spot power density readings. With a homogeneous light source and power density measured from the total output delivered, divided by the area of the spot, complete responses were obtained with doses ranging from 20 joules per cm^2 to 30 joules per cm^2. Doses greater than this resulted in excessive necrosis and pain in white patients. Straight-tipped fibers were nonhomogeneous and could result in overtreatment of the central area with necrosis and pain and in undertreatment of the periphery. The reaction to photodynamic therapy given 2 days after injection was greater than at 3 days. The reaction from 3 to 6 days appeared to be clinically similar. The laser light itself could cause hyperthermia, depending on the power density.

These data show that photodynamic therapy for cutaneous and subcutaneous cancers can provide a complete response, in some cases for up to 5 years.

▶ Although photodynamic therapy is an exciting development in the treatment of poorly accessible visceral tumors, using fiber delivery systems, its role in dermatology is not yet clear. As far as one can tell from the variable follow-up data in this study, photodynamic therapy can be used successfully in the treatment of a variety of difficult primary and secondary cutaneous malignancies.—R.W. Gange, M.D.

A Hypothetical Explanation for the Aging of Skin: Chronologic Alteration of the Three-Dimensional Arrangement of Collagen and Elastic Fibers in Connective Tissue

Imayama S, Braverman IM (Yale Univ)

Am J Pathol 134:1019–1025, May 1989 15–21

The age-related changes in human skin are best correlated with the 3-dimensional organization of collagen and elastic fibers. With a new method for preparing fibers in the connective tissue for scanning electron microscopy, the 3-dimensional arrangement and chronologic alterations of the fibrous components of the connective tissue of rats aged 2 weeks to 24 months were studied.

In the 2-week-old rat the elastic fibers were arranged in a multilayered, ordered meshwork of relatively straight fibers, whereas the collagen fiber bundles were curled randomly within the elastic meshwork. With postnatal growth the collagen and elastic fibers were dynamically rearranged, resulting in an ordered arrangement of mature collagen bundles attained by distorting the elastic fiber meshwork. During adulthood there was subsequent tortuosity of the distorted elastic fibers and incomplete rebuilding of the elastic fiber network laid down in a form to interlock with the collagen bundles.

These changes may explain the laxity, sagging, and wrinkling of the aged skin. The tortuosity of the elastic fibers implies that they have been stretched and have lost their original elasticity and ability to restitute short and straight. The interlocking of the collagen and elastic fibers does not allow these 2 fibrous systems to function independently, as they normally should, and thus decreases tissue compliance.

▶ This paper is a superb visual presentation of scanning electron microscopic photographs of the changes in collagen and elastic tissue that occur with aging. Most important, however, is the use of a perfusion technique fixation to preserve the 3-dimensional view of the dermis. It would be interesting indeed if these authors were to perfuse an isolated limb using the same technique in skin previously irradiated with radiant energy to follow the changes that occur using different parts of the spectra, i.e., ultraviolet radiation and infrared.—T.B. Fitzpatrick, M.D., Ph.D.

Physiological Consequences of Human Skin Aging

Balin AK, Pratt LA (Rockefeller Univ; Cornell Univ Med Ctr)

Cutis 43:431–436, May 1989 15–22

Skin disease may require different treatment in the older patient because of the anatomical changes in aging skin. Knowledge of these changes should aid in the recognition of skin disease among the elderly and facilitate treatment decisions.

The stratum corneum has a lower moisture content with advancing age, resulting in rougher, more brittle skin. The longer renewal time of the epidermis in aged persons means that irritating substances remain longer on the skin and medications applied to the skin require longer treatment to be successful. Epidermal rete ridges are decreased, reducing the area of contact between the dermis and epidermis. Thus the epidermis peels off readily as a result of simple trauma in an elderly person and epidermal wound healing is prolonged. Decreases in Langerhan's cells and melanocytes also characterize the aging epidermis.

The number of cells in the dermis decreases with age and the dermis becomes thinner. Collagen fibers are no longer deposited in an orderly manner as they are in younger skin. Changes in elastic tissue contribute to fine wrinkling and loss of resiliency. A decrease in small blood vessels leads to a lowered inflammatory response, delayed wound healing, and impaired thermal regulation. Pallor is a visible sign of the decreased vasculature among the elderly. Growth of nails and hair is slowed in elderly persons; similarly, eccrine, apocrine, and sebum secretions are reduced (table).

Skin diseases may not have the same presenting signs that are typical in

Decreases in Cutaneous Physiologic Functions Caused by Intrinsic Aging

Epidermal renewal
Wound healing, tissue repair
Hair growth
Nail growth
Eccrine and apocrine gland secretion
Sebum secretion
Immune surveillance
Antigen presentation
Inflammatory response
Vascular supply
Absorption
Response to heat and cold
Tactile sensitivity
Pain perception
Vitamin D synthesis
Photoprotection

(Courtesy of Balin AK, Pratt LA: *Cutis* 43:431–436, May 1989.)

younger skin, and medications may be absorbed at a slower rate through elderly skin. All of these age-related changes must be taken into account in the treatment and prevention of skin disease in the elderly.

▶ Re-reviews the observations of others about changes that occur with aging and sun exposure.—R.S. Stern, M.D.

Histopathologic Characteristics and Ultrastructure of Aging Skin
Smith L (Univ of Washington)
Cutis 43:414–424, May 1989 15–23

The visible effects of aging on skin include roughness, wrinkles, and uneven pigmentation. Many variables affect these outward signs of aging: structural alterations in the skin, environmental influences, altered health, nutritional status, and activity level. Skin appears different not only because of age but according to sex, skin type, and body region. Analysis of biopsy specimens obtained from young and older persons reveals that many age-associated changes in skin are related to the mechanical, biochemical, and physiologic changes of advancing age.

In the furrows of the skin deepening and broadening occur. Fine furrows are shallower and plateau areas larger. The result is greater coarseness and less flexibility, changes that may appear as wrinkles. Skin is normally thinner in women than in men, although age-related thinning occurs sooner in men than in women. In both sexes, subcutaneous fat increases around the abdomen and waist and is lost in the hands and feet.

Aging causes the epidermis to become thinner and flatter (Fig 15–3).

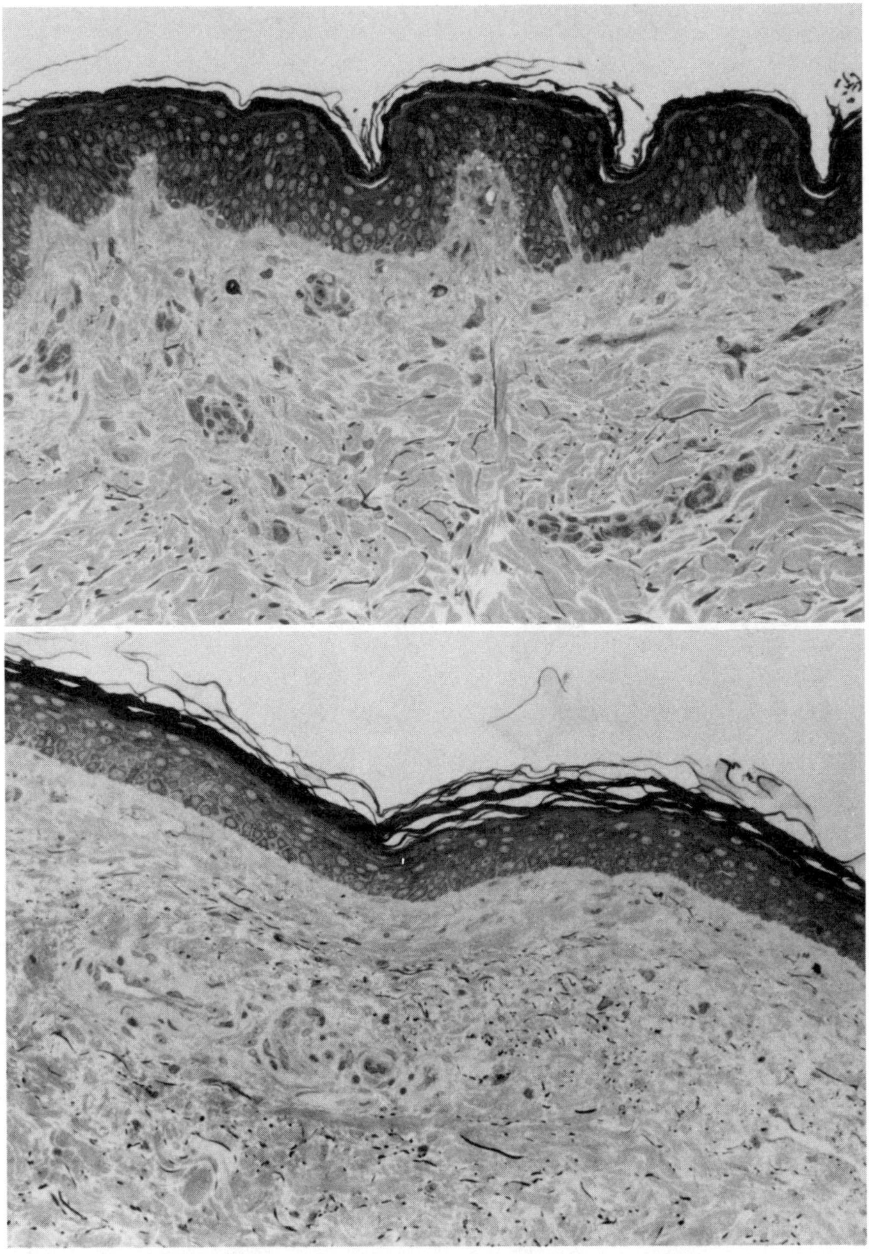

Fig 15–3.—Light micrographs of skin from the upper arms of a 23-year-old man (**top**) and a 72-year-old man (**bottom**). Surface contours of 23 years display regular furrows compared to the flattened external surface at 72 years. (Richardson's blue stain.) (Courtesy of Smith L: *Cutis* 43:414–424, May 1989.)

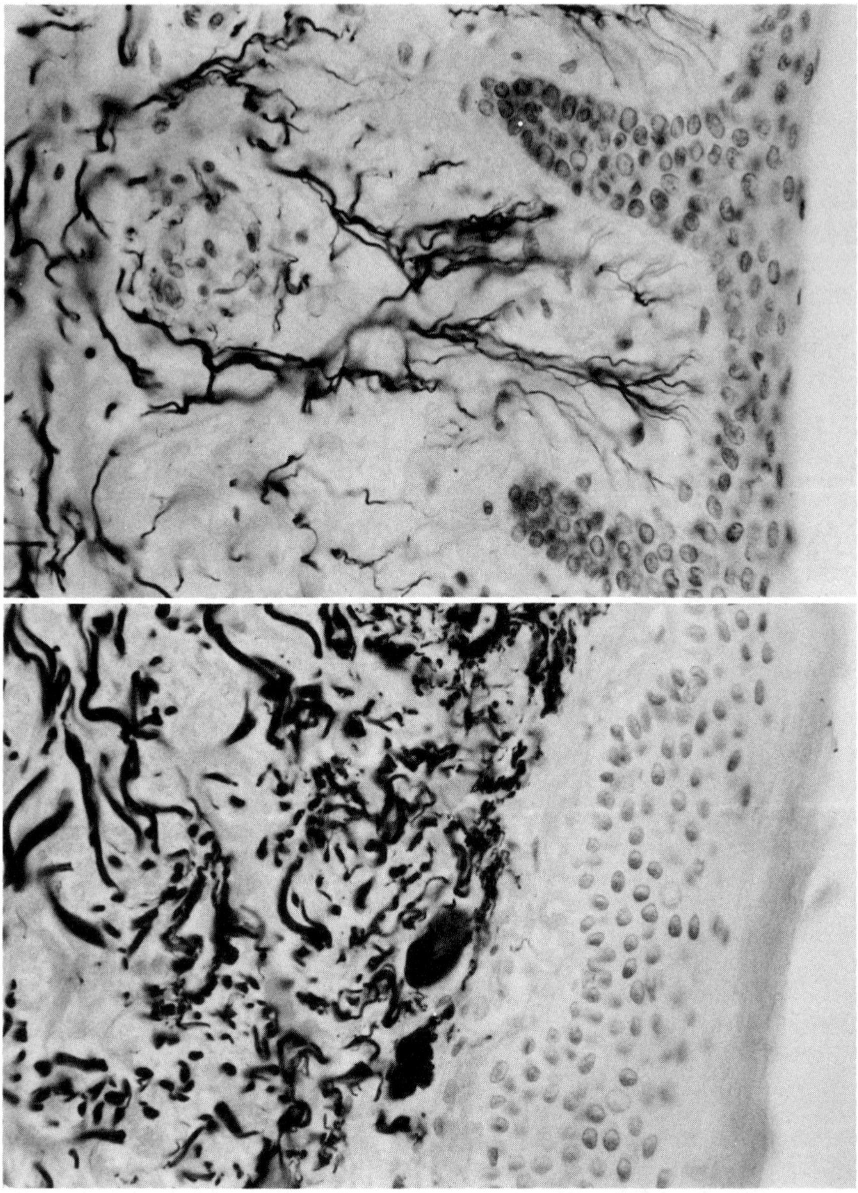

Fig 15–4.—Light micrographs of skin at 35 years (**top**) and 59 years of age (**bottom**) stained with elastic-specific stain. The elastic tissue in younger adult skin shows fine fibers perpendicular to the dermal-epidermal junction linked to the elastic fiber network in the papillary and intermediate dermis. (Orcein stain.) (Courtesy of Smith L: *Cutis* 43:414–424, May 1989.)

The numbers of melanocytes steadily decrease and pigment production is diminished. The pigmented spots common on the skin of the elderly result from a progressively uneven distribution of heavily pigmented cells. Because the immune response is impaired by a decrease in Langerhans' cells, autoimmune skin disorders appear more frequently.

The dermal-epidermal junction is flattened when epidermal projections into the dermis are retracted. The older dermis also contains a reduced amount of collagen, with resultant thinning of the skin. Even more dramatic are age-related changes in elastic fibers, which may become frayed, porous, and matted together (Fig 15–4). Visible signs of elastic fiber changes include sagging and fine wrinkling. These changes are heightened with increasing sun exposure. Blood vessels show a reduced density with aging, and hair follicles, sebaceous glands, and sweat glands exhibit reduced production and alterations in structure. All of these changes vary significantly from one person to another because of the skin's response to internal and external factors.

Topical Tretinoin and Photoaged Skin
Goldfarb MT, Ellis CN, Weiss JS, Voorhees JJ (Univ of Michigan)
Cutis 43:476–482, May 1989 15–24

Both open and double-blind trials show that topical tretinoin is successful in reversing some of the histologically and clinically apparent changes of photoaging. Fine wrinkling improved the most followed by pinkness, coarse wrinkling, and tactile roughness. Histologically, there is an increase in epidermal thickness, an increased mitotic rate in the epidermis, compaction of the stratum corneum, reduction of epidermal dysplasia, and decreased melanocytic hypertrophy and hyperplasia. The dermis also contains more active fibroblasts and fine new collagen; formation of small blood vessels occur. Functional studies show increased blood flow, increased transepidermal water loss, and greater permeability and reactivity.

Optimal improvement is achieved by using tretinoin 0.1% cream to the limit of tolerance daily. Some patients may note improvement as early as 2 weeks of treatment. A decrease in fine wrinkling can be observed after 2–4 months of treatment. After a year of therapy most patients see further improvement and treatment may then be maintained by 3–4 applications per week. Although clinical improvement may be modest, most patients are pleased with the result. The majority of patients experience retinoid dermatitis but are usually able to tolerate the treatment. Retinoid dermatitis is most severe during the first month of therapy and exacerbated by exposure to ultraviolet light, excessive heat and sweating, and occlusion of the tretinoin under jewelery or a watchband. The patient should be advised to decrease the frequency of application and avoidance of exacerbating factors. By carefully discussing with the patient the application of the medication, the possible occurrence of initial dermatitis, and the type of improvement to expect, compliance with and tolerance of tretinoin therapy are greatly enhanced.

▶ Topical tretinoin changes the clinical and histologic appearance of photoaged skin. Proof that it makes the skin young or truly reverses photoaging is still lacking.—R.S. Stern, M.D.

16 Pigmentary Disorders

Penile Melanosis
Revuz J, Clerici T (Hôp Henri Mondor, Paris)
J Am Acad Dermatol 20:567–570, April 1989 16–1

Distinctive macular pigmented lesions of the penis, or penile melanosis, were seen in 5 patients in a period of 10 years. All 5 underwent punch biopsy, and specimens were stained with hematoxylin-eosin and saffron; Fontana's stains were also performed. All patients were white. The age at diagnosis ranged from 17 to 70 years, and had been present from 1 to 10 years. No preexisting lesions, local trauma, or inflammation were reported.

The lesions were composed of macular hyperpigmentation of the penile shaft and/or glans. Histologic examination showed only hyperpigmentation of the basal cell layer. There was no melanocytic hyperplasia. During follow-up of 3–13 years, some lesions enlarged, but all conditions remained benign. The principal differential diagnostic dilemma was in ruling out acral lentiginous melanoma.

Penile melanosis appears to share clinical and microscopic features with Laugier-Hunziker syndrome of the buccal mucosa and vulvovaginal melanosis. These 3 disorders may be classified as essential melanotic hyperpigmentation of the mucosa.

▶ The histology of these 5 cases of genital pigmentation was demonstrated to be melanosis rather than melanocytosis. However, more sensitive methods for detecting melanocytes other than routine histology were not used in assessment, i.e., dopa sections, electron microscopy, S-100, or other melanocyte markers. Other studies describe a similar gross morphology that consists of melanocytic hyperplasia. It seems reasonable to follow such patients photographically after histologic documentation of melanosis or "benign" melanocytosis rather than subjecting them to mutilating excision and possibly destruction or partial loss of function. More such cases need to be studied using the most sensitive methods available for assessing melanocyte number and morphology.—A.R. Rhodes, M.D., M.P.H.

Hyperpigmentation of the Clavicular Zone: A Variant of Friction Melanosis
Magaña-Garcia M, Carrasco E, Herrera-Goepfert R, Pueblitz-Peredo S (Hosp Gen de Mexico; Hosp Gen "Dr. Manuel Gea González"; Univ Nacional Autónoma de Mexico, Mexico City)
Int J Dermatol 28:119–122, March 1989 16–2

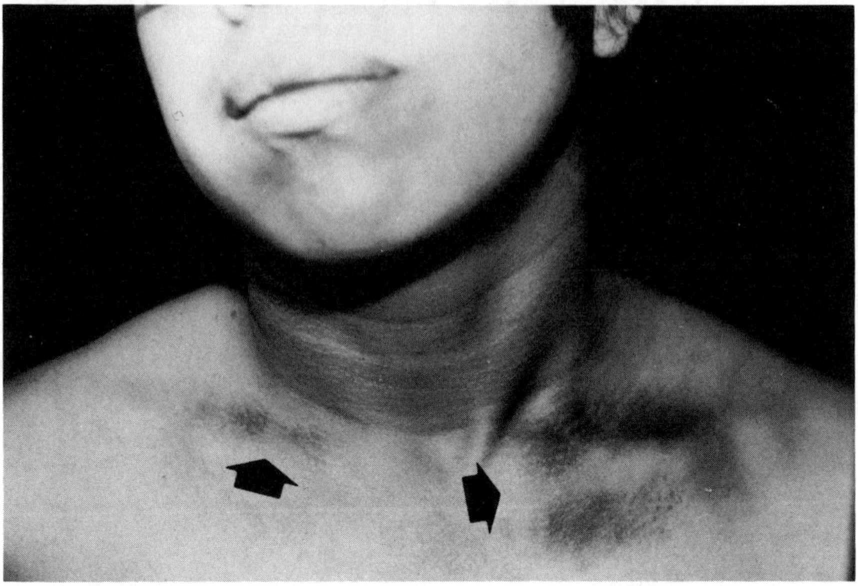

Fig 16–1.—Idiopathic hyperpigmentation of the clavicular zone. (Courtesy of Magaña-Garcia M, Carrasco E, Herrera-Goepfert R, et al: *Int J Dermatol* 28:119–122, March 1989.)

An idiopathic form of hyperpigmentation of the clavicular zone was investigated in 10 females of Mexican ancestry aged 16–22 who had skin type V. The lesions consisted of well-circumscribed, glistening, pigmented areas in the clavicular zones (Fig 16–1). In 2 patients the lesions extended to the lateral aspects of the neck. All had been present from 1 to 5 years and were asymptomatic. Histologic examination showed focal to extensive necrosis of the epidermis, focal areas of junctional cleavage, and melanin deposition principally within the epidermis and also in the dermis, and melanophages.

This entity is in the group of brown hypermelanoses. It appears that friction with clothing or scrubbing with pads made of sedge (a common practice) against the clavicular protuberances is fundamental in its pathogenesis. This lesion should be differentiated from macular amyloidosis and other pigmentary disorders.

▶ Physical trauma stimulates melanin hyperpigmentation. The degree of hyperpigmentation that develops with trauma depends on an individual's constitutive (genetic) and facultative (ultraviolet radiation or hormone) pigmentation capacity. Posttraumatic and postinflammatory hyperpigmentation is a common complaint of persons with brown or black skin. If the physical trauma is vigorous and localized to one area there will be localized hyperpigmentation, as described in this report. This is a common phenomenon in persons with skin phototype V who rub their skin with "scrub pads" or stiff brushes (see the 1989 YEAR BOOK OF DERMATOLOGY, p 301), although the patients described here did not give such a history. Also, the clavicle is a common site of so-called macular amyloidosis. Hori and Kobori (1), in their chapter, include a photograph in color (Fig 7) that shows hypermelanosis on the clavicle identical to the appearance in Figure 16–1. Amyloid is not always present in macular amyloidosis. In the patients reported here, amyloid was not stated to be present, but it was not clear whether it was carefully looked for using electron microscopy.

In summary, this is probably not a special, previously undescribed type, but, rather, falls into the category of hyperpigmentation from putative trauma in these patients; this would fit into the classification of macular amyloidosis sine amyloid—a not uncommon clinical situation. We see several patients each year with pruritic areas on the back, especially in which there is macular hyperpigmentation, pigment incontinence, and dermal melanophages, but amyloid may or may not be present.—T.B. Fitzpatrick, M.D., Ph.D.

Reference

1. Hori Y, Kobori T, in Fitzpatrick TB, et al (eds): *Biology and Diseases of Dermal Pigmentation.* Tokyo, Univ of Tokyo Press, 1981, ch 28.

Pigmented Macules in Patients Treated With Systemic 5-Fluorouracil

Cho KH, Chung JH, Lee AY, Lee YS, Kim NK, Kim CW (Seoul Natl Univ, Korea)
J Dermatol 15:342–346, August 1988 16–3

Mucocutaneous complications are commonly seen when 5-fluorouracil (5-FU) is given. During a study of cutaneous complications of cancer che-

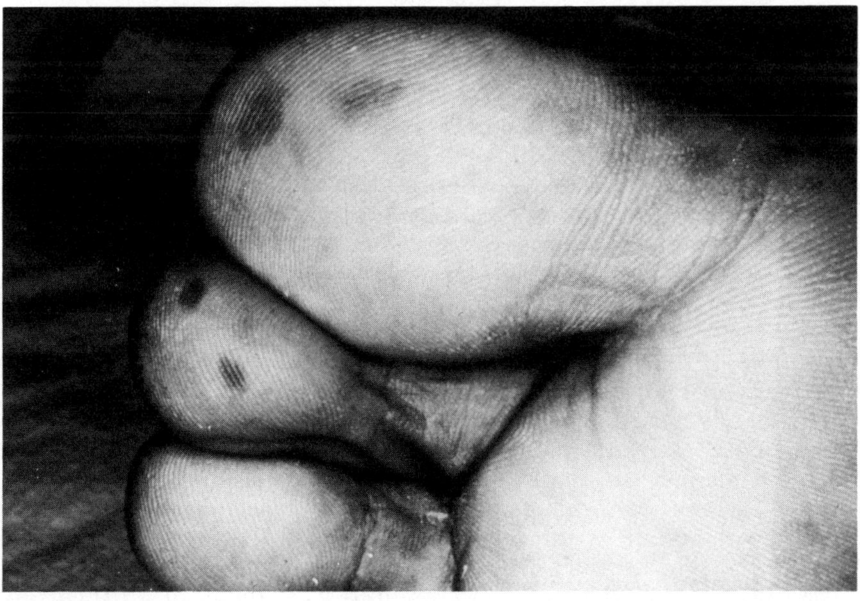

Fig 16–2.—Pigmented macules on the volar side of the toes. (Courtesy of Cho KH, Chung JH, Lee AY, et al: *J Dermatol* 15:342–346, August 1988.)

motherapy, macular, dark brown pigmented spots were noted in 72 of 137 patients (52.6%) treated with systemic 5-FU.

The pigmented macules usually appeared on the palms and soles (Fig 16–2), and they were found in patients who received 5-FU in combination with other chemotherapeutic regimens and in patients who received only 5-FU. The incidence of macular pigmentation was proportional to the number of chemotherapy cycles. Histologic examination showed a slight increase in melanin pigmentation in the epidermis without any change in the melanocyte number.

The multiple pigmented macules observed in some patients treated with 5-FU have not been reported previously. The pigmented macules may have developed as a result of increased melanogenesis.

▶ These pigmented lesions are probably lentigo simplex. Microscopic study of lentigines reveals an increased number of melanocytes in the basal layer, an elongation of the rete ridges, and increased melanin in melanocytes and in basal keratinocytes. Although an increased number of melanocytes was not observed in this report, it would be necessary to perform split DOPA preparations and obtain actual counts of the melanocytes.

It should be noted that these authors have commented on the incidence of pigmented similar macules on the hands and feet in normal Koreans not receiving chemotherapy. It is possible that there exist latent genetically programmed melanocytes that do not become clinically apparent until stimulated by chemotherapy. Lentigo-like hyperpigmented macules have recently been observed in children receiving chemotherapy for leukemia (1). Again, there may be "latent" melanocytes that become clinically visible only when stimulated to increased melanogenesis.—T.B. Fitzpatrick, M.D., Ph.D.

Reference

1. Hughes BR, et al: *Br Med J* 299:88, 1989.

Observations and Proposed Mechanism of N,N′,N″-Triethylenethiophosphoramide (Thiotepa)-Induced Hyperpigmentation

Horn TD, Beveridge RA, Egorin MJ, Abeloff MD, Hood AF (Johns Hopkins Hosp; Univ of Maryland)

Arch Dermatol 125:524–527, April 1989 16–4

A patterned hyperpigmentation may occur in women receiving N,N′,N″-triethylenethiophosphoramide (thiotepa) and cyclophosphamide intravenously as treatment for metastatic adenocarcinoma of the breast. The potential mechanism of this side effect was investigated.

After thiotepa and cyclophosphamide were given intravenously to 5 women with cancer of the breast, a patterned hyperpigmentation confined to the skin occluded by adhesive-containing materials (Fig 16–3) developed in all 5. Thiotepa concentrations were found in 3 patients in occluded and nonoccluded skin, plasma, bandage with adhesive, and

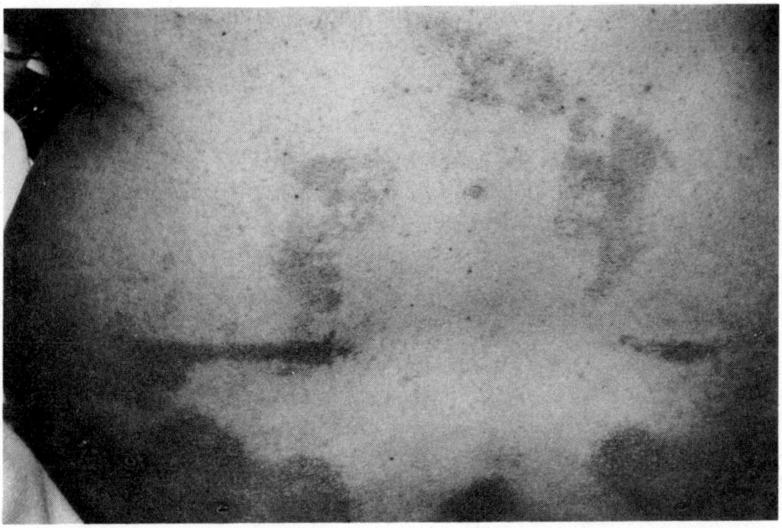

Fig 16–3.—Hyperpigmentation underneath bandages placed on lower back. (Courtesy of Horn TD, Beveridge RA, Egorin MJ, et al: *Arch Dermatol* 125:524–527, April 1989.)

gauze containing sweat. It may be that thiotepa is excreted onto the skin surface in sweat, accumulates beneath adhesive-containing bandages and ECG pads, and exerts a local toxic effect, resulting in the observed hyperpigmentation.

The mechanisms of most cutaneous drug eruptions are not known definitively. This study provided evidence that the patterned hyperpigmentation induced by thiotepa may result from a direct local toxic effect of the drug arising from excretion and concentration in sweat, with subsequent occlusion. Such a mechanism may underlie other eruptions as well, such as the flagellate hyperpigmentation caused by bleomycin and acral erythema induced by cytarabine.

▶ This is a direct "hit" on the melanocytes, much like the action of psoralen and ultraviolet A (UVA), which results in striking hyperpigmentation when given topically, orally, or in oil of bergamot after exposure to the UVA in sunlight. The melanin hyperpigmentation can occur without any preceding erythema. Patients with berlock pigmentation do not come to the dermatologist complaining of erythema but of hyperpigmentation. Biopsy of berlock hyperpigmentation reveals that the melanocytes are in mitosis, a rare event in normal melanocytes. Therefore, there is not only proliferation of melanocytes but an increase in the production of melanosomes; in addition, the melanosomes become larger in size and remain as nonaggregated single particles in the keratinocyte—they become similar to the large melanosomes present normally in the melanocytes of persons with brown and black skin and in the matrix of brown and black hair. These same observations (increased number of melanosomes and presence of nonaggregated melanosomes in the keratinocytes) were also made in this study reported from Johns Hopkins. It would be interesting to follow up these patients and observe the duration of the thiotepa effect on induction of hyperpigmentation. Pigmentation from psoralens can persist for months.—T.B. Fitzpatrick, M.D., Ph.D.

Exogenous Ochronosis: An Epidemiological Study

Hardwick N, Van Gelder LW, Van Der Merwe CA, Van Der Merwe MP (Univ of Pretoria; South African Med Research Council)

Br J Dermatol 120:229–238, February 1989 16–5

Skin lightening preparations are widely sold throughout the world. A survey was done to investigate the relationship between the use of these preparations and ochronosis among black patients in 2 South African hospitals. For a period of 3 months, blacks were randomly selected for examination from among persons attending outpatient clinics at 2 hospitals. Patients seeking treatment for skin problems were excluded. When relevant, male and female patients were studied separately. Patients underwent clinical examination and questioning about the use of skin lighteners. If possible, the preparations were identified by specific names.

Fifteen percent of males and 42% of females had exogenous ochrono-

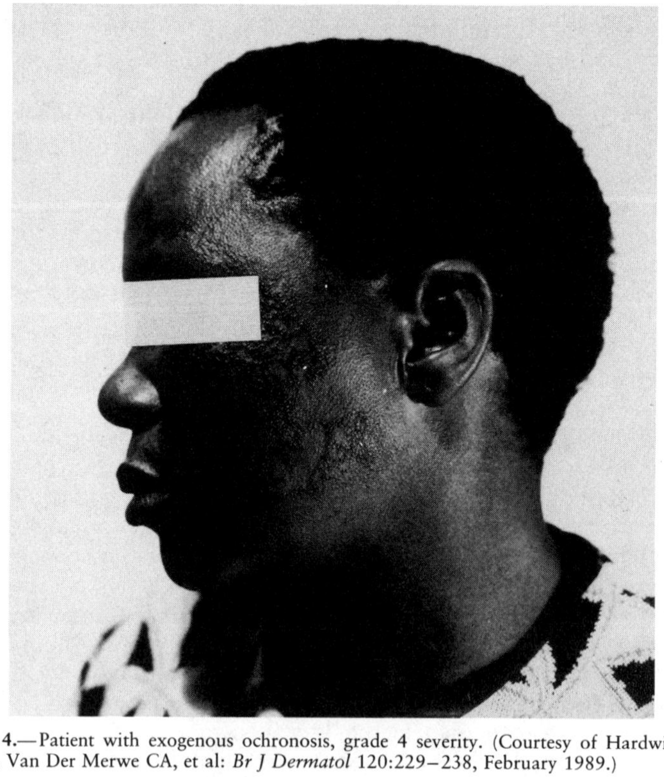

Fig 16–4.—Patient with exogenous ochronosis, grade 4 severity. (Courtesy of Hardwick N, Van Gelder LW, Van Der Merwe CA, et al: *Br J Dermatol* 120:229–238, February 1989.)

sis (Fig 16–4). Among users of skin lighteners, the prevalence was 69%. Education and ochronosis were inversely related. Even products that contained 2% hydroquinone, or less, as well as a sunscreen, caused ochronosis.

The results confirm the link between exogenous ochronosis and the topical use of hydroquinone, even in small concentrations. South Africa has planned legislation to ban over-the-counter sales of products containing hydroquinone. Other countries should follow this lead.

▶ These authors state that hydroquinone-containing skin lightening agents have become a part of the black South African culture along with canned soft drinks and cigarettes. This is somewhat true in the black population of the United States. In drug stores in black neighborhoods in the United States several commercial preparations are available as skin lightening agents, or "skin tone" creams. There is a very large market for hydroquinone among the brown and black populations of the world (estimated at more than $4.5 million in South Africa). Several commercial preparations are available in the United States, mostly in a 2% concentration, but there are 2 preparations with higher concentrations: a prescription drug containing 3% and another, an over-the-counter (OTC) cream containing 4%. Hydroquinone, in our experience, does not cause permanent white macules, similar to what is frequently seen when using MBH (see below for discussion.) The high incidence of exogenous ochronosis noted in this study may be related to the high concentrations of hydroquinone that are available only in South Africa, some as high as 10%. The authors state that even a 2% concentration produced exogenous ochronosis. However, it is impossible to monitor the patients and to know precisely what they have used; many may have used higher concentrations in addition to 2%. We have not seen exogenous ochronosis caused by topical hydroquinone in concentrations of 2% and 3%. Until this is observed we will continue to use 2% or 3% hydroquinone preparations.

Boyle and Kennedy (1) have emphasized the major side effects of topical hydroquinone (ochronosis-like blue pigmentation and poikiloderma-like patches) occur when concentrations of more than 2% are used. Higher concentrations (i.e., 4% and 5%) are more effective but also more irritating as primary irritants—but not, in our clinical experience, as allergic sensitizers.

It is interesting that topical hydroquinone was first introduced as a depigmenting agent in the United States. The introduction of hydroquinone came a few years after the first use of the *monobenzyl ether* of hydroquinone (MBH), which was advocated for the treatment of brown melanin hyperpigmentation, especially melasma, in 1953 (2). It was then used throughout world as an OTC bleaching agent. However, a few years after the introduction of MBH as an OTC depigmenting agent for the treatment of melasma, some patients, especially in South America and Asia, noted the development of irreversible small white macules in the areas of the melasma where the MBH had been applied. This strikingly disfiguring depigmentation remained after applications of MBH were stopped. This untoward reaction of MBH led to a withdrawal of the product from the Japanese market, and a change in the regulations in the United States, and MBH became a prescription drug.

It is now available for the permanent depigmentation of the skin, and it is a valuable therapeutic drug for the treatment of patients with vitiligo. *It is used in patients with extensive vitiligo in whom the areas of pigment loss are so extensive and disfiguring that it is better to depigment the normal skin than to attempt to repigment the vitiligo skin with PUVA.* This method of depigmenting the normal skin with MBH, although requiring about 1 year of topical applications, is very effective and patients are pleased with the results. The stark white skin color that results from this treatment with MBH is, in fact, not very apparent; furthermore, the skin color can be modified by ingestion of commercially available (Solatene) beta-carotene, which provides a less white skin that is more acceptable to most people; it is not advisable to use OTC betacarotene because of its low potency and questionable purity. We have used MBH depigmentation in more than 200 patients with excellent results. We have never seen any evidence of an exogenous ochronosis as noted with hydroquinone, but the preparations are usually used only for a year, which is the time it takes to completely depigment the "normal" skin in vitiligo patients.—T.B. Fitzpatrick, M.D., Ph.D.

References

1. Boyle J, Kennedy CTC: *Br J Dermatol* 114:501, 1986.
2. Lerner AB, Fitzpatrick TBJ: *JAMA* 152:577, 1953.

Hypomelanosis of Ito: Spectrum of the Disease

Glover MT, Brett EM, Atherton DJ (Hosp for Sick Children, London)
J Pediatr 115:75–80, July 1989 16–6

More than 70 cases of hypomelanosis of Ito have been reported, most of which are sporadic. Nineteen patients, 10 of whom had neurologic abnormalities, were reviewed. None had a family history suggestive of hypomelanosis of Ito.

Two patients had alterations at birth. The hypopigmentation was macular and difficult to discern in some white patients; ultraviolet illumination was helpful (Fig 16–5). Hypopigmentation often took the form of linear bands, but circumscribed nonlinear zones sometimes were present. Fifteen patients had bilateral lesions.

Twelve children were significantly delayed developmentally. Three had ocular abnormalities, and 4 had obvious hemihypertrophy, which, however, was not related to the laterality of hypopigmentation. Three children had syndactyly. In 4 patients CT of the brain revealed abnormal neuronal migration, and in 3 there was cerebral atrophy. Eleven of 17 electroencephalograms revealed abnormalities. Results of all 10 karyotyping studies were negative.

The precise criteria for the diagnosis of hypomelanosis of Ito remain uncertain. Careful evaluation of the eyes and of hearing is important. In addition, epilepsy may develop, and developmental delay is not uncommon.

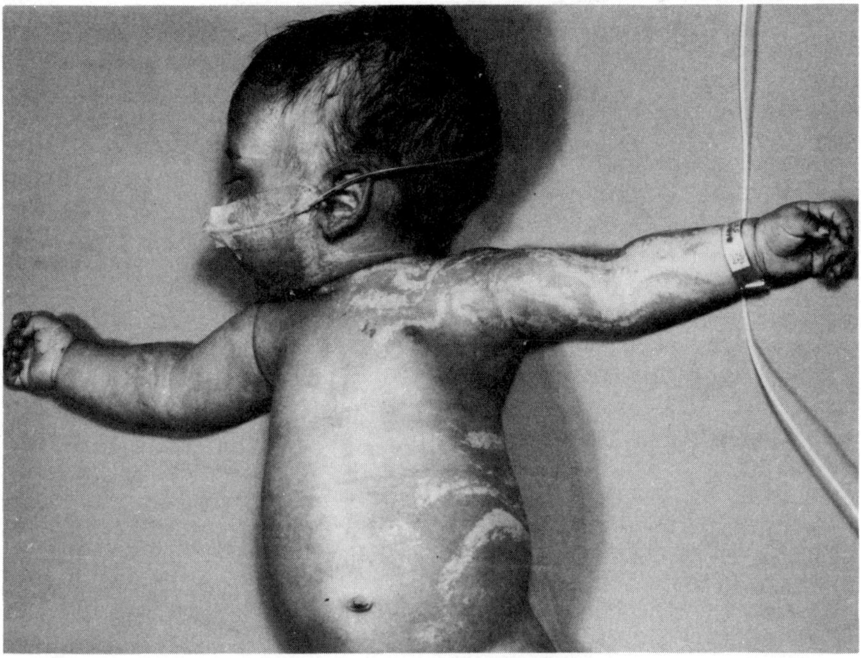

Fig 16–5.—Patient photographed with ultraviolet illumination to demonstrate hypopigmentation more clearly. (Courtesy of Glover MT, Brett EM, Atherton DJ: *J Pediatr* 115:75–80, July 1989.)

▶ This is the most complete summary of this important neurocutaneous disorder since Jelinek's summary in 1973 (1). Ito's hypomelanosis could be confused with tuberous sclerosis because of the striking similarities, especially hypomelanosis with the presence of melanocytes and associated anomalies of the nervous system. Other features permit a diagnosis between the 2 disorders (Tables 1, 2, pp 286–287). The outstanding feature of Ito's hypomelanosis is the striking distribution pattern of Blaschko's lines, a pattern never seen in my experience in tuberous sclerosis. Prof. A. Blaschko described these lines based on the empirical average of a large number of systematized nevi (2).

Chromosomal mosaicism has been reported in Itos's hypomelanosis in dermal fibroblasts and peripheral blood lymphocytes. It has been proposed by Donnai et al. (3) that in patients with pigmentary anomalies and chromosomal mosaicism or chimerism there are 2 clones of cells having different pigment potential that, if established in the early stages of embryonic development (primitive streak stage), will be randomly distributed neural crest cells that become melanoblasts.—T.B. Fitzpatrick, M.D., Ph.D.

References

1. Jelinek JE, et al: *Arch Dermatol* 107:596, 1973.
2. Blaschko A: *Die Nervenverteilung in der Haut in ihrer Beziehung zu den Erkrankungen der Haut.* Vienna, Braumiuller, 1901.
3. Donnai D, et al: *Lancet* 1:1443, 1986.

TABLE 1.—Comparison of Tuberous Sclerosis and Ito's Hypomelanosis

	Tuberous Sclerosis	**Ito's Hypomelanosis**
Heredity	Autosomal dominant	Probably autosomal dominant
Epidemiology		
Race	All	All
Sex	Equal incidence	2.5:1 female/male ratio
History		
Onset of hypomelanosis	Birth, very rarely during infancy	Birth, early infancy, or childhood
Associated Systemic Abnormalities	See Précis	More than 75% have seizures, mental retardation, and an abnormal EEG
Skin Examination		
Type of lesion	Hypomelanotic macules	Hypomelanotic macules
Size, shape, arrangement	Polygonal, lance-ovate ("ash-leaf"), scattered, discrete	Whorled or streaked in Blaschko's lines (see Figures)
Distribution	Trunk, extremities	Trunk, extremities
Laboratory and Special Examinations		
Light and electron microscopy	Decreased dopa reaction, number of melanocytes, and melanosome size	Same as tuberous sclerosis
Wood's light	Hypomelanosis, but less "whiteness" than in vitiligo macules	Same as tuberous sclerosis
Differential Diagnosis	"White spots" may occur in tuberous sclerosis, vitiligo, piebaldism, nevus depigmentosus, and postinflammatory leukoderma, but Ito's hypomelanosis is unique among these because of its distribution pattern in Blaschko's lines	

(Courtesy of Fitzpatrick TB, Parrish JA, Gonzalez E, et al: *Dermatologic Capsule Comment* 8:1–11, November–December 1986.)

TABLE 2.—Precis of the Diagnosis of Tuberous Sclerosis

	Epidemiology
Incidence	In institutions, 1:100–1:300; general population, 1:20,000–1:100,000
Inheritance	Autosomal dominant
	History
Skin Signs	White macules present at birth or may appear in infancy
	Angiofibromata and shagreen patches, which usually appear after 4 yrs
	Ungual fibroma
Constitutional Symptoms	Seizures (infantile spasms), 86% incidence; the earlier the onset of seizures the more severe the mental retardation
Mental Status	Mental retardation (40% incidence) or normal intelligence

Physical Examination

Skin (96% incidence)	
Type of lesion	Hypomelanotic macules—not pure but off-white, one or many Papules/nodules—red and skin-colored Plaques (shagreen patch)—skin-colored Ungual fibromas (22% incidence)
Shape, size, arrangement	White macules (86% incidence): *polygonal* ("thumbprint") 0.5–2.0 cm; *lance-ovate* ("ash-leaf") 3–4 cm (1.0–12.0 cm). *Tiny white macules* ("confetti") on legs or on both legs and arms Angiofibromatous papules (many), 50% incidence, 1–2 mm; or nodules (few), 1.0 cm on the face Plaques (shagreen patches), 20% incidence, usually isolated, soft, single, or rarely multiple
Distribution	White macules occur* on the trunk (56%), lower extremities (32%), upper extremities (7%), and head and neck (5%) Angiofibromatous papules on the face Shagreen patches, most often on the posterior trunk or buttocks
Associated Systems	Central nervous system (tubers producing seizures), eye (gray or yellow retinal plaques, 50% incidence), heart (benign rhabdomyomas), kidney, liver, thyroid, testes, and gastrointestinal system (hamartomas of mixed-cell type)

Laboratory and Special Examinations

Light and Electron Microscopy	Decreased dopa reaction, number of melanocytes, and melanosome size; melanization
Wood's Light	Hypomelanosis, dull white or off-white—not as white as in vitiligo
Radiography	CT or NMR for determining location, size, and shape of calcifications and presence of gliomas; especially necessary in children with white spots and seizures and in parents (of childbearing age) of patients with tuberous sclerosis with or without skin signs, seizures, or mental retardation

Differential Diagnosis

White spots: vitiligo, piebaldism, nevus depigmentosus, postinflammatory leukoderma

Note: In infancy, tuberous sclerosis may be suspected by white spots and by seizures. In young children with tuberous sclerosis, there may or may not be angiofibromata, ungual fibromata, shagreen patches, and mental retardation; white spots are present in 86% of patients, however.

*Based on 65 patients cited by Soter NA, Fitzpatrick TB, Mosher DB, et al: Disorders of pigmentation, in Fitzpatrick TB, et al (eds): *Dermatology in General Medicine,* ed 3. New York, McGraw-Hill, 1987, p. 794.

(Courtesy of Fitzpatrick TB, Parrish JA, Gonzalez E, et al: *Dermatologic Capsule Comment* 8:1–11, November–December 1986.)

Transplantation of In Vitro-Cultured Epidermis Bearing Melanocytes for Repigmenting Vitiligo

Falabella R, Escobar C, Borrero I (Univ of Valle, Cali, Colombia)

J Am Acad Dermatol 21:257–264, August 1989 16–7

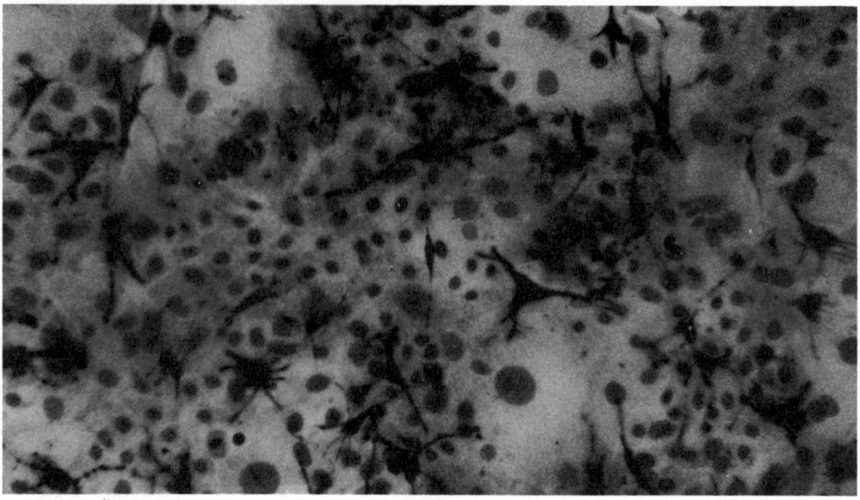

Fig 16–6.—Microscopic appearance of in vitro-cultured epidermis bearing melanocytes disclosing numerous dopa-positive polydentritic melanocytes intermingled with keratinocytes. (Dopa counterstained with Wright's stain; original magnification, ×150.) (Courtesy of Falabella R, Escobar C, Borrero I: *J Am Acad Dermatol* 21:257–264, August 1989.)

Vitiligo is an acquired depigmenting disorder of unknown cause in which melanocytes are damaged. A new method of repigmenting vitiliginous skin involves the transplantation of in vitro-cultured epidermis-bearing melanocytes, after denuding the vitiliginous skin with liquid nitrogen. Epidermal tissue is taken from a skin strip 4 × 1.5 cm in size from the infragluteal region. Epidermal sheets were harvested 3 weeks after plating (Fig 16–6). The grafting technique was similar to that used for suction blister grafts.

Satisfactory repigmentation was achieved in 3 patients managed in this way. Slightly hyperpigmented spots occurred in 2 patients and small achromic areas persisted around and between grafts in 1. This approach holds promise for selected patients having large depigmented areas or refractory lesions in acral zones. Larger transplants to extensive areas in a single session require replication by serial subculturing.

▶ This technique appears to be feasible and reasonably successful, especially in segmental vitiligo. Segmental vitiligo frequently does not respond very well, if at all, to oral or topical PUVA photochemotherapy. Possibly, segmental vitiligo is a special type of leukoderma different from vitiligo vulgaris in which the depigmentation process is strictly localized to the area of the segmental vitiligo. Vitiligo vulgaris exhibits a depigmentation in "normal" skin after induction with a needle. This isomorphic phenomenon may not be present in segmental vitiligo, but this has not been tested in a sufficient number of patients with this disease. The area of depigmentation in segmental vitiligo could be a somatic mutation, similar to segmental neurofibromatosis. It would be desirable to undertake to induce the isomorphic phenomenon in a series of patients with segmental vitiligo to prove this hypothesis of a localized anomaly limited to the area of the leukoderma in segmental vitiligo (see also the 1989 YEAR BOOK OF DERMATOLOGY, p 306).—T.B. Fitzpatrick, M.D., Ph.D.

Tattooing for the Management of White Patches
Vadodaria SJ, Vadodaria BS (Bombay)
Ann Plast Surg 23:81–83, July 1989 16–8

A white patch is a social taboo in Indian society, as it is considered a sign of bad luck, is correlated with leprosy, and is believed to be inherited. Although white patches are not contagious, patients who have them encounter considerable problems in social situations. The 3 main conditions that cause white patches are vitiligo, leukoderma, and nevus anemicus. When a white patch remains static despite conservative treatment, it can be camouflaged by tattooing. In this procedure, inert pigments are matched to the natural skin color and impregnated into the intradermal plane. Only static white patches are considered for tattooing, as the procedure does not prevent the progress of underlying disease.

Tattooing of white patches is done as an office procedure under local anesthesia. The patient does not have to miss work in the postoperative period because the procedure is relatively painless. All patients were evaluated 1 week and 6 weeks after treatment.

None of the patients studied experienced allergic or photosensitive reactions. Although a 100% color match with the surrounding skin was not achieved, patients were generally satisfied with the overall camouflage of the white patch. A few patients required some touch-up work because the patches were still too light at the 6-week follow-up. A biopsy of the tattooed skin was performed during the retattooing of 1 patient. Histologic examination of the biopsy specimen confirmed pigment retention within the intradermal plane. Tattooing of white patches is simpler and less expensive than melanocyte transfer.

▶ Many persons with brown or black skin are virtually devastated by the presence of isolated white macules on regions of the body that are exposed to the public. This technique may be good for the truly stable leukodermic macules such as occur following trauma, or heat burns. A possible problem in using tattooing in vitiligo vulgaris is that the macules are not unpredictably stable; this means that an area tattooed may enlarge. Furthermore, the trauma associated with the procedure can induce new white macules as a consequence of the isomorphic phenomenon.—T.B. Fitzpatrick, M.D., Ph.D.

17 Psoriasis and Related Disorders

Feelings of Stigmatization in Patients With Psoriasis
Ginsburg IH, Link BG (Columbia Univ)
J Am Acad Dermatol 20:53–63, January 1989 17–1

The concept of stigma is important in the attempt to understand how patients experience psoriasis. Stigma is defined as a biological or social mark that sets a person apart from others, is discrediting, and disrupts interactions with others. To clarify the specific content of the stigma experience as it relates to psoriasis, 100 psoriasis patients aged 20–70 years, 75% of whom had moderate to severe psoriasis, were surveyed. Of the 100 patients, 51 were hospitalized for treatment of their psoriasis, 18 were clinic outpatients, and 31 were private outpatients. Eleven other hospitalized patients refused to participate, for reasons suggesting anxiety.

The patients completed a detailed questionnaire regarding 6 dimensions of the stigma experience: anticipation of rejection, feelings of being flawed, sensitivity to others' attitudes, guilt and shame, secretiveness, and positive attitudes. Each answer was scored on a 6-point scale from strongly agree to strongly disagree. For interpretation, weights were assigned to each answer according to the importance of the item in relation to each of the underlying 6 dimensions of the stigma experience.

Different predictors emerged from different dimensions of the stigma experience. Being older was a mitigating force for some aspects of stigma, but not for others. Of all the aspects measured, bleeding was the strongest predictor of feelings of stigma and despair. Bleeding of lesions may result from noncompliance and scratching. Because stigma dimensions correlated strongly with despair, afflicted patients who experience despair may fail to moisturize their skin, fail to sunbathe, or not comply with treatment in other ways, possibly worsening the disease status. Therefore, an understanding of the feelings of stigma in patients with psoriasis is important for their clinical management.

▶ This paper deals essentially with internally generated stress—how the disease affects patient attitudes and emotions. Among the clinical messages here are 2 that we can readily utilize in practice:

1. Younger patients may be more sensitive about their disease and deserve a little more of our time, patience, understanding, and reassurance.
2. Bleeding is an indication of stigma and despair and should prompt additional inquiry about feelings and also about compliance with the therapeutic program.—R. Masters, M.D.

A Psychocutaneous Profile of Psoriasis Patients Who Are Stress Reactors: A Study of 127 Patients

Gupta MA, Gupta AK, Kirkby S, Schork NJ, Gorr SK, Ellis CN, Voorhees JJ (Univ of Michigan)

Gen Hosp Psychiatry 11:166–173, May 1989 17–2

In approximately 40% of cases, psychosocial stress appears to play a role in the onset or exacerbation of psoriasis. However, it is difficult to identify patients who should receive psychosocial treatment.

Findings in 64 patients who reported exacerbation of psoriasis with stress were compared with those in 63 patients who reported no association between psoriasis and stress. All patients underwent a standard course of treatment for psoriasis. Researchers designed 2 test instruments to measure minor daily stressful events, i.e., the Hassle Scale, and psoriasis-related daily stress, i.e., the Psoriasis Life Stress Inventory (PLSI). Patients also underwent clinical evaluation of the extent and severity of their disease.

High-stress reactors were younger than low-stress reactors, but the groups were otherwise not distinguishable demographically. High-stress reactors had higher Hassle ratings and higher PLSI scores, indicative of greater disease-related stress. High-stress reactors had more severe psoriasis on the scalp, face, neck, forearms, hands, and genital region. In particular, the disease-related stress score correlated with the severity of psoriasis in these "emotionally charged" body areas. Interpersonal dependency correlated with overall severity of disease. In low-stress reactors, intensity of anger correlated with the total severity of psoriasis; the PLSI score correlated directly with the severity of disease in the emotionally charged body regions.

High-stress reactors can be differentiated clinically from low-stress reactors. Appropriate psychosocial interventions may reduce the morbidity associated with psoriasis and may lessen the number of major flare-ups in psoriatics who are high-stress reactors.

▶ The authors have studied the relationship between psychosocial stress and psoriasis. Most psoriatics can tell whether stress makes their disease worse. The authors point out that psoriasis in exposed areas and in the genital region is itself a source of stress. Those who are more affected by stress are more interpersonally dependent and do not handle anger well. For these patients the authors suggest that psychotherapy and assertiveness therapy may be helpful.

In general, a calm, encouraging, supportive attitude would seem to be helpful. We must listen more to the patient—the act of listening is itself supportive.—R. Master, M.D.

Active and Inactive Edges of Psoriatic Plaques: Identification by Tracing and Investigation by Laser-Doppler Flowmetry and Immunocytochemical Techniques

Macdonald Hull S, Goodfield M, Wood EJ, Cunliffe WJ (Leeds Gen Infirmary; Univ of Leeds, England)
J Invest Dermatol 92:782–785, June 1989 17–3

Although histologic and biochemical differences between psoriatic lesions and normal or uninvolved skin are well documented, the initiating factor for new psoriatic lesions has not yet been identified. That psoriatic plaques move and change shape is known from clinical observation, but very early changes in plaque movement have not been investigated. A method was designed by which 82 moderately severe, untreated chronic plaques in 15 patients and 38 treated plaques in 6 patients were traced over a 3-week period to identify their advancing edge. Laser Doppler flowmetry was used to measure cutaneous blood flow at a point immediately adjacent to the plaque perimeter at its most active site and at a similar point on its inactive edge.

Movement of the plaque edge was observed in 75 (91.4%) of the 82 untreated plaques and in 37 (97.3%) of the 38 treated plaques. Of the 75 untreated plaques with movement, 49 moved asymmetrically, enlarging consistently in 1 direction only, whereas 26 moved symmetrically, enlarging in all directions. Of the 37 treated plaques with movement, 21 were reduced asymmetrically and 16 were reduced symmetrically.

Punch biopsy specimens obtained at the study sites revealed no epidermal changes or excess T lymphocyte activity. This finding suggests that the earliest change in a developing psoriatic plaque is increased blood flow, probably associated with an as yet unidentified initiating factor that accumulates at the active edge of the psoriatic plaque, where it stimulates transformation of normal skin to psoriatic plaque.

▶ The search for the initial event in psoriasis is the premier grail of dermatology. This work provides additional support for the notion that, whatever it is, the cutaneous vasculature is pretty close to where it takes place.—J.D. Bernhard, M.D.

Guttate Psoriasis Associated With Perianal Streptococcal Disease

Honig PJ (Univ of Pennsylvania; Children's Hosp of Philadelphia)
J Pediatr 113:1037–1039, December 1988 17–4

Acute guttate psoriasis may occur in association with streptococcal infection of the upper respiratory tract. Four children had psoriatic skin changes in association with group A β-hemolytic streptococcal infection of the perianal skin. The 3 boys and 1 girl had persistent anal pruritus associated with inflammation of the perianal skin and a psoriasiform eruption. The psoriatic eruption appeared 9 months after onset of perianal inflammation in 2 children.

Examination revealed an erythematous, papulosquamous, guttate eruption on the trunk and extremities. A skin biopsy specimen showed changes compatible with psoriasis. All children had intense erythema of the anal mucosa and perianal skin, and culture of this area grew group A β-hemolytic streptococcus. The streptococcal perianal dermatitis responded to penicillin, and the psoriasiform skin changes cleared within 14 to 35 days after therapy.

A psoriasiform eruption may occur as a result of skin infection with group A β-hemolytic streptococcus. These cases provide further evidence of the relationship between streptococcal infection and the induction of acute guttate psoriasis.

▶ The role of pharyngeal group A β-hemolytic streptococcus infection in the pathogenesis of flares or appearance of guttate-pattern psoriasis is well accepted (1–3). Rosenberg believes that localized infection by *Pityrosporum, Candida albicans,* and bacteria other than streptococcus can trigger psoriasis flares as well (4). Although the mechanism of microbial-associated flares is unknown, these authors hypothesize that bloodborne microbial antigen is fixed in the skin, resulting in koebnerization of psoriasis.

This report by Honig informs us that the perianal area should also be examined and cultured for the streptococcus. Streptococcal perianal disease has been reported as an entity only in the past few years (5, 6). Psoriatic involvement of the intergluteal cleft might provide a better milieu for impetiginization by streptococcus. As with guttate psoriasis flares associated with streptococcal pharyngitis, antibiotic treatment might also be expected to clear streptococcal perianal disease-associated guttate psoriasis.—R.A. Johnson, M.D.

References

1. Norrlind R: *Acta Derm Venereol (Stockh)* 28:571, 1948.
2. Chalmers RJG, et al: *Arch Dermatol* 118:141, 1982.
3. Chalmers RJG, et al: *Arch Dermatol* 119:956, 1983.
4. Rosenberg EW, Noah PW: *J Am Acad Dermatol* 18:151, 1988.
5. Kokx NP, et al: *Pediatrics* 80:659, 1987.
6. Rehder PA, et al: *Arch Dermatol* 124:702, 1988.

Antipsoriatic Effects of Zidovudine in Human Immunodeficiency Virus-Associated Psoriasis

Kaplan MH, Sadick NS, Wieder J, Farber BF, Neidt GW (Cornell Univ)
J Am Acad Dermatol 20:76–82, January 1989 17–5

Psoriasis may complicate HIV type 1 infection. Zidovudine (ZVD) was used in the treatment of 4 men aged 30–35 years with confirmed HIV infection and psoriasis. The dose was 200 mg every 4 hours. Within 2–6 weeks the psoriasis improved dramatically in all 4 patients. The ameliorating effect was sustained for more than 1 year in 2 patients despite worsening helper T cell depletion. In 1 patient the antipsoriatic effect was sustained despite continued p24 antigenemia. One patient, a drug addict who stopped taking ZVD, had a relapse of psoriasis that again resolved when he resumed taking the drug.

The antipsoriatic effect of ZVD apparently is associated with the production of a significant macrocytic effect on red blood cells and appears dose dependent. The drug is clearly effective in the treatment of HIV-associated psoriasis. Topically applied ZVD should be tested in non-HIV-associated psoriasis to determine whether it has some antipsoriatic effect in less severe forms of the disease.

▶ Psoriasis vulgaris as well as Reiter's syndrome occur with increased frequency of HIV-infected patients. Some patients are more resistant to common antipsoriatic therapies. Because of the immunosuppressant effects of topical corticosteroids and ultraviolet light irradiation, these modalities of therapy are not used as aggressively as in non-HIV-infected patients. Methotrexate is also contraindicated because of its effect on the immune system. Early in the HIV epidemic, HIV-infected patients with psoriasis were treated with methotrexate, resulting in either rapid progression or the appearance of Kaposi's sarcoma. Once methotrexate was discontinued, Kaposi's sarcoma either regressed to its previous involvement or disappeared completely. There are several reports of ZVD therapy (200 mg orally every 4 hours) having an antipsoriatic effect. It remains to be learned whether ZVD has a direct antipsoriatic effect, or whether it improves the status of the immune system with resultant improvement of psoriasis. In that ZVD is now given at a reduced dose of 100 mg every 4 hours to patients whose CD4 counts are less than 500 cells per mm^3, it will be of interest to know whether this dose has antipsoriatic effects as well. Newer antiretroviral agents, 2′,3′-dideoxycytidine and 2′,3′-dideoxyinosine are currently undergoing large-scale clinical trials; these agents might also prove to have antipsoriatic effects.—R.A. Johnson, M.D.

The Effect of Supplementation With Selenium and Vitamin E in Psoriasis

Fairris GM, Lloyd B, Hinks L, Perkins PJ, Clayton BE (Royal South Hants Hosp; Southampton Gen Hosp, England)

Ann Clin Biochem 26:83–88, January 1989 17–6

Psoriasis patients have decreased selenium concentrations in whole blood, plasma, and leukocytes as well as decreased activity of selenium-dependent glutathione peroxidase (GSH-Px). Selenium supplementation was given to 60 adults with moderate or severe psoriasis. They were randomly assigned to receive daily, on a double-blind basis, 600 μg of selenium-enriched yeast alone or with 600 IU of vitamin E, or placebo for 12 weeks.

Before supplementation the patient's had significantly lower concentrations of selenium in whole blood and plasma than controls; however, erythrocyte GSH-Px activity was normal. After 12 weeks of selenium supplementation they had significantly increased selenium concentrations in whole blood and plasma, GSH-Px activity in platelets, and vitamin E in plasma, but the mean selenium concentration in skin and the erythrocyte GSH-Px activity failed to increase. Selenium levels rose significantly in leukocytes only in the selenium group not receiving vitamin E. The mean area of psoriasis and the mean severity index were similar in both supplementation groups and in the placebo group. Selenium toxicity did not occur.

Selenium in this form is not effective in the treatment of psoriasis. Selenium concentrations in whole blood or plasma may not be the only indications of selenium status.

▶ I had never thought of psoriasis as a selenium-deficiency disease. I am still not convinced it is. Further, supplementation with selenium and vitamin E is not helpful.— R.S. Stern, M.D.

Efficacy of Topical Treatment in Psoriasis With MC 903, a New Vitamin D Analogue

Staberg B, Roed-Petersen J, Menné T (Gentofte Hosp, Copenhagen)
Acta Derm Venereol (Stockh) 69:147–150, April 1989 17–7

Psoriasis may respond to topical or systemic active vitamin D metabolites, but there is a potential risk of hypercalcemia and hypercalciuria. The antipsoriatic effect of MC 903, a synthetic vitamin D analogue associated with a much lower risk of inducing hypercalcemia, was studied in 10 inpatients with chronic plaque-type psoriasis. In 2 symmetrically located psoriatic plaques, topical treatment with MC 903 cream, containing 1.2 mg of MC 903 per gram of cream, was compared with placebo cream in a double-blind, controlled, left-right, randomized fashion during 6 weeks of therapy.

Clinical improvement was significant after 1 week of treatment with MC 903 compared with baseline, and after 4 weeks of MC 903 therapy in lateral comparison with the placebo cream base treatment. Further, the lesions cleared completely during 6 weeks of MC 903 therapy in 3 patients. Measurement of skin blood flow by laser Doppler technique was not superior to objective clinical assessment of disease activity. No adverse reactions were observed.

The vitamin D analogue MC 903 is potentially useful in the treatment of psoriasis. It has potent effects on cell proliferation and cell differentiation with minimal effects on calcium metabolism.

▶ This study is part of the search for vitamin D analogues that improve psoriasis but do not affect calcium metabolism. Although vitamin D is significantly effective, this study and others show that the degree of improvement with vitamin D is usually relatively modest. Still, vitamin D and its analogues remain potentially helpful agents in the treatment of psoriasis.— R.S. Stern, M.D.

Psoriasis and Vitamin D_3: A Review of Our Experience

Morimoto S, Yoshikawa K (Osaka Univ, Japan)
Arch Dermatol 125:231–234, February 1989 17–8

Psoriasis is characterized by an abnormally exaggerated turnover of epidermal cells. Although the etiology of psoriasis is unknown, it is believed that it is caused by loss of the normal regulatory mechanism of the cell cycle. Recent studies have shown that the calcitrophic hormone calcitriol (1,25-dihydroxyvitamin D_3) regulates the terminal differentiation of epidermal keratinocytes.

The clinical efficacy of active metabolites of vitamin D_3 in the treatment of psoriasis vulgaris was evaluated in 40 patients, 17 of whom were randomly assigned to oral administration of 1-α-hydroxyvitamin D_3 for 6 months, 4 to oral administration of calcitriol for 6 months, and 16 to topical administration of calcitriol for 8 weeks. To assess the correlation between serum levels of calcium-related factors and disease severity, calcium serum levels were measured in 34 other psoriasis patients.

Significant improvements were obtained in 13 of the 17 patients treated with 1-α-hydroxyvitamin D_3 for 6 months, 1 of the 4 patients treated with oral calcitriol for 6 months, and in 16 of the 19 patients treated with calcitriol applied topically for 8 weeks. None of the topically treated patients had improvement in contralateral skin lesions that had been treated only with vehicle for control. There was a significant negative correlation between the severity of psoriasis and calcitriol serum levels, but not between disease severity and other calcium-related parameters.

Topically applied active forms of vitamin D_3 appear to be effective in the treatment of psoriasis. Endogenous calcitriol may also be involved in the development of the disease.

▶ More evidence that vitamin D may make a difference in the treatment of psoriasis. We need more studies before this agent's place is defined.—R.S. Stern, M.D.

Interleukin 2 and Psoriasis

Lee RE, Gaspari AA, Lotze MT, Chang AE, Rosenberg SA (Natl Cancer Inst, Bethesda)

Arch Dermatol 124:1811–1815, December 1988 17–9

Immunotherapy with interleukin-2 alone or in conjunction with lymphokine-activated killer (LAK) cells is under investigation as a treatment for cancer not amenable to conventional therapy. Toxic reactions associated with this therapy involve multiple organ systems, including the skin. Dermatologic complications generally consist of erythema and pruritus, followed by mild desquamation. Complete resolution of these skin reactions may require up to 3–4 weeks. A review was made of the dermatologic complications in 3 men aged 29–62 with metastatic cancer and preexisting psoriasis who were treated with interleukin-2.

All 3 patients had renal cell carcinoma that had metastasized to the cervical lymph nodes in 1 and to the lungs in the other 2. During immunotherapy all 3 patients experienced acute exacerbation of psoriasis that was generalized in 2 patients and localized to the groin in 1. In all 3, the psoriatic flare resolved on discontinuation of interleukin-2 therapy and with standard topical treatment for psoriasis. The exacerbation of psoriasis did not affect the response to immunotherapy.

Histologic analysis of serial skin biopsy specimens available for 2 of the 3 patients revealed psoriasiform changes in involved skin as well as epidermal spongiosis and a perivascular mononuclear cell infiltrate. Of the 3 patients, 2 were not being treated for their psoriasis before immunotherapy. Therefore, the exacerbation in these 2 patients could not be attributed to interruption of treatment. The third patient was being treated for his psoriasis with methotrexate and topical steroid, but treatment was discontinued during interleukin therapy. In this case, discontinuation of the psoriasis treatment may have contributed to the subsequent exacerbation. However, psoriasis need not be considered an absolute contraindication to immunotherapy with interleukin-2, as topical treatment effectively induced remission in all 3 men.

▶ Interferon appears to "upregulate" the epidermal proliferation in patients with psoriasis and hence worsen the disease.—R.S. Stern, M.D.

---

311 nm UVB Phototherapy—An Effective Treatment for Psoriasis

Green C, Ferguson J, Lakshmipathi T, Johnson BE (Univ of Dundee, Scotland)

Br J Dermatol 119:691–696, December 1988 17–10

Well-established treatment modalities for psoriasis include phototherapy with ultraviolet B (UVB) and psoralen photochemotherapy (PUVA). Both give satisfactory results, but greater remission is obtained with PUVA. The main concern with PUVA is its potential carcinogenicity. A new experimental fluorescent lamp (Philips TL-01), which emits a narrow band at 311 and a minor peak at 305 nm, was shown to be less carcinogenic in mice than the conventional broad-band UVB TL-12 lamps. The efficacy of these new lamps was determined in 52 patients with psoriasis.

Patients were treated 3 times weekly and subdivided into 3 groups: plaque, plaque/guttate, and guttate psoriasis. The results of a previous study of 25 patients with psoriasis who were treated by conventional UVB phototherapy were used for comparison. The same inclusion criteria, treatment schedule, and assessment criteria were used with 1 exception: Because of burning, the UVB-treated patients were seen twice daily.

With the experimental lamp a satisfactory response was obtained in 92% of those with plaque psoriasis and 100% of those in the plaque/guttate and guttate groups. The incidence of burning was 10%. One year after cessation of therapy, 38% of the patients remained in remission. When the group given conventional UVB phototherapy was compared with the experimental group, both the time taken to achieve a satisfactory response and the total duration of therapy were significantly less in the experimental group, with cumulative exposure doses on the same order of magnitude in each group. In the conventional group, the rate of burning was 28% despite the twice-weekly treatment schedule. Also, only 5% in the conventionally treated group remained in remission 1 year after treatment, compared with 38% in the experimental group.

Knowledge that the retinoids have an anticancer effect has stimulated research with these drugs in combination with both UVB and PUVA with successful results. The new TL-01 lamp also is associated with less risk in terms of UV carcinogenesis and should be studied in combination with 1 of the oral retinoids.

---

311 nm UVB Lamps in the Treatment of Psoriasis With the Ingram Regimen

Karvonen J, Kokkonen E-L, Ruotsalainen E (Univ Central Hosp, Oulu, Finland)

Acta Derm Venereol (Stockh) 69:82–85, March 1989 17–11

Treatment with ultraviolet-B (UVB) phototherapy is commonly used for psoriasis; however, conventional broad-band UVB lamps pose an increased risk of skin cancer. A lamp emitting only therapeutic UVB but not short-wave UVB might solve the problem. The experimental fluorescent Philips TL 01 lamp has an emission spectrum with a narrow peak at 311 nm. This lamp was compared with a conventional broad-band lamp in the treatment of 20 psoriatic patients according to the Ingram regimen. In each patient, 1 arm was treated with the new lamp and 1 arm with the conventional lamp. A second trial was performed on another 40 patients.

In the first trial results were similar in both arms of 12 patients, but in 8 patients the new lamp was more effective. In the second trial 53% of 17 patients treated with the experimental lamp had good results, compared with 30% of 23 patients treated with the conventional lamp.

The 311-nm UVB lamp is at least as effective as conventional broadband UVB lamps in the treatment of psoriasis according to the Ingram regimen. Theoretically, the new lamp should be safer than conventional lamps, but no long-term data on the safety of the 311-nm lamp in humans are available.

▶ Both of these studies (Abstracts 17–10 and 17–11) appear to confirm that 311-nm radiation can be used successfully to treat psoriasis.—R.W. Gange, M.D.

Are Topical Corticosteroids Useful in Phototherapy for Psoriasis?

Dover JS, McEvoy MT, Rosen CF, Arndt KA, Stern RS (Beth Israel Hosp, Boston; Massachusetts Gen Hosp, Boston)

J Am Acad Dermatol 20:748–754, May 1989 17–12

Ultraviolet B (UVB) radiation is a well-established treatment of moderate and severe plaque-type psoriasis. A prospective, randomized, double-blind, placebo-controlled trial evaluated the effect of a potent topical corticosteroid cream used with UVB phototherapy on time to clearing and duration of remission in 53 outpatients with psoriasis. The patients received suberythemogenic UVB phototherapy 3 times a week plus topical corticosteroid or placebo emollient cream to be applied twice a day until clearing.

Nine patients in each group were noncompliant. A trend toward a slightly more rapid response was noted in the treatment group, but no significant differences were seen between groups in early response to therapy, number of treatments, and UVB dose required to achieve clearing. Patients treated with the topical corticosteroid remained in remission longer than controls. Life-table analysis predicted that 62% of controls would have flaring of disease within 6 months of clearing, compared with only 42% of topical corticosteroid-treated patients.

The use of a potent topical corticosteroid cream in conjunction with UVB therapy appears to have no substantial effect on the time required to clear psoriasis, even in patients whose psoriasis is moderate. A trend toward longer remission may exist in patients treated with the corticosteroid as opposed to those treated with placebo, but this finding did not reach significance even in this large series.

▶ In contrast, other studies have indicated shorter remission times from UVB therapy when concomitant steroid treatment is used (1, 2). In a lengthy discussion the authors present possible reasons for these differences. Our own preference is for the use of UVB plus emollients without general topical steroid treatment, although the latter is often used in difficult localized areas.—R.W. Gange, M.D.

References

1. Larko O, et al: *Acta Derm Venereol (Stockh)* 64:151, 1984.
2. Horowitz SN, et al: *J Am Acad Dermatol* 13:784, 1985.

Double-Blind Comparison of a Dithranol and Steroid Mixture With a Conventional Dithranol Regimen for Chronic Psoriasis

Grattan CEH, Christopher AP, Robinson M, Cowan MA (Gen Hosp, Birmingham, England)

Br J Dermatol 119:623–626, November 1988 17–13

Previous studies of a dithranol and steroid regimen and a tar and steroid regimen for psoriasis found an earlier relapse when steroid was included. However, 1 of these studies had serious methodologic flaws. A double-blind comparison of a dithranol and steroid mixture with a conventional dithranol regimen for chronic psoriasis was done in 24 patients. Dithranol in Lasser's paste and dithranol and fluocinonide in Lassar's paste were used.

A more rapid reduction in severity of the psoriasis was noted on the side treated with the combined dithranol and fluocinonide preparation, but there was no difference in the final time to clearance between the 2 sides. Fewer burning episodes and greater staining of the skin occurred on the side treated with dithranol plus fluocinonide. Twenty patients were followed for as long as 3 months. Eleven had more relapses on the side treated with dithranol and fluocinonide, and 2 had more on the side treated with dithranol alone. In 7 patients no appreciable difference was evident.

These findings confirm that the addition of a topical steroid to a dithranol regimen results in significantly earlier relapse. However, patients treated with dithranol plus fluocinonide had fewer burning episodes and a more rapid clinical response. Therefore, this mixture has a place in the management of patients who experience burning with low concentrations of dithranol, enabling them to tolerate treatment during the early stages before changing to dithranol in Lassar's paste.

▶ Earlier relapses of psoriasis have been noted in steroid-treated groups after a variety of combination therapies using topical steroids combined with other modalities.—R.W. Gange, M.D.

Sulfasalazine: A Potential Psoriasis Therapy?

Gupta Ak, Ellis CN, Siegel MT, Voorhees JJ (Univ of Michigan)

J Am Acad Dermatol 20:797–800, May 1989 17–14

Sulfasalazine is effective in treating inflammatory bowel disease and rheumatoid arthritis, diseases characterized by abnormal arachidonic acid metabolism with increased 5-lipoxygenase pathway activity. Sulfasalazine may act in part as a 5-lipoxygenase inhibitor. Its use has been reported in pustular psoriasis and psoriatic arthritis but not psoriasis vulgaris. An open trial was carried out involving 32 patients with moderate to severe stable plaque psoriasis to investigate the efficacy of the drug in the treatment of psoriasis vulgaris. Patients were treated with 3 g of sulfasalazine daily for 8 weeks.

Of the 24 patients who completed the trial, 3 had a poor response; their dosage was increased to 4 g/day with only slight improvement. Two patients were essentially clear at the end of treatment. A marked response was noted in 10 patients, a modest response in 7, and a minimal response in 5. Of the 8 patients who did not finish the trial, 4 were dropped after a generalized, apparently drug-induced macular eruption developed, and 1 dropped out because of nausea and fatigue. Side effects generally were mild and transient among the patients who completed therapy. These side effects included nausea in 7 patients, fatigue in 4, indigestion in 2, diarrhea in 1, and a macular eruption with a photosensitive distribution in 2. The eruptions resolved within a week.

Nineteen of 24 patients in this series had modest to marked improvement or clearing of psoriasis after 8 weeks of sulfasalazine therapy. If these results are confirmed by a double-blind study, sulfasalazine may become an alternative treatment in some patients.

▶ As with so many open studies, the results here are promising. What we need now is a double-blind control trial. If the results are confirmed, it would be further evidence that the immune system is important as primary modulator of psoriasis. We have learned, however, that at least in tissue culture, cyclosporine also has an antiproliferative effect.—R.S. Stern, M.D.

Palmoplantar Psoriasis: Experience With 8-Methoxypsoralen Soaks Plus Ultraviolet A With the Use of a High-Output Metal Halide Device

Coleman WR, Lowe NJ, David M, Halder RM (Univ of California, Los Angeles; Howard Univ Hosp, Washington, DC)

J Am Acad Dermatol 20:1078–1082, June 1989 17–15

Palmoplantar psoriasis often is resistant to traditional topical measures. An uncontrolled study of 8-methoxypsoralen water bath soaks at 2.5 mg/L plus ultraviolet A (UVA) exposure was undertaken in 11 patients with moderate to severe involvement whose disease had resisted topical treatment. Hand or foot soaks were carried out for 30 minutes, 2 or 3 times a week, followed by UVA radiation.

The mean number of treatments required for peak improvement was 28, and the mean peak UVA dose was 10 J/cm^2. Patient responses averaged 55%; 1 patient had complete clearing, 7 had a good response, and 3 had no significant response. In no patient did disease become worse during treatment. Five patients had erythema and 1 had pruritus and vesiculation.

This is a relatively effective and well-tolerated treatment. Peak serum levels of 8-methoxypsoralen were 3 ng/mL, suggesting that systemic side effects can be avoided. The treatment may be especially useful in patients who do not tolerate systemic psoralen and in those for whom systemic retinoids are contraindicated.

▶ Both 8-methoxypsoralen (methoxsalen) and trimethylpsoralen (trioxsalen) are very insoluble in water. Yet there is enough solubility to use both of these photoactive psoralens in bath or soak regimens. The PUVA bath has been used on a large scale by Dr. Torkel Fisher in Sweden, who pioneered this therapy beginning in 1976 (1), not long after the discovery of oral PUVA photochemotherapy in 1974 for the treatment of psoriasis. The treatment regimen consists of 50 mg of trioxsalen (prepared by dissolving 0.25% trioxsalen in ethanol) and a bath prepared by using 20 mL of the trioxsalen-alcohol solution in 150 L of water. The patient is immersed, except for the head, for 10–15 minutes and is irradiated within 15 minutes after the bath. The starting doses are very low; 0.1–0.2 J/cm^2. The maximum dose, which is usually reached within 6–8 weeks, is 1.0–2.0 J/cm^2. The details of the trioxsalen bath treatment are given in a long chapter (2). Following patients for 14 years, Fisher did not discover any skin cancer in 149 of them.

The psoralens are highly potent photoactive agents, and the PUVA bath technique is very effective indeed. We have treated 32 patients using the Torkel Fisher method, with FDA approval. Thirteen of these patients had recalcitrant pustular psoriasis of the palms and soles. In this group, 55% of the patients cleared after an average of 26 treatments and a total cumulative UVA dose of 70 J/cm^2. There were 4 failures and only mild phototoxicity. These results are about the same as reported in the abstract by Coleman et al. using 8-methoxypsoralen soaks in palmoplantar psoriasis. The treatment is cumbersome, however, and there are logistics problems, especially having a bath available near a UVA radiator.

Psoralen soaks are indicated in the following clinical settings: (1) Children under 12 years who cannot be given oral PUVA and in whom UVB has failed; (2) patients who must give up oral PUVA because of severe side effects (nausea); (3) patients who have no options, i.e., in whom UVB and oral PUVA have failed and who cannot take methotrexate because of contraindications or youth; and (4) those patients with generalized psoriasis who have had clearing with PUVA except for the last 5%, which is resistant to PUVA photochemotherapy.—T.B. Fitzpatrick, M.D., Ph.D.

References

1. Fisher T, et al: *Acta Derm Venereol (Stockh)* 56:383, 1976.
2. Fisher T: *Topical psoralen ultraviolet radiation,* in Roenigk HH, Maibach HI (eds): *Psoriasis.* New York, Dekker, 1985.

Acitretin and Etretinate in the Treatment of Palmoplantar Pustulosis: A Double-Blind Comparative Trial

Lassus A, Geiger J-M (Univ Central Hosp, Helsinki; F Hoffmann-La Roche & Co Ltd, Basle, Switzerland)

Br J Dermatol 119:755–759, December 1988 17–16

Acitretin, an acid form of the ethyl ester etretinate, is effective in the treatment of psoriasis. Palmoplantar pustulosis can be cleared or much improved by etretinate treatment. The advantage of acitretin is its rapid elimination from the body. The therapeutic effects of acitretin and etretinate in palmoplantar pustulosis were determined in a randomized, double-blind study.

Sixty patients (18 men and 42 women aged 22–76 years) were randomly allocated to 1 of the 2 retinoid treatment groups. During the first 4 weeks of treatment the patients received 3 10-mg capsules daily. In the following 8 weeks the number of capsules varied according to clinical improvement.

After 12 weeks of treatment in both groups the mean number of pustules was reduced from 57.8 to 3.9 in the group given acitretin and from 57.1 to 5.7 in those given etretinate. The number of pustules was not significantly different before treatment or at the end of treatment in either group. No significant differences were found in scores with regard to erythema, infiltration, scaling, or involved area. The areas of the palms and soles that were affected were comparable in both groups before and after treatment. Palmar lesions, however, responded better to retinoid treatment than did plantar lesions. All patients had adverse reactions of

Clinical Adverse Events in Both Groups

	Acitretin ($n = 30$)		Etretinate ($n = 29$)	
	No. of patients	%	No. of patients	%
Dry lips/cheilitis	30	100%	29	100%
Dry mouth	22	73%	18	62%
Dry skin	21	70%	12	41%
Dry nose	18	60%	10	34%
Scaling (palms/soles)	18	60%	14	48%
Scaling (elsewhere)	14	47%	7	24%
Dry eyes/conjunctivitis	6	20%	7	24%
Hair loss	6	20%	4	14%
Pruritus	3	10%	2	7%
Nail fragility	2	7%	2	7%
Other	7*	23%	1†	3%

*Localized infections, 2; erythema, 1; retinoid dermatitis, 1; purpura, 1; dysuria, 1; nausea, 1.
†Sticky skin, 1.
(Courtesy of Lassus A, Geiger J-M: *Br J Dermatol* 119:755–759, December 1988.)

the hypervitaminosis A type (table). Adverse reactions were more frequent in the acitretin-treated group than in the group given etretinate.

Acitretin is effective in the treatment of palmoplantar pustulosis. The effectiveness and tolerance of acitretin and etretinate do not differ significantly.

▶ Further evidence for the approximate therapeutic equivalency of acitretin and etretinate. There was a trend toward more mucocutaneous side effects in the acitretin-treated group.—R.S. Stern, M.D.

A Modified Dosage Schedule for Increased Efficiency in PUVA Treatment of Psoriasis

Carabott FM, Hawk JLM (St Thomas' Hosp, London)
Clin Exp Dermatol 14:337–340, September 1989 17–17

Combined therapy consisting of orally administered psoralen with ultraviolet A radiation (PUVA) is commonly used in the treatment of psoriasis, but the optimal UVA dose increments for achieving the most rapid clearing of rash using the smallest total radiation dose have not yet been established. Conventional dosage schedules are formulated to simplify operator calculations and minimize patient side effects. An attempt was made to maximize the efficiency of PUVA therapy while reducing the risk for skin cancer.

Ten patients with chronic widespread plaque psoriasis underwent PUVA therapy in which the UVA dosage schedule was modified but the psoralen formulation and doses unchanged. All 10 patients had previously experienced complete clearance of psoriasis with conventional

PUVA therapy 3 times a week for 6–8 months. None had received systemic treatment for psoriasis before entry into the study.

Psoralen was administered orally 2 hours before UVA treatment. The initial and incremental UVA doses were maximized to near-erythemogenic levels as determined by weekly testing for minimal phototoxic dose treatment. Each patient's minimal phototoxic dose was assessed 72 hours after UVA irradiation until psoriasis had fully cleared.

With the modified schedule there was a 55% geometric mean reduction in the duration of treatment when compared to treatment duration with the last previous conventional UVA course. The reduction in total cumulative UVA treatment dose from the last previous conventional course was 31%. Six of the 10 treated patients were still in remission after a mean of 5.7 months; the other 4 relapsed after a mean of 3.9 months.

Increasing the initial and incremental UVA doses in PUVA treatment of psoriasis to near-erythemogenic levels as determined by weekly minimal phototoxic dose testing substantially reduces treatment duration and cumulative UVA dose when compared with conventional treatment schedules.

▶ This study attempts to maximize the efficiency of PUVA treatment using weekly minimal phototoxic dose testing as a guide to weekly UV dose increments. The authors claim substantial advantages from this logical approach, which is presumably now standard practice in their units. The results of treatment of larger numbers of patients are awaited with interest. A split-body comparison with standard PUVA would also add weight to the findings, which used retrospective controls.—R.W. Gange, M.D.

Comparison of Therapeutic Efficacy of Topical PUVA, Oral Etretinate, and Combined PUVA and Etretinate for the Treatment of Psoriasis and Development of PUVA Lentigines and Antinuclear Antibodies

Takashima A, Sunohara A, Matsunami E, Mizuno N (Nagoya City Univ Med School, Japan)

J Dermatol 15:473–479, December 1988 17–18

The combination of oral PUVA and etretinate is more effective in the treatment of psoriasis than oral PUVA alone. The combination of etretinate and topical PUVA (Re-PUVA) was compared with topical PUVA alone during a 7-year study period in which 117 patients were treated. All had relatively severe psoriasis involving more than 20% of the whole-body area. Sixty-two patients were treated with PUVA alone and 38 with Re-PUVA. In addition, 17 patients received monotherapy with oral etretinate for 32 weeks.

In both the PUVA and the Re-PUVA groups, 50% of the patients began to improve after 6 treatments within 6 weeks. To clear psoriasis completely in 50% of the patients, PUVA alone required 63 treatments or 63 weeks. The addition of etretinate reduced the number of PUVA

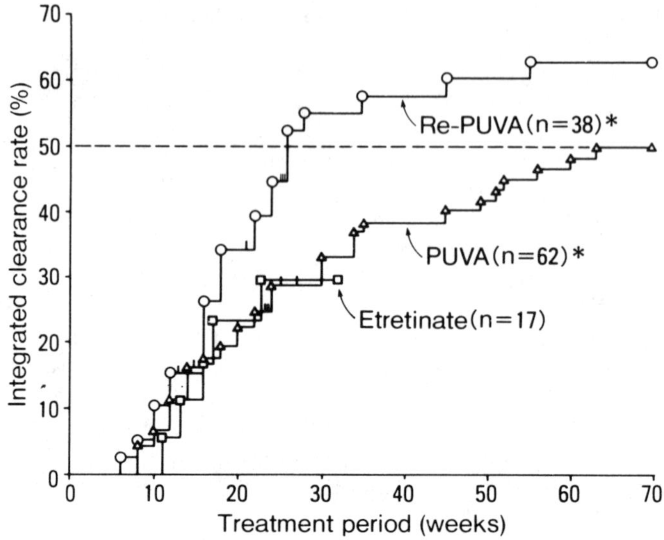

Fig 17–1.—Complete clearance and duration of treatment. The integrated rate of patients with complete clearance of psoriatic eruptions is plotted as a function of the treatment period. *Spikes,* patients who discontinued treatment; *asterisks,* statistically significant difference ($P < .05$). (Courtesy of Takashima A, Sunohara A, Matsunami E, et al: *J Dermatol* 15:473–479, December 1988.)

treatments required to achieve the same efficacy to 26 (Fig 17–1). The integrated clearance rate in 70 weeks was 63% in the Re-PUVA group, compared with 50% in the PUVA group (a statistically significant difference). The addition of etretinate failed to inhibit the production of PUVA lentigines, but clearly suppressed the expression of antinuclear antibody. Patients in both groups gradually relapsed after treatment was discontinued. Psoriasis recurred in 50% of the patients after 4 months and in 85% after 1 year. Of 17 patients treated with etretinate monotherapy, 13 began to improve within 9 weeks but relapsed within 6 months after discontinuation of treatment. The other 4 patients had no response to oral monotherapy.

The findings support the contention that the combination of topical PUVA and oral etretinate is more effective in the treatment of psoriasis than topical PUVA alone.

▶ This is a nonrandomized, small study, difficult to interpret. It supports investigations in Europe and the United States that show that etretinate plus PUVA does clear most patients' psoriasis more rapidly than PUVA alone.—R.S. Stern, M.D.

Acitretin (Ro 10–1670) in the Treatment of Severe Psoriasis: A Randomized Double-Blind Parallel Study Comparing Acitretin and Etretinate

Ledo A, Martín M, Geiger JM, Marrón JM (Ramón y Cajal Hosp, Madrid; F Hoffmann-La Roche, Basel, Switzerland; Productos Roche SA, Madrid)

Int J Dermatol 27:656–660, November 1988 17–19

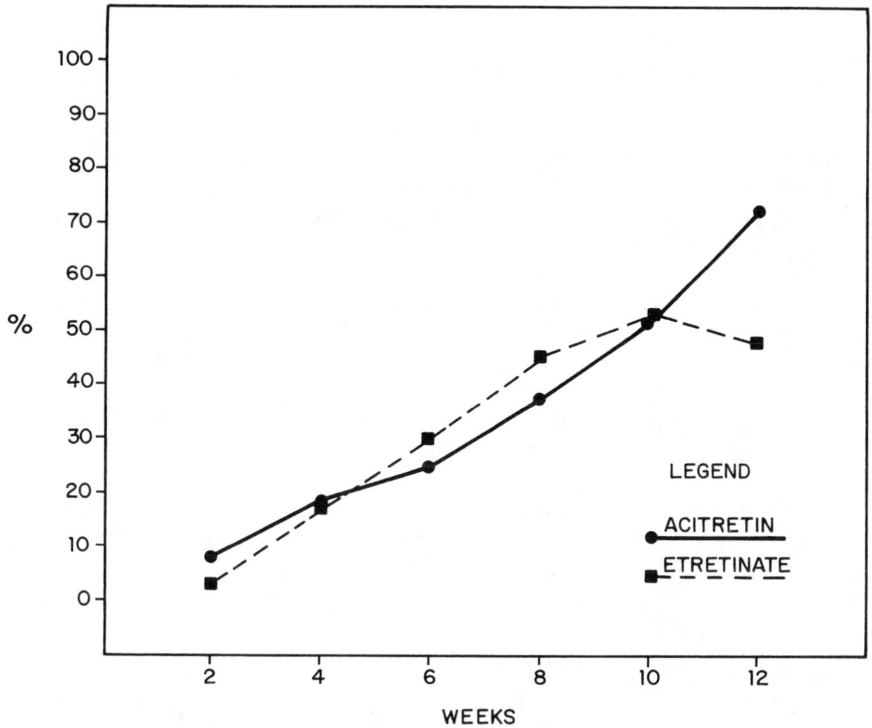

Fig 17–2.—Score improvements in patients treated with acitretin or etretinate (median values). (Courtesy of Ledo A, Martín M, Geiger JM, et al: *Int J Dermatol* 27:656–660, November 1988.)

Etretinate is effective in the symptomatic treatment of severe psoriasis; however, the drug is eliminated from the body only slowly. Acitretin appears to have similar antipsoriatic properties, but its terminal elimination half-life is 2–4 days. A comparison was made of the 2 drugs in 20 patients. Nineteen had psoriasis vulgaris with more than 20% of the skin surface involved, and 1 had palmoplantar pustular psoriasis. In each treatment group 1 patient had a psoriatic arthropathy.

The patients were treated with 30 mg/day for 8 weeks, after which the dose was individualized, the maximum dose not to exceed 80 mg/day. The treatment lasted for 12 weeks. Patients were examined every 2 weeks, and laboratory tests were performed initially and at 4-week intervals thereafter. The mean dose at the conclusion of the study was slightly less in the group given acitretin than in the group given etretinate. Both groups had a 50% improvement in symptoms at week 10. Differences in results at the end of the study were not significant (Fig 17–2).

Acitretin and etretinate do not differ significantly in their effectiveness or in adverse effects in the treatment of psoriasis. Acitretin, however, has a shorter period of potential teratogenicity after treatment has been discontinued.

▶ Neither drug appeared to be particularly effective, with only a 50% improvement after 10 weeks. Because retinoids are most commonly used in combination with phototherapy, a trial with concomitant UV would perhaps have been more interesting.—R.W. Gange, M.D.

A Double-Blind Comparison of Acitretin and Etretinate in the Treatment of Severe Psoriasis: Results of a Nordic Multicentre Study

Kragballe K, Jansén CT, Geiger J-M, Bjerke JR, Falk ES, Gip L, Hjorth N, Lauharanta J, Mork N-J, Reunala T, Rosén K, Schmidt H, Thune PO, Vahlquist C (Marselisborg Hosp, Aarhus, Denmark; Central Hosp, Turku, Finland; F Hoffmann-La Roche & Co Ltd, Basel, Switzerland; Haukeland Hosp, Bergen, Norway; Tromsö Hosp, Norway, et al)

Acta Derm Venereol (Stockh) 69:35–40, March 1989 17–20

Although etretinate is effective in the treatment of severe psoriasis, it is extremely lipophilic, as most of the drug is stored in fatty tissues. Its terminal elimination half-life has been estimated at up to 120 days. Acitretin, the free acid of etretinate, is less lipophilic, and its terminal half-life is only 2–4 days. Thus acitretin may represent an important therapeutic alternative to etretinate in women of childbearing age. The antipsoriatic effect and tolerability of acitretin and etretinate were compared in 168 pa-

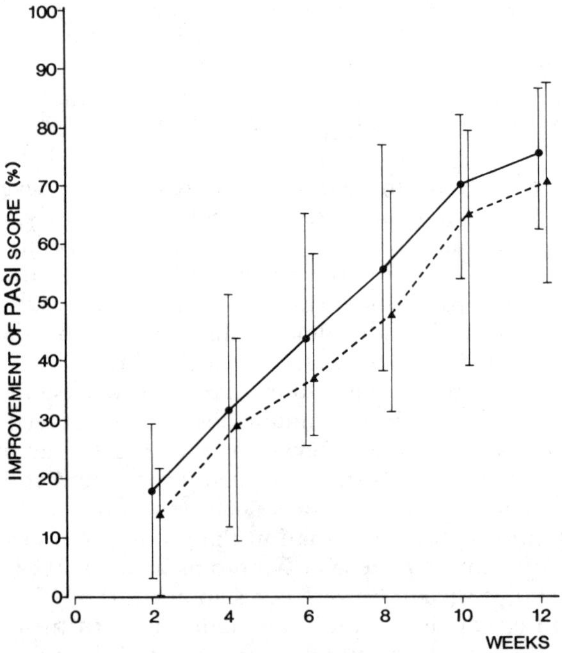

17–3.—Percent improvement of PASI scores in psoriatic patients who completed the study. **Circles,** 99 patients given acitretin; **triangles,** 24 patients given etretinate. Values are medians and interquartile range. (Courtesy of Kragballe K, Jansén CT, Geiger J-M, et al: *Acta Derm Venereol (Stockh)* 69:35–40, March 1989.)

tients with longstanding, severe psoriasis; 127 were treated with acitretin and 41 with etretinate.

The dose of each drug, 40 mg daily for the first 4 weeks, was adjusted individually in the subsequent 8 weeks. All patients were evaluated at biweekly intervals on the Psoriasis Area and Severity Index (PASI) rating scale. Twenty-one etretinate-treated patients and 99 acitretin-treated patients completed the study. The average daily dose of acitretin was 0.54 mg/kg, and of etretinate, 0.65 mg/kg. (The difference was statistically not significant.)

The PASI scores improved in parallel in the 2 treatment groups (Fig 17–3). At week 12 the PASI score improvement was 75.8% in the acitretin-treated group and 70.8% in the etretinate-treated group. However, the PASI score had not reached a plateau at completion of the study. Marked or total clearance of psoriatic lesions was obtained in 84% of the acitretin-treated patients and in 80% of the etretinate-treated patients. All patients experienced mucocutaneous side effects. Assessments of overall tolerability by investigators and patients showed a statistically significant difference in favor of etretinate.

Acitretin and etretinate are equally effective in the treatment of psoriasis. Although acitretin was not as well tolerated as etretinate, it has the important advantage of having a much shorter terminal half-life. Therefore, acitretin is preferred for women of childbearing potential.

▶ Acitretin is the carboxylic acid derivative of etretinate. The 2 drugs appear to have approximately equal efficacy. Acitretin's main advantage is its shorter half-life. As a result, within weeks of cessation of therapy detectable levels of drug are no longer present. This would permit the use of this drug in women with childbearing potential, providing they use adequate contraconception during therapy and for a brief period thereafter. This allows the therapeutic benefits of retinoids to be offered to psoriatic women of childbearing potential. Great care should be taken when prescribing this drug to women to inform them about the need for contraception during treatment and in the immediate posttreatment interval.— R.S. Stern, M.D.

Tin-Protoporphyrin and Long Wave Length Ultraviolet Light in Treatment of Psoriasis

Emtestam L, Berglund L, Angelin B, Drummond GS, Kappas A (Karolinska Inst, Stockholm; Rockefeller Univ)

Lancet 1:1231–1233, June 3, 1989 17–21

Tin-protoporphyrin, a synthetic heme analogue, in conjunction with ultraviolet A (UVA) radiation might prove useful in treating psoriasis. Ten patients with plaque-type psoriasis who failed to respond to standard topical or systemic treatment received a combination of tin-protoporphyrin and intermittent long-wavelength UV light therapy. Patients received tin-protoporphyrin, 2 μmol/kg, for 1 day and 3 weeks of UVA light treatment. The average cumulative UVA dose was 98 J/cm^2.

Tin-protoporphyrin lowered the UVA light threshold in all patients. All 10 patients had a positive clinical response, and some had nearly complete clearance of lesions. No adverse side effects were noted. The serum bilirubin levels decreased by approximately 35% for 8–10 days. Increased solar sensitivity did not lead to discomfort. No patient had rebound disease activity. The clinical effect appeared to last for at least 6 weeks after the 3-week trial.

Combined treatment with tin-protoporphyrin and UVA light may be helpful in the treatment of resistant plaque-type psoriasis.

▶ The management of generalized psoriasis (>20% body area) is at present very difficult as there are few choices: UVB phototherapy, PUVA photochemotherapy, and methotrexate. These treatments can be combined with adjuvants such as oral retinoids with PUVA and UVB. More recently, cyclosporine has been introduced, but it is doubtful if this will be used as a monotherapy; it will probably be combined with PUVA. Treatment with UVB plus tar (Goeckermann regimen) is an inpatient treatment and is not now an option for treatment because of the new restrictions by third-party carriers; day-care centers are able to use the Goeckermann regimen, but this is available in only a few centers in the United States.

There is considerable research at present to develop a new agent for psoriasis. If this is effective only as a topical chemical, it will not be practical to use in patients with generalized psoriasis. Pending some striking breakthrough (as, for example, patients with the use of oral zinc to completely control the disease acrodermatitis enteropathica) any new agent will have effects on all cells and its action will not be limited to skin cells. This local action has been the marvelous advantage of PUVA photochemotherapy: It is a "local" therapy but given orally; the therapeutic action on DNA occurs only when UVA interacts with psoralens in the skin. No toxicity associated with PUVA photochemotherapy on the kidney, bone marrow, or liver has been reported. Photochemotherapy—using nonionizing radiation such as UVA that has little or no deep penetration and virtually no biological action alone (in the doses used)—in combination with a drug given orally is an ideal treatment. The problem is that PUVA binds to DNA, and this has led to concern regarding a long-term carcinogenic effect. It has been used in tens of thousands of patients now for more than 16 years and only a small number of PUVA-induced squamous cell carcinomas have been reported; almost all of these PUVA-induced cancers have not thus far been aggressive tumors.

The photochemotherapy proposed in this report from Sweden has one clear and important advantage over PUVA photochemotherapy—its action is most probably not on the DNA of the epidermal cells (although these authors did not speculate on the mechanism of action). Porphyrins interacting with light have their pharmacologic action principally on cell membranes. Thus it would not alter DNA, and there would not be a risk of skin cancer as a result of tin-protoporphyrin plus UVA.

This therapy, however, has some limiting factors: It must be given intravenously, and even more impractical is that the photosensitivity persists for days, which makes it impossible for the physician to control the light exposures.

(Psoralens are excreted within a few hours, and there is virtually no photosensitivity after 6 hours, and none at all after 12 hours.) When hematoporphyrins were given for the treatment of lung cancer, patients remained photosensitive for weeks and severe phototoxic effects (erythema, edema of the face and neck) occurred, even in winter in Northern latitudes with the only light exposure obtained being that while going to and from the hospital for x-ray treatments.

This site of action on cell membranes rather than on DNA is what we should seek in a new drug-light treatment for a chronic disease such as psoriasis; porphyrins probably would not do.—T.B. Fitzpatrick, M.D., Ph.D.

Topical Methotrexate Therapy for Psoriasis

Weinstein GD, McCullough JL, Olsen E (Univ of California, Irvine; Duke Univ)
Arch Dermatol 125:227–230, February 1989 17–22

Because the systemic administration of methotrexate is associated with a significant risk of hepatic fibrosis and cirrhosis, the widespread use of this drug in the treatment of patients with only minimal psoriasis is contraindicated. Certain theoretical and experimental evidence suggests that methotrexate may be effective when applied topically. However, efforts to treat psoriasis locally by intralesional injection or topical application have been unsuccessful.

To increase the percutaneous penetration of methotrexate, the drug was given in concentrations of 0.1%, 0.5%, and 1% in 3% laurocapram gel. It was tested topically in a double-blind clinical trial that included 42 patients with psoriasis vulgaris. None of the patients had received systemic or topical antipsoriatic therapy for at least 1 month before the study. Either the drug formulations or vehicle alone were applied twice daily to a small area of lesional skin for a total of 6 weeks. In each patient 2 different randomly assigned preparations were evaluated in bilaterally distributed plaques. Lesions were scored weekly for scale, erythema, and elevation.

After 6 weeks of treatment, overall improvement of 50% or more in the combined scores for scale, erythema, and elevation was achieved in 64% of the patients given the 0.1% formulation, in 59% of those given the 0.5% formulation, and in 56% of those given the 1% formulation. Only 25% of the patients improved when the vehicle was used alone. Only 2 patients had total clearing of the test sites treated for 6 weeks with 0.1% and 1% methotrexate. However, 1 week after therapy was discontinued the vehicle-treated sites did not differ from the methotrexate-treated sites.

These preliminary findings suggest that methotrexate preparations may have a beneficial effect in the treatment of psoriasis if they provide adequate percutaneous absorption.

▶ The search for a topically effective antimitotic agent for psoriasis continues. This study suggests that new formulations may help us use an old agent, methotrexate, in this way.—R.S. Stern, M.D.

Methotrexate Dosage in Patients Aged Over 50 With Psoriasis

Fairris GM, Dewhurst AG, White JE, Campbell MJ (Royal South Hants Hosp; Southampton Gen Hosp, England)

Br Med J 298:801–802, March 25, 1989 17–23

To test whether psoriasis in elderly patients can be controlled with less than the recommended dose of methotrexate (10–25 mg once a week), studies were made in 23 patients older than 50 years. The minimal therapeutic dose of methotrexate was established by reducing the weekly dose until the disease relapsed. The dose was then increased at intervals of 1 or 2 months until psoriasis was controlled to the patient's satisfaction.

The minimal therapeutic dose of methotrexate needed to control the disease was correlated significantly with both predicted creatinine clearance and age. The weekly therapeutic dose of methotrexate was decreased with decreasing predicted creatinine clearance and increasing age. The progressive deterioration in creatinine clearance associated with the natural aging process may account for the reduced therapeutic dose of methotrexate among the elderly.

▶ This paper provides a clear lesson: Be sure that you determine creatinine clearance in older patients before beginning methotrexate therapy, or, alternatively, begin at lower doses. Because methotrexate is cleared by the kidneys, dosage needs to take into account any diminution in renal function.—R.S. Stern, M.D.

The Role of Liver Biopsies in Psoriatic Patients Receiving Long-Term Methotrexate Treatment: Improvement in Liver Abnormalities After Cessation of Treatment

Newman M, Auerbach R, Feiner H, Holzman RS, Shupack J, Migdal P, Culubret M, Camuto P, Tobias H (New York Univ)

Arch Dermatol 125:1218–1224, September 1989 17–24

The potential development of hepatotoxic reaction remains a major issue in long-term methotrexate therapy. In all, 364 liver biopsy specimens were obtained from 168 patients with psoriasis, many of whom received long-term methotrexate therapy.

Of the 83 patients who underwent liver biopsy before starting methotrexate therapy, 14 had 1 or more risk factors predictive of liver abnormality. All of these patients had normal pretreatment biopsy specimens. Seventeen patients had abnormal biopsy specimens before methotrexate therapy, but only 1 had an identifiable risk factor and 5 had abnormal liver function test results. Thirty-one patients had biopsies before and after methotrexate treatment and 86 had biopsy only after treatment. In these patients the probability of a normal biopsy specimen dropped below 50% at cumulative doses of 3,115 mg and 5,776 mg of methotrexate, respectively. The significant difference found was mainly because patients who had biopsy before and after methotrexate treatment received most of their medication by the parenteral rather than the oral route. Biopsy grade after methotrexate treatment correlated significantly with obesity. Other risk factors and liver chemistry did not correlate with biopsy grade. In 11 patients fibrosis or cirrhosis was seen in liver biopsy specimens; 8 had meaningful improvement in biopsy grade, and none had progression of abnormalities after withdrawal of methotrexate therapy for 6 or more months.

Pathologic fibrotic changes in the liver associated with methotrexate therapy are potentially reversible after withdrawal of treatment. A period of 12 months should be allowed after withdrawal of methotrexate treatment before repeating the liver biopsy in anticipation of possible resumption of therapy.

▶ Because of the nonrandomized nature of this follow-up study, conclusions based on comparing patients with and without pretreatment liver biopsies may not be valid. In contrast to the findings reported in Abstract 17–25, these data suggest that blood tests are poor predictors of liver biopsy results. The apparent improvement in subsequent biopsies among patients with fibrosis or cirrhosis probably reflects sampling variation rather than true improvement. Fibrosis and cirrhosis are unlikely to improve but early on may only involve focal areas. Because a liver biopsy samples only a small piece of the liver, a repeat biopsy may give a quite different picture from that seen in an earlier sample. I do not believe that this paper provides strong evidence that withdrawal of methotrexate reverses fibrotic or cirrhotic changes in the liver.— R.S. Stern, M.D.

Detection of Hepatotoxicity Associated With Methotrexate Therapy for Psoriasis

O'Connor GT, Olmstead EM, Zug K, Baughman RD, Beck JR, Dunn JL, Seal P, Lewandowski JF (Dartmouth-Hitchcock Med Ctr, Hanover, NH)

Arch Dermatol 125:1209–1217, September 1989 17–25

The role of liver function tests and clinical and demographic information in the detection of methotrexate-associated hepatotoxicity was evaluated in a retrospective study of 147 liver biopsy specimens obtained from 78 psoriatic patients treated with the drug. The joint sensitivity of aspartate aminotransferase (AST), alkaline phosphatase (ALP), and total bilirubin values to detect abnormal results from a posttreatment liver biopsy specimen was .86, and the predictive value of a negative test was .93. Logistic regression analysis demonstrated that ALT, ALP, and total bilirubin values correlated positively with the presence of an abnormal liver biopsy specimen, even after adjusting for the confounding effects of age and history of cholecystitis. The concordance index was .92 (perfect, 1.0).

The probability of an abnormal result from a posttreatment liver biopsy specimen could be calculated using the logistic regression model and specific patient information. The mathematical model calculates the independent weight associated with each of the 6 variables, including age, gender, AST value, ALP value, history of cholecystitis, and cumulative dose of methotrexate in relation to the coefficients derived from the regression equation. The model was a highly significant predictor of liver biopsy specimen grade.

A multivariate risk estimation model can predict the likelihood of positive findings from liver biopsy specimens in the detection of methotrexate-associated hepatotoxicity. The clinical use of this model awaits further validation.

▶ An excellent use of mathematical modeling to determine the predictive value, positive and negative, of various laboratory tests in the detection of methotrexate-associated hepatic toxicity. Before this model can be applied to patients with confidence, however, it needs verification in a larger and more heterogeneous population.—R.S. Stern, M.D.

Relapse Rates in Moderately Severe Chronic Psoriasis Treated With Cyclosporin A

Higgins E, Munro C, Marks J, Friedmann PS, Shuster S (Royal Victoria Infirmary, Newcastle Upon Tyne, England)

Br J Dermatol 121:71–74, July 1989 17–26

Cyclosporine A is an effective systemic treatment for psoriasis. Relapse reportedly occurs rapidly on cessation of cyclosporine therapy, but this could be explained by the natural history of the very severe psoriasis in some patients. If clearance were followed by a reasonable remission period and toxicity were negligible, moderately severe psoriasis could be managed with infrequent short courses of cyclosporine. Relapse in psoriasis as it commonly appears in patients with less severe disease was studied in 17 individuals.

All 17 patients had chronic psoriasis, but none had more than 2 attacks severe enough to merit hospitalization in any previous year. Cyclosporine A, 5 mg/kg, was administered daily. Of the 17 patients, 12 had clearing within a mean of 9.25 weeks. By 6 months, 5 of 12 patients had relapsed; this rate was not significantly different from that reported previously with dithranol or psoralens plus ultraviolet A therapy. Continuing cyclosporine for up to 4 weeks after clinical clearance did not offer any advantage. There were no significant adverse effects on renal function or blood pressure.

Common psoriasis requiring hospital treatment responds to cyclosporine A without a rapid relapse after cessation of treatment. The high relapse rates with CsA reported previously were probably related to the severity and natural history of the disease in those patients.

▶ Because patient selection and the definition of flare are such important determinants of time to relapse, open uncontrolled studies on this topic are almost impossible to interpret. The wisdom of the use of cyclosporine in patients with chronic stable psoriasis for whom so many other less toxic therapies are available, even in the short term, would seem to be open to serious question.—R.S. Stern, M.D.

Long-Term Cyclosporin for Psoriasis

Griffiths CEM, Powles AV, McFadden J, Baker BS, Valdimarsson H, Fry L (St Mary's Hosp, London; Landspitalinn, Reykjavik, Iceland)

Br J Dermatol 120:253–260, February 1989 17–27

Cyclosporine is an effective treatment for psoriasis; however, most studies have been of short duration. Because psoriasis can recur relatively quickly on cessation of the drug, it is important to determine the effectiveness and safety of low-dose cyclosporine for long-term maintenance treatment. Thirteen patients with persistent psoriasis unresponsive to other treatment were treated with cyclosporine for periods ranging from 12 to 25 months (mean, 18 months). Doses ranged from 1 to 4 mg/kg/day (mean, 2.8 mg).

At the end of 1 month there was a 72% decline in the mean psoriasis area and severity index (PASI). The reduction was 81% when the study was concluded. There was no tachyphylaxis to cyclosporine in any patient. All patients thought the drug was the most effective treatment they had had and reported fewer side effects with it than with other drugs or photochemotherapy. Topical steroids, given as adjuvant treatment after 3 months, had beneficial effects in 11 of 13 patients; 6 patients became mildly to moderately hypertensive. Hypertension was controlled in 3 with a reduction in cyclosporine dosage; the others received hypotensive agents. The mean serum creatinine level rose from 72 to 90 μM/L during the study. In 7 patients hypertrichosis developed.

Low-dosage cyclosporine appears to be effective in clearing psoriasis and maintaining benefits over the long term. Moderate nonprogressive nephrotoxicity can probably be expected, however.

▶ With the short duration of follow-up for such a toxic drug in such a chronic disease, this cannot be considered to be long-term follow-up. The proportion of patients with side effects, including hypertrichosis, hypertension, and renal function measured by less than the most sensitive methods, strongly suggests that even if this drug works, its chronic toxicity may make its long-term utility quite limited. Even in this small group a squamous cell carcinoma developed in 1 patient 6 months after starting cyclosporine. Recently, more sensitive measurements of renal function suggest that cyclosporine-related renal toxicity may be even greater than is suggested in this article. See the article by Gilbert et al. (1).—R.S. Stern, M.D.

Reference

1. Gilbert, S.C., et al: *J Am Acad Dermatol* 21:470, 1989.

Effectiveness of Cyclosporine Treatment in Severe Psoriasis: A Clinical and Immunologic Study

Finzi AF, Mozzanica N, Cattaneo A, Chiappino G, Pigatto PD (Univ of Milan, Italy)

J Am Acad Dermatol 21:91–97, July 1989 17–28

Cyclosporine is a potent immunosuppressive agent and as such might be useful in the treatment of immune skin diseases. A previous study reported that cyclosporine, even at low doses, is effective in the treatment of psoriasis. An open clinical trial was carried out to assess the efficacy of short-term cyclosporine administration in 13 patients aged 30–67 years hospitalized with severe, diffuse plaque-type psoriasis. Those with pustular or erythrodermic psoriasis were excluded, but 2 patients studied had psoriatic arthropathy of the joints of the hands and feet.

The Psoriasis Area and Severity Index (PASI) was determined before and after the trial. Cyclosporine was given in doses of 3–5 mg/kg/day for the first 3 weeks. If no response was observed, the dose was increased to 5 mg/kg/day for 1–2 weeks. Treatment was stopped at remission or after 5 weeks of treatment. All patients were followed monthly for up to 6 months after cyclosporine therapy was discontinued. Seven patients underwent punch biopsy before and 15 days after the start of cyclosporine therapy.

Within 3–4 weeks of treatment, psoriasis in 12 patients went into remission, and 1 patient had significant improvement. The mean PASI score decreased by 82%; the 1 patient who did not have remission had a 56% decrease in the PASI score. There were no significant changes after the first 7 days of therapy, but within 10 days there was conspicuous improvement in most cases. Cyclosporine also considerably relieved the pain and improved joint function in the 2 patients with articular disease. There were no major side effects. Skin infections developed in 3 patients, but most infections regressed spontaneously after cyclosporine treatment was discontinued. Two other patients had biochemical evidence of slight transient renal dysfunction.

Immunohistologic studies done in 7 patients revealed that psoriatic plaques contain an infiltrate composed mainly of activated helper T lymphocytes. After 15 days of cyclosporine treatment the number of CD4+ cells in the epidermis and dermis decreased significantly, and Langerhans cells were more evenly distributed within the epidermis. Although cyclosporine at low doses was effective in the treatment of severe psoriasis, its potential nephrotoxic side effects limit its use to those patients who can be monitored carefully.

▶ Another study indicating that cyclosporine works but is associated with substantial risks.—R.S. Stern, M.D.

Intralesional Cyclosporin in Psoriasis: Effects on T Lymphocyte and Dendritic Cell Subpopulations

Baker BS, Powles AV, Savage CR, McFadden JP, Valdimarsson H, Fry L (St Mary's Hosp, London; Landspitalinn, Reykjavik, Iceland)
Br J Dermatol 120:207–213, February 1989 17–29

Patients with psoriasis who are treated systemically with cyclosporine A have fewer epidermal and dermal CD4+, CD8+, and DR+ CD8+ T cells before recovery. The effect of the intralesional injection of cyclosporine A on T cells in the plaques was determined in 10 psoriatic patients. Two symmetric plaques in each patient were chosen. One plaque was injected with 3.3–8.3 mg of cyclosporine A, and the other was injected with saline on 6 occasions over 12 days. Two days later, biopsy specimens were obtained double blind and examined with the double-labeling immunofluorescent technique.

The cyclosporine-treated plaques cleared significantly better. Total CD4+, CD8+, and DR+ CD4+ T cells were significantly fewer in the treated plaques than in the control plaques. Also, T lymphocytes were significantly decreased in the dermis of treated plaques. Total numbers of dendritic cells were not decreased with cyclosporine treatment; however, DR+CD1– dendritic cells were decreased significantly, and DR–CD1+– dendritic cells were increased significantly in treated plaques.

The intralesional injection of cyclosporine A appears to be effective in the treatment of psoriatic plaques, and T lymphocytes appear to be implicated in the mechanism of cyclosporine action. A topical application of cyclosporine that could penetrate lesions would be a successful treatment that would avoid the side effects of systemic cyclosporine.

▶ The authors believe that the effect of intralesional cyclosporine is a result of its effects on T lymphocytes. Although cyclosporine does affect T lymphocytes, it also has antiproliferative effects in keratinocytes in culture.—R.S. Stern, M.D.

Cyclosporine in the Treatment of Psoriatic Arthritis

Gupta AK, Matteson EL, Ellis CN, Ho VC, Tellner DC, Voorhees JJ, McCune WJ (Univ of Michigan)
Arch Dermatol 125:507–510, April 1989 17–30

The prevalence of arthritis among patients with psoriasis has been estimated to be 5% to 7%, but it may be as high as 39% in hospitalized patients with psoriasis. Anecdotal reports have suggested that oral cyclosporine may be effective in the treatment of psoriatic arthritis. The short-term efficacy of cyclosporine in the treatment of psoriatic arthritis was evaluated in an open study.

Six patients with moderately severe to severe psoriatic arthritis were given cyclosporine orally, 6 mg/kg/day for 8 weeks. Significant improvement was noted in all patients within 2–4 weeks. Rheumatologic assessment at the end of therapy revealed certain trends in disease activity.

There was a reduction in the number of tender joints, the joint tenderness index, and duration of morning stiffness; an increase in grip strength was observed. There was also a reduction in the number of swollen joints, the joint swelling index, and the time needed to walk 50 ft. Overall, psoriatic arthritis was significantly improved, as independently assessed by the patient and physician. Both psoriasis and psoriatic arthritis worsened within 4 weeks of discontinuation of therapy.

Short-term, low-dose cyclosporine therapy may be an effective treatment in patients with psoriasis and psoriatic arthritis. Larger double-blind studies are needed to confirm these preliminary findings and to determine the relationship of therapeutic benefit to toxicity.

▶ Cyclosporine is effective in rheumatoid arthritis. Therefore, improvement of psoriatic arthritis, as documented in the study, is not surprising. This is a suppressive, not a remitting, agent. In most cases, less toxic therapy can be utilized.—R.S. Stern, M.D.

Systemic Therapy With Fumaric Acid Derivates: New Possibilities in the Treatment of Psoriasis

Nieboer C, de Hoop D, van Loenen AC, Langendijk PNJ, van Dijk E (Free Univ Hosp, Amsterdam; Stichting Ziekenhuisvoorzieningen Gelderse Vallei, Ede-Bennekom, The Netherlands)

J Am Acad Dermatol 20:601–608, April 1989 17–31

Fumaric acid (FA) therapy is a popular treatment for psoriasis in western Europe. Some studies show poor therapeutic results and serious side effects, however. To clarify the situation, several controlled studies were undertaken with derivatives of FA: monoethylfumaric acid ester (MEFAE) sodium and dimethylfumaric acid ester (DMFAE).

Six different studies were conducted. All patients had stable nummular and plaque psoriasis with at least 10% involvement of the body surface. Study 1 was an open study with FA compound therapy (FACT); study 2 was a controlled study with MEFAE sodium *vs.* placebo; study 3 was a controlled study with DMFAE *vs.* placebo. Study 4 compared therapy with 720 mg of MEFAE sodium with 240 mg of MEFAE sodium. Study 5 was a continuation study with DMFAE, and study 6 was a controlled study with topical MEFAE applied in different concentrations.

Treatment with MEFAE sodium in dosages of up to 240 mg daily was ineffective in the treatment of psoriasis. Daily dosages of 720 mg brought a significant decrease in scaling and itching but did not affect extension of the eruption. In 240-mg daily dosages, DMFAE produced a significant reduction in symptoms and prevented extension. Side effects of FA treatment included diarrhea, nausea, general malaise, and severe stomachache. With the 720-mg dosage of MEFAE and with the 240-mg dosage of DMFAE, there were mild disturbances of liver and kidney function. Also, a relative lymphopenia with a selective decrease of suppressor T lymphocytes was found in 50% of patients treated with DMFAE.

Oral treatment with FA derivatives should still be considered an experimental treatment of psoriasis. However, this therapy deserves further study.

▶ A bit confusing: So many treatment groups, each of which is so small it is hard to draw reliable inferences from the data. Given the level of efficacy and side effects demonstrated, these compounds do not seem all that promising for psoriasis therapy.—R.S. Stern, M.D.

Antipsoriatic Effect of Semi-Occlusive Treatment: O_2-Consumption, Blood Flow, and Temperature Measurements Compared to Clinical Parameters

Broby-Johansen U, Kristensen JK (Univ of Copenhagen)

Clin Exp Dermatol 14:286–288, July 1989 17–32

Measured by transcutaneous polarographic electrodes, oxygen consumption might relfect the clinical activity of psoriasis and the efficacy of treatment. The effects of a semiocclusive hydrocolloid dressing were monitored by changes in oxygen consumption, skin temperature, and cutaneous blood flow in 10 patients with chronic plaque-type psoriasis.

Daily treatment with crude coal tar was used, sparing the areas under study. The patients had a general relapse with involvement of 30% to 90% of the body surface. Cutaneous blood flow was measured with a laser-Doppler flowmeter.

A clinical effect was evident from the first day of treatment, although several patients had a slight reduction in ratings for untreated test sites. Only 2 patients remained in complete remission after 3 months. Clinical improvement was not associated with significant change in any of the objective measures.

▶ This very interesting study shows that almost complete occlusion (hydrocolloids are almost completely occlusive) works as well as tar in the therapy of psoriasis. The true semiocclusive thin film membranes will not work. I tried this myself about 7 years ago. Because the mechanism is not elucidated here, more research needs to be done. I would suggest looking at a variety of growth factors, particularly the angiogenesis factor, as normalization of the papillary cutaneous vasculature seems to be a key factor in psoriasis improvement.—J.C. Alper, M.D.

18 Urticaria and Mast Cell Disorders

The Effect of Psoralen Photochemotherapy (PUVA) on Symptomatic Dermographism

Logan RA, O'Brien TJ, Greaves MW (St John's Hosp for Diseases of the Skin, London)

Clin Exp Dermatol 14:25–28, January 1989 18–1

Treatment of symptomatic dermographism with antihistamine is ineffective in some patients. Because the symptoms are distressing, an alternative treatment is desirable.

Fourteen adults with symptomatic dermographism poorly controlled with antihistamines received treatment with photochemotherapy to the whole body 3 times a week for 4 weeks. Two hours before irradiation, oral 8-methoxypsoralen, 0.6 mg/kg, was given. Initial doses of ultraviolet A (UVA) were based on the patient's skin type. Doses of UVA were increased weekly at varying rates, depending on the patient's tolerance. A control area on the upper back was covered with aluminum foil during treatment. Patients were evaluated before treatment, after 2 weeks of treatment, and at the end of the course.

Five patients had clinically significant reductions in itching, but 4 of them had relapses to pretreatment levels of itching within 3 months of the final treatment. Even among patients who experienced symptomatic relief there was no significant change in skin reactivity between the wheal and flare responses in treated skin and those in control skin.

Photochemotherapy may temporarily bring symptomatic relief in some patients with symptomatic dermographism. However, results do not justify its use in most of these patients.

► Dermographism is present in 25% of the "normal" population. The word is *"symptomatic"* dermographism—a level of discomfort that affects the patient adversely; causes are said to be thyroid disorders, pregnancy, menopause, diabetes, food allergens, drugs (penicillin), during infestations, and after wasp and bee stings; yet in a large study there was no association with systemic diseases, food allergens, atopic diathesis, or medications (1). Curiously, dermographism is not necessarily present in chronic urticaria, although 50% of patients studied by Winkelmann (2) had chronic or acute urticaria.

This negative study of the effect of PUVA photochemotherapy on dermographism emphasizes the necessity of careful investigation of patients and use of control sites: there was no change in skin reactivity between the wheal and flare responses in PUVA-treated skin compared to control, although the patients had symptomatic relief. It would be interesting to repeat this study using placebo PUVA (i.e., oral placebo capsules plus UVA) to see if there is symptomatic relief.—T.B. Fitzpatrick, M.D., Ph.D.

References

1. Breathnach SM, et al: *Clin Exp Dermatol* 8:463, 1983.
2. Winkelmann RK: *J Cutan Pathol* 12:485, 1985.

Therapy of Chronic Idiopathic Urticaria With Nifedipine: Demonstration of Beneficial Effect in a Double-Blinded, Placebo-Controlled, Crossover Trial

Bressler RB, Sowell K, Huston DP (Baylor College of Medicine; Methodist Hosp, Houston)

J Allergy Clin Immunol 83:756–763, April 1989 18–2

Chronic idiopathic urticaria is usually treated symptomatically. Nifedipine may inhibit the release of inflammatory mediators from mast cells and therefore may be beneficial in the management of this disorder. Ten patients with chronic urticaria of unknown origin refractory to maximally tolerated doses of H_1 and H_2 antihistamines were evaluated in a double-blind, placebo-controlled, crossover trial. Patients were treated with placebo or nifedipine for 4 weeks and then crossed over to the other treatment for another 4 weeks.

Seven patients completed the study. All 7 clearly demonstrated a therapeutic effect of nifedipine, and all 7 experienced significant improvement in weekly hive count, weekly hive index, and weekly itch index. None of these parameters improved significantly with placebo. The endpoint hive index and itch index were also significantly improved with nifedipine as compared to placebo. The drug was well tolerated.

Nifedipine appears to be a safe and effective adjunct to antihistamine therapy in patients with chronic idiopathic urticaria. This finding is particularly important in that a significant number of patients continue to have disease despite treatment with maximally tolerated doses of antihistamine.

▶ The therapeutic benefit of nifedipine, a calcium channel antagonist, in the treatment of chronic idiopathic urticaria should be confirmed in other controlled trials. Of theoretical importance is the effect of this agent on histamine release from mast cells and on the proliferation of lymphocytes. Each of these cell types is increased in number in the lesional skin of patients with chronic idiopathic urticaria (1).—N.A. Soter, M.D.

Reference

1. Elias J, et al: *J Allergy Clin Immunol* 78:914, 1986.

Clinical Evaluation of Ketotifen for Chronic Urticaria: Multicenter Double-Blind Comparative Study With Clemastine

Kamide R, Niimura M, Ueda H, Imamura S, Yamamoto S, Yoshida H, Kukita A (Jikei Univ, Tokyo; Fujita Gakuen Health Univ, Aichi Prefecture; Kyoto Univ; Hiroshima Univ; Nagasaki Univ; et al)
Ann Allergy 62:322–325, April 1989 18–3

Urticaria, a common problem, usually appears as itching and wheals accompanied by sudden local redness. It frequently disappears completely within several hours. Histamine release from cutaneous mast cells around the capillaries undoubtedly plays an important role in the development of ordinary urticaria. A multicenter double-blind comparative study was made of ketotifen and clemastine in the treatment of chronic urticaria.

Patients with chronic urticaria who had repeated eruptions of unknown origin for at least 1 month, as well as itching and maculae, were given either a ketotifen capsule or a clemastine tablet. Of 305 patients who began the study, 151 receiving ketotifen and 137 receiving clemastine were included in the analysis. Both treatment groups had marked reductions in the severity of maculae, but the decreases were significantly greater in the patients given ketotifen by the end of the second week. The intensity of itching rapidly lessened in both groups, but the decrease was greater in the ketotifen-treated group. When cases considered moderately improved or better were considered, the final global improvement ratings in the ketotifen- and clemastine-treated groups were 70.2% and 57.7%, respectively. When the final global improvement and safety ratings were combined, the utility rating for ketotifen was significantly higher than that of clemastine.

Ketotifen is significantly more effective and safer than clemastine, a standard antihistamine, in the treatment of chronic urticaria. Ketotifen may also be useful in preventing recurrence.

▶ Ketotifen is an antiallergic therapeutic agent that has several mechanisms of action, including the prevention of mast cell histamine release induced by IgE and compound 48/80 in vitro, inhibition of passive cutaneous anaphylaxis in vivo, antagonism of histamine at the H1 receptor site, and calcium channel blockade. In addition, it can diminish the wheal-and-erythema reaction induced by platelet-activating factor in vivo (1). Ketotifen also has been reported to control the cutaneous symptoms of urticaria pigmentosa (2).—N.A. Soter, M.D.

References

1. Chung KF, et al: *J Allergy Clin Immunol* 81:1192, 1988.
2. Czarnetski BM, et al: *Br J Dermatol* 105:563, 1981.

Comparative Study of Astemizole and Terfenadine in the Treatment of Chronic Idiopathic Urticaria: A Randomized Double-Blind Study of 40 Patients

Paul E, Bödeker R-H (Universität Giessen, West Germany)
Ann Allergy 62:318–320, April 1989 18–4

Terfenadine, a new type of histamine H_1-receptor blocker, has become widely accepted in the treatment of chronic urticaria and other allergic disorders. The drug is beneficial and produces slight or no sedative effects. Terfenadine was tested as a reference substance against another new antihistamine, astemizole, in a randomized, double-blind study.

Forty patients with chronic urticaria were treated with terfenadine or astemizole. Patients quantified and documented the intensity of their symptoms every day. Both terfenadine and astemizole resulted in reduction of the intensity of pruritus and the severity of wheals. Side effects were rare and generally not serious with both antihistamines. Among patients taking astemizole, 2 complained of headaches and 1 of constipation. Among those taking terfenadine, 1 patient complained of "congestion in the head" and 1 of dry mouth.

Both terfenadine and astemizole affect the intensity of pruritus and the severity of wheals in patients with chronic urticaria. Neither antihistamine produced sedative side effects in this series.

▶ Low-sedating H_1 antihistamines are a welcome addition in the treatment of dermatologic disorders. At the present time, terfenadine and astemizole are the 2 agents available in the United States, although others will become available in the future. Although these agents are comparable in terms of efficacy and lack of side effects, their pharmacokinetics differ in that terfenadine has a rapid onset of action and astemizole a delayed onset of action.—N.A. Soter, M.D.

Treatment of Chronic Idiopathic Urticaria With Astemizole

Huerter CJ, Bergfeld WF, Wagner WO, Dijkstra JWE (Cleveland Clinic Found)
Cleve Clin J Med 56:263–266, May 1989 18–5

Astemizole is a long-acting H_1 receptor antagonist that has proven effective in the treatment of chronic idiopathic urticaria; it does not cause the typical antihistaminic side effects. In an open clinical trial 20 patients received astemizole for 8 weeks to assess the efficacy of the drug in reducing symptoms of chronic idiopathic urticaria as well as to assess the side effects.

Seventeen patients completed the study; 1 withdrew at 4 weeks because of the drug's ineffectiveness; another withdrew because of side effects, and the third because of protocol violation. Astemizole significantly reduced the signs and symptoms of urticaria, as well as its severity, by anatomical location. Five patients reported complete clearing. No patient reported sedation or anticholinergic effects, but a significant weight gain was observed.

Astemizole appears to be effective in treating chronic idiopathic urticaria. Its major drawback appears to be weight gain. Although further studies are warranted, astemizole may allow the reduction or discontinuation of systemic corticosteroids in patients who require chronic steroid therapy for control of urticaria.

▶ This open trial with astemizole in the treatment of chronic idiopathic urticaria confirms previous studies. Astemizole, one of several new low-sedating H_1 antihistamines, is effective in the treatment of urticaria.—N.A. Soter, M.D.

Rubber Contact Urticaria: Allergenic Properties of 19 Brands of Latex Gloves

Turjanmaa K, Laurila K, Mäkinen-Kiljunen S, Reunala T (Univ of Tampere, Helsinki)

Contact Dermatitis (Copenhagen) 19:362–367, November 1988 18–6

Contact urticaria from latex (natural rubber) surgical and cleaning gloves appears to be a common condition that is not detected easily. The diagnosis can be confirmed with prick tests, and specific IgE antibodies can be demonstrated by the latex radioallergosorbent test. Differences between skin reactivity to various laser surgical and cleaning gloves were examined by prick test in 40 persons, 26 of whom were sensitized to surgical and 14 to cleaning latex gloves.

Six of 17 surgical gloves and 1 of 2 cleaning gloves (table) produced positive reactions in more than 87% of allergic persons. The frequencies

Trade Names and Manufacturers of the 21 Gloves Examined

Latex surgical gloves

1. Ansell Gammex, Ansell Rubber Co. Ltd., Malacca, Malaysia
2. Ansell No Powder, Ansell Rubber Co. Ltd., Malacca, Malaysia
3. Eudermic, Becton Dickinson, New Jersey, USA
4. Exona, Semperit, Vienna, Austria
5. Glads, Ansell Rubber Co. Ltd., Bangkok, Thailand
6. Micro-Touch, Johnson & Johnson, Arlington, Texas, USA
7. Neutralon Brown, Johnson & Johnson, Arlington, Texas, USA
8. Opett, Semperit, Vienna, Austria
9. Opett Comf. Powderfree Brown, Semperit, Vienna, Austria
10. Opett Derma, Semperit, Vienna, Austria
11. Perry microptic, Smith & Nephew, Massilon, Ohio, USA
12. Perry orthopedic, Smith & Nephew, Massilon, Ohio, USA
13. Perry white latex, Smith & Nephew, Massilon, Ohio, USA
14. Puritee, The Puritee Medical Company Ltd., Slough, Berks, UK
15. Sempermed, Semperit, Vienna, Austria
16. Travenol Ultralan, Travenol Laboratories SA, Lessines, Belgium
17. Triflex, Travenol Laboratories SA, Lessines, Belgium

Latex cleaning gloves

18. Marigold, LRC Products Ltd., London, England
19. Natura, Vascongada de Gaucho y Latex, Spain

Non-latex control gloves

20. Elastyren, Danpren Gloves A/S, Albertslund, Denmark
21. Triflex vinyl, Travenol Laboratories SA, Lessines, Belgium

(Courtesy of Turjanmaa K, Laurila K, Mäkinen-Kiljunen S, et al: *Contact Dermatitis (Copenhagen)* 19:362–367, November 1988.)

of positive reactions to 4 other surgical latex gloves were as low as 8% to 21%, suggesting that not all surgical gloves are equally allergenic. Control prick tests with 1 synthetic rubber and 1 polyvinyl chloride glove were negative for all persons. Two surgical latex gloves that produced either a high or low number of positive prick tests in allergic persons were analyzed by high-pressure liquid chromatography. Similar allergenic protein fractions revealed protein peaks at molecular weights of 2,000, 5,000, and 30,000 daltons. Corresponding proteins were noted in 1 latex cleaning glove and in natural rubber.

All 19 latex gloves produced positive prick tests, confirming that they contain an allergen. However, the frequencies of positive test reactions ranged from 100% to 8%, suggesting that there are differences in the composition or amount of latex allergen eluting from these gloves.

Clinical Observations on Delayed Pressure Urticaria

Warin RP (Bristol Royal Infirmary, England)

Br J Dermatol 121:225–228, August 1989 18–7

Several aspects of delayed pressure urticaria (DPU) necessitate prolonged study of individual patients. Many tests designed to produce experimental wheals in DPU are not satisfactory for outpatients, including the usual method of pressing the dermographometer point hard onto the skin and then observing the results 4–6 hours later. A new approach was developed.

Method.—A glass sphere 1.5 cm in diameter is used to concentrate the pressure on the outer aspect of the forearm beneath a cuff to which a plastic bag containing various household materials is attached to make up the approximate weight. The patient carries out the test 4–10 hours before each appointment.

Repeated pressure tests at regular intervals were done on 48 patients with DPU. There were considerable variations in response, with periods of positive testing ranging from a few days to months or years. All 48 patients had chronic urticaria or angioedema, or both, although some had only minor and occasional attacks. Pressure tests were also done at regular intervals on 7 patients with chronic urticaria who had wheals at pressure sites but no history of pressure-induced wheals. These wheals coincided with positive pressure tests. Probably, these patients had DPU, but only for a short time.

Delayed dermographism was studied in 8 patients with DPU. A good correlation in time and degree was noted between positive pressure tests and delayed dermographism, which confirms that delayed dermographism is in fact DPU provoked by a slightly different mode of pressure.

Most patients with DPU tend to have the condition for a prolonged time, although the disease fluctuates. Many patients clearly have phases when DPU is apparent and when the tests are positive. These phases can last for only a few days or for years and may recur at intervals, often coinciding with an increase of any chronic urticaria or angioedema. This variability in response may be responsible for negative results of tests in patients with a history of DPU.

▶ This study points out some of the nuances in evaluating patients with chronic forms of urticaria. Most of the patients with DPU also experienced chronic idiopathic urticaria. Patients without a history of pressure-induced lesions may have positive reactions after pressure challenges. The observation that delayed dermographism was associated with positive pressure tests leads to the suggestion that delayed dermographism is a form of pressure urticaria, a concept that has been proposed previously (1) but is not universally accepted (2).—N.A. Soter, M.D.

References

1. Dover JS, et al: *J Am Acad Dermatol* 18:1289, 1988.
2. Shuster S: *J Am Acad Dermatol* 21:588, 1989.

The Oak Processionary Caterpillar (*Thaumetopoea processionea* L) and Man: Urticating Apparatus and Mechanism of Action

Lamy M, Novak F, Duboscq MF, Ducombs G, Maleville J (Univ of Bordeaux, France)

Ann Dermatol Venereol 115:1023–1032, 1988 18–8

In 1985 and 1986, a well-known tourist spot in France, the Poitou-Charentes area, had significant swarming of the oak processionary caterpillar (OPC). This influx was accompanied by a significantly greater incidence of serious skin reactions. The venom secreted by the hair glands of the OPC has long been known to cause urticaria in humans. The pine processionary caterpillar (PPC) has been well described, but the OPC has not.

Hairs removed from the backs of OPCs under ether anesthesia were studied with electron microscopy to assess their morphology. The hairs were also analyzed with electrophoresis on acrylamide gel to identify the proteins responsible for the urticating properties of the secreted venom. The findings were compared with thaumetopoein, the known urticating protein secreted by the PPC.

Electron microscopy showed that the structure of the hairs and hair sacs of the OPC is similar to that of the PPC, and that the nomenclature used to describe the PPC may also be applied to the OPC. Comparison of the electrophoretograms of both caterpillar species revealed that OPC hair glands secrete a thaumetopoein-like protein that has a structure similar to that of the protein secreted by the PPC. The proteins from both species were found on biologic testing to be equally toxic and to have similar histamine-releasing effects.

Oak processionary caterpillars are the most urticating when they are in their last larval stage, which occurs between the end of June and the middle of July. The contact dermatitis caused by the OPC's venom is clinically similar to that caused by the PPC. Persons who come into contact with the OPC venom, perhaps while camping, usually have characteristic orange papules 3–5 mm in size on the upper extremities. Most signs and symptoms disappear within 48 hours after administration of an antihistamine preparation.

The urticating apparatus of both the OPC and the PPC species remains in the forest environment all year long while the caterpillar itself completes its transformation into a butterfly. Its ever-present venom constitutes a permanent risk for painful skin reactions.

▶ In the United States the gypsy moth caterpillar *Lymantria dispar* has been associated with urticaria as well as, at times, rhinitis, eye irritation, and shortness of breath. Wheal-and-flare reactions occur after scratch tests with lyophilized extracts of the caterpillar, and histamine has been measured in the hairlike setae. The cutaneous lesions may be caused by contact with free, wind-blown setae or by direct contact with setae on the caterpillar (1).—N.A. Soter, M.D.

Reference

1. Shama SK, et al: *N Engl J Med* 306:1300, 1982.

Hematopathology of the Bone Marrow in Pediatric Cutaneous Mastocytosis: A Study of 17 Patients

Kettelhut BV, Parker RI, Travis WD, Metcalfe DD (Natl Inst of Allergy and Infectious Diseases, Bethesda, Md; Clinical Ctr, NIH, Bethesda)

Am J Clin Pathol 91:558–562, May 1989 18–9

Systemic mastocytosis can be diagnosed in patients with adult-onset urticaria pigmentosa (UP) by identifying characteristic focal collections of mast cells in bone marrow biopsy specimens. Detailed studies of bone marrow from adults with UP and systemic mastocytosis have been reported, but similar studies have not been performed on bone marrow specimens from children. Sixteen bone marrow aspirates and 15 trephine core biopsy specimens from 17 children with documented cutaneous mastocytosis were assessed for evidence of mast cell infiltrates and other bone marrow abnormalities.

Fifteen specimens showed up; 2 showed diffuse cutaneous mastocytosis. Eight bone marrow aspirates from 8 children and 23 trephine core bone marrow biopsy specimens from 16 children, examined for hematologic abnormalities not associated with cutaneous mastocytosis, comprised a control group. Eosinophilia was prominent in 9 of the specimens of cutaneous mastocytosis. Elevated mast cell numbers in bone marrow aspirates were noted in 5 children with cutaneous mastocytosis and in 2 controls. Evaluation of the trephine core bone marrow biopsy specimens revealed focal perivascular and paratrabecular aggregates, consisting of mast cells, eosinophils, and early myeloid cells, in 10 of 15 children. Similar lesions were found in trephine core bone marrow biopsy specimens from 3 control patients. The focal mast cell lesions that characterize adult systemic mastocytosis were not seen.

Cutaneous mastocytosis in children typically resolves by adulthood and is rarely associated with definitive bone marrow findings suggestive of systemic mast cell disease.

▶ The authors confirm the impression that bone marrow involvement in pediatric cutaneous mastocytosis is usually absent, consistent with the observations that pediatric mastocytosis is most commonly a self-limited disease whose symptoms, if any, are likely related to the release of mediators (e.g., histamine) from the cutaneous mast cells themselves. Bone marrow aspirates and biopsies in children should be restricted to those with unexplained anemia, leukocytosis, thrombocytopenia, or hepatosplenomegaly.— R. Masters, M.D.

Solid and Hematologic Malignancies in 60 Patients With Systemic Mast Cell Disease

Travis WD, Li C-Y, Bergstralh EJ (Mayo Clinic and Found, Rochester, Minn)
Arch Pathol Lab Med 113:365–368, April 1989 18–10

It is recognized that solid and hematologic malignant tumors occur in patients with systemic mast cell disease (SMCD), but the nature of the

Temporal Relationship of Malignancies to Systemic Mast Cell Disease (SMCD)

Time	No. of Cases
Group 1	
Before SMCD	
Lymphoma (well-differentiated lymphocytic type)	1
Breast carcinoma	2*
Total	**3**
Concurrent with SMCD	
Lymphoma (well-differentiated lymphocytic type)	1*
Acute nonlymphocytic leukemia	2
Refractory anemia with excess blasts in tranformation	1
Total	**4**
After SMCD (1 d to 5 mo)	
Pancreatic adenocarcinoma	1
Acute nonlymphocytic leukemia	2
Gastric adenocarcinoma	1
Small-cell carcinoma of the lung	1
Total	**5**
After SMCD (6 to 11 mo)	
Acute nonlymphocytic leukemia	3
Group 2	
After SMCD (>12 mo)	
Transitional cell carcinoma of the bladder	1
Breast adenocarcinoma	1
Malignant lymphoma (diffuse large-cell type)	1
Pleural mesothelioma	1*
Total	**4**

*One patient with breast carcinoma also had a pleural mesothelioma; another patient with breast carcinoma also had a well-differentiated lymphocytic type of lymphoma.

(Courtesy of Travis WD, Li C-Y, Bergstralh EJ: *Arch Pathol Lab Med* 113:365–368, April 1989.)

relationship is not well understood. Patients with SMCD may be at increased risk for the development of malignancy. Solid vs. hematologic malignancies may also be significant in patients with SMCD. Sixty patients with SMCD were reviewed for signs and symptoms of mastocytosis, the presence of malignancy, and family history or other risk factors for malignancy. Slides were reviewed in each case.

Nineteen malignancies were found in 17 patients. There were 8 solid tumors, 7 acute nonlymphocytic leukemias, 3 malignant lymphomas, and 1 refractory anemia with excess blasts in transformation. Of 17 patients, 13 had malignancies either before or within 12 months of SMCD diagnosis (table). Statistical analysis showed that patients with SMCD are not at increased risk for malignancy following the diagnosis of SMCD. The variety of solid malignancies indicated a random distribution; in contrast, the hematologic malignancies appeared to principally affect the myeloid cells.

Most associated neoplasms appear before or within 1 year of the diagnosis of SMCD; therefore, patients with SMCD may not have an increased risk of malignancies developing after the diagnosis of SMCD. Both solid and hematologic malignancies may have an adverse effect on the prognosis in patients with SMCD, but the distribution of solid tumors appears to be random, whereas the predominance of myeloid hematologic disorders suggests that SMCD may represent a myeloproliferative disorder.

▶ The authors are careful to suggest that their data indicate that patients with SMCD may not be at increased risk for other malignancies. They conclude their paper by citing 3 additional cases of SMCD associated with 4 malignancies (2 solid tumors and 2 dysmyelopoietic syndromes), which appeared after their statistics were completed. I don't think the last word is in on this subject.—R. Masters, M.D.

19 Vascular Disorders

Intralesional Corticosteroid Therapy for Infantile Hemangiomas
Sloan GM, Reinisch JF, Nichter LS, Saber WL, Lew K, Morwood DT (Childrens Hosp of Los Angeles; Univ of Southern California, Los Angeles)
Plast Reconstr Surg 83:459–466, March 1989 19–1

Successful management of infantile hemangiomas with systemic corticosteroids has been reported. Because of the potentially serious adverse effects of systemic corticosteroids, intralesional corticosteroid treatment, primarily for eyelid hemangiomas, has been explored. Direct intralesional corticosteroid therapy for infantile hemangiomas in a variety of locations was investigated.

Intralesional corticosteroid injections were performed in 31 hemangiomas in 30 infants aged 1–10 months at the time of the first injection. One to 5 injections were given 6 weeks apart in each case. Lesions were located in the head and neck region, except for 1, which was on the buttock. A betamethasone acetate and triamcinolone acetonide mixture was used. Four lesions (13%) virtually disappeared. Ten lesions (32%) had a more than 50% reduction in volume, and another 10 showed a definite but less than 50% reduction in volume. Seven lesions (23%) decreased only little or not at all. None of the lesions showed further growth. All of the injections were given without anesthesia. There were no significant complications.

Intralesional corticosteroid injections are a reasonably safe, effective treatment for hemangiomas in properly selected infants. Because any therapeutic modality has potential complications, this approach is recommended only for rapidly growing, symptomatic, or particularly deforming lesions.

▶ This study documents the usefulness of intralesional corticosteroid therapy in 30 infants and 31 "hemangiomata." A good or excellent response was reported in 45% of cases. Unfortunately, it is difficult to determine if the poor response in half the cases was related to unique features of the hemangiomata treated, method of treatment, or misclassification. There was no clear definition provided to distinguish true hemangiomata (endothelial proliferation) from vascular malformation (abnormal, dilated vessels). Vascular malformations do not seem to respond to corticosteroid therapy. Corticosteroid therapy in this series was fraught with the usual complications, so the indications for its use should be clearly documented.—A.R. Rhodes, M.D., M.P.H.

Clinical Parameters and Transcutaneous Oxygen Measurements for the Prognosis of Venous Ulcers

Nemeth AJ, Eaglstein WH, Falanga V (Univ of Pittsburgh)

J Am Acad Dermatol 20:186–190, February 1989 19–2

Transcutaneous oxygen pressure ($TcPO_2$) monitoring is a simple, rapid, noninvasive technique for determining local tissue oxygen delivery through the skin. Whether the measurement of $TcPO_2$ levels at the ulcer site in patients with venous skin ulcers would be useful as a prognostic tool was evaluated in 4 men and 10 women with venous ulcers in 14 limbs who were studied prospectively. The mean age was 69.6 years, and ulcers had been present for a mean duration of 15.6 months before referral. All 14 patients underwent extensive evaluation, which included $TcPO_2$ studies. The mean follow-up period was 10.5 months.

During the follow-up period the ulcers of 4 patients (29%) healed with conservative treatment after a mean healing time of 4.8 months. Treatment consisted of topical and systemic antibiotics and conventional and occlusive dressings. None of the other 10 patients had ulcer healing. One ulcer that had been healed for 5 months later recurred. Only 1 of the 7 patients who had more than 1 ulcer had an ulcer that healed.

In all patients the mean ulcer $TcPO_2$ level was significantly reduced when compared with the control chest site. However, there was no significant difference between the mean ulcer $TcPO_2$ levels in healed and unhealed ulcers. Thus $TcPO_2$ levels may not be predictive of the response to therapy in venous ulcers.

▶ This is a very important study. There are those investigators of wound healing who believe that oxygen tension at the base of wounds is one of the most important factors to measure when assessing the ability of certain devices to help improve the ability to heal. It is important for other laboratories to confirm these data.—J.C. Alper, M.D.

Enhancement of Wound Healing by Topical Treatment With Epidermal Growth Factor

Brown GL, Nanney LB, Griffen J, Cramer AB, Yancey JM, Curtsinger LJ III, Holtzin L, Schultz GS, Jurkiewicz MJ, Lynch JB (Emory Univ; Vanderbilt Univ; Univ of Louisville)

N Engl J Med 321:76–79, July 13, 1989 19–3

Epidermal growth factor (EGF) accelerates epidermal regeneration of skin graft donor sites and partial-thickness burns in animals. In a prospective, randomized, double-blind study the effect of topically applied EGF on the healing rate of skin graft donor sites was tested in 12 patients who required skin grafting for reconstructive surgery or burns. Paired donor sites were prepared for each patient: 1 was treated with silver sulfadiazine cream alone and the other was treated with the cream combined with biosynthetic EGF, 10 μm/mL. Healing was assessed by planimetric studies of daily photographs.

Treatment with cream containing EGF lessened the average time to reach 25% and 50% healing by about 1 day and the time to reach 75% and 100% healing by about 1.5 days. These results were supported by punch biopsy sections taken from the donor sites 3 days after healing began. Follow-up a maximum of 1 year later showed no evidence of complications, including neoplasia, in the healed donor sites.

When EGF is topically applied to partial-thickness donor sites, it accelerates the healing rate in human beings. This ability could be of clinical value in patients with a large wound area but limited donor area. The full clinical implications of these observations remain to be explored.

▶ This study unquestionably shows that EGF-treated *clean* donor sites heal, on the average, about 1.5 days faster than those treated with silver sulfadiazine (SSD) cream. The real questions, however, are these: (1) Is the 1.5 days worth the very significant cost difference between EGF and SSD: (2) Will the same effect occur in chronic, bacterially contaminated wounds? (3) What subgroups of wounds might benefit from such an expensive type of therapy?—J.C. Alper, M.D.

Treatment of Skin Ulcers With Cultured Epidermal Allografts

Phillips TJ, Kehinde O, Green H, Gilchrest BA (Boston Univ; Harvard Med School)

J Am Acad Dermatol 21:191–199, August 1989 19–4

Treating skin ulcers in elderly, diabetic, paraplegic, or other debilitated patients can be difficult. Because keratinocytes from neonates are more responsive to mitogens than those from older donors, the response of skin ulcers to treatment with cultured epidermal allografts derived from neonatal foreskin was investigated.

Thirty-six nonhealing skin ulcers in 23 patients were treated with cultured allogeneic epidermal sheets derived from neonatal foreskin. Complete healing occurred in 73% of the ulcers within 8 weeks, with a mean healing time of 3.3 weeks. In the remaining 27% of ulcers there was a decrease in size of 35% to 93% within 8 weeks. Pain was markedly relieved within 24 hours of grafting in 30 painful ulcers. The cultured epidermal sheets acted by stimulation of host keratinocytes to divide and migrate instead of by permanent acceptance of the allograft. Of the 26 ulcers that healed within 8 weeks, 88.5% remained healed for 10–18 months, with an overall mean duration of healing of 13 months (Fig 19–1).

Cultured allografts derived from neonatal foreskin can be helpful in the treatment of difficult skin ulcers. Such allografts offer the advantages of rapid growth in culture and immediate availability. They obviate skin biopsies, are simple to apply, and can be stored for future use; also, grafting procedure is painless.

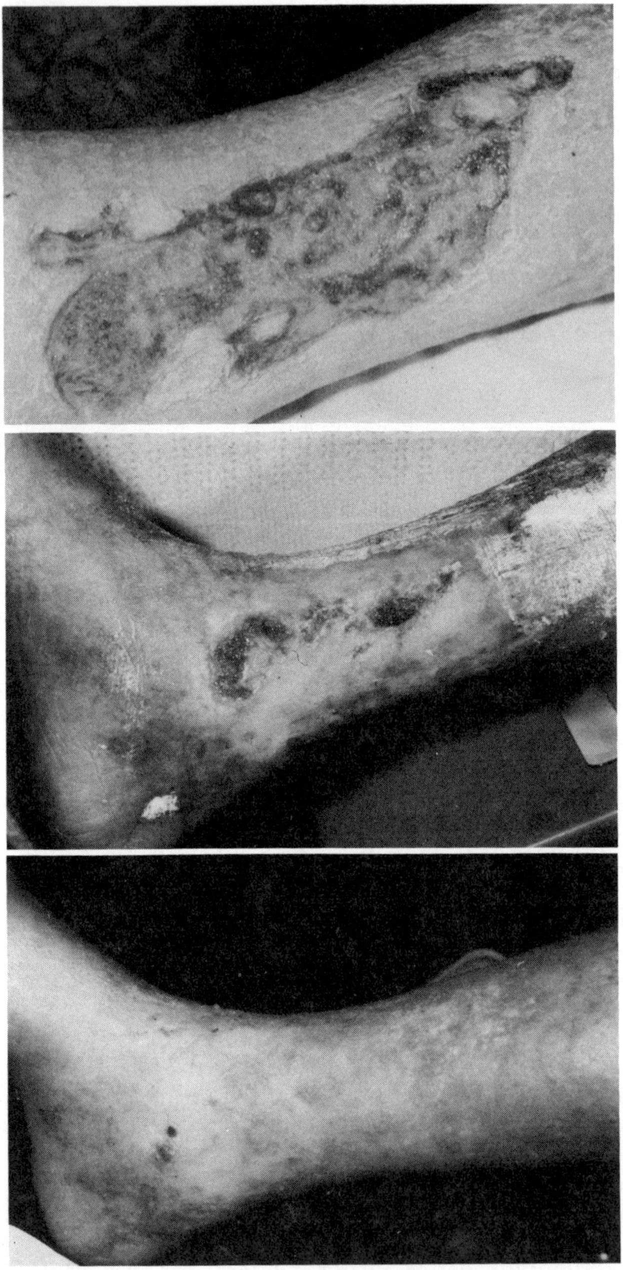

Fig 19–1.—Nonhealing ulcer (40 cm^2) of 6 years' duration on medial aspect of right leg of 84-year-old woman. **Top,** appearance of ulcer immediately before application of cultured allografts. **Center,** 10 days after application of cultured allograft; considerable reduction in ulcer area to 3.9 cm^2. **Bottom,** at 6 weeks, ulcer healed completely. (Courtesy of Phillips TJ, Kehinde O, Green H, et al: *J Am Acad Dermatol* 21:191–199, August 1989.)

▶ This is an interesting study and shows potential for the use of cultured skin allografts in certain situations. These situations, however, remain to be defined. As the authors state, the study is uncontrolled. It is mentioned that previous therapy included only saline dressings. The study would have been more convincing if one of the semiocclusive dressings had been used first and had failed. An even more persuasive argument could be made for the cultured skin dressings if they had been compared to one of these occlusive dressings, particularly in the few patients with bilateral ulcers. Because of the high cost of cultured skin allograft dressings, it is hoped that such studies are planned for the future.—J.C. Alper, M.D.

Sustained Compression and Healing of Chronic Venous Ulcers

Blair SD, Wright DDI, Backhouse CM, Riddle E, McCollum CN (Charing Cross and Westminster Med School, London)

Br Med J 297:1159–1161, Nov 5, 1988 19–5

Chronic venous ulcers are traditionally treated with adhesive plaster compression bandages. It has been calculated that an external pressure of 35 mm Hg to 40 mm Hg at the ankle is required to prevent capillary transudation in legs severely affected by venous disease. A bandaging system was designed that would achieve and sustain this level of compression for at least 1 week. It was tested as part of a larger randomized trial of 5 different dressings.

The study population consisted of 126 patients (mean age, 71 years) who had chronic venous ulceration of 148 legs. These ulcers had not responded to bandaging with gauze impregnated with zinc and adhesive plaster during a mean treatment period of 27.2 months. Of these patients, 22 had a history of deep vein thrombosis. The ulcerated legs were randomly assigned to treatment with 1 of 5 dressings: 43 patients were treated with a nonadhesive dressing, 25 with a pinch skin graft, 26 with a hydrocolloidal dressing, 28 with a porcine dermis, and 26 with silver sulfadiazine. The traditional plaster bandage and the 4-layer system were then sequentially applied to 20 consecutive patients. Pressures were measured 4, 8, and 24 hours, and 7 days after bandaging. Ulcers were cleaned with saline before weekly rebandaging. In patients with ulcers that had not healed at 12 weeks, treatment was considered a failure and surgery was recommended.

The 4-layer bandage achieved an initial mean pressure of 42.5 mm Hg at the medial malleolus, compared with 29.8 mm Hg achieved with adhesive plaster bandaging. However, the initial pressure achieved with the adhesive plaster bandage dissipated rapidly to 10.4 mm Hg at 24 hours, whereas the 4-layer bandage sustained the pressure for at least 1 week. By completion of the 12-week study, 110 (74%) of the 148 leg ulcers had healed completely, a rate comparing favorably with recent reports of 45% healing attained with elastic bandages.

Sustained compression of more than 40 mm Hg results in rapid healing of chronic venous leg ulcers. The newly designed 4-layer bandaging system is capable of maintaining the required pressure.

▶ Probably, any physician who cares for patients with leg ulcers knows that if the edema is not controlled, the ulcer doesn't heal. This study very elegantly proves this dictum. After reading the method of bandaging these patients with the 4-layer technique, however, I don't think that it is very practical, at least not in the United States. Some bright engineering type needs to design a stocking that is easy to put on, cosmetically acceptable, and effective. I wonder why no one has accomplished this yet.—J.C. Alper, M.D.

Use of Topical Ketanserin in the Treatment of Skin Ulcers: A Double-Blind Study

Janssen PAJ, Janssen H, Cauwenbergh G, De Doncker P, De Beule K, Lewi P, Tytgat HF, Lapière CM (Janssen Research Found, Beerse, Belgium; MS Clinic, Melsbroek; Univ of Liège, Belgium)

J Am Acad Dermatol 21:85–90, July 1989 19–6

Ketanserin is a serotonergic antagonist that competitively and selectively blocks S_2-serotonergic receptors. Because serotonin has a role in the peripheral circulation of patients with peripheral vascular diseases, a randomized, double-blind, clinical trial was initiated to assess the effect of a 2% ketanserin ointment formulation on decubitus wounds, venous ulcers, and ischemic skin ulcers.

Of 74 patients, 25 had decubitus ulcers, 37 had venous ulcers, 6 had ischemic ulcers without diabetes, and 6 had ischemic ulcers with diabetes. Thirty-six patients (mean age, 65 years) were randomly assigned to treatment with ketanserin ointment and 38 patients (mean age, 68 years) to placebo. The study lasted for a minimum of 2 weeks and a maximum of 8 weeks. One placebo-treated patient and 1 ketanserin-treated patient, both with venous ulcers, dropped out of the study. All patients with decubitus ulcers were hospitalized at the time of treatment. Patients were scored on granulation tissue and epithelialization on a scale of 0–3.

After 2 weeks of treatment the average covering of the wound in ketanserin-treated patients was significantly better than that in placebo-treated patients. The difference became even more pronounced after 4 weeks of treatment and persisted throughout the study. The initial wound area in the ketanserin group was decreased by 50% after 2.6 weeks of treatment, compared with a 50% reduction in wound area obtained after 6.6 weeks of placebo treatment. No statistical difference was observed in terms of granulation, epithelialization, or wound closure as a function of the pathogenesis of the ulcer.

▶ This is a very impressive study, particularly as it lasted only for a maximum of 8 weeks and significant healing occurred during that time. My only problem with the study design is that a bland control substance such as petrolatum was not used. It is possible that the vehicle (control substance) without ketanserin inhibits wound healing and the effect is only that of suspending such inhibition. I agree that is unlikely. It's too bad that no photos were included in the paper. I look forward to more confirmatory studies.—J.C. Alper, M.D.

Multicenter Trial of Cadexomer Iodine to Treat Venous Stasis Ulcer

Holloway GA Jr, Johansen KH, Barnes RW, Pierce GE (Harborview Med Ctr; Univ of Washington; Virginia Commonwealth Univ, Richmond; Univ of Kansas)

West J Med 151:35–38, July 1989 19–7

Cadexomer iodine is a topical polymeric starch bead similar to dextranomer but with iodide, 0.9% weight per weight. It allows hygroscopic removal of wound secretions as well as bacteria in the fluid; at the same time, the bonded iodine becomes bactericidal. The efficacy of cadexomer iodine in accelerating the healing of venous stasis ulcer was studied in a prospective, randomized, crossover trial. Seventy-five patients randomly received either cadexomer iodine or standard saline wet-to-dry compressive dressing.

Both cadexomer iodine and standard treatment were effective in reducing ulcer size and promoting healing. However, ulcers healed more than twice as rapidly with cadexomer iodine than with standard treatment. In addition, there was a trend toward less pain, exudate, pus, and debris and more rapid development of granulation tissue with cadexomer iodine than with the standard treatment. Seven of 12 patients crossed over from standard treatment to cadexomer iodine therapy had healing; in contrast, no patient switched from cadexomer iodine to control therapy. Neither treatment was superior in reducing bacterial numbers. Except for mild local burning in wounds treated with cadexomer iodine, no significant adverse effects were noted. Topical cadexomer iodine may be a useful addition in the treatment of venous stasis ulcers.

▶ A couple of very important pieces of data were left out of the abstract summary. Statistical significance was achieved only at 2 of the 3 centers in the study. Also, there was significance only if the overall healing rate of the treatment vs. the control groups was calculated. If the healing rate calculated as a proportion of the baseline ulcer circumference was examined, there was no statistical significance at all. Because this latter measurement is the most important, my interpretation of these results is that treatment with cadexomer iodine is no better than saline wet-to-dry dressings. This is not surprising, as just above every study that has analyzed the effect of iodine on wound healing has shown that it inhibits epithelialization of the wound surface.—J.C. Alper, M.D.

Malignant Fibrous Histiocytoma: A New Complication of Chronic Venous Ulceration

Berth-Jones J, Graham-Brown RAC, Fletcher A, Henderson HP, Barrie WW (Leicester Royal Infirmary, England)

Br Med J 298:230–231, Jan 28, 1989 19–8

Malignant fibrous histiocytoma has not been reported previously in association with chronic venous ulceration. Three women aged 77, 80, and 81 years, respectively were seen with this lesion. The first woman had an ulcer over the left medial malleolus, the second had an ulcerated mass over the right medial malleolus, and the third had a large ulcer over the medial aspect and front of the right lower leg.

In all 3 tumors histologic analysis revealed pleomorphic spindle cells with occasional multinucleated cells and mitotic activity ranging from 1 to 4 mitoses per high-power field. A storiform pattern was noted in 2 ulcers and was less pronounced in the third. The first patient had areas of necrosis and hemorrhage. In all 3, malignant fibrous histiocytoma was diagnosed morphologically and with the aid of immunocytochemistry. None of the lesions had staining to intracellular cytokeratin antigens by antibodies CK 1 or CAM 5.2. All 3 tumors stained positively for vimentin but not for desmin or leukocyte common antigen. The main differential diagnosis, spindle cell squamous carcinoma, was excluded in all 3 patients.

Predisposing factors to malignant fibrous histiocytoma are radiotherapy and trauma. None of the 3 patients described had a history of radiotherapy, and only 1 had a history of minimal trauma. Malignancy should be considered by all physicians managing chronic venous ulcers. A biopsy should be performed promptly when needed.

▶ This paper adds another malignant tumor to the list of those that should always be kept at the front of the mind of any physician treating chronic ulcers. Any ulcer that does not heal or grows larger after several months of appropriate therapy should be thoroughly investigated for evidence of malignancy and osteomyelitis.—J.C. Alper, M.D.

Sclerotherapy: A Personal Appraisal

Bodian EL (New York Univ)

J Dermatol Surg Oncol 15:156–161, February 1989 19–9

Sclerotherapy is now widely accepted for treatment of varicosities. Hypertonic saline causes no allergic side effects and is the sclerosant of choice. Cramping may occur, but it disappears within minutes. Polidocanol does not sclerose veins as rapidly as saline, but it is less painful on injection. Allergic reactions are rare. Many anaphylactic reactions have been reported with sodium morrhuate, and it should not be used to treat sunburst varicosities. Sotradecol can cause severe local reactions, but it rarely induces systemic problems.

Recanalization of a sclerosed venule is a rare complication. Telangiectatic matts occur in up to 15% of patients, usually appearing on the medial and anterior surfaces of the thigh. They usually disappear within 3–6 months, but occasionally they become permanent. Ulceration is often the result of poor technique, especially inserting the needle too deeply so that it is positioned below the venule. When pigmentation occurs, it can be as unattractive as the original sunburst varicosities.

Proper injection technique is most important. The syringe should suit the size of the hand, and the needle should be sharp. The site should be magnified. It is essential to watch the needle point to avoid perforating the tiny blood vessel once the needle is in the vein. The needle should be aimed parallel to the vein, not under it. A small bolus of air should be injected before the sclerosing solution to reduce chances of side effects. To keep the air in front of the solution, the needle should be tilted up.

Excellent results can be obtained with sclerotherapy of sunburst varicosities if proper procedures are followed. Diagrams of the legs help to identify sites for treatment and for assessment of previous therapy.

▶ Pearls from one of the experts in the field, who is an advocate of hypertonic saline. Great photos.—J.L. Fewkes, M.D.

Injection Sclerotherapy for Spider Telangiectasias: A 20-Year Experience With Sodium Tetradecyl Sulfate

Tretbar LL (Univ of Missouri, Kansas City)

J Dermatol Surg Oncol 15:223–225, February 1989 19–10

A 20-year experience with the treatment of spider veins using multiple small injections was reviewed. Sodium tetradecyl sulfate (Sotradecol) was used to treat 1,426 legs with spider telangiectasias. If the patient had an allergic history, a test dose of Sotradecol was given. During the first 18 years under review, a 1% solution of Sotradecol was injected directly into the spider vein (group 1). In the 19th year (group 2) one-third percent solution was used. In the final year (group 3) one-third percent solution was injected into associated blue feeder veins rather than into the spinder veins themselves.

No local or systemic major complications were observed. All patients had 80% to 90% clearing of spider veins regardless of the treatment method. In up to 70% of the patients treated with a 1% solution at least 1 ulcer developed. Ulceration was decreased dramatically in group 2, and those ulcers that did occur were smaller, less painful, and produced less scarring. In approximately 33% of patients in group 1 pigmentation developed that remained for as long as 2 years. Pigment developed in only 5% of small veins and in 10% of larger veins in group 2. When only blue feeder veins were injected, neither pigmentation nor ulceration occurred. Capillary blush developed in only 5% of patients and only in those having direct spider injections.

Both concentrations of Sotradecol can eliminate spider telangiectasias effectively. The incidence and severity of side effects are reduced when the lower concentration is used. Injection of the subcutaneous blue veins treats the source of the venous hypertension rather than the result. Spider veins that do not resolve spontaneously within 1 month after blue vein injection may be injected directly.

▶ The main reason for objection to this FDA-approved sclerosant is the reportedly high incidence of allergic, including anaphylactoid, reactions. If you're searching for your ideal sclerosant, this article must be read.—J.L. Fewkes, M.D.

Treatment of Essential Telangiectasia: Effects of Increasing Concentrations of Polidocanol

Norris MJ, Carlin MC, Ratz JL (Cleveland Clinic Found)

J Am Acad Dermatol 20:643–649, April 1989 19–11

Superficial telangiectasia on the thighs, legs, and ankles is a common occurrence among women between the ages of 30 and 50. Although these spider veins are generally asymptomatic, they are considered unattractive. Sclerotherapy has been gaining in popularity as a simple and effective treatment for essential telangiectasias. Of the commonly used sclerosants worldwide, only sodium morrhuate and sodium tetradecyl sulfate have been approved by the Food and Drug Administration. Polidocanol has not yet been approved for use as a sclerosant in the United States, but it is widely available in Europe.

The effects of increasing concentrations of polidocanol in the treatment of essential telangiectasias were evaluated in 20 women aged 30–57 who had bilaterally symmetric telangiectasias of the legs and thighs. The legs were divided into 4 quadrants with approximately equivalent numbers and sizes of vessels. Each quadrant was treated with a maximum of 2 mL of the same solution at each visit. Each patient received polidocanol injections in concentrations of 0.25%, 0.5%, 0.75%, or 1% every 4 weeks until all involved vessels had cleared or for a maximum of 6 visits.

The mean time to clearing of the superficial veins ranged from 2.9 treatments for the 0.75% solution to 3.7 treatments for the 0.25% solution. The best clearing rate (70.6%) was obtained with polidocanol 0.5%, followed by a clearing rate of 62.5% with the 1% polidocanol solution, 56.3% with the 0.75% solution, and 35.3% within the 0.25% solution. The differences were not statistically significant. There were no allergic reactions to polidocanol, and none of the women had superficial ulceration or necrosis. However, polidocanol 0.75% and 1% caused more side effects and more hyperpigmentation than did the 2 solutions having lower concentrations of the sclerosant. Thus concentrations of polidocanol greater than 0.5% are not necessary to achieve fast, successful sclerosis.

Polidocanol 0.5% solution in the treatment of essential telangiectasias is extremely safe, effective, and well-tolerated. The treatment would be a valuable alternative to the FDA-approved sclerosants.

▶ This is an overly complete clinical study of polidocanol by physicians who prefer it. It should be balanced by reading articles by other experts who prefer hypertonic saline (Abstract 19–9) or sodium tetradecyl sulfate (Abstract 19–10).—J.L. Fewkes, M.D.

Polidocanol (Aethoxyskerol) for Sclerotherapy of Superficial Venules and Telangiectasias
Goldman PM (Univ of California, Los Angeles)
J Dermatol Surg Oncol 15:204–209, February 1989 19–12

Polidocanol, a urethane, is unique among local anesthetics in its lack of an aromatic ring. It was developed in the 1950s as a topical, local, and epidural anesthetic. It was first used as a sclerosant in Germany in the late 1960s. Polidocanol induces sclerosis via endothelial damage, interfering with cell-surface lipids and disposing to thrombus formation and later fibrous cord formation. It probably is a weaker detergent-type of sclerosant than is sodium tetradecyl sulfate. A disposable 30-gauge needle was used for sclerotherapy. Injections usually began above and continued downward from the largest to the smallest vessels. Postsclerotherapy compression was advantageous.

About 5,000 sclerotherapy procedures in 1,500 patients in the past decade have given generally satisfactory results without significant complications. Most patients with telangiectasias and superficial venules were adequately treated with 0.25% polidocanol. Only 5 small superficial ulcerations occurred. There were no true allergic reactions. Most adverse effects were temporary, probably the most troublesome being pigmentation. Polidocanol may eventually be viewed as being close to the ideal sclerosant.

▶ This is an excellent and complete review of this sclerosant in the hands of one of the masters. Too bad there are no photos.—J.L. Fewkes, M.D.

Noninvasive Examination of the Venous System in the Leg: Presclerotherapy Evaluation
Fronek HS (Scripps Clinic and Research Found, La Jolla, Calif)
J Dermatol Surg Oncol 15:170–173, February 1989 19–13

The history and examination can rule out serious venous disease in patients seeking treatment of varicose veins and telangiectasia. Subtly visible varicosities proximal to or underlying the veins to be treated, as well as incompetent deep or perforating veins and deep venous thrombosis, need to be identified. Merely injecting distal telangiectasia will not solve the problem permanently if the source of venous reflux is proximal.

Simple examination with a tourniquet helps to assess the overall adequacy of venous outflow from the leg, and the Trendelenburg test can demonstrate an insufficient valve at the proximal end of the greater saphenous vein. Plethysmography can help to detect deep venous thrombosis and reveals the general state of the deep venous valves. Several deep veins are accessible to Doppler examination, and venous signals can be augmented by limb compression. The Doppler examination can detect incompetent perforating veins by demonstrating bidirectional flow resulting from insufficient valve. Doppler examination is easy to perform, inexpensive, and particularly well suited for presclerotherapy evaluation, although other methods also are useful.

▶ This article is a "must read" for anyone doing any type of venous sclerotherapy. It demonstrates how to screen patients to get the best cosmetic result.—J.C. Alper, M.D.

Sclerotherapy: Review of Results and Complications in 200 Patients

Puissegur Lupo ML (Tulane Univ)

J Dermatol Surg Oncol 15:214–219, February 1989 19–14

Sclerotherapy has become popular as a treatment for the destruction of superficial "spider" and varicose veins of the legs. A review of this procedure in 200 cases noted certain complications.

Patients were treated with either 20% sodium chloride (NaCl) and heparin, 23.4% NaCl or polidocanol .5% to 1%. The volume of sclerosing fluid injected varied with the length and caliber of the vessel, with a total volume up to 6 cc in severe cases. Patients were instructed to wear self-adhesive bandages for 24 hours after injection. Normal activity, but not vigorous exercise, was encouraged. Retreatment, if necessary, was performed at intervals of 4–8 weeks to prevent reinjection of an area that had not yet faded to its maximal extent.

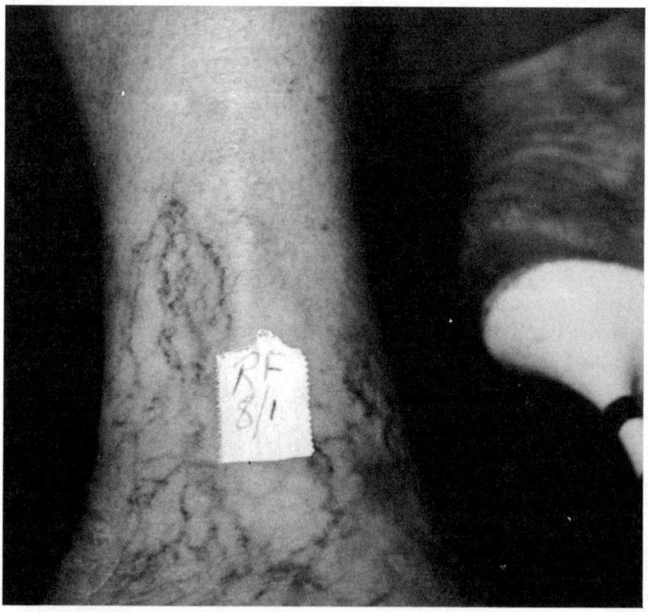

Fig 19–2.—Pretreatment view of lateral right ankle. (Courtesy of Puissegur Lupo ML: *J Dermatol Surg Oncol* 15:214–219, February 1989.)

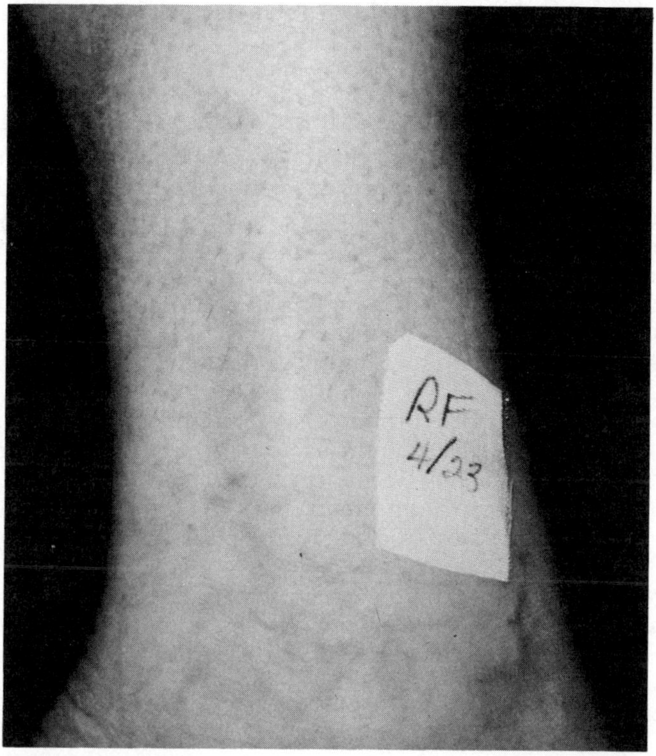

Fig 19–3.—Lateral right ankle 8 months and 2 treatments later, using 20% NaCl and 100 units of heparin/cc. (Courtesy of Puissegur Lupo ML: *J Dermatol Surg Oncol* 15:214–219, February 1989.)

The success rate was 95% (Figs 19–2 and 19–3), and patient satisfaction was 98%. In the 2% of patients who were dissatisfied, treatment had failed. Some patients were treated with both polidocanol and NaCl. Most believed that saline was superior because of the rapid resolution, but more than half of these preferred polidocanol because it was painless and usually brought results eventually. Complications included temporary bruising, burning or cramping with injection, and ankle edema associated with treatment of that area. In somc patients a network of tiny bright pink vessels developed that blanched with pressure; 1% of the patients experienced skin slough, ulceration, and eventual scarring. Temporary hyperpigmentation was another side effect. The choice of treatment did not appear to be related to complications.

Sclerotherapy for spider veins has an extremely high success rate. Rapid fading and less cramping are produced with 20% saline than the stronger saline solution. Because fading is slower, polidocanol might be reserved for patients with an intolerance for discomfort.

▶ This article from one clinician reporting on personal experience in the past 4 years with 200 patients adds nothing new to better studies.—J.L. Fewkes, M.D.

Compression in the Treatment of Leg Telangiectasia: Theoretical Considerations

Goldman MP (Univ of California, San Diego)
J Dermatol Surg Oncol 15:184–188, February 1989 19–15

Women with telangiectasias of the leg most often request treatment for cosmetic reasons, and any measures used should be very safe. Sclerotherapy remains the most effective approach, and the results may be enhanced by postsclerosis compression. Adequate compression can lead to direct aposition of the walls of the treated vein to produce more effective fibrosis with less strong sclerosing solutions. Thrombus formation is discouraged, and postsclerosis pigmentation is less likely. In addition, a graduated compression stocking improves the function of the calf muscle pump.

Because a significant proportion of smaller spider veins communicate directly with larger varicose or reticular superficial veins, compression of "feeders" should reduce flow to the smaller connected vessels. The optimal compression pressure is uncertain, but the use of narrow foam rubber pads under compression stockings can increase cutaneous pressure up to 50%.

The proper duration of compression also is open to debate. A medium-strength compression stocking having effective compression of 30 mm to 40 mm Hg at the ankle may be useful. Blood is not totally emptied from the veins, but any compression reduces the effective vein diameter and minimizes the risk of thrombus formation.

▶ This is a *very* detailed recap of the scientific literature behind the rationale for compression after sclerotherapy. The bottom line is, use it.—J.L. Fewkes, M.D.

Systemic Vasculitis in Association With Human Immunodeficiency Virus Infection

Calabrese LH, Estes M, Yen-Lieberman B, Proffitt MR, Tubbs R, Fishleder AJ, Levin KH (Cleveland Clinic Found)
Arthritis Rheum 32:569–576, May 1989 19–16

Infection with HIV can cause a number of immunologic events in addition to AIDS. The clinical, pathologic, virologic, and immunologic features of severe vasculitis were evaluated in a patient with HIV infection. In some cases, HIV and necrotizing vasculitis may be related etiologically.

Biopsy specimens of muscles and nerves were obtained from the living patient and studied with light microscopy. After the patient died, specimens of the heart, lung, and liver were similarly studied. Researchers also performed extensive laboratory studies.

Muscle specimens showed lymphocytic vasculitis; the appearance of the lymphocytes was morphologically consistent with activated T cells.

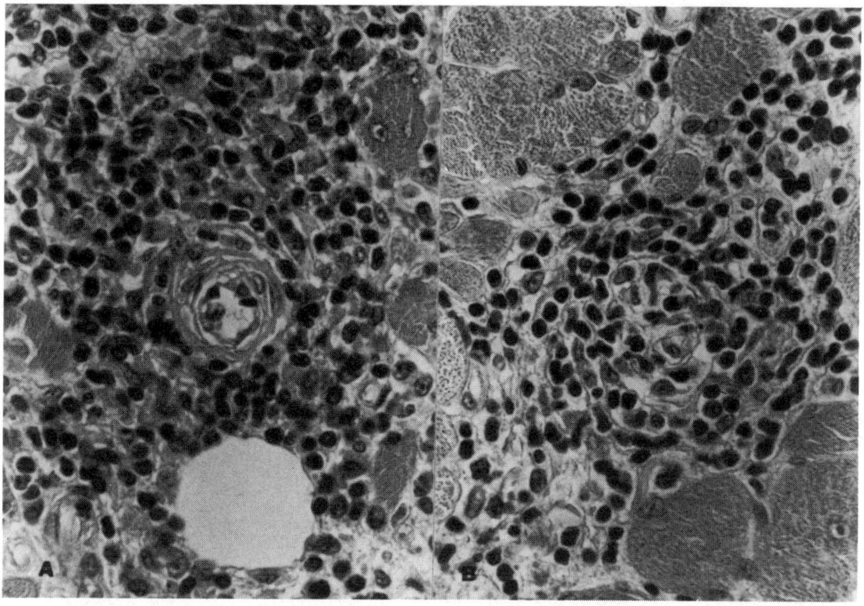

Fig 19–4.—Sections of skeletal muscle from a patient with severe vasculitis and HIV infection. **A**, infiltration of the arterial wall by a lymphoplasmacytic infiltrate. **B**, compression of the vessel lumen secondary to vasculitis. (Courtesy of Calabrese LH, Estes M, Yen-Lieberman B, et al: *Arthritis Rheum* 32:569–576, May 1989.)

Many blood vessels were obliterated (Fig 19–4). Lung, kidney, and myocardium samples were less inflamed but showed the same pattern of angiocentric lymphocytic infiltrates. Kidney specimens revealed a marked interstitial nephritis with preservation of the glomeruli. There was no evidence of viral antigens in inflammatory infiltrates. Immunologic evaluation showed that infiltrating cells were predominantly CD3+, CD8+, and CD4−. Lymphocytes demonstrated a significant deletion of T cell antigen receptor determinants.

Some patients with HIV infection may also have lymphoproliferative disorders with angiocentric features consistent with systemic necrotizing vasculitis. Clinicians should be aware of this possibility in the differential diagnosis.

▶ To date, only 14 cases of vasculitis associated with HIV infection have been reported: 4 resembled polyarteritis nodosa, 4 were lymphomatoid granulomatosis, 2 were granulomatous angiitis restricted to the CNS, and in 1 patient each, leukocytoclastic vasculitis, polyangiitis or overlap syndrome, and eosinophilic necrotizing vasculitis of the temporal arteries. Two mechanisms are thought to be responsible for viral-induced vasculitis: direct viral replication within vascular walls, and immune mechanisms directed at or caused by viral infection. The authors believe that both mechanisms were involved in their patient, with a vascular inflammatory disease occurring as part of an immunoproliferative disorder.—R.A. Johnson, M.D.

A Cutaneous Sign of IgA-Associated Small Dermal Vessel Leukocytoclastic Vasculitis in Adults (Henoch-Schönlein Purpura)

Piette WW, Stone MS (Univ of Iowa Hospitals and Clinics)

Arch Dermatol 125:53–56, January 1989 19–17

In the course of evaluating patients with lesions of palpable purpura, several patients were identified who had distinctive clinical lesions consisting of plaques of palpable purpura. Affected vessel walls contained substantial granular deposits of IgA in all cases. The characteristic appearance of these clinical lesions was predictive of IgA deposition.

Seven patients had lesions characteristic of classic palpable purpura, but they also had unique lesions not seen with other types of leukocytoclastic vasculitis. The distinctive lesions consisted of plaques containing multifocal areas of hemorrhage or necrosis, usually in a livedoid pattern. The lesion margins typically had a retiform configuration. Biopsy specimens from all patients were obtained for routine light microscopy study and direct immunofluorescent staining. All patients had small dermal vessel vasculitis associated with preponderant or prominent IgA vascular or perivascular deposition. Leukocytoclastic vasculitis was proved in all patients but 1 (table).

The distinctive cutaneous lesions in these patients may be evidence of the presence of IgA deposition in patients with small vessel leukocytoclastic vasculitis and may suggest a different pathogenesis for lesion development in some patients with IgA-associated vasculitis.

▶ This observation of a distinctive cutaneous sign for Henoch-Schönlein purpura in the form of plaques with purpura or necrosis in a livedoid pattern must be confirmed.—N.A. Soter, M.D.

Erythermalgia, A Rare Syndrome of the Extremities: Thirteen Cases

Lazareth I, Fiessinger JN, Priollet P (Hôp Broussais, Paris; Hôp Saint-Joseph, Paris)

Presse Méd 17:2235–2239, Nov 26, 1988 19–18

Erythermalgia is a rare vascular acropathy that affects the feet more often than the hands. It is characterized by paroxysmal attacks during which the extremities become red, hot, and extremely painful. Exposure to heat and exertion may precipitate an attack, whereas exposure to cold, rest, and, often, aspirin administration typically relieve the symptoms. Erythermalgia may develop as a primary disorder or secondary to a myeloproliferative syndrome.

During a 5-year study period erythermalgia was diagnosed in 17 women and 10 men, 23 of whom were reexamined and reevaluated on the basis of 3 major criteria and 4 minor criteria. The 3 major criteria were paroxysmal attacks, burning pain in the extremities, and redness of the involved area during an attack. The 4 minor criteria were the typical precipitating factors of heat and exertion, elevated local temperature dur-

Morphological Differences Found in Leukocytoclastic Vasculitis

Clinical Category	Classic Palpable Purpura	Present Series	SLE, PAN, and Mixed Cryoglobulins
Vessel size	Small	Small	Small and medium
Lesion diameter, cm	Small (0.5-1.0)	Large (>2) and small	Large (>2) and small
Depth of involvement	Superficial (dermis)	Superficial (dermis)	Deep (dermis and fat)
Hemorrhage	Confluent	Patterned accentuation	Confluent
Necrosis	Necrosis variably present, not patterned	Marked superficial necrosis or ulceration, livedoid pattern	Deep necrosis, not patterned
Margins	Smooth	Retiform	Usually smooth

Abbreviations: SLE, systemic lupus erythematosus; *PAN*, polyarteritis nodosa.
(Courtesy of Piette WW, Stone MS: *Arch Dermatol* 125:53–56, January 1989.)

ing an attack, the typical relieving factors of exposure to cold and rest, and response to aspirin administration. The diagnosis of thermalgia was retained if reexamined patients met all 3 major criteria and at least 2 of the 4 minor criteria. The diagnosis of thermalgia was retained in 13 of the 23 patients.

Of these, 4 patients (median age, 64 years) had erythermalgia secondary to essential thrombocytopenia in 2 and to Vaquez' disease in 2. The remaining 9 patients (median age, 41 years) had primary erythermalgia. Of the 13 patients, 12 had bilateral symptoms. The hands were involved in 5 patients and the feet in 12. The disease was judged minimally disabling in 7 patients and disabling in 4—2 with secondary and 2 with primary erythermalgia. Capillaroscopy was normal in 6 patients, nonspecific in 1, and indicative of acrocyanosis in 6. At follow-up all 4 with secondary erythermalgia were cured. Of the 9 patients with primary disease, 1 was cured, 3 were stable, 4 were improved, and 1 was worse.

In addition to the fact that patients with secondary erythermalgia were generally older than those with the primary form, some of these patients had unilateral symptoms; their symptoms were less severe and always resolved when the underlying disease was cured. In contrast, patients with primary erythermalgia always had bilateral involvement with more severe symptoms of longer duration.

▶ The authors classify erythermalgia (erythromelalgia) as primary or secondary. The latter is related to essential thrombocytopenia, lupus erythematosus, a myeloproliferative syndrome, or drugs. The 2 drugs implicated were nifedipine and bromocriptine; withdrawal of these led to resolution of the erythermalgia, which recurred on reinstitution of drug therapy.

Primary erythermalgia may be treated successfully with aspirin (5 of 9 cases) or, if that, fails by a β blocker.—R. Masters, M.D.

The Treatment of Chilblains With Nifedipine: The Results of a Pilot Study, a Double-Blind Placebo-Controlled Randomized Study and a Long-Term Open Trial

Rustin MHA, Newton JA, Smith NP, Dowd PM (Middlesex Hosp; St Thomas' Hosp, London)

Br J Dermatol 120:267–275, February 1989 19–19

Perniosis, or chilblains, is a cold-related cutaneous disorder that may have a vascular etiology. To determine whether nifedipine, a vasodilator drug, may be effective in the treatment of perniosis, 10 patients were given the drug, in a 5-mg dose initially, until the effective or maximal tolerated dose was reached, treatment was for 6 weeks. The lesions completely resolved in 7 patients within 14 days of treatment with nifedipine, 60 mg daily.

In a subsequent double-blind, placebo-controlled, randomized study, 10 patients with severe recurrent acral perniosis received nifedipine-retard, 20 mg, or placebo 3 times daily for 6 weeks and then were crossed over to the alternate medication for another 6 weeks. The lesions cleared completely in 7 patients within a mean of 8 days, and no new lesions developed during nifedipine therapy. Pain, soreness, and irritation were also reduced.

In a long-term, open trial, the modal dose of nifedipine-retard among the 31 patients who completed the 2-month treatment schedule was 60 mg. A comparison of the pretreatment and posttreatment skin biopsy specimens showed resolution of the dermal edema and epidermal necrosis and reduction in the perivascular infiltrate. Laser Doppler velocimetry showed an increase in cutaneous blood flow after administration of nifedipine. Adverse side effects included headache and facial flushing.

Nifedipine appears to be effective in the treatment of chilblains. The increased digital cutaneous blood flow with nifedipine may, in part, be mediated by inhibition of the α_1-adrenoreceptor-mediated vasoconstriction.

▶ Calcium channel blockers have proven to be sometimes helpful in the treatment of Raynaud's phenomenon (1). This study suggests that chilblains is also aided by this drug.—R.S. Stern, M.D.

Reference

1. Smith CR, Rodeheffer RJ: *Am J Cardiol* 55:154B–157B, 1985.

Arterio-Venous Shunt Dermatitis in Chronic Renal Failure Patients on Maintenance Haemodialysis

Goh CL, Phay KL (Middle Road Hosp, Singapore)

Clin Exp Dermatol 13:379–381, November 1988 19–20

Cutaneous complications affecting arteriovenous (A-V) shunt sites in patients receiving chronic hemodialysis are unusual. The prevalence and causes of dermatitis affecting A-V shunt sites were evaluated in 88 patients in chronic renal failure treated by hemodialysis.

Of the group, 7 patients (8%) had dermatitis confined to areas around the site of entry of the A-V shunt needles. The lesions consisted of lichenified, scaly patches with pigmentary changes. All represented cumulative insult irritant contact dermatitis from soaps, disinfectants, and alcohol used for skin cleansing during hemodialysis. The mean duration of dialysis was longer in patients with dermatitis (4 years) than in patients without dermatitis (3 years). None of the patients with dermatitis had a history of atopy, whereas its prevalence was 19% in patients without dermatitis. Generalized pruritus was more common in patients with dermatitis (29%) than in those without it (17%). All 5 patients with dermatitis who were patch tested had negative responses. Four patients with A-V shunt dermatitis responded to treatment with mild topical steroids and substitution of normal saline for skin cleansing before hemodialysis.

Patients receiving chronic hemodialysis may experience irritant contact dermatitis at the A-V shunt site caused by cumulative insult from soaps, alcohol, and disinfectants used for skin cleansing. These patients should use the minimal necessary disinfectant to prevent irritant dermatitis.

▶ In addition to the obvious external local factors, the localization of a higher concentration of whatever substance is responsible for uremic pruritus at the site of an A-V anastomosis may also play a role in some cases (1).—J.D. Bernhard, M.D.

Reference

1. Monk BE, Sarkany I: *Br J Dermatol* 105:92, 1981.

20 Viral Infections

Warts in Fish Handlers

Rüdlinger R, Bunney MH, Grob R, Hunter JAA (Univ Hosp, Zürich; Royal Infirmary, Edinburgh; Univ of Zürich)

Br J Dermatol 120:375–381, March 1989 20–1

Because fish handlers frequently have warts, an attempt was made to identify which viruses cause these lesions. Questionnaires were sent to 93 commercial fish merchants, 41 of whom replied. Thirteen (38%) reported having employees with hand warts. Ten fish handlers and 1 fisherman with multiple hand warts subsequently underwent clinical examination, during which a sample was taken from the warts. The duration of the warts varied from 3 months to 24 years. The back of the fingers was the most frequently affected site.

Samples were examined by Southern blot and reverse blot analysis. No DNA was detected in the sample from 1 patient, 1 type of human papillomavirus (HPV) DNA was found in 6 samples, and 2 types of HPV DNA were found in 4 samples; HPV_4 was found in 1 sample, HPV_1-related virus in 3 samples, a virus hybridizing with HPV_{27} and HPV_2 in 5 samples, and HPV_7 in 7 samples.

A previous study had demonstrated HPV_7 in warts on the hands of butchers and meat handlers; that study proposed that butcher meat might be a possible source of HPV_7. However, this study showed that fish handlers also have warts caused by HPV_7, suggesting that HPV_7 is unlikely to originate from animal sources. Rather, environmental conditions may be a factor in the clinical manifestation of HPV_7 infection.

▶ The findings of HPV types 1, 2, and 7 in fish handlers' warts are similar to the findings of HPV types in butchers' warts. Type 1 has been linked with plantar warts and type 2 with common warts. The mode of transmission of HPV type 7, the cause of occupational warts in butchers and fish handlers, is unclear.—R.A. Johnson, M.D.

Human Papillomavirus Typing of Penile Condyloma

O'Brien WM, Jenson AB, Lancaster WD, Maxted WC (Georgetown Univ)

J Urol 141:863–865, April 1989 20–2

Papillomavirus infection is responsible for genital condyloma and is a significant risk factor for uterine cervical neoplasia. Although these viruses have been extensively studied in women, less attention has been paid to this infection in men. Papillomavirus infection was studied in 37 men, 9 with infected sexual partners and 28 who noticed a genital lesion on themselves.

Samples were sufficient for DNA analysis of papilloma type in 26 of the 37 patients. Lesions were caused by human papillomavirus types 6, 11, and 31 and by an uncharacterized type, except for 1 infection caused by type 16. In addition to penile shaft condyloma, urethral condyloma was present in 5 cases; more than 1 type of virus was present in 4 of these patients. The papillomavirus type could not be predicted from clinical or histologic features.

Human papillomavirus types 6 and 11 are believed to have low cervical oncogenic potential, and type 31, not much higher. The uncharacterized viral type remains a cipher. Male infection with these types of virus places the female sexual partner at risk for condyloma, without substantially increasing the risk of cervical cancer.

▶ The 5 patients reported had penile intraepithelial neoplasia (PIN) 1 (mild dysplasia) occurring either on the penis or within the urethra; these lesions were associated with HPV types 6a, 11a, 16, and 31. Cervical intraepithelial neoplasia (CIN) is usually associated with HPV types 16, 18, and 31. It is of interest that 3 of the 5 cases of PIN were associated with HPV types 6 and 11. Previously, PIN (bowenoid papulosis) has been associated with HPV types 16 and 18, specific types known for their oncogenic potential. Penile intraepithelial neoplasia associated with HPV types 6 and 11 probably has even less potential for evolution to invasive squamous cell carcinoma than does PIN associated with types 16 and 18. Also of interest was the finding that 4 patients appeared to be infected with more than 1 HPV type. In addition to other reasons, male patients with known genital HPV infections should use condoms with a new HPV-infected partner to protect against infection with other HPV types.—R.A. Johnson, M.D.

Cytological Screening to Detect Subclinical Anal Human Papillomavirus (HPV) Infection in Homosexual Men Attending Genitourinary Medicine Clinic

Haye KR, Maiti H, Stanbridge CM (The Royal Infirmary, Manchester; St Mary's Hosp, Manchester, England)

Genitourin Med 64:378–382, December 1988 20–3

During the past decade the incidence of genital human papillomavirus (HPV) infection in men and women has at least doubled. A previous study in a cohort of homosexual men showed that anal warts were 7 times more common than penile warts. Because the increase in anal HPV infection may also affect the incidence of anorectal neoplasia, particularly in immunocompromised patients, the importance of anal cytologic screening in the detection of subclinical HPV infection among homosexual men was assessed.

During a 2-year study period, 264 unselected homosexual men underwent proctoscopy to obtain anal and perianal smears for cytologic screening. All patients had had more than 1 sexual partner, and all had been exposed to anal sex. For comparison, anal and perianal smears were obtained from 11 men who underwent proctoscopy for conditions other than sexually transmitted diseases.

Satisfactory smears were obtained from 221 patients. Forty-three smears were excluded because they were technically unsatisfactory. All smears from the 11 control patients were negative for HPV infection, as were smears from 148 (67%) of the 221 study patients. Of the 73 patients with abnormal smears, only 18 had anal or perianal warts at presentation. Thus anal cytologic screening identified subclinical lesions in 55 patients (31%) who had no macroscopic evidence of anal or perianal warts. In 11 of the 55 patients clinical warts subsequently developed.

Of the 73 abnormal smears, 45 were rated borderline as they had some cellular atypia suggestive of HPV infection, 21 were abnormal with warty atypical cells (Fig 20–1), and 7 had cellular atypia plus dyskaryosis suggestive of intraepithelial neoplasia. All 73 patients whose smears were ab-

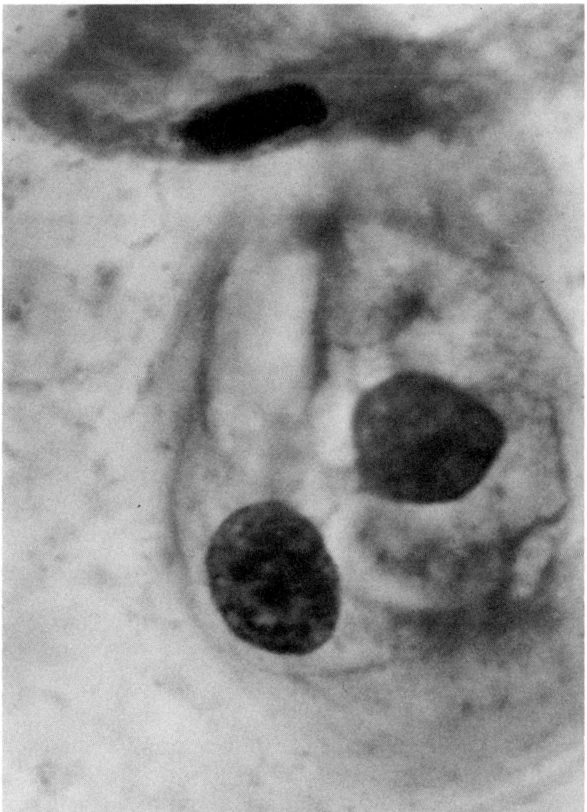

Fig 20–1.—Binucleate squamous cell from anal smear showing koilocytotic atypia. Papanicolaou stain. (Courtesy of Haye KR, Maiti H, Stanbridge CM: *Genitourin Med* 64:378–382, December 1988.)

normal were asked to return for repeat cytologic testing within 2–3 months, but only 40 patients complied.

In view of the fact that abnormal findings were detected by cytologic screening in 31% of this population without clinical evidence of anal or perianal warts, anal cytologic testing should be incorporated into the evaluation of homosexual men attending genitourinary clinics.

▶ The finding that 73 of 221 (33%) of homosexual males with a history of anal sex had cytologic evidence of HPV infection is, at first, surprising. Only 18 of these 73 (25%) had clinical evidence of anal or perianal warts, i.e., 55 of the 221 homosexual men (25%) had subclinical HPV anal/perianal infection. Subsequent follow-up examinations revealed that clinically apparent warts developed subsequently in 11 of the 55. These findings are, however, similar to findings in a group of heterosexual male partners of women with condyloma; 90% of the men had histologic evidence of HPV infection, but only 18% of these had clinical evidence of condylomata (1). In that 33% of anal squamous cell carcinomas have detectable HPV DNA (2), anal cytologic testing seems reasonable for the comprehensive care of homosexual men.— R.A. Johnson, M.D.

References

1. Sedlacek TV, et al: *Am J Obstet Gynecol* 154:494, 1986.
2. Beckman AM, et al: *Int J Cancer* 43:1042, 1989.

Personality Factors as Predictors of Therapeutic Response to Cryosurgery in Patients With Warts

Kalivas L, Penick E, Kalivas J (Univ of Kansas)

J Am Acad Dermatol 20:429–432, March 1989 20–4

Although warts are caused by viruses, occasionally they may disappear with suggestion therapy or hypnosis. This phenomenon suggests that psychological factors might influence the host response to the viral lesion, possibly through mediating the immune response. The role of personality characteristics in the treatment of warts with cryosurgery was analyzed.

Researchers administered the Tennessee Self-Concept Scale to 50 patients with various kinds of warts just before cryosurgery. After cryosurgery patients were separated into 2 groups according to the success or failure of the cryosurgery. Groups were compared as to sociodemographic and clinical data as well as on the basis of their responses to the scale.

Clinical follow-up data were available for 42 patients. Treatment succeeded in 23 patients and failed in 19. There were no significant differences in clinical, sociodemographic, or personality characteristics that differentiated successfully treated patients from those with failed treatments. Only 1 personality characteristic, psychological harmony— self-satisfaction, had possible significance. A total of 8 questions showed possibly significant differences between the way the 2 treatment groups answered. The answers to 2 questions: "I should trust my family more" and "I should have more sex appeal" might be useful in predicting future success and failure rates. A patient who answered "mostly true" to the first question and "completely false" to the latter would have a 91% chance of success with cryosurgery for warts, whereas one who answered "mostly true" to the first question but "completely true" to the latter could expect a 100% probability of failure.

Certain personality factors apparently influence a patient's response to cryosurgery for warts. Further research could determine the predictive value of personality factors in the general population contemplating wart cryosurgery.

▶ It would be interesting to compare the results obtained after a follow-up period of longer than 1 month, also the relationship between treatment outcome and the patient's expectations.—R.W. Gange, M.D.

Salicylic Acid in Karaya Gum Patch as a Treatment for Verruca Vulgaris

Bart BJ, Biglow J, Vance JC, Neveaux JL (Univ of Minnesota)
J Am Acad Dermatol 20:74–76, January 1989 20–5

TRANS-VER-SAL is a topical transdermal system that delivers salicylic acid for the treatment of verruca. This treatment modality acts by continuous passive diffusion of dissolved salicylic acid molecules from an epicutaneous reservoir into the infected tissue. A double-blind trial was undertaken to assess the therapeutic efficacy of this delivery system in 61 healthy volunteers with confirmed verruca vulgaris on the hands.

All warts were present for less than 1 year, and none were larger than 12 mm in diameter. No more than 3 warts per patient were treated. None of the patients had undergone treatment for their warts during the 4 weeks before the trial. Patients were assigned randomly to treatment with medicated patches containing salicylic acid 15% dispersed in a karaya gum, polyethylene glycol-300, and propylene glycol matrix. Control patches contained the same ingredients except for salicylic acid. All patients were scheduled for follow-up examinations on weeks 4, 8, and 12. Fifty-three patients completed the trial. Eight patients, 2 in the treatment group and 6 in the placebo group, were dropped because of noncompliance with the study protocol.

Of the 28 patients, 19 (68%) who completed 12 weeks of treatment with patches containing the active ingredient and 7 (28%) of 25 patients who received placebo patches had complete clinical resolution of the warts. Thirty-one of 45 warts treated with medicated patches and 14 of 40 warts treated with placebo patches had complete resolution. The high drop-out rate in the placebo group was thought to be caused by failure of the warts to clear. None of the patients had any indications of systemic toxicity or topical infection.

The higher cure rate among patients treated with medicated patches containing salicylic acid was attributed to the effective delivery of the drug to the wart under occlusion. The occluded environment provided by the karaya gum may have been responsible for the significant resolution among those using control patches.

▶ A major problem for the TRANS-VER-SAL delivery system of 15% salicylic acid in karaya gum is the need for daily changing of the patches, i.e., removing the old patch, abrading the wart with an emery board, moistening it with water, trimming the transdermal patch to the size of the wart, applying the new karaya patch, and, finally, covering the patch with surgical tape, for up to 84 days. Unless the patient is highly motivated and compulsive, compliance with these directions will be low. Of interest also was the efficacy in cure of the placebo karaya gum patch in 35% of patients as opposed to the medicated patch in 69%.—R.A. Johnson, M.D.

Patient-Applied Podofilox for Treatment of Genital Warts

Beutner KR, Conant MA, Friedman-Kien AE, Illeman M, Artman NN, Thisted RA, King DH (Univ of California, San Francisco; Sutter Solano Med Ctr, Vallejo, Calif; Oclassen Pharmaceuticals, Inc, San Rafael, Calif; New York Univ; Univ of Chicago)

Lancet 1:831–834, Apr 15, 1989 20–6

The incidence of genital warts is increasing. Patient-applied podofilox reportedly is a safe, well-tolerated treatment that is as effective as office-based therapy in the treatment of genital warts. Results of the first multicenter, placebo-controlled trial of patient-applied podofilox treatment were evaluated.

The series included 109 men with clinically diagnosed genital warts who were randomly assigned to a treatment group to self-administer 0.5% podofilox in lactate-buffered alcohol or a placebo group that administered the vehicle only. Baseline characteristics were comparable in both groups. Medications were applied in treatment cycles: twice daily for 3 days followed by 4 days of no treatment. Patients were evaluated at the end of each treatment cycle. The minimal number of treatment cycles was 2, and the maximum was 4. Treatments were evaluated for both efficacy and safety.

There was a marked decrease in the mean percentage of visible warts and wart area in the podofilox group. At the end of treatment, 73.6% of all podofilox-treated warts had disappeared, but only 8.3% of placebo-treated warts had resolved. The total wart area was reduced by 82.3% in treated patients but by only 4.2% in the placebo group. Almost half of the patients in the podofilox group were completely free of warts at some time during treatment, whereas no placebo-treated patients were wart free.

Inflammation and skin erosion were common in podofilox-treated patients, as were burning and pain to a lesser degree, but there were no clinically important systemic reactions, and local reactions were transient and reversible. The convenience and relatively lower cost compared with other promising treatments make podofilox therapy attractive for many patients.

▶ The results of this study, i.e., disappearance of 73.6% of all podofilox-treated warts compared to 8.3% of placebo-treated warts, are very impressive indeed. Only patients considered reliable were allowed to participate in the study. Podofilox was applied twice daily for 3 days, followed by no treatment for 4 days; this cycle was repeated 2 to 4 times. The reported local discomfort from podofilox seems comparable to that experienced with currently used modalities of physician-applied podophyllin in benzoin, cryosurgery, or electrosurgery. Patient-applied podofilox for genital warts warrants further investigation, because of its efficacy and cost efficiency; however, careful patient selection for reliability is imperative.—R.A. Johnson, M.D.

Intralesional Interferon Alfa-2b Treatment of Condylomata Acuminata Previously Resistant to Podophyllum Resin Application

Boot JM, Blog FB, Stolz E (Univ Hosp Rotterdam-Dijkzigt, Rotterdam)

Genitourin Med 65:50–53, February 1989 20–7

There is as yet no consistently effective form of treatment for condylomata acuminata, as the existing therapies are often associated with recurrence after initial resolution. However, recent trials of human recombinant interferon have yielded promising results. The safety and efficacy of intralesionally injected interferon α_{2b} in the treatment of resistant genital warts was assessed in 7 men and 3 women aged 19–55, who had no response to treatment with podophyllum resin applied for 4–10 months.

Three warts on each patient were injected intralesionally 3 times a week with 10^6 IU of interferon α_{2b} for 3 weeks. Follow-up was conducted for another 13 weeks. All patients were asked not to take any medication that could interfere with the treatment or modify the natural course of the disease.

Intralesional injection of interferon α_{2b} resulted in a highly significant reduction in the mean size of the treated warts by week 16. In 6 of the 10 patients, both test and control condylomata cleared completely. However, 1 patient had a relapse after initial clearing, and in 2 patients condylomata that had shrunk began to increase in size during 7 and week 12. Condylomata remained refractory in the other 4 cases. There were no serious side effects; 6 patients had mild, nondisabling influenza-like symptoms.

Only half of the patients in this trial had complete resolution of their genital warts. Additional studies need to be done to find the optimal doses and schedules for this treatment modality.

▶ Intralesional injection of interferon appears to be effective in eradication of clinically apparent human papillomavirus infection in some patients with genital warts (1–4). Its efficacy is probably equal to that of cryosurgery and more than that of podophyllin therapy. Some authors find intralesional interferon more effective when combined with cryosurgery. The major deterrent to intralesional interferon therapy is the expense of the drug itself, combined with the frequency of patients visits (9 visits, i.e., 3 times weekly for 3 weeks, compared to 1 visit in 3 weeks for cryo- or electrosurgery). In an economic climate of cost containment, the frequency of visits necessary for intralesional interferon therapy is an overwhelming deterrent.—R.A. Johnson, M.D.

References

1. Friedman-Kien AE, et al: *JAMA* 259:533, 1988.
2. Kirby PK, et al: *Am J Med* 85:183, 1988.
3. Kirby P: *JAMA* 259:572, 1988.
4. Reichman RC, et al: *Ann Intern Med* 108:675, 1988.

Comparative Study of Systemic Interferon Alfa-nl and Isotretinoin in the Treatment of Resistant Condyloma Acuminata

Olsen EA, Kelly FF, Vollmer RT, Buddin DA, Weck PK (Duke Univ; Burroughs Wellcome, Research Triangle Park, NC)

J Am Acad Dermatol 20:1023–1030, June 1989 20–8

A systemic form of treatment for condyloma acuminata may be effective in completely eradicating the human papillomavirus, thus resulting in more lasting remissions, than local therapy. Intereron alfa-nl and isotretinoin were evaluated as primary therapy in 17 healthy men with histologically confirmed refractory condylomata acuminata. Patients were randomly assigned to receive interferon alfa-nl, 5 million units, subcutaneously daily for 2 weeks, then twice weekly for 4 weeks, or isotretinoin, 1 mg/kg orally daily for 6 weeks.

Five men (56%) treated with interferon alfa-nl had an objective clinical response (≥50% clearance of the baseline lesion area); 1 patient had a complete response. The mean reduction from baseline was 52%. In contrast, none of the patients who received isotretinoin had an objective response. Four partial responders and 2 of 3 minimal responders to interferon alfa-nl received interferon therapy 3 times weekly in combination with daily isotretinoin for 6 weeks; all had further regression of warts, with responses ranging from 64.7% to 98.9% clearing from baseline. Seven patients were switched from isotretinoin therapy to interferon alfa-nl 3 times weekly for 6 weeks; only 2 had objective responses. Side effects were common and generally predictable for each drug but were generally not exacerbated when interferon and isotretinoin were used in combination.

Parenteral interferon alfa-nl is an effective alternative treatment for patients with refractory condyloma acuminata. Side effects are common but are generally well tolerated.

▶ Interferon therapy, whether intralesional or parenteral, reduces the size of genital warts (1). Oral retinoids have a similar effect on human papillomavirus (HPV)-induced lesions of common warts, epidermodysplasia verruciformis (2), and laryngeal papillomatosis (3). The rationale for the use of systemic therapy for genital warts seems reasonable in that much of HPV infection is subclinical and cannot be detected even using acetowhitening. In this study, the efficacy of parenteral interferon and isotretinoin was low, especially compared with the flulike side effects experienced by most interferon-treated patients. There may be a role for parenteral interferon, or interferon combined with isotretinoin, in immunodeficient patients with HIV infection, or in transplant patients with extensive HPV infection.— R.A. Johnson, M.D.

References

1. Gall SA, et al: *Obstet Gynecol* 67:643, 1986.
2. Lutzner MA: *N Engl J Med* 302:1091, 1981.
3. Alberts DS, et al: *J Biol Response Mod* 5:124, 1986.

Immunotherapy of Genital Warts With Inosine Pranobex and Conventional Treatment: Double Blind Placebo Controlled Study

Davidson-Parker J, Dinsmore W, Khan MH, Hicks DA, Morris CA, Morris DF (Prince of Wales' Hosp, London; Royal Victoria Hosp, Belfast, Northern Ireland; Leighton Hosp, Crewe; District Gen Hosp, Barnsley; Royal Shrewsbury Hosp, Shrewsbury, England)

Genitourin Med 64:383–386, December 1988 20–9

Several treatments are available for genital warts, but the persistent of such warts may be associated with a defective immune response. Inosine pranobex is reportedly effective in patients with human papillomavirus infection of the genital areas. A prospective, multicenter, double-blind, placebo-controlled study was done to confirm whether inosine pranobex improves the efficacy of the conventional treatment of patients with genital warts.

Fifty-five patients who had genital warts for at least 1 year underwent a 4-week course of inosine pranobex, 3 g/day. This treatment improved the clinical response to conventional treatment. More patients given inosine pranobex had improvement than those given placebo, but the difference in general response between the groups was not significant. When numbers of warts and extent of lesions were considered, however, patients receiving inosine pranobex did significantly better.

For patients with a long history of genital warts, a 4-week course of 3 g of inosine pranobex daily can significantly improve the efficacy of conventional treatment. More patients given this treatment than patients given placebo had a reduction in both the number of warts and extent of the lesions and showed overall clinical improvement.

► Inosine, a nucleoside xanthione β-D-ribofuranoside, is an intermediate in the formation of adenosine monophosphate (AMP). Its nucleotide inosine monophosphate (IMP) is formed by deamination of AMP. Pranobex is 2-hydroxypropyldimethyl-ammonium 4-acetamidobenzoate. Isosine pranobex is marketed in the United Kingdom as Immunovir (Leo), where it is prescribed for herpes simplex infection, genital warts, and in disorders of immunodeficiency such as HIV disease. A dose of 1 g 3 times daily is given for 14–28 days as an adjunct to traditional treatment for genital warts. In spite of the study by Davidson-Parker and coworkers, the efficacy of inosine pranobex is yet to be proven.—R.A. Johnson, M.D.

Human Herpesvirus-6 Infection (Exanthem Subitum) Without Rash

Suga S, Yoshikawa T, Asano Y, Yazaki T, Hirata S (Fujita Gakuen Health Univ, Toyoake, Aichi; Mino Municipal Hosp, Mino, Gifu, Japan)
Pediatrics 83:1003–1006, June 1989 20–10

Exanthem subitum, a common infectious disease of infancy, usually occurs in children aged 6 months to 3 years. It typically begins with an abrupt temperature rise; skin eruptions coincide with the subsidence of fever on the third or fourth day. In many infants the disease occurs as an inapparent infection or febrile illness without skin eruption. Without specific tests, however, diagnosis has been difficult to confirm. Exanthem subitum with an atypical clinical course, confirmed by virus isolation and specific diagnostic tests, occurred in a 7-month-old boy and a 6-month-old girl.

The patients had been in good health until they had a 3-day febrile episode. Exanthem subitum was suspected, but there was no skin eruption after the fever subsided. The virus was isolated from peripheral blood mononuclear cells in the acute stage, identified by the cytopathic effects of infected cells and the specific immunofluorescent staining of the cells with convalescent sera from exanthem subitum. The virus could not be isolated from cells in the convalescent stage.

The virus isolates displayed large cell formation of infected mononuclear cells, specific immunofluorescent staining of infected cells with convalescent serum of the disease, and herpesvirus morphology by electron microscopy. In both patients, there were seroconversions against the representative strain of the causative agent of exanthem subitum.

▶ The tally of human herpesviruses was 6 at the last count: herpesvirus type 1, herpesvirus type 2, varicella-zoster virus, cytomegalovirus, Epstein-Barr virus, and the most recently discovered, human herpesvirus-6 (previous known as B lymphotropic herpesvirus). The majority of adults have had infection with these 6 herpesviruses, as indicated by seroprevalence studies. Primary infection may or may not cause clinical illness. These viruses are immortalized in our tissues. As is evidenced by the immunodeficiency of HIV disease, the first 5 herpesviruses can reactivate as function of the T helper cells declines, causing significant morbidity and mortality. In that human herpesvirus-6 is only recently discovered, it will be of great interest to observe what other disease states are associated with human herpesvirus-6, other than exanthem subitum.—R.A. Johnson, M.D.

Sequential Genital Infections With Herpes Simplex Virus Types 1 and 2

Al Samarai AM, Shareef AA, Kinghorn GR, Potter CW (Basrah Med College, Iraq; Sheffield Univ Med School, England)

Genitourin Med 65:39–41, February 1989 20–11

Concurrent oral and genital infections with an identical herpes simplex virus (HSV), either type 1 (HSV 1) or type 2 (HSV 2), may occur in the same person. Previous oral herpes infections caused by HSV 1 do not protect against subsequent genital infection with HSV 2. Although exogenous reinfection in patients with asymptomatic recurrent genital herpes is considered uncommon, during a 3-year study period 5 patients were seen with acquired sequential infections caused by genital HSV 1 and HSV 2.

The patients, 2 men and 3 women aged 19–37, were enrolled in a clinical trial of antiviral therapy for genital herpes. During the trial swabs from genital lesions were sent routinely for HSV tissue culture. All HSV isolates were identified by an enzyme-linked immunosorbent assay, using either a monoclonal or a polyclonal antibody technique. To differentiate between primary and nonprimary infection, the patients' serum samples were analyzed with the microneutralization test. Samples taken at the acute phase that showed titers of less than 1/10 for both virus types were considered indicative of primary infection.

Genital reinfection may occur in patients of either sex, and either HSV 1 or HSV 2 may be the initial virus type. However, HSV 1 and HSV 2 isolates from the same person have different sensitivities to antiviral drugs. To avoid incorrect conclusions about the effect of the antiviral study drug on the development of resistance of HSV to that drug, the type and strain of all HSV isolates should be monitored continuously in any therapeutic efficacy study.

▶ This report points out that, although infected with 1 type and strain of HSV, we are not protected immunologically against superinfection with the other type of HSV, or a different HSV strain. Presumably, depending on exposure to new HSV-infected sexual partners, patients might become infected with 2, 3, or even more strains of HSV type 2. Condom use should be emphasized to patients to protect not only against HSV infection but also against HIV infection. Genital ulcer disease (e.g., genital herpes) places the patient at increased risk for HIV infection.— R.A. Johnson, M.D.

Increasing Incidence of Eczema Herpeticum: Analysis of Seventy-Five Cases

Bork K, Bräuninger W (Johannes Gutenberg Univ, Mainz, West Germany)

J Am Acad Dermatol 19:1024–1029, December 1988 20–12

Eczema herpeticum is a rare herpes simplex virus infection with disseminated skin involvement. Recently, the incidence of this infection has apparently been increasing. Researchers analyzed 75 cases occurring between 1969 and 1986 to determine the incidence rates and reasons for development. Patients had no preexisting disease other than atopic dermatitis that resulted in the development of generalized herpes simplex infection. No case of eczema vaccinatum was observed during the study period.

The 75 patients had 12 recurrences appearing at intervals ranging from several months to 6 years. After 1980 there was a marked increase in the incidence of eczema herpeticum: 15 patients were seen in 1985 and 12 in 1986. In contrast, between 1969 and 1976 there were no more than 2 cases per year. The mean age at development of the disease was 22.7 years; slightly more than half of the patients were women. Of 63 patients, 9 had recurrent herpes labialis before the onset of eczema herpeticum; 15 patients had preceding facial-oral herpes simplex.

Thirty-eight patients were treated with acyclovir, which led to rapid improvement. Treatment with immunoglobulins, immunostimulating agents, or antibiotics did not influence the duration of the disease.

The findings show a greatly increased incidence of eczema herpeticum. In this study affected patients were not predominantly infants, as had been found previously. Acyclovir was the most effective treatment used in these patients.

▶ Disseminated cutaneous herpes simplex virus infection occurs most commonly in patients with atopic dermatitis, i.e., eczema herpeticum, but it also occurs in patients with mycosis fungoides, keratosis follicularis (Darier's disease), thermal burns, pemphigus folliaceus, Sézary syndrome, and congenital ichthyosiform erythroderma. Eczema herpeticum is a potentially fatal infection (1), frequently complicated by superinfection by *Staphylococcus aureus* and/or group A β-hemolytic streptococci. Other estimates of mortality rates for eczema herpeticum range from 6% to 10%. Currently, death complicating eczema herpeticum is uncommon, mainly because of the use of antibiotics and acyclovir, which can be administered either orally or intravenously (2–4).—R.A. Johnson, M.D.

References

1. Sanderson IR, et al: *Br Med J* 294:693, 1987.
2. Nimura M, Nishikawa T: *Am J Med* 85 (suppl 2A):49, 1988.
3. Atherton DJ, Harper JI: *J Am Acad Dermatol* 18:757, 1988.
4. O'Neill JF, Norvell SS: *J Assoc Milit Dermatol* 15:11, 1989.

Grappling With Herpes: Herpes Gladiatorum

Becker TM, Kodsi R, Bailey P, Lee F, Levandowski R, Nahmias AJ (Univ of New Mexico, Albuquerque; Emory Univ; Princeton Univ)

Am J Sports Med 16:665–669, November–December 1988 20–13

Herpes gladiatorum is a skin infection, often found in college wrestlers, that is caused by herpes simplex virus (HSV). The members of 4 college wrestling teams were surveyed and high school and college athletic trainers nationwide were samples. Serum samples from 1 college wrestling team also were studied for HSV antibodies.

Of 48 college wrestlers studied, 9 reported histories of herpes gladiatorum. Only 1 of these had a history of oral HSV infection, but 7 had at least 1 match with an opponent who had cold sores or a vesiculopapular skin rash. Clinical manifestations of herpes gladiatorum in the 9 included a vesiculopapular rash on the face, upper arm, and/or trunk. All had tingling or burning sensations before the appearance of the rash; 1 athlete was hospitalized with fever, malaise, and pain after the first occurrence. The number of recurrences ranged from 1 to 8. All wrestlers were treated symptomatically.

Of 12 members of 1 team, 5 with herpes gladiatorum had serum antibody titers to HSV-1; no HSV-2 antibodies were found. None of the 5 had histories of cold sores or other HSV infections. Of the 94 college wrestling teams surveyed, 64.9% reported at least 1 episode of HSV skin infection during the 1984–1985 season; of 69 high schools, 24.6% had episodes. Athletic trainers reported that 7.6% of college wrestlers and 2.6% of high school wrestlers had HSV skin infections.

Wrestlers exposed to opponents with cutaneous HSV lesions are at high risk for the development of herpes gladiatorum. Early recognition and diagnosis of HSV skin infection, and immediate exclusion of the infected wrestler from competition and practice, are the best means of prophylaxis.

▶ The variable incidence of herpes gladiatorum was reported previously not only in wrestlers but also in rugby players (1, 2). A recent report attributed an epidemic of herpes gladiatorum to skin abrasions caused by new coarse-textured shirts issued to wrestlers; when these shirts were no longer worn, the epidemic of herpetic infections abated (3). Certainly, players with new herpetic outbreak can be excluded from participation. Alternatively, if an HSV lesion is diagnosed, the player can be treated with acyclovir, 200 mg orally every 4 hours (5 doses per day) for 5 days. Twenty-four hours after beginning treatment the player would no longer be contagious and could thus continue competition.—R.A. Johnson, M.D.

References

1. Selling B, Kilbrick S: *N Engl J Med* 270:979, 1964.
2. Mare JB, et al: *S Afr Med J* 54:752, 1978.
3. Strauss RH, et al: *N Engl J Med* 320:599, 1989.

Viral Activity in Skin Lesions of Herpes Zoster

Hata S, Sugai T, Asoh S, Asada Y, Nishijima S, Soh Y, Doi A, Baba K (Osaka Rosai Hosp; Osaka Kaisei Hosp; Kansai Med Univ; Tsukaguchi Hosp of Hyogo Prefecture; Kobe Municipal Central Hosp, Osaka, Japan; et al)

J Dermatol 15:448–450, October 1988 20–14

Viral activity in the herpes zoster rash is an important factor in determining the period of isolation. Virus materials were obtained from 59 patients with herpes zoster to assess viral activity throughout the course of the rash.

Varicella-zoster virus (VZV) was isolated in 41 of 53 patients on the first to ninth days after the rash. The virus concentration was highest on days 1 and 2 of the rash and gradually decreased to day 9. The isolation rate correlated with the condition of the skin lesions rather than with the days of illness. The virus concentration was high in vesicular fluids and decreased in the roofs, and virus was also isolated in the crust.

These data support the importance of herpes zoster as the source of VZV infections and the reliability of virus isolation for the diagnosis of herpes zoster.

▶ Varicella-zoster virus is highly contagious; it well known that persons without a history of varicella can be infected with VZV from a patient with zoster without direct contact (1, 2). This was well documented recently when a hospitalized patient contracted zoster; subsequently, 3 nurses from the ward that housed the patient had varicella (3). Two of the nurses had no direct contact with the patient, implying that airborne transmission of VZV had occurred.—R.A. Johnson, M.D.

References

1. Hyams PJ, et al: *Am J Infect Control* 12:2, 1984.
2. Gustafson TL, et al: *Pediatrics* 70:550, 1982.
3. Josephson A, et al: *J Infect Dis* 158:238, 1988.

Detection of Herpes Simplex Virus DNA in Cutaneous Lesions of Erythema Multiforme

Brice SL, Krzemien D, Weston WL, Huff JC (Univ of Colorado)

J Invest Dermatol 93:182–187, July 1989 20–15

Herpes simplex virus (HSV) has been associated with erythema multiforme (EM) since 1813, but the pathogenesis of EM, including herpes-associated EM (HAEM) is still unclear. The hypothesis that HAEM involves an immune-mediated response against cutaneous HSV-specific antigens was investigated. The DNA from lesion samples of 13 cases of HAEM and 9 cases of idiopathic EM were amplified using the polymerase chain reaction and tested for the presence of HSV DNA sequences; the results were compared with those of 6 bullous pemphigoid lesions. Localization experiments involving in situ hybridization using an HSV-specific ^{35}S RNA probe also were performed.

Southern analysis showed the presence of HSV DNA in 9 cases of HAEM and 6 cases of idiopathic EM. Herpes simplex virus DNA was not detected in any bullous pemphigoid lesions. In situ hybridization showed predominant localization of HSV nucleic acids to epidermis. No hybridization of HSV nucleic acids was found in chronic dermatitis lesions.

Herpes simplex virus DNA is found in lesions of both HAEM and idiopathic EM, primarily in the epidermis. These results support the hypothesis that HAEM involves an immune-mediated response against HSV present in the epidermis.

▶ In an additional study published from the same laboratory, Huff and Weston (1) provide further evidence in their very careful report of an episode of recurrent EM in 22 subjects, linking HSV as the etiologic factor for the recurrence. Detection of type-common HSV glycoprotein gB on or in keratinocytes is further evidence as to the herpetic etiologic of recurrent EM. They considered that the immunologic reaction in recurrent EM HSV-specific, and the host immune response may be directed against HSV antigens expressed on keratinocytes. Further evidence for the role of HSV in recurrent EM is the efficacy of oral acyclovir prophylaxis in prevention. Acyclovir, 200–600 mg/day, continually has proven extremely effective in preventing the recurrence of HSV infection and of HAEM. When HAEM occurs only a few times yearly, it can be treated episodically with oral acyclovir begun at the first indication of a new herpetic outbreak. In that HAEM typically follows within 1–3 weeks, most recurrences can be prevented by early treatment of the HSV outbreak.—R.A. Johnson, M.D.

Reference

1. Huff JC, Weston WL: *Medicine* 68:133, 1989.

Prevalence and Clinical Spectrum of Skin Disease in Patients Infected With Human Immunodeficiency Virus

Coldiron BM, Bergstresser PR (Univ of Texas, Dallas)

Arch Dermatol 125:357–361, March 1989 20–16

The prevalence and severity of skin disease was evaluated in 100 patients receiving care in a rural outpatient immunodeficiency clinic. All were serologically reactive to human immunodeficiency virus (HIV) by enzyme-linked immunosorbent assay and Western blot assay.

Skin disease was present in 92% of the patients. Seborrheic dermatitis, candidiasis, xerosis, and dermatophysis were the most common skin disorders, followed by folliculitis, molluscum contagiosum, warts, chronic ulcerative herpes, and psoriasis. None of the patients given zidovudine had *Candida* infection. Neither the prevalence nor severity of skin diseases differed among the clinical subgroups of patients with acquired immunodeficiency syndrome (AIDS), those with AIDS-related complex, or those who were asymptomatic. However, the prevalence of skin disease, except for dermatophytosis, in these HIV-positive patients was significantly higher when compared with a historical control population.

There is a high prevalence of skin disorders in HIV-positive patients.

Examination by a dermatologist should be a part of the initial evaluation and continuing care of these patients.

▶ Patients infected with HIV should be scrutinized by the dermatologist even more carefully than the patient at risk for melanoma. The entirety of the mucocutaneous surfaces, including the oropharynx and the perineal epithelium, should be observed on each and every dermatologic examination. Few of these patients escape 1 or more of the ever-expanding list of cutaneous diseases to which these immunodeficient patients are vulnerable. During 1989, two excellent comprehensive dermatologic atlases were published covering the mucocutaneous manifestations of HIV infection (1, 2).—R.A. Johnson, M.D.

References

1. Friedman-Kien AE: *Color Atlas of AIDS*. Philadelphia, WB Saunders Company, 1989.
2. Ansary MA, et al: *A Colour Atlas of AIDS in the Tropics*. London, Wolfe Medical Publications Ltd, 1989.

Pruritic Skin Lesions: A Common Initial Presentation of Acquired Immunodeficiency Syndrome

Liautaud B, Pape JW, DeHovitz JA, Thomas F, LaRoche AC, Verdier RI, Deschamps M-M, Johnson WD (Haitian Study Group on Kaposis Sarcoma and Opportunistic Infection, Port-au-Prince, Haiti; Cornell Univ Med College, New York)

Arch Dermatol 125:629–632, May 1989 20–17

Nearly half of a series of 134 Haitians with AIDS seen in an 18-month period in 1983–1984, had intensely pruritic skin lesions of unknown origin. The lesions were a presenting feature of AIDS in 79% of the 62 affected patients. The lesions appeared 8 months on average before the diagnosis of Kaposi's sarcoma or opportunistic infection. Siblings and friends of the patients did not have pruritic eruptions; all 6 sex partners of patients who did have eruptions were seropositive for HIV.

Numerous erythematous or hyperpigmented macules and papules 2–8 mm in size were present, often with 5- to 10-mm dermal or subcutaneous nodules. Vesicles commonly were associated with the papules. The pruritic lesions usually appeared first on the extensor surfaces of the arms and spread to the lower limbs, trunk, and forehead. In 80% of the patients the lesions persisted until death. Many treatments, including systemic antibiotics and steroids, were tried, but none was successful. Examination of biopsy specimens showed acute polymorphonuclear leukocyte infiltration with eosinophils prominent and destruction of pilosebaceous and sweat glands.

Insect bites, immune complex disease, and vasculitis are not likely causes of this eruption. Nor did it appear that the lesions were a cutaneous manifestation of the systemic infection. The possibility should be considered that they represent primary HIV infection of the skin.

▶ Not discussed in detail in this paper but an issue of major importance is the nature of the so-called AIDS or HIV exanthem related to acute infection and often associated with a "glandular fever"-like illness (1). Dermatologists are also referred to several excellent books (1–4).—J.D. Bernhard, M.D.

References

1. Brehmer-Andersson E, Torssander J: *Acta Derm Venereol (Stockh)* 70:85, 1990.
2. Friedman-Kien AE: *Color Atlas of AIDS.* Philadelphia, WB Saunders, 1989.
3. Weismann K, et al: *Skin Signs in AIDS.* Copenhagen, Munksgaard, 1988.
4. Penneys NS: *Skin Manifestations of AIDS.* Philadelphia, JB Lippincott Co, 1990.

Chronic Diffuse Dermatitis and Hyper-IgE in HIV Infection

Lin RY (Metropolitan Hosp, New York)

Acta Derm Venereol (Stockh) 68:486–491, 1988 20–18

Human immunodeficiency virus causes a variety of cutaneous abnormalities. Chronic dermatitis and markedly elevated concentrations of serum IgE, an association not previously noted in HIV infection, were found in 3 men who were seropositive for the HIV antibody.

Man, 25, a black from Honduras, was hospitalized with fever and malaise that had persisted for 18 months. He reported shortness of breath of a month's duration. Findings included oral thrush and prominent inguinal adenopathy. The following year he was readmitted with fever and painful adenopathy. In addition, lichenification and focal areas of hyperpigmented papules had developed on all extremities and the thorax (Fig 20–2). The patient improved spontaneously and was discharged. Within 2 months he was readmitted with fever and a productive cough. Bronchoscopic lavage findings were herpes simplex and α streptococcus. The patient was discharged to a clinic 2 weeks later and underwent skin biopsy. The serum IgE level was 6,262 IU/mL; antibody to HIV-1 was positive, but antibody to HIV-2 was not found. The patient was treated successfully for his skin condition with zidovudine, 200 mg every 4 hours.

All 3 patients had significant hyperkeratosis and variable parakeratosis, as well as mixed dermal infiltrates. Histopathology did not reveal characteristics of classic psoriasis. The IgE level was greater than that reported in patients with AIDS or AIDS-related complex. Depletion of T helper cells was present without invasive opportunistic infection, and no immediate hypersensitivity to common aeroallergens was discovered. Some patients with HIV infection may manifest a unique hyper-IgE syndrome in association with chronic diffuse dermatitis.

▶ Production of IgE by B cells involves antigen presentation via antigen-presenting cells, T helper cells, and stimulation of B cells. Locally produced IgE first sensitizes local mast cells; then, if produced in sufficient quantity, it enters the circulation and binds to receptors on both circulating basophils and tissue-fixed mast cells throughout the body. In this report, all 3 patients appeared to

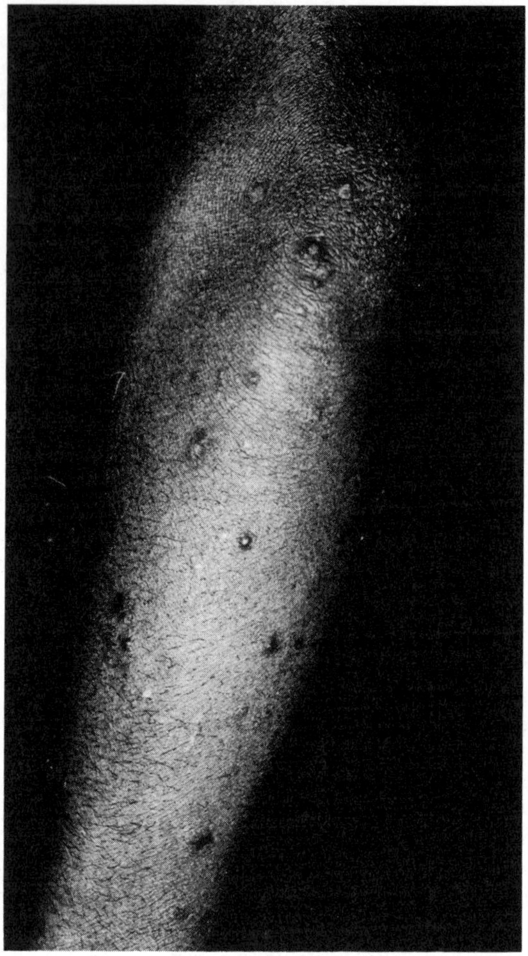

Fig 20–2.—Hyperpigmented papules on left arm. (Courtesy of Lin RY: *Acta Derm Venereol (Stockh)* 68:486–491, 1988.)

have had atopic dermatitis. It is possible that the IgE was produced in response to some unidentified infectious agent. More likely, however, the hyper-IgE-emia was related to HIV-induced immunodysregulation, which is supported by the observation that the patients improved clinically after zidovudine therapy was begun.—R.A. Johnson, M.D.

Comparison of the Efficacy of Surgery and Acyclovir Therapy in Oral Hairy Leukoplakia

Herbst JS, Morgan J, Raab-Traub N, Resnick L (Mt Sinai Med Ctr, Miami Beach; Univ of North Carolina)

J Am Acad Dermatol 21:753–756, October 1989 20–19

Oral hairy leukoplakia, which results from permissive infection of the epithelial cells by Epstein-Barr virus (EBV), occurs almost solely in patients with HIV infection. It is highly predictive for the development of AIDS. In most patients it is asymptomatic, although some complain of pain or burning. Therapeutic responses to surgical excision and orally administered acyclovir were compared in a group of patients with oral hairy leukoplakia.

Forty-five men who were seropositive for HIV participated in the 3-month open-label trial. Fourteen patients underwent surgical excision. Pain was relieved in the 4 symptomatic patients, and there were no recurrences in the areas of excision (Fig 20–3). However, new foci of leukoplakia developed in 10 patients after 3 months. Sixteen patients were given oral acyclovir therapy. Twelve had a clinical regression, but all had recurrences after 3 months. Three patients had relief of pain while receiv-

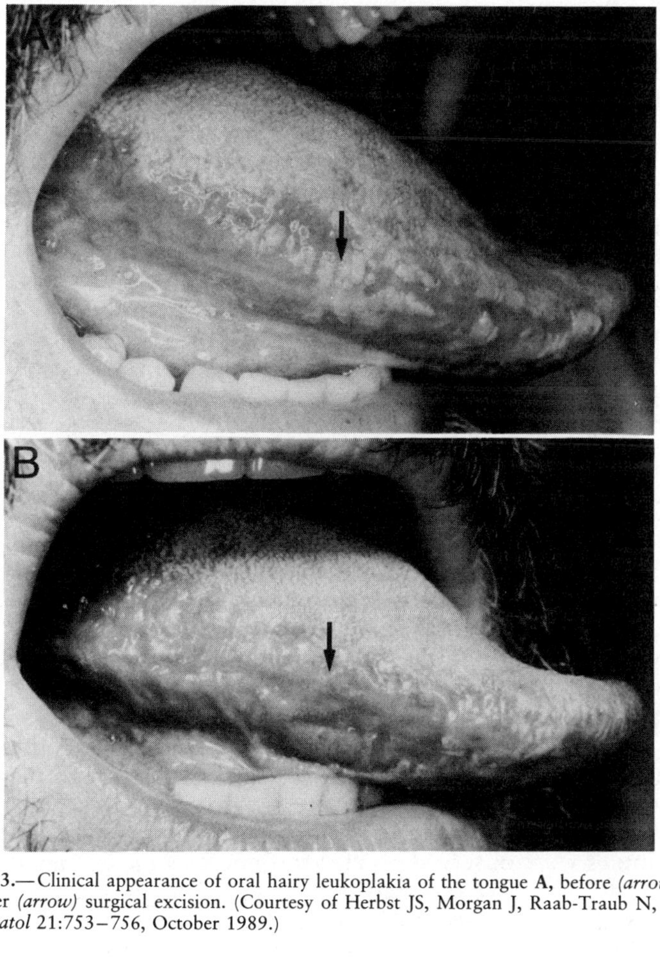

Fig 20–3.—Clinical appearance of oral hairy leukoplakia of the tongue **A**, before *(arrow)* and **B**, 3 months after *(arrow)* surgical excision. (Courtesy of Herbst JS, Morgan J, Raab-Traub N, et al: *J Am Acad Dermatol* 21:753–756, October 1989.)

ing acyclovir, but the pain recurred in 2 of them after acyclovir treatment was discontinued.

Acyclovir therapy produces leukoplakia regression by inhibiting the replication of EBV. Because new foci of leukoplakia may continue to appear, repeated excisions may be needed.

▶ Oral hairy leukoplakia is an EBV-induced epithelial hyperplasia occurring on the lateral and underside of the tongue, and occasionally on the buccal or soft palatal mucosa. Most patients are unaware of its presence. In a few patients it is yet another visible stigma of their HIV-induced immunodeficiency. Most HIV-infected patients with complaints of intraoral pain or burning have concomitant oral candidiasis, which is much more likely to cause symptoms than oral hairy leukoplakia. If observed on a daily basis, the severity, and even the presence, of oral hairy leukoplakia varies considerably. When given for other indications, oral acyclovir and zidovudine and intravenously administered ganciclovir have been reported to cause regression of oral hairy leukoplakia (1–3). Surgical excision of this asymptomatic evanescent epithelial hyperplasia is contraindicated, because of its lack of extended therapeutic efficacy, unexceptable morbidity to the patient, and risk to the surgeon.—R.A. Johnson, M.D.

References

1. Resnick L, et al: *JAMA* 259:384, 1988.
2. Newman C, et al: *Ann Intern Med* 107:348, 1987.
3. Kessler HA, et al: *Arch Intern Med* 148:2496, 1988.

Human Parvovirus B19 Infection Among Hospital Staff Members After Contact With Infected Patients

Bell LM, Naides SJ, Stoffman P, Hodinka RL, Plotkin SA (Univ of Pennsylvania; Univ of Iowa)

N Engl J Med 321:485–491, Aug 24, 1989 20–20

In 1975 human parvovirus B19, a small, single-stranded DNA virus, was discovered in asymptomatic blood donors. It was later found to be associated with aplastic crisis in patients with chronic hemolytic anemia, and with erythema infectiosum, hydrops fetalis, rheumatoid-like arthritis, and chronic suppression of the bone marrow in immunocompromised patients. Among health workers this viral agent has not been recognized as a nosocomial infection hazard.

Unsuspected parvovirus B19 infections in 2 hospitalized adolescents with sickle cell disease resulted in 2 separate outbreaks of erythema infectiosum among nurses. Both patients had aplastic crisis with unsuspected parvovirus infection. In both patients tests for IgM and IgG antibodies to parvovirus B19 were positive, and parvovirus-like particles in the early serum samples were observed on electron microscopic examination.

Forty health care workers had been exposed to the infected patients. Of these, twelve (30%) became infected, 2 (5%) were possibly infected, 8 (20%) had evidence of past infection with B19, and 18 (45%) remained seronegative. In the first outbreak the attack rates were 36% in susceptible contacts, and in the second outbreak, at least 38%. Clinical symptoms included malaise, rash, and joint pain, which began a mean of 12.6 days after exposure. All symptomatic infected persons had joint pain and swelling, which were often cited as the reason for missing work. The joint pain lasted for a mean of 12 days.

Hospital workers are at risk of contracting nosocomial erythema infectiosum from patients with parvovirus-associated aplastic crisis. Therefore, all patients with hereditary hemolytic anemias who are admitted with febrile illness should be evaluated for aplasia. If aplastic crisis is suspected, these patients should be placed promptly in respiratory and contact isolation.

▶ The seroprevalence of parvovirus B19 varies from 30% to 60% in adult populations. Many primary infections are subclinical and asymptomatic. In most patients with symptomatic illness, the clinical disease is erythema infectiosum, a mild febrile illness characterized by a "slapped cheek" facial rash and a reticulated or lacelike rash on the trunk and extremities some patients, especially adults, experience a self-limited arthropathy. There are, however, 3 groups of patients who experience significant morbidity from parvovirus B19 infection: patients with chronic hemolytic anemias (e.g., sickle cell disease, hemoglobin SC disease, hereditary spherocytosis, β-thalassemia, autoimmune hemolytic anemia) can experience transient aplastic crisis and severe anemia; immunodeficient patients (patients receiving maintenance chemotherapy for acute lymphocytic leukemia, patients with congenital immunodeficiencies, those with HIV-related immunodeficiency) can experience severe chronic anemia associated with red cell aplasia; and the fetus of pregnant women can experience hydrops fetalis and fetal death (1). It would be wise for the dermatologist to determine whether patients with erythema infectiosum or their contacts are in these risk groups and to avoid contact with such individuals.—R.A. Johnson, M.D.

Reference

1. *MMWR* 38:81, 1989.

21 Dermatologic Surgery Including Laser

The Stretched Scar: The Benefit of Prolonged Dermal Support
Elliot D, Mahaffey PJ (St Andrew's Hosp, Billericay, Essex, England)
Br J Plast Surg 42:74–78, January 1989 21–1

The rate of scar stretching after surgery is maximal for 6 months then continues at a slower rate. Dermal support with a nonabsorbable suture for the whole of this 6-month period of maximal scar stretching may reduce scar stretching.

Eighty-six skin wounds of the arm and forearm resulting from elliptical excisions of tattoos were studied after 1 year and 3 comparisons were made. In a group of 31 wounds there was a highly significant and numerically considerable reduction (37.5%) of scar stretching with the subcuticular polypropylene (Prolene) suture remaining in situ for 6 months as compared to the conventional percutaneous nylon suture. In another group of 26 wounds, a significant reduction in scar width (15.7%) was noted when the subcuticular Prolene suture remained in situ for 6 months rather than 3 weeks. In another 29 wounds the subcuticular polyglycolic acid (Dexon) suture achieved no reduction in scar width when compared with conventional interrupted sutures.

Scar stretching after surgery is no longer an uncontrollable factor. It appears that Prolene sutures allow significantly and numerically less scar stretching than conventional interrupted nylon sutures. A study to compare scar stretching with polyglyconate (Maxon), the newer generation of absorbable suture with complete absorption at 180 days, with polypropylene is needed.

▶ The authors note that PDS and Maxon, absorbable sutures that are longer lasting than Dexon or Vicryl, were not available at the time of this study but need to be tested. This is an important article noting the *benefit* of subcutaneous sutures, the *importance* of correctly choosing the suture to be used, and the *practicality* of certain sutures.—J.L. Fewkes, M.D.

The Bilobed Flap for Nasal Reconstruction
Zitelli JA (Montefiore Hosp, Pittsburgh)
Arch Dermatol 125:957–959, July 1989 21–2

The bilobed flap is particularly suitable for nasal reconstruction. An improvement in the standard design of the bilobed flap has minimized the

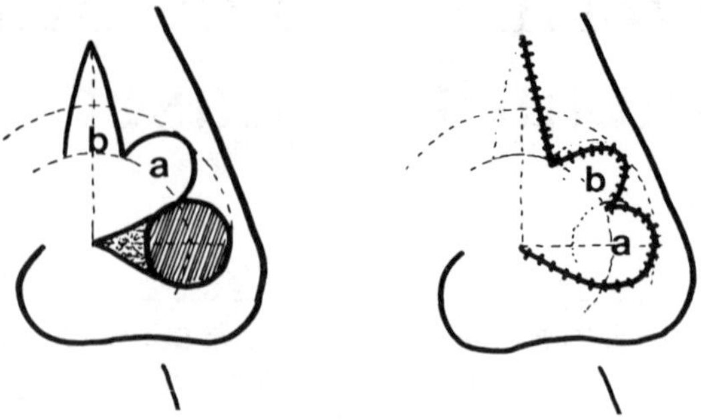

Fig 21–1.—Improved design. These changes minimize dog ear formation and reduce the chance of trapdoor or pincushion formation. (Courtesy of Zitelli JA: *Arch Dermatol* 125:957–959, July 1989.)

problems of pincushioning and tissue protrusions. The bilobed double transposition flap is accomplished with each flap rotating along an arc and transposed only 45 degrees (total, 90–100 degrees), with a Burow's triangle included in the initial design at the point of rotation (Fig 21–1). The excess skin for this flap is ultimately recruited from the lax skin of the upper side wall of the nose.

Four hundred consecutive surgical wounds were studied for wound management, including 192 consecutive nasal reconstructions after skin cancer surgery. The bilobed double transposition flap was the most commonly used flap. Twenty wounds were repaired with the bilobed flap, and most of these were located on the lower third of the nose. Cosmetic results were good or excellent in all of these patients. There was no wound infection, dehiscence, or pincushioning. Color match and texture match were excellent in all patients, and none required surgical revision for scarring or tissue protrusion.

The bilobed double transposition flap is most useful on defects of the lower third of the nose, especially those involving the lateral tip, supratip, or ala near the tip. It is most practical for defects less than 1.5 m in diameter. It can be designed with its base medial or lateral. Flaps based laterally on the side wall of the nose are most useful for reconstruction of defects near the nasal tip, whereas medially based flaps are more useful for repair of alar defects.

▶ This is a very useful flap and fun to do once the principles of flap rotation are learned. Dr. Zitelli gives some very useful tips. However, this is not the first flap to learn to do.—J.L. Fewkes, M.D.

Cryosurgical Management of Myxoid Cysts

Böhler-Sommeregger K, Kutschera-Hienert G (Univ of Vienna)

J Dermatol Surg Oncol 14:1405–1408, December 1988 21–3

Numerous treatments have been proposed for the permanent cure of digital mucoid cysts. Radical surgical excision has a high cure rate, but it may also be complicated by loss of motion or joint stiffness. Multiple needle punctures and injection with steroids or sclerosing agents have had high failure rates. Treatment of digital mucoid cysts and cysts of the oral mucosa with liquid nitrogen cryosurgery was evaluated.

Eighteen patients with digital mucoid cysts and 31 with mucoceles of the oral mucosa underwent treatment by cryosurgery using an intermittent open spray. Surgeons first punctured digital lesions and voided the mucous contents. Oral cysts were not pretreated. Freeze time was 15–30 seconds, after which the frozen area was allowed to thaw before another freeze-thaw treatment was administered. Ten digital cysts and 22 oral cysts were treated twice. Postcryosurgery treatment for digital lesions included application of cold compresses 3 times daily. Bacitracin powder and ointment were applied until the lesions healed completely. For oral lesions the only follow-up treatment was repeated rinsing with sage tea.

Healing time ranged between 21 and 30 days. Cosmetic and functional results were excellent. Postoperative pain was minimal and was easily managed with oral analgesics. At 3-year follow-up there had been 7 recurrences of digital cysts, with an average 9.4 months to recurrence. In all but 1 recurrence, which developed occurred very late, patients with recurrences had had only 1 freeze-thaw treatment cycle. Five recurrences were successfully retreated with a course of 2 freeze-thaw cycles. In 1 oral lesion there was relapse after 3 months; the remainder showed complete clinical healing, regardless of whether 1 or 2 freeze-thaw cycles were used.

Liquid nitrogen spray cryosurgery is an effective treatment for mucous cysts. Two freeze-thaw cycles are recommended for patients with digital mucoid cysts; for oral cysts, 1 cycle appears to be sufficient.

▶ With relatively low cure rates of mucoid cysts with various treatments, this technique is certainly worth trying to see if it is as effective in other hands. I was surprised that there was not more impressive scarring and discomfort noted by patients with digital lesions.—J.L. Fewkes, M.D.

Neoplasms of the Conchal Bowl: Treatment With Mohs Micrographic Surgery

Clark DP, Hanke CW (Univ of Missouri; Indiana Univ, Indianapolis)
J Dermatol Surg Oncol 14:1223–1228, November 1988 21–4

Cancers located in the conchal bowl are potentially dangerous lesions. Rates of local recurrence, distant metastases, and mortality vary but up to 18% of patients with squamous cell carcinoma arising in the external ear are found to have metastases at surgical treatment (table). Thirty-four tumors of the conchal bowl were treated with Mohs' micrographic surgery.

Procedure.—Twenty-six patients had basal cell carcinoma and 8 had squamous cell carcinoma. Mohs' micrographic surgery was performed as outpa-

Incidence of Metastasis From Squamous Cell Carcinoma of the External Ear

Author	Number of Cases	Number (% of Metastases)
Afzelius et al.	69	13 (16.8%)
Pless	177	10 (6.0%)
Schewe and Pappalardo	335	23 (6.9%)
Blake and Wilson	81	10 (12.0%)
Lederman	110	20 (18.0%)
Robins and Nix	78	0 (0%)
Ceilley et al.	29	0 (0%)
Fredricks	27	2 (7%)
Bailin et al.	18	0 (0%)
Goodwin and Jesse	46	4 (8%)

(Courtesy of Clark DP, Hanke CW: *J Dermatol Surg Oncol* 14:1223–1228, November 1988.)

tient surgery. One percent lidocaine with epinephrine was locally infiltrated, and a 1- to 2-mm-thick layer of tissue was excised. A tissue map was developed, and the excised tissue was color coded. Horizontal frozen sections were processed, and the peripheral and deep surgical margins were examined microscopically. The process was repeated until the surgical margins were free of tumor.

Initial treatment with Mohs' micrographic surgery resulted in a tumor-free wound in all but 1 patient, who had extensive involvement of the external ear canal with invasion of cartilage and middle ear. That patient was referred to an otolaryngologist for further treatment. In the remaining patients, wounds were allowed to heal by second intention. One patient required a delayed split-thickness graft after 4 weeks. The other patients had excellent functional and cosmetic results with healing by second intention. There was no significant stenosis of the external ear canal. Two episodes of cellulitis were treated successfully.

Treatment with Mohs' micrographic surgery provides the best chance of tumor removal with maximal conservation of normal tissue. Complete tumor removal is essential in high-risk areas such as the conchal bowl and external auditory canal. Allowing conchal bowl wounds to heal by second intention achieves excellent cosmetic results with minimal morbidity.

▶ This is a good article to remind us of the difficulties of treating conchal bowl tumors as well as the potential for serious complications. Mohs is certainly the treatment of choice, but all patients need to be examined clinically and/or radiologically for metastases and followed carefully.—J.L. Fewkes, M.D.

Interpretation of Mohs Micrographic Frozen Sections: A Peer Review Comparison Study

Grabski WJ, Salasche SJ, McCollough ML, Berkland ME, Gutierrez JA, Finstuen K (Brooke Army Med Ctr, Fort Sam Houston, Texas)
J Am Acad Dermatol 20:670–674, April 1989 21–5

Mohs surgeons receive intense training in histopathologic interpretation during their fellowship training because acting as one's own pathologist is an integral part of the Mohs fresh-tissue micrographic technique. However, the competence of Mohs surgeons to interpret the frozen sections generated during micrographic surgery has never been critically evaluated.

A total of 1,000 randomly selected Mohs micrographic slides were reviewed retrospectively and interpreted by a Mohs surgeon. The Mohs surgeon's interpretations were compared with those provided by general pathologists. Any disputed slides were then matched with an equal number of uncontested control slides from the same patient and reviewed in a blind manner by a Mohs surgeon and a Mohs fellow, a board-certified pathologist and a third-year resident in pathology, and a board-certified dermatopathologist. After independent review of the disputed slides by each of these 3 groups, the same slides were then reviewed by all 3 groups sitting at a multiheaded microscope. The dermatopathologist's interpretation was used as the standard.

There was agreement on interpretations of 913 of the 1,000 slides reviewed and disagreement on 87. The difference in interpretations of 52 of the 87 disputed slides would have resulted in a change in treatment. However, on review, the pathologist revised his interpretation of 76 of the 87 disputed slides. His revised analysis reduced the number of patients who would have been treated differently to 2. Of the remaining contested 11 slides, 4 were resolved in favor of the Mohs surgeon and 2 in favor of the pathologist. The other 5 contested slides lacked objective findings, and the dispute could not be resolved. The agreement index was 97.7% for the Mohs surgeon and 94.3% for the pathologist. The total overall agreement on interpretation between the 3 groups was 98.9%.

The 98.9% agreement in interpretation among these 3 groups confirms that Mohs surgeons are highly skilled in reading fresh-tissue slides, and that they have intimate knowledge of the spectrum of the normal anatomy for each subsite at varying depths.

▶ This article delineates all of the salient points to support the expertise that Mohs surgeons have in interpreting their own slides. Anyone not doing so is not doing Mohs and therefore cannot expect to have the excellent cure rates.—J.L. Fewkes, M.D.

Pseudoepitheliomatous Hyperplasia Following Mohs Micrographic Surgery

Weber PJ, Johnson BL, Dzubow LM (Fort Lauderdale, Fla; Univ of Pennsylvania)
J Dermatol Surg Oncol 15:557–560, May 1989 21–6

Pseudoepitheliomatous hyperplasia (PH) can occur secondarily in several cutaneous disorders. One such instance of PH was noted after Mohs micrographic surgery (MMS) for squamous cell carcinoma of the left brow.

Woman, 73, had a left-brow squamous cell carcinoma for at least 8 months. After biopsy and curettage, excessive granulation tissue was noted at the site of the wound. Several silver nitrate applications were needed for complete healing. Suspicious bumpiness later developed around the scar, and multiple biopsies were done. Four stages of MMS were needed to remove the moderately well-differentiated squamous cell carcinoma. The margin was freshened by removing several fragments of circumferential skin 2–3 mm in width and the defect was grafted. Pathologic analysis of the fragments indicated that all 4 margins had foci of necrosis, ulceration, and foci of infiltrating well-differentiated squamous cell carcinoma. Comparison of the frozen section obtained at the initial MMS with the subsequent fragments revealed dissimilar processes. The entire graft and a 5-mm margin were removed to the periosteum, and another reconstructive graft was done. Mohs histologic assessment revealed no residual tumor.

This growth was at first considered a benign histologic curiosity, but its ultimate effect was not benign.

▶ Bravo to the surgeons for following up on a case that did not have a routine reconstruction. However, I'm still not sure what to do with this entity if it is found. Nevertheless, it's good to know that it exists, so that the problems as noted in this case report can be avoided.—J.L. Fewkes, M.D.

Monopolar and Bipolar Treatment

Sebben JE (Univ of California, Davis)

J Dermatol Surg Oncol 15:364–366, April 1989 21–7

In the context of electrosurgery, the terms *monopolar* and *monoterminal* and *bipolar* and *biterminal* are often confused and used interchangeably. However, the principles underlying these techniques are markedly different.

Some forms of non–high-frequency electrosurgery, such as electrolysis and surgical galvanism, are truly polar because they use direct current. In polar treatment the negative pole becomes the treatment electrode. The negative pole releases electrons, which split water into hydrogen gas and hydroxide used for the chemical destruction of tissue.

High-frequency electrosurgery uses alternating current, which does not have positive and negative poles. In high-frequency electrosurgery, the electric energy alternately enters and exists the tissue through the treatment electrode. Because the treatment electrode is not polar, it should be referred to as a terminal. The terms *monoterminal* and *biterminal* are therefore technically more correct than the terms *monopolar* and *bipolar* when referring to high-frequency electrosurgical procedures. However, the *-polar* suffix is more commonly used than the *-terminal* suffix.

The prefix *-mono* in the term *monopolar* refers to only 1 electrode actively destroying the tissue. Monopolar treatment can be accomplished without a dispersive electrode if the voltage is high and only small amounts of current are delivered. Applications include electrocoagulation, electrofulguration, and electrodesiccation. However, cutting tissues usually requires lower voltage and larger amounts of current, in which case the use of a dispersive electrode is essential. When both a treatment electrode and a dispersive electrode are used, the treatment is still technically monopolar.

True bipolar treatment occurs when tissue destruction is accomplished with 2 treatment electrodes originating from separate sides of the electrosurgical circuit. Bipolar forceps are the most common application of bipolar treatment.

For consistency in nomenclature, the term *monopolar* should be reserved for a description of electrosurgical treatment in which a single treatment electrode is used, either with or without a dispersive electrode. The term bipolar should be used only to describe electrosurgical treatment in which 2 separate treatment electrodes are used.

▶ The article briefly and effectively explains a complex set of terms.—J.L. Fewkes, M.D.

Frigipoint: A New Cryosurgical Instrument
Karakashian GV, Sweren RJ (Monmouth Beach, NJ; Baltimore)
J Dermatol Surg Oncol 15:514–517, May 1989 21–8

Cryosurgery is the destruction of tissue by withdrawing heat from a biological system. Despite new advances in cryosurgery, liquid-nitrogen-saturated, cotton-tipped applicators remain the most commonly used instruments. A handheld dipstick cryoprobe, Frigipoint, was developed that

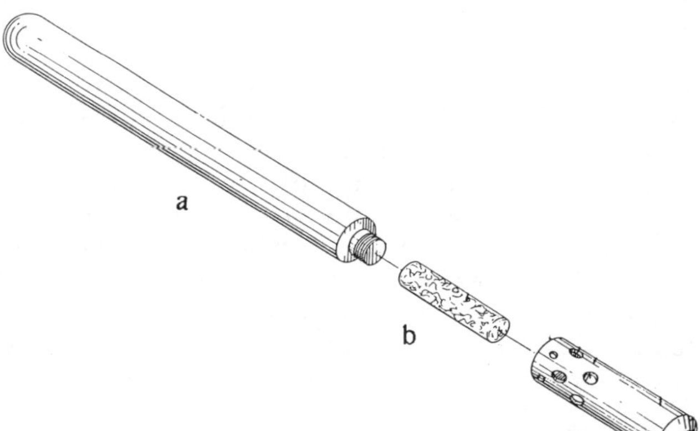

Fig 21–2.—Schematic drawing of Frigipoint. **A,** nonthermoconductive handle. **B,** cryogen absorbent member. **C,** applicator tip. (Courtesy of Karakashian GV, Sweren RJ: *J Dermatol Surg Oncol* 15:514–517, May 1989.)

has 3 components: a thermal conductive housing chamber tapered to tips with diameters of 2–10 mm, a cryogen absorbent member in the housing chamber, and a low-thermal conductivity handle that is threaded onto the housing chamber (Fig 21–2).

Laboratory experiments using a gelatin medium demonstrate that the delivery of the cryogen is uniform over the region of application, producing a flat-bottom ice ball. Animal studies indicate that liquid nitrogen spray produces greater depth of destruction and inflammation than Frigipoint. In preliminary clinical trials, 68 lesions in 16 patients were treated, including actinic keratosis, molluscum contagiosum, verruca plana, solar lentigo, seborrheic keratosis, and verruca vulgaris. After cryosurgery with Frigipoint, all but 1 lesion resolved.

Frigipoint is an effective, safe, portable instrument having a wide range of dermatologic applications. It provides efficient and well-controlled focal cryosurgical treatment of many lesions with 1 immersion of the probe in liquid nitrogen. It also has met with high patient and physician acceptance.

▶ This article was nicely done with both clinical and scientific evaluation. Unfortunately, it did not compare the Frigipoint with the cotton-tipped applicators, with which it is most similar. At this point, I do not see any great advantage.—J.L. Fewkes, M.D.

Lipodystrophy and Its Treatment

Ketterings C (St Clara Hosp, Rotterdam)

Ann Plast Surg 21:536–543, December 1988 21–9

Lipodystrophy, which occurs almost exclusively in women, is characterized by a normal or slender upper body and an extraordinarily massive lower body having enormous amounts of subcutaneous fat. Patients with lipodystrophy often have psychological problems; other complaints are painful, heavy legs, edema, and varicose veins. Most patients have alimentary adiposity.

Subcutaneous lipectomy by the Ilouz method can provide good results. Weight loss is advised; after sufficient weight loss, only liposuction of the trochanteric area and the medial side of the knee is required. There is no unpleasant scarring of the legs. Older patients often require skin reduction. Surgery in the lower legs usually provides good to excellent results (Fig 21–3). Results in the upper legs may be disappointing, however, especially if the patient gains weight after surgery. Given this possibility, the recommended treatment is liposuction of the lower legs, medial side of the knee, and the trochanteric area. Skin reduction without lipectomy is indicated only when the skin is ptotic on the medial side of the upper legs.

Younger patients with lipodystrophy have principally psychological complaints; older patients are troubled by pain and leg weariness. Treatment consists of dieting, subcutaneous lipectomy by liposuction, and prescription of elastic stockings.

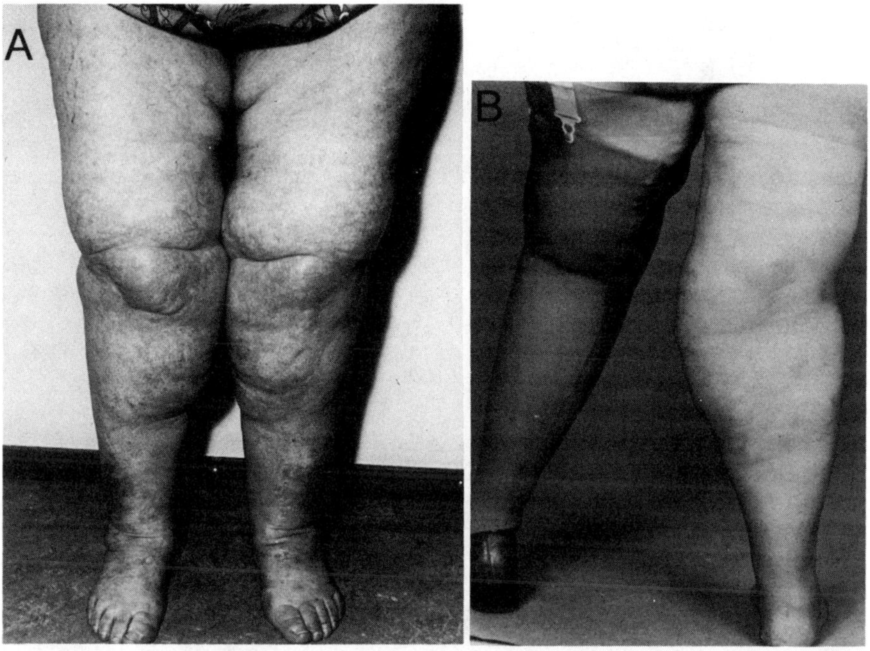

Fig 21–3.—**A,** in this patient experiencing pain and weariness of the legs, a dermal backflow was seen and dermolipectomy on the medial aspect of the knees was performed. **B,** after the operation she was able to wear stockings. (Courtesy of Ketterings C: *Ann Plast Surg* 21:536–543, December 1988.)

▶ This article is for the advanced expert in liposuction. The treatment of these patients almost utilizes a vascular surgery approach.—J.L. Fewkes, M.D.

Aging Hands: A Technique of Hand Rejuvenation by Laser Resurfacing and Autologous Fat Transfer
Abergel RP, David LM (Univ of California, Los Angeles; Inst of Laser and Cosmetic Surgery, Hermosa Beach, Calif)
J Dermatol Surg Oncol 15:725–728, July 1989 21–10

The hands are primary targets for actinic damage and premature aging. Successful hand rejuvenation entails treatment of the sun-damaged skin and subcutaneous atrophy. A simple technique, which combines fat transfer and laser resurfacing, is described to effectively rejuvenate hands and erase the signs of aging.

Technique.—Local anesthesia is used. Seborrheic and actinic keratoses and other cutaneous lesions are vaporized with a carbon dioxide laser, whereas lentigines are resurfaced. Subcutaneous atrophy is addressed by fat harvesting and injection. About 20 cc of fat, which can fill both atrophied hands, is harvested, often from the abdomen, with a 14-gauge needle on a 5-cc syringe. Fat is then injected at the wrist on a line crossing the longitudinal axis of the third phalanx.

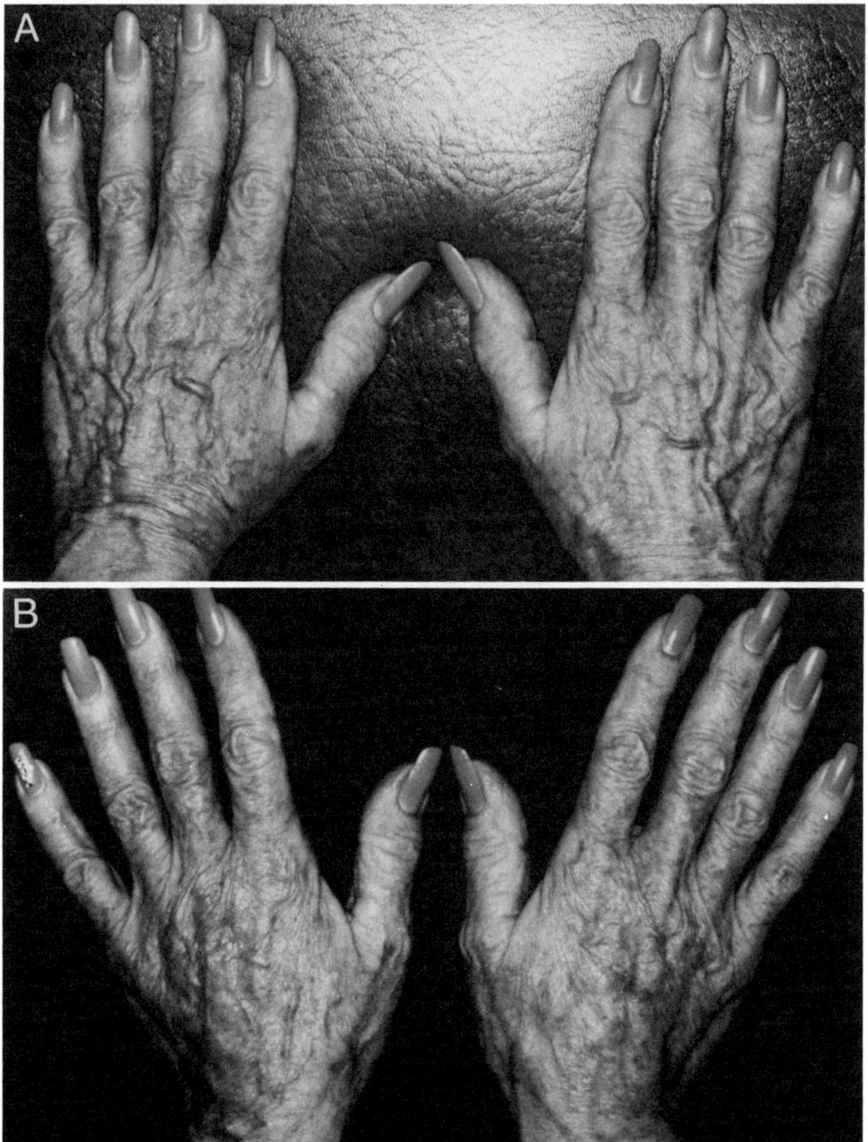

Fig 21–4.—**A,** preoperative view showing extreme atrophy of the skin ans subcutaneous tissue, with veins and tendons protruding on the dorsum of the hands. **B,** final results at 1 month is a smoother aspect of the hands with veins and tendons dissimulated as a result of the subcutaneously injected fat. Laser-treated sites have healed without scarring or pigmentary changes. (Courtesy of Abergel RP, David LM: *J Dermatol Surg Oncol* 15:725–728, July 1989.)

An adhesive bandage is placed over the injection site, and prophylactic antibiotics are given.

This technique provides good results with no pigmentary changes and no scarring (Fig 21–4). Treatment is fast, and results are evident immediately. The simplicity of this technique should make it popular, but the long-term results of fat transfer need to be addressed.

▶ Some of the most cosmetically successful fat transfers are in the hand. However, improvement may last for only 3 months. Anyone attempting the techniques described in this article should first receive adequate instruction.— J.L. Fewkes, M.D.

The Treatment of Multiple Lipomas by Liposuction Surgery

Spinowitz AL (State Univ of New York, Brooklyn)

J Dermatol Surg Oncol 15:538–540, May 1989 21–11

Lipomas may be small and barely visible or large and disfiguring. A rare hereditary pattern of lipomas is known as familial multiple lipomatosis. Angiolipoma is a multiple, tender, and often painful variant. Liposuction surgery has recently been included as an alternative treatment to surgical excision in the management of lipoma.

Case 1.—Man, 68, had many disfiguring nodules measuring 1–7.5 cm on his trunk and upper extremities, some of which were painful and tender. Because his father had a similar condition, he was believed to have familial multiple lipomatosis. He underwent suction-assisted lipectomy under local anesthesia, during which 9 lipomas 2–7.5 cm in size were removed from the right upper extremity through 3 incisions, each 5 mm in size. Approximately 50 cc of blood-tinged fat was removed during the procedure. In addition, many small, firm, encapsulated lipomas were loosened with the liposuction cannula and then milked or massaged out through an incision site a few centimeters away. The patient had no recurrence during a 12-month follow-up.

Case 2.—Man, 78, had multiple painful nodules on both the upper and lower extremities and lower back. He first noticed these nodules at age 37. There was no family history of similar lesions. Examination revealed a total of 34 lesions, most of which were located on the upper extremities. Excisional biopsy confirmed a diagnosis of angiolipoma. He underwent suction-assisted lipectomy, during which 6 angiolipomas ranging in size from 3 cm to 8.5 cm were removed from the left upper extremity through 3 incisions, each 5 mm in size. Approximately 30 cc of blood-tinged fat was removed during the procedure. As in the first patient, several small, firm, encapsulated angiolipomas were also loosened and removed. The patient subsequently underwent a similar procedure on the contralateral upper extremity. He had no recurrence during his 18-month follow-up.

Lipomas less than 3–4 cm in size still usually are removed by surgical excision. When the lipoma reaches 4 cm or more in size, or in the case of multiple lipomas, liposuction offers an excellent alternative to excisional surgery.

▶ Liposuction is a great aid for *multiple* lipomas when done by someone with adequate training.—J.L. Fewkes, M.D.

The Role of Skin Testing in the Use of Collagen Injectable Materials
Elson ML (Dermatology Ctr, Nashville)
J Dermatol Surg Oncol 15:301–303, March 1989 21–12

Greatly improved materials for soft tissue augmentation have been introduced in the last 10 years; however, allergic reactions still sometimes occur despite initial negative skin testing. To prevent local reactions after treatment, it has been proposed that the number of skin tests or the interval between them be varied.

The first 200 patients were evaluated with a single test dose of Zyderm I to the volar forearm before soft-tissue augmentation. The next 200 patients underwent a similar test. If the test was positive at 72 hours, the patient was dropped from the study. Otherwise, the patient underwent a second skin test 14 days later. Both skin tests were interpreted 4 weeks after the initial test. When both tests were negative, patients underwent augmentation.

The hypersensitivity rate to the first skin test was 2.5% in both the single-test and double-test groups. Of 195 patients receiving treatment after a single negative skin test, 3.1% had hypersensitivity reactions at the treatment sites. In the double-skin test group, 7 patients who had negative reactions to the first test had positive reactions to the second test. There were no allergic reactions in the 171 treated patients who had 2 negative skin tests.

All patients under consideration for soft-tissue augmentation with bovine collagen injectable materials should undergo double skin testing before treatment. The additional exposure may significantly reduce the number of patients experiencing allergic reactions at treatment sites.

▶ The current recommendations of the Collagen Corporation are for double skin testing spaced 2 weeks apart. Therefore, the first injection is 6 weeks after the first skin test.—J.L. Fewkes, M.D.

Capillary Hemangioma (Strawberry Mark) of Infancy: Comparison of Argon and Nd:YAG Laser Treatment
Achauer BM, Vander Kam VM (Univ of California, Irvine; Beckman Laser Inst;

Children's Hosp of Orange County)
Plast Reconstr Surg 84:60–69, July 1989 21–13

Because capillary hemangiomas of infancy have a tendency to regress, treatment is generally limited to patients with impaired function; however, in some patients, psychosocial factors may indicate treatment. Argon laser treatment was compared with neodymium:yttrium/aluminum/garnet (Nd:YAG) laser treatment in 55 pediatric patients with these birthmarks.

The children were from 2 weeks to 5 years old. Hemangiomas were photographed and measured before treatment. Only patients with functional impairment or psychosocial problems were treated. Thirty patients received 31 argon laser treatments and 25 received 26 Nd:YAG laser treatments.

Poor results were more common with the argon laser than with the Nd:YAG laser, but both lasers were more effective when the lesions were small (Fig 21–5). For larger lesions the Nd:YAG laser was consistently more effective. There were no excellent results with lesions larger than 1.5 cm.

Although it was less effective, there were fewer and less severe complications with the argon laser. Overall, 12% of patients had complications, 9% of which were associated with the Nd:YAG laser. Complications included postoperative bleeding, delayed healing, and hypertrophic scar-

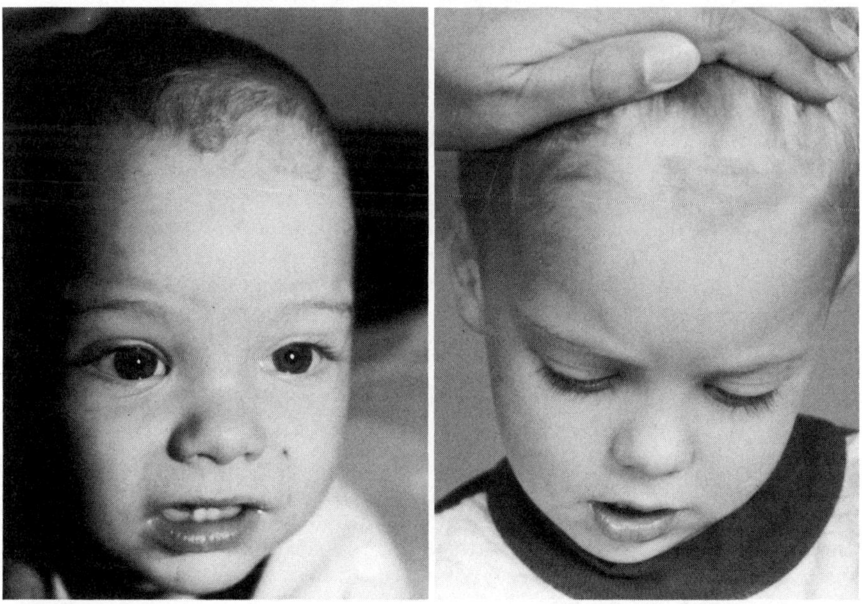

Fig 21–5.—**A,** preoperative view of flat, red hemangioma. **B,** excellent result of argon laser treatment 1 year after treatment. The lesion disappeared immediately after treatment and healing was not delayed. (Courtesy of Achauer BM, Vander Kam VM: *Plast Reconstr Surg* 84:60–69, July 1989.)

ring. Both the Nd:YAG and the argon lasers have roles in the management of strawberry hemangioma of infancy.

▶ As the authors acknowledge, the study is limited in value as a comparison between the 2 types of laser treatment. However, they do document fairly successful responses of bulky lesions to Nd:YAG treatment, although the incidence of complications and scarring was high.—R.W. Gange, M.D.

Argon Laser Treatment of Port Wine Stain

Malm M, Jurell G, Glas J-E (Karolinska Hosp, Stockholm; Sabbatsberg Hosp, Stockholm)

Scand J Plast Reconstr Surg 22:245–248, 1988 21–14

Port-wine stain is a form of nevus flammeus that grows proportionally with the child and shows no tendency to fade. Treatment of port-wine stain with the argon laser has been promising, but exposure times, power outputs, aperture sizes, and distance from laser handpiece to skin have varied considerably. These parameters were studied in 84 patients who had port-wine stains, mostly on the face and neck.

Punch biopsy was used to establish the diagnosis; biopsy specimens were classified according to the degree of fullness—$>15\%$, $>3\%$ $<15\%$, or $\leq 3\%$—of vessels containing luminal erythrocytes. The predicted response to laser treatment was excellent, desirable, or undesirable, respectively, for each category. Scarring was calculated separately. The argon laser was used in a continuous 10-second mode with an average output of 0.7 W. The dermaprobe was hand held perpendicular to and 1.5 cm above the skin, with a spot size of 1 mm. Energy density was kept between 40 and 50 J/cm^2. Two experienced plastic surgeons evaluated the results from slides.

Results were excellent in 45% of patients. Either excellent or desirable results were achieved in 80% of patients whose preoperative biopsy specimens were classified as predicting excellent results; 32% of patients whose preoperative biopsies were judged to predict undesirable results also had excellent results. Scarring was not predictable by biopsy; vessel biopsy specimens from 5 of 6 patients with hypertrophic scarring had been classified as excellent and 1 as desirable. The plastic surgeons differed in their evaluations in only 4 of 84 cases and never by more than 1 grade.

The preoperative punch biopsy specimen is a good predictor of probable treatment results, but some patients with undesirable predictions from biopsies may also benefit from treatment. Patients should always undergo test treatment; those with favorable results are good candidates for argon laser treatment, regardless of biopsy classification. Scarring cannot be predicted by biopsy classification.

▶ This study confirms the value of argon laser treatment, and further documents the predictive significance of biopsy with respect to treatment outcome. The 7% incidence of hypertrophic scarring noted in this study could not be predicted on biopsy and is one of the main reasons for the growing popularity of the tunable dye laser, which very rarely scars.—R.W. Gange, M.D.

Continuous Wave (CW) Dye Lasers Vs. CW Argon Laser Treatment of Port Wine Stain (PWS)

Malm M, Rigler R, Jurell G (Karolinska Hosp and Inst, Stockholm)
Scand J Plast Reconstr Surg 22:241–244, 1988 21–15

Many surgeons have successfully used the continuous wave (CW) argon laser for treatment of port-wine stains; however, poor results and scarring are common in younger patients with pink lesions and small, relatively bloodless vessels. Favorable results with a pulsed dye laser have been reported. Results of treatment with the CW 577-nm dye laser were compared to results with the CW argon laser to determine whether wavelength influenced the outcome and whether energy density was important in regular argon laser treatment.

Twenty patients with port-wine stains were randomly assigned to receive either CW argon laser or CW dye laser treatment, followed by treatment with the other laser after at least 1 week. Preoperative punch biopsy specimens were classified as excellent, desirable, or undesirable on the basis of prediction of results of laser treatment. The argon laser was used in a continuous 10-second mode, with an output power of 0.7 W and spot size of 1 mm. An additional 30 J/cm^2 area was treated with a 0.45 W output in 5 patients. Rhodamine 6G was incorporated in the dye laser, which was used in continuous mode and pumped by a 6 W argon laser. The power was set at 577 nm, and spot size was 1 mm. Output was generally 0.45 W. Treatment was performed with at least 2 different energy densities for each laser.

Fourteen patients had the same results with the argon laser as with the dye laser; 3 had better results with the dye laser, and 3 had better results with the argon laser. Ten of 11 patients with biopsy predictions of excellent response to treatment had excellent results regardless of the laser used.

Treatment with a 577-nm dye laser yielded results comparable to those with argon laser, probably because the thermal relaxation time is more important than the specificity of the wavelength. Further study could provide standardized subjective evaluations that would increase the accuracy of comparisons among results of different studies.

▶ As the authors indicate in their discussion, the results of this careful and well-documented study are not surprising. A comparable study using argon and pulsed dye lasers would be of interest.—R.W. Gange, M.D.

Treatment of Children With Port-Wine Stains Using the Flashlamp-Pulsed Tunable Dye Laser

Tan OT, Sherwood K, Gilchrest BA (Boston Univ)
N Engl J Med 320:416–421, Feb 16, 1989 21–16

Many different approaches to the treatment of port-wine stains have been tried, but most are only minimally effective. For 10 years the argon laser has been used with good to excellent results in about 80% of adult patients. Hypertrophic scarring occurs in fewer than 5% of adults, but in children, argon-laser therapy produces cosmetically unacceptable scars in up to 40%. Promising early results with a flashlamp-pulsed tunable dye laser prompted a clinical trial to assess its efficacy in 35 white children aged 3 months to 14 years with disfiguring port-wine stains of the head and neck ranging in size from 4 cm^2 to 200 cm^2. Three had bilateral lesions. A flashlamp-pulsed tunable dye laser emitting energy at a wavelength of 577 nm with a pulse duration of 360 μsec was used.

All 35 children had complete clearing of the port-wine stains after an average of 6.5 laser treatments to each lesional area; 33 (94.3%) had complete clearing without hypertrophic scarring; 2 (5.7%) had small, isolated depressed scars in areas accidentally traumatized within 24 hours of laser treatment. Transient hyperpigmentation was noted in 20 children, but the discoloration cleared completely within 3–4 months. Lesions overlying bony prominences such as the forehead, temple, and nose required an average of 3.7 laser treatments, whereas lesions on the cheek and lips required an average of 7.5 treatments. Children younger than 7 years required fewer treatments for optimal response than did older children.

The excellent results obtained with the flashlamp-pulsed tunable dye laser in 33 of 35 children treated for disfiguring port-wine stains strongly suggest that this laser is superior to the argon laser for use in this age group.

▶ These investigators obtained complete clearing of port-wine stains in all children, the oldest of whom was 14 years. Other than age, it is not clear from the paper what features distinguished this group to allow such good results, which differ radically from the general experience in older patients.—R.W. Gange, M.D.

Preliminary Study of the Vascular Dynamics of Port-Wine Hemangioma With Therapeutic Implications for Argon Laser Treatment

Apfelberg DB, Smith T, White J (Palo Alto Med Found, Calif)
Plast Reconstr Surg 83:820–827, May 1989 21–17

The etiology of port-wine hemangiomas is unknown, and the causes of progressive change are unclear. The vascular dynamic physiology of port-wine stains also is confusing. A preliminary study of the vascular dynamics was performed on 10 patients aged 17–38 years with port-wine hemangiomas of the face and extremities. A laser Doppler velocimeter was used to study differential perfusion and blood flow.

Port-wine hemangiomas did not always have different perfusion than normal skin but did respond less vigorously to heat challenges. Port-wine hemangioma vessels showed no uniform response to cooling. Xylocaine plus epinephrine injection resulted in significantly reduced perfusion and vasoconstriction. Argon laser treatment did not uniformly alter laser Doppler perfusion. Laser Doppler velocimeter flow studies were unable to predict future good or bad results of laser treatment.

▶ It is unfortunate that there is no noninvasive method of predicting the outcome of laser treatment. Although biopsies may be helpful, there are wide variations of response in the same individual.—R.W. Gange, M.D.

Treatment of Perifolliculitis Capitis Abscedens et Suffodiens With the Carbon Dioxide Laser

Glass LF, Berman B, Laub D (Univ of California, Davis)

J Dermatol Surg Oncol 15:673–676, June 1989 21–18

Perifolliculitis capitis abscedens et suffodiens is a chronic disease of the scalp seen mainly in black men. Numerous firm or fluctuant nodules and abscesses intercommunicate by sinus tracts on the occiput and vertex of the scalp. Hair is easily removed, and a severe scarring alopecia frequently develops. In the early stages, treatment has included moist compresses and Burow's soaks, topical or intralesional steroids, and systemic antibiotics. Treatment was carried out with the carbon dioxide (CO_2) laser in a 36-year-old man.

Man, 36, had abscedens et suffodiens. The lesions were refractory to previous conservative management, including systemic antibiotics and 8 weeks of 13-cis-retinoic acid, 1 mg/kg/day. He had intractable pain and continuous drainage. Surgical intervention was proposed. The most fluctuant nodule, about 6 cm^2 in area, was selected for CO_2 laser therapy. After local anesthesia as obtained, the CO_2 laser in the focused mode at 31,830 W/cm^2 was used to incise the deep dermis around the nodule border. The entire lesion was excised with sweeping motions of the focused laser beam, and retraction of the tissue was facilitated with the tissue forceps. Hemostasis was attained by defocusing the laser beam to vaporize the base. A sterile compression dressing was applied. Wound care involved daily cleansing with 3% hydrogen peroxide and application of bacitracin ointment. The patient was seen every 2 weeks until complete reepithelialization occurred. Healing by second intention was complete in 6 weeks, and there was no evidence of recurrence after 4 months.

Carbon dioxide laser excision is a useful treatment modality for isolated lesions of perifolliculitis capitis abscedens et suffodiens. The role of this treatment, alone and in conjunction with other modalities, requires further study.

▶ The CO_2 laser is useful for facilitating surgery in areas where bleeding interferes with scalpel surgery.—R.W. Gange, M.D.

Pearly Penile Papules: Treatment With the Carbon Dioxide Laser
Magid M, Garden JM (Santa Cruz, Calif; Northwestern Med School, Chicago)
J Dermatol Surg Oncol 15:552–554, May 1989 21–19

Pearly penile papules occur frequently over the corona and sulcus of the penis. These asymptomatic lesions are acral angiofibromas. Some men, however, are disturbed by their presence and request their removal. Two patients were successfully treated with the carbon dioxide (CO_2) laser.

In both men the lesions had been present since puberty and were asymptomatic. Physical examination showed multiple pearly white to normal skin-toned papules 1–2 mm in diameter in single or double rows over the corona of the penis. Pearly penile papules, diagnosed in both patients, were removed because of significant associated psychological distress.

Procedure.—In both patients, the glans of the penis was prepared and anesthetized locally with 1% lidocaine. Using a defocused beam that was about the diameter of each papule, the lesions were treated with the CO_2 laser set at 0.1 second and 5 W. The procedure was well tolerated. The patients were told to wash the area twice daily with hydrogen peroxide and apply a topical antibiotic ointment. The treated regions healed without skin texture or pigmentary changes; all treated lesions were ablated.

▶ This seems like a reasonable approach for those individuals who cannot be persuaded to live with their papules. The "lesions" illustrated in this article seem to have been very small.—R.W. Gange, M.D.

Outcome of Carbon Dioxide Laser Therapy for Persistent Cutaneous Viral Warts
Logan RA, Zachary CB (St John's Hosp for Diseases of the Skin, London)
Br J Dermatol 121:99–105, July 1989 21–20

A small group of otherwise normal patients have persistent cutaneous viral warts, sometimes for many years, that may cause considerable discomfort and embarrassment. Eighteen adults with persistent warts were treated with the CO_2 laser. Twelve had plantar warts and 6 had lesions on the hands. The median duration of warts before treatment was 5 years. The laser was used as a last resort for both symptomatic and cosmetic indications.

Five patients with plantar warts and 5 with finger warts were cured, for an overall rate of 56%. Both atrophic and hypertrophic scars were seen. Fourteen patients described severe posttreatment pain that lasted for a median of 3 weeks. Analgesics were required by 17 patients for an average of 2 weeks. Only 4 patients had a history that suggested postoperative infection. Bleeding was not a significant problem. One patient had persistent contracture of a treated finger and resultant poor grip. Four patients with plantar warts were unable to walk for an average of 13 days after treatment. Eight patients were satisfied that the treatment had improved their eventual clinical status, 9 believed they were worse off after treatment, and 1 patient was undecided.

More than half of these patients with persistent warts were cured by CO_2 laser treatment. Long-term studies comparing laser treatment with modalities such as bleomycin or interferon are needed.

Benefits of the CO_2 Laser for Verruca Resistant to Other Modalities of Treatment

Apfelberg DB, Druker D, Maser MR, White DN, Lash H, Spector P (Palo Alto Med Found, Calif)

J Dermatol Surg Oncol 15:371–375, April 1989 21–21

The efficacy of the CO_2 laser in the treatment of verruca is recognized, but most studies have used CO_2 laser treatment as a primary therapy and few have evaluated its efficacy in the treatment of verruca resistant to other forms of therapy. During a 64-month study period, 33 patients aged 12–56 years whose warts had been treated from 1 to 5 times without eradication were treated with the CO_2 laser. Six patients had undergone more than 5 unsuccessful treatments.

Eight patients were unavailable for follow-up. Of the remaining 25 patients, 8 reported complete success, for a 32% cure rate. Another 5 reported partial to 95% success, i.e., most of the warts were eradicated but some had recurred. Twelve patients (48%) reported total failure, i.e., persistence and recurrence of all warts.

Although the CO_2 laser is useful in the treatment of warts recalcitrant to other therapies, almost half of the patients in this series were not improved. Despite this high failure rate, the CO_2 laser should still be strongly considered when other treatment modalities have been unsuccessful.

▶ These 2 papers (Abstracts 21–20 and 21–21) present comparable and rather disappointing results of CO_2 laser treatment of resistant warts. The findings confirm that the honeymoon period for the CO_2 laser treatment for warts is over, and that careful patient selection is very important. Few would now use the CO_2 laser as first-line treatment. The incidence of severe pain in the series reported by Logan et al. (severe in 14 of 18 patients, lasting for a median of 3 weeks) is surprisingly high compared with our own experience.—R.W. Gange, M.D.

Infectious Papillomavirus in the Vapor of Warts Treated With Carbon Dioxide Laser or Electrocoagulation: Detection and Protection

Sawchuk WS, Weber PJ, Lowy DR, Dzubow LM (Natl Cancer Inst, Bethesda, Md; Univ of Pennsylvania)

J Am Acad Dermatol 21:41–49, July 1989 21–22

A recent report indicates that papillomavirus DNA can be isolated from the vapor (smoke plume) of warts treated with the CO_2 laser. Prompted by concerns for operator safety, the relative amounts of virus isolated from the vapor of human and bovine warts treated with laser and with electrocoagulation were investigated. In addition, the use of a surgical mask to protect operators against potential virus exposure was evaluated. The vapor from each therapy was collected with a dry filter vacuum apparatus and was analyzed for the presence of papillomavirus.

Among the human plantar warts treated, human papillomavirus DNA was detected in 5 of 8 laser-derived vapors and 4 of 7 electrocoagulation-derived vapors. Because there is no reproducible in vitro infectivity assay for human papillomavirus particles, bovine warts were used to determine whether the papillomavirus in the vapor was infectious. With a bioassay, infectious bovine papillomavirus was readily detected in the vapor from bovine warts treated with either modality, and more virus was present in the laser-derived vapors. Placing a surgical mask in front of the collection filter inhibited the passage of virtually all laser- or electrocoagulation-derived virus.

Papillomavirus DNA can be detected in the vapor derived from warts treated with CO_2 and electrocoagulation. The potential risk from inhalation may be reduced markedly by wearing a surgical mask. Laser treatment may pose a greater theoretical hazard than electrocoagulation.

▶ These investigators have confirmed the recent observation of Garden et al. (1) regarding the CO_2 laser plume and its potential infectivity. The findings reinforce the need for efficient smoke evacuation and properly fitted and tied masks. Other lasers may also liberate particulate material from the surface of the skin.—R.W. Gange, M.D.

Reference

1. Garden JM, et al: *JAMA* 259:1199, 1988.

An Effective Cosmetic Treatment for Ota's Nevus

Cosman B, Apfelberg DB, Druker D (Palo Alto Med Found, Calif)

Ann Plast Surg 22:36–42, January 1989 21–23

A cosmetic treatment may be effective for Ota's nevus, a congenital facial melanocytic lesion.

Method.—Snowy dry ice is used for facial skin, excluding eyelids. It is applied until the skin turns white, and the adjacent lesional skin is then treated similarly.

After 24 hours the elevated blebs and epithelium are peeled under local anesthesia. Topical antibiotics are applied to the area daily. The treatment is repeated monthly, usually 6–10 times, until marked clearing of the dark pigment is achieved. The eyelid skin is blanched with the argon laser under local anesthesia.

This treatment was used in 5 women with Ota's nevus in the cheek, eyelid, and forehead. An average of 8 snowy dry ice treatments and 2.5

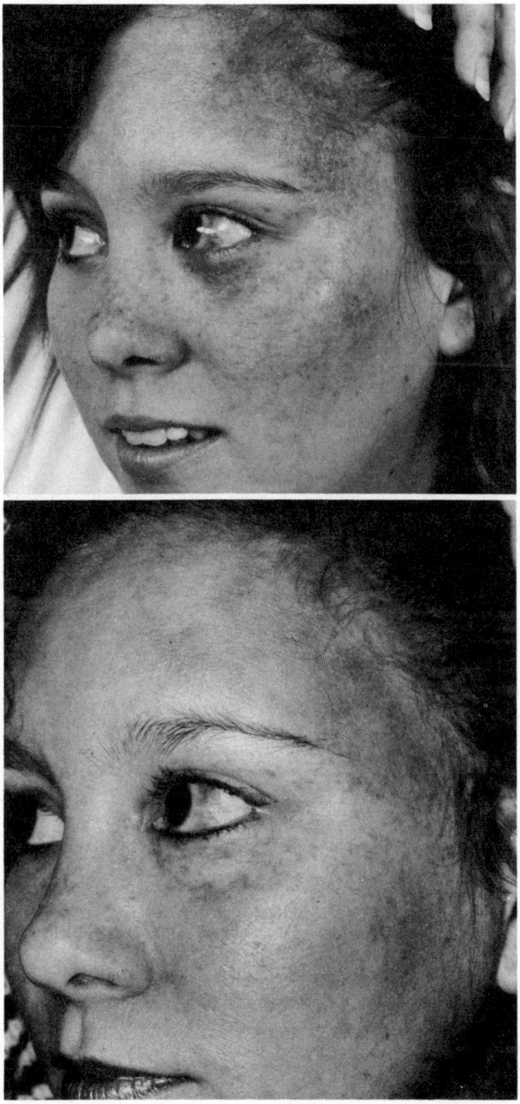

Fig 21–6.—A, nevus of forehead and temple before treatment. **B,** good lightening without scar or recurrence on forehead and temple after treatment. Patient underwent 11 snowy dry ice/epithelial peeling treatments. (Courtesy of Cosman B, Apfelberg DB, Druker D: *Ann Plast Surg* 22:36–42, January 1989.)

laser treatments were given. Excellent results (marked lightening, no scars) were achieved in 1 patient and good (partial lightening) in 4 (Fig 21–6).

The combination of snowy dry ice and epithelial peeling and argon laser for Ota's nevus is for cosmetic ablation only. These patients are still at risk with regard to the local and systemic complications of Ota's nevus, such as secondary open-angle or angle-closure glaucoma.

▶ We have asked Dr. Charles Taylor to comment on this article.

▶ This case series describes a cosmetic treatment for nevus of Ota, a congenital facial melanocytic lesion. It is not uncommon for this disease to be treated with 1 method exclusively, usually with less than successful results. Our own experience using a Q-switched ruby laser has been disappointing. Although the numbers are small in this report, the suggestion of combination techniques for this therapeutic problem is appealing and reflects the growing trend toward construing nevus of Ota as 2 disorders rather than 1, namely, the problem of both superficial and deep pigment. As the authors suggest, Ohshiro has also reported success with snowy dry ice and epithelial peeling followed by the ruby laser (1). A controlled comparison of these 2 techniques (i.e., argon vs. ruby laser following snowy dry ice and epithelial peeling) is eagerly awaited.—C. Taylor, M.D.

Reference

1. Ohshiro T: *Laser Treatment for Nevi.* Tokyo, Medical Laser Research, Nippon Laser Association, 1980, pp 128–137.

22 Dermatopathology

Tufted Angioma (Angioblastoma): A Benign Progressive Angioma, Not to Be Confused With Kaposi's Sarcoma or Low-Grade Angiosarcoma

Jones EW, Orkin M (St John's Hosp for Diseases of the Skin, London)
J Am Acad Dermatol 20:214–225, February 1989 22–1

Twenty patients with confirmed tufted angioma were encountered in 23 years; 12 presented before age 5 years and 6 in the first year of life, but only 3 patients had a blemish at birth. The neck, upper chest, and shoulder were the most frequent sites. The lesions varied widely in size and appearance, but dull red macules with a mottled appearance were most frequent; they usually were 2–5 cm.

A focal arrangement of tightly packed capillaries was seen at varying dermal levels, often in rounded or ovoid tufts that occasionally coalesced to form tracts of angiomatous tissue. The tufts sometimes indented lymph vessels to produce a glomerularlike appearance. The tufts consisted chiefly of hypertrophied endothelial cells. Mucinous material was not much increased. In 1 patient there was a small area of lymphatic-like proliferation. Cell marker studies confirmed the presence of endothelial and perithelial cells.

Tufted angioma is a distinctive lesion that must be distinguished from other vascular pathologies occurring in young persons. Despite progressive spread, the lesion behaves in a benign way. Histologic study is necessary to rule out more serious lesions.

▶ Tufted angiomas are uncommon, but not rare, vascular lesions of the skin. These lesions are important in that they are benign and should not be misdiagnosed as Kaposi's sarcoma. The differential diagnosis of this lesion includes various benign and malignant hemangioendotheliomas. This paper nicely illustrates the important features of this lesion.—T.J. Flotte, M.D.

Malignant Endovascular Papillary Angioendothelioma (Dabska Tumor): A Case Report and Review of the Literature

Morgan J, Robinson MJ, Rosen LB, Unger H, Niven J (Mt Sinai Med Ctr of Greater Miami, Miami Beach, Fla; Univ of Miami)
Am J Dermatopathol 11:64–68, 1989 22–2

Dabska described a vascular tumor in the skin of children consisting of anastomosing vascular channels with intraluminal papillary or tuftlike projections of endothelial cells, possibly with cytologic atypia. The prognosis appears to be relatively good.

Boy, 10 years, was first seen with a 1.1-cm pink-tan nodule in the skin over the left scapula that had been present for about a year. It gradually increased in size. Shave biopsy led to a diagnosis of malignant endovascular papillary angioendothelioma, and the rest of the nodule was excised conservatively. The patient was well 22 months later. Oval to spindled cells with an increased nuclear-cytoplasmic ratio were present. The nuclei were hyperchromatic and mildly pleomorphic; mitotic figures were rare. Electron microscopy demonstrated features of endothelial cells. Immunoperoxidase staining with C3.1 antigen was strongly positive in the endothelial cells of both the glomeruloid and anastomosing channel parts of the lesion.

This tumor must be distinguished from vegetant intravascular hemangioendothelioma, epithelioid hemangioendothelioma, and low-grade angiosarcoma. The differential diagnosis also includes malignant hemangioendothelioma and acquired tufted angioma.

▶ The AIDS epidemic has generated a great deal of interest in vascular tumors. The Dabska tumor was first described in 1969. Since that time very few cases have been reported. The position of this lesion in the nosology of vascular tumors is uncertain, but it most likely represents a unique entity. It is interesting that Dr. Dabska reviewed the diagnosis and concurred with the authors. It will be interesting to see, as more of these cases accumulate, what the final disposition of these tumors will be.—T.J. Flotte, M.D.

Glomus Tumours: An Immunohistochemical Profile of 11 Cases

Dervan PA, Tobbia IN, Casey M, O'Loughlin J, O'Brien M (Mater Misericordiae Hosp; Univ College, Dublin)

Histopathology 14:483–491, May 1989 22–3

Glomus tumors usually appear as single, painful skin nodules. Ultrastructural studies have suggested that these tumor cells are modified smooth muscle cells. To investigate the origin of these cells, 11 glomus tumors were examined immunohistochemically with a group of connective tissue, epithelial, and muscle-specific antibodies.

Most tumors contained nerve fibers, which accounts for the pain frequently experienced by patients. All tumors reacted with monoclonal antibody HHF 35, which reacts only with muscle-specific actin. All tumors stained positively for vimentin (Fig 22–1). Staining for cytokeratins, desmin, myoglobin, S-100 protein, neurofilaments, and factor VIII-related antigen produced negative results in all 11 glomus tumors.

These immunohistochemical results confirm that glomus tumors are composed of modified smooth muscle cells. Immunohistochemical analysis can be used to distinguish these tumors from other types in cases for which microscopic diagnosis proves inadequate.

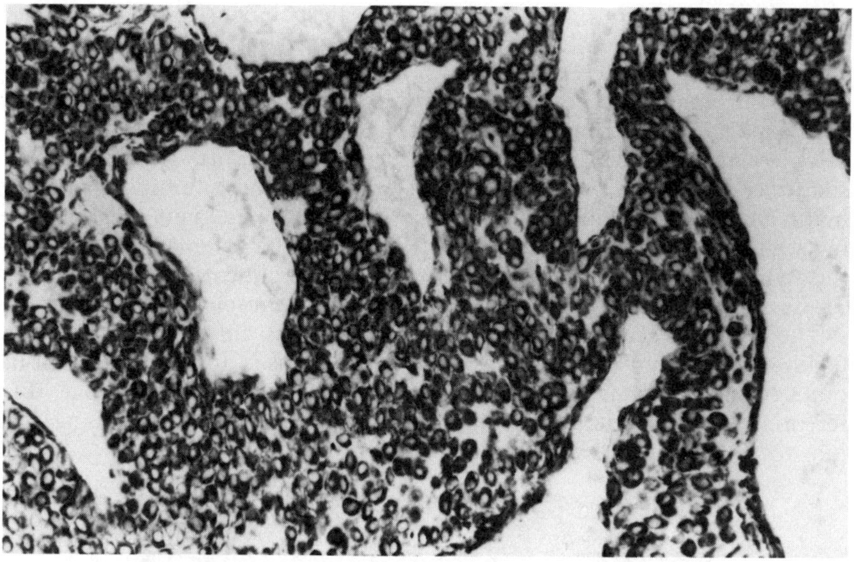

Fig 22–1.—Intense staining for vimentin in glomus cells surrounding dilated vascular channels. Original magnification, ×500. (Courtesy of Dervan PA, Tobbia IN, Casey M, et al: *Histopathology* 14:483–491, May 1989.)

▶ This article demonstrates that the immunohistochemical profile of a positive reaction with muscle-specific actin and vimentin with a negative reaction to cytokeratin, factor VIII, and S100 protein should distinguish glomus tumors from most other tumors in the differential diagnosis. In addition, they have confirmed the presence of nerve fibers present within the tumors, which may account for the pain associated with them.—T.J. Flotte, M.D.

Pleomorphic Fibroma of the Skin: A Benign Neoplasm With Cytologic Atypia: A Clinicopathologic Study of Eight Cases
Kamino H, Lee JY-Y, Berke A (New York Univ Med Ctr)
Am J Surg Pathol 13:107–113, February 1989 22–4

Nuclear atypia is usually considered characteristic of malignant neoplasms, but it also occurs in several benign simulators of malignant neoplasms, including pleomorphic lipoma, pleomorphic leiomyoma, ancient schwannoma, and pseudosarcomatous dermatofibroma. The most common skin lesions (e.g., fibroepithelial polyps and fibromas) usually are not associated with nuclear atypia. Sections of 9 skin biopsy specimens from 8 patients, including 1 recurrence after partial surgical removal, were studied by light microscopy and immunohistochemical staining. Prominent nuclear atypia and rare mitotic figures were observed.

All lesions were asymptomatic, solitary, and slow growing. They were flesh-colored, nonulcerated, high-dome-shaped papules or polypoid lesions, measuring from 4 to 16 mm in greatest dimension. The patients were men and women aged 33–67 years. Five lesions were on the extremities, 1 on the face, and 2 on the trunk. The clinical diagnoses were nevus, fibroma, fibrokeratoma, neurofibroma, hemangioma, and polyp. All neoplasms were characterized histologically by sparse cellularity and thick collagen bundles randomly oriented amid spindle- and irregularly shaped cells (Fig 22–2). Most cells had large, pleomorphic, and hyperchromatic nuclei with small nucleoli. Many multinucleated giant cells, including some with multilobed nuclei, were present. The cytoplasm of most of the atypical spindle and giant cells was positive for vimentin staining, and in 3 cases spindle-shaped cells were positive for anti-muscle actin staining.

The lesions described are a variant of cutaneous fibromas. Researchers believe that the nuclear atypia seen in these lesions is analogous to that in other benign mesenchymal neoplasms. On the basis of the histologic differentiation, cytologic atypia, and benign clinical course, it is suggested that these lesions be termed "pleomorphic fibromas."

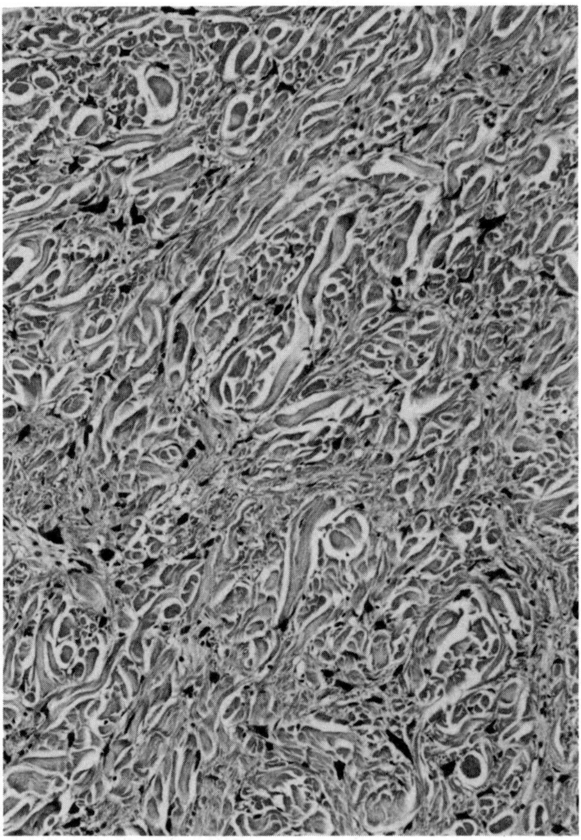

Fig 22–2.—Low-power examination shows sparse cellularity and thick collagen bundles in a haphazard array. (Courtesy of Kamino H, Lee JY-Y, Berke A: *Am J Surg Pathol* 13:107–113, February 1989.)

▶ The authors describe a new entity that they entitle "pleomorphic fibroma of the skin," which is an uncommon but not rare lesion. It is important for histopathologists to recognize this lesion because the first time one sees an example, it can be disturbing.—T.J. Flotte, M.D.

Fibrous Hamartoma of Infancy: Eight Additional Cases and a Review of the Literature

Paller AS, Gonzalez-Crussi F, Sherman JO (Children's Mem Hosp, Chicago; Northwestern Univ)

Arch Dermatol 125:88–91, January 1989 22–5

Fibrous hamartoma of infancy is a benign, persistent soft tissue tumor that appears in the first 2 years of life. The lesion is not clinically distinctive, but histopathologic examination of affected tissue demonstrates the characteristic elements of fibrous, adipose, and myxoid mesenchymal tissue.

Girl, 2 months, had a nodule that developed on the right buttock at the site of her first immunization just after it was given. The lesion was initially considered to be a resolving hematoma, an abscess, or a foreign body reaction. One year later, however, it had increased in size. Palpation of the skin-colored lesion showed it to be a firm, nontender, movable nodule with irregular borders and a

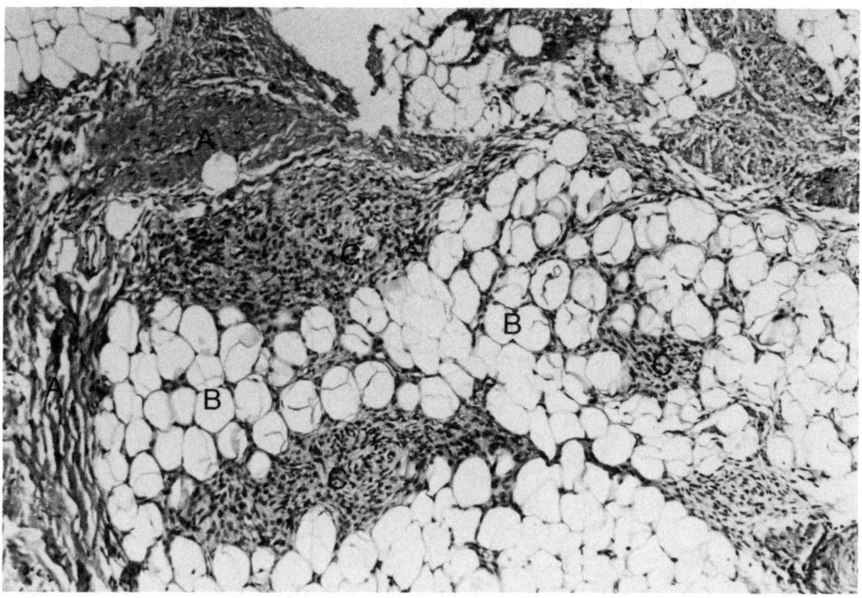

Fig 22–3.—Typical histologic appearance of fibrous hamartoma of infancy. Occurrence of dense collagenous tracts (A), adipose tissue (B), and foci of myxoid, primitive-appearing mesenchyme (C) is considered diagnostic. Hematoxylin-eosin; original magnification, ×75. (Courtesy of Paller AS, Gonzalez-Crussi F, Sherman JO: *Arch Dermatol* 125:88–91, January 1989.)

Locations of 78 Lesions of Fibrous Hamartoma of Infancy

Locations	No.
Axillary	20
Abdomen, inguinal, groin, buttocks, perianal	15
Arm, wrist	13
Chest wall, breast	11
Shoulder, back	10
Neck	3
Face, scalp	3
Foot	1
Pharynx	1
Unknown	1
Total	**78**

(Courtesy of Paller AS, Gonzalez-Crussi F, Sherman JO: *Arch Dermatol* 125:88–91, January 1989.)

lobulated surface. The infant was otherwise healthy. When the patient was examined at 17 months of age, the lesion had grown larger and a biopsy was done. Histopathologic evaluation revealed the 3 types of tissue that characterize fibrous hamartoma of infancy: dense fibrocollagenous areas, often appearing as bands or septa coursing in different directions; mature adipose tissue; and foci of collagen-poor, moderately or densely cellular myxoid mesenchymal tissue (Fig 22–3).

Sixty-seven cases of fibrous hamartoma of infancy have been described previously, although few have been described in the dermatologic literature. Eight new cases have been added, and the clinical statistics of all 75 were compiled (table). Only 3 of the children had more than 1 tumor.

▶ As this is a tumor of infancy that doesn't spontaneously regress and, in fact, may grow larger, it is important to differentiate it from a malignant tumor. Also, there does not seem to be a distinct clinical appearance, so the only method of diagnosis is a biopsy.—J.C. Alper, M.D.

Plexiform Fibrohistiocytic Tumor Presenting in Children and Young Adults: An Analysis of 65 Cases

Enzinger FM, Zhang R (Armed Forces Inst of Pathology, Washington, DC; Research Lab of Tumor Pathology and Cancer Hosp, Shanghai)
Am J Surg Pathol 12:818–826, November 1988 22–6

An unusual and hitherto undescribed neoplasm with morphological features resembling cutaneous fibrous histiocytoma and fibromatosis was found in 65 children and adults. The mean age was 16.2 years (range, 2 months to 71 years), and two thirds of the patients were younger than 20. The female:male ratio was almost 3:1.

The tumor presented as a slow-growing, poorly demarcated dermal or subcutaneous mass that rarely exceeded 3 cm in diameter. All but 1 was solitary. Its most common location was the upper extremity (63%), particularly the shoulder and forearm . The microscopic appearance varied from case to case, ranging from distinct aggregates of rounded histiocytic-like cells and giant cells (fibrohistiocytic type) to a predominantly plexiform fibroblastic pattern (fibroblastic type).

Of the 32 patients for whom follow-up information was available, 20 were alive and well after local excision. Twelve had recurrence, including 2 with metastases to regional lymph nodes. Metastasis to the lung or other organs was not observed. There was no correlation between biologic behavior and any specific clinical or morphological parameter.

This tumor represents a specific entity that has characteristic clinical and easily identifiable histologic features. It bears some resemblance to cutaneous fibrous histiocytoma and fibromatosis but differs in its multinodular or plexiform growth pattern and its frequent occurrence in children and young adults. Other differential diagnoses include plexiform neurofibroma and benign and malignant giant cell tumor.

▶ This paper by Drs. Enzinger and Zhang is a beautifully illustrated description of a new entity.—T.J. Flotte, M.D.

Juvenile Xanthogranuloma: Clinical and Pathologic Correlation

Tahan SR, Pastel-Levy C, Bhan AK, Mihm MC Jr (Massachusetts Gen Hosp, Boston)

Arch Pathol Lab Med 113:1057–1061, September 1989 22–7

The clinical, microscopic, and some immunohistochemical features of juvenile xanthogranuloma (JXG) were investigated in 34 patients. One or more JXG lesions were present in patients ranging in age from birth to 50 years, peaking in incidence before age 1 year and between ages 20 and 30 years. The male:female ratio was 4:1. Most of the lesions occurred singly, usually in the cephalic area. Occasional multiple lesions were papulonodular, penetrating the reticular dermis or panniculus, or both. Varied architectural patterns (e.g., xanthogranulomatous, xanthomatous, fibrohistiocytic, and combined) were seen. The cellular constituents included foamy histiocytes, lymphocytes, epithelioid monocytes, eosinophils, Touton giant cells, and spindle cells in 2 forms (dendritic and fusiform). The S100-positive dendritic cells comprised a minor but important component of expansion zones and were found in all lesions tested.

Juvenile xanthogranuloma represents a complex interaction of cells and messengers in a dynamically evolving process. Because of the antigen-processing abilities of dendritic S100-mononuclear cells, the clustering of these cells at the peripheral expanding zones suggests that antigen interaction occurs at the peripheral growth zones.

▶ This paper presents little new information regarding these lesions; however, it does present a very carefully done clinial and histologic description of this entity, which is also well illustrated.—T.J. Flotte, M.D.

Epithelioid Cell Histiocytoma: A New Entity

Jones EW, Cerio R, Smith NP (Guy's and St Thomas' Hosps; St John's Hosp for Diseases of the Skin, London)
Br J Dermatol 120:185–195, February 1989 22–8

Dermatofibroma, or histiocytoma, can have many different histologic appearances. A previously unrecognized variation of histiocytoma was observed.

Researchers found 19 examples of epithelioid cell histiocytomas among 103,540 specimens received for histologic examination (table). All patients were adults, with women slightly outnumbering men. All but 1 lesion occurred on the limbs, mostly in the lower extremities, the thigh being the most common site. Most lesions were firm, sessile, or polypoid nodules or papules, ranging from 0.5 to 1.5 cm in diameter. Most were circular or ovoid with smooth surfaces. Generally, the tumor tissue was in direct or close contact with the overlying epidermis. Lesions had been present for a few months to 3 or more years. One patient had a recurrence, and 1 had multiple lesions.

Immunohistochemical findings were similar to those of ordinary histiocytomas. About half of the constituent cells labeled with a polyclonal antibody directed against factor XIIIa, an antibody that labels dermal-fixed connective tissue cells and cells in typical histiocytoma but does not label cells of Spitz or common melanocytic nevi.

The epithelioid cell variant of histiocytoma should be considered in the differential diagnosis when a superficial nodule containing large, plump, angulated cells is encountered. These lesions tend to occur as elevated vascular nodules that could stimulate pyogenic granulomas.

▶ This article presents a well-illustrated description of a lesion that the authors would like to become a new entity. The histologic pattern seems to be a reasonably common one, and most authors, I think, would classify this as a dermatofibroma. It is not clear that there is any advantage to identifying this lesion as distinct.—T.J. Flotte, M.D.

Hair Shafts in Epidermoid Cysts

Aloi FG, Tomasini CF (Univ of Turin, Italy)
Dermatologica 179:29–31, 1989 22–9

Keratinous cysts of the skin are common but few contain hair shafts. In a 10-year period 17 cases of epidermoid cysts that contained hair shafts were found among 964 epidermoid cysts. The median age of the 10 women and 7 men was 56.5 years. Twelve patients had a solitary lesion 0.5–1.5 mm in diameter in various anatomical sites. Five patients had small, closely set lesions, most often on the eyelids. The lesions had been present for 1–3 years.

Biopsy Specimens and Patient Details

Patient no.	Sex	Age at presentation	Site of lesion	Duration prior to excision	Suspected clinical diagnosis
1	M	24	Left arm	'Many years'	Resembled pyogenic granuloma
2	F	36	Right upper thigh	?	Resembled pyogenic granuloma
3	F	51	Left thigh	4 years	Resembled fibrous histiocytoma
4	M	25	Forearm	?	Glomus tumour
5	F	29	Left shoulder	2 months	Melanotic lesion
6	F	23	Left inside knee	4 years	Histiocytoma/malignant melanoma
7	M	56	Right calf	3 months	Pyogenic granuloma/histiocytoma
8a*	F	31	Dorsum of left hand	1 month	Pyogenic granuloma
8b*	F	33	Dorsum of left hand	3 months later re-excision	Pyogenic granuloma
9	F	63	Posterior thigh	12 months	Basal cell epithelioma/wart/ malignant melanoma
10	F	31	Leg	2 months	Pyogenic granuloma
11	M	41	Right upper arm	6 months	Vascular histiocytoma
12	F	25	Leg	6 months	Pyogenic granuloma/angioma
13	F	44	Left thigh	10 years	Papilloma
14	M	32	Leg	2 years	—
15	F	24	Right leg	1 year	Histiocytoma
16	M	61	Left thigh	3–4 years	—
17	M	63	Left side of foot	8 months	Eccrine poroma/pyogenic granuloma
18	F	34	Left thigh	8 years	Histiocytoma
19	F	60	Thigh	?	Pyogenic granuloma

*Patient 8 had 2 biopsies.
(Courtesy of Jones EW, Cerio R, Smith NP: *Br J Dermatol* 120:185–195, February 1989.)

The 12 solitary, isolated cysts were found in the mid-dermis, and in 4 cases a porelike connection with the epidermal surface was seen. The cyst wall consisted of stratified squamous epithelium. In 9 of the 12 solitary dermal cysts a hair follicle was found in the cyst wall. The 5 grouped lesions were more superficial and smaller than the isolated cysts. In each case some of the cyst walls had a connection with a hair follicle. As in the solitary lesions, the lumen contained lamellar keratinous material (Fig 22–4).

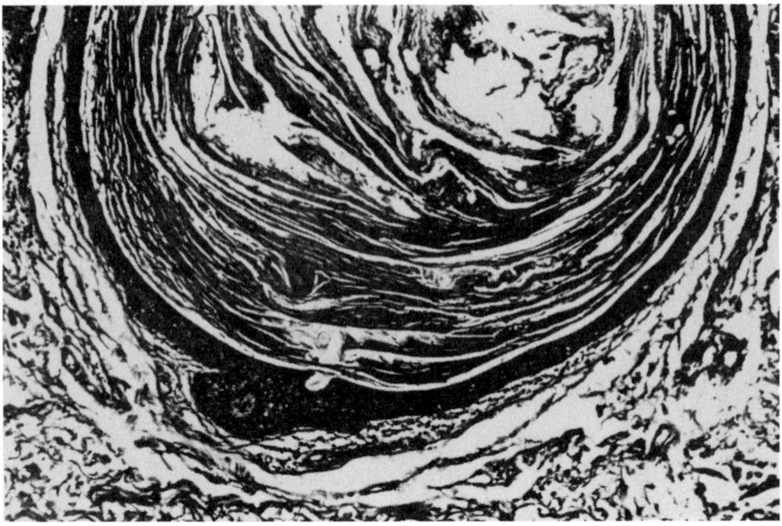

Fig 22–4.—Part of cyst containing many hair shafts. A rudimentary hair follicle is seen in connection with cyst wall. Hematoxylin-eosin; original magnification ×100. (Courtesy of Aloi FG, Tomasini CF: *Dermatologica* 179:29–31, 1989.)

The solitary type of cyst may be considered a solitary counterpart of the eruptive vellus hair cyst.

▶ Everything you might ever want to know concerning epidermal cysts containing hair, but will probably never use.—J.C. Alper, M.D.

Idiopathic Scrotal Calcinosis: A Possible Aetiology Reaffirmed

Akosa AB, Gilliland EA, Ali MH, Khoo CTK (Wexham Park Hosp, Berkshire, England)

Br J Plast Surg 42:324–327, May 1989 22–10

Usually, dystrophic calcinosis cutis is idiopathic. It is disputed whether scrotal calcinosis is idiopathic, however, or if calcification occurs in the epithelium of preexisting cysts. Five patients were seen with scrotal calcinosis. Four had multiple scrotal nodules and 1 had a solitary nodule. The patients were otherwise healthy and had no signs of other systemic metabolic disease. In all 5 patients the lesions, which were excised and examined histologically, were diagnosed clinically as sebaceous cysts.

Microscopic examination of the lesions revealed multifocal aggregates of basophilic calcium deposits within the dermis of the scrotal skin (Fig 22–5). The collections were surrounded by epithelioid cells, sclerotic fibrous tissue without an epithelial lining, and foreign body giant cells. One patient had remnants of a ruptured epidermal cyst with florid granulation tissue and a foreign body giant cell reaction to keratin. There was

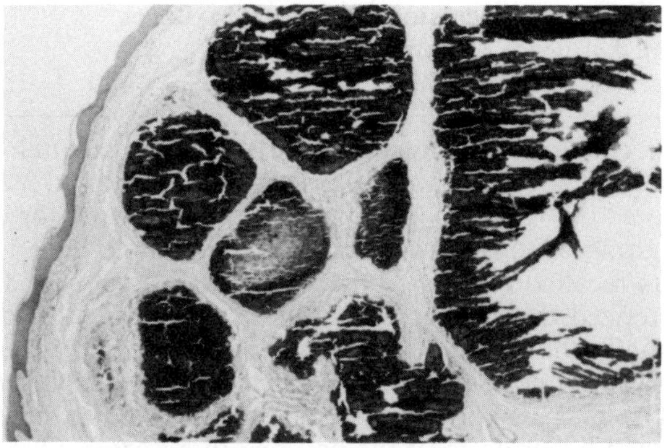

Fig 22–5.—Multifocal aggregates of calcium deposited within the dermis of the scrotal skin. Hematoxylin-eosin; original magnification, ×25. (Courtesy of Akosa AB, Gilliland EA, Ali MH, et al: *Br J Plast Surg* 42:324–327, May 1989.)

a separate nodule of amorphous calcium surrounded by fibrous connective tissue without an inflammatory reaction. In another patient typical epidermal cysts showed normal maturation of lining squamous epithelium with central laminated layers of keratin. Calcium stains revealed both central and peripheral calcium deposits (Fig 22–6). In 1 cyst there was thinning and attenuation of the epithelial lining over part of the surface.

The findings indicate that scrotal calcinosis results from dystrophic calcification of epidermal cysts. The nodules are usually asymptomatic, but when symptoms occur the lesions may be excised under local anesthetic.

▶ It would be interesting to know whether scrotal epidermal cysts calcify more often than epidermal cysts in other locations and, if so, why.—J.D. Bernhard, M.D.

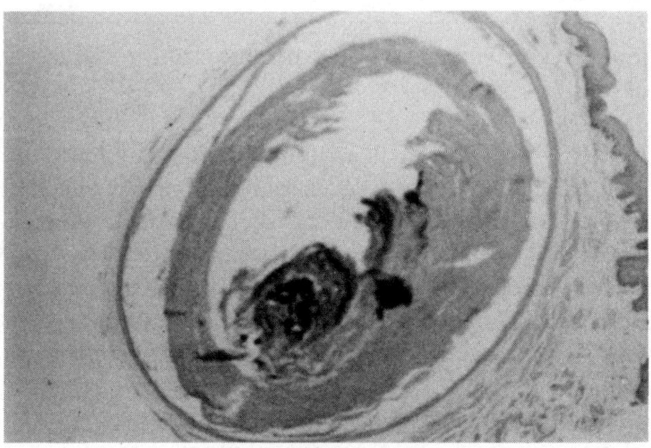

Fig 22–6.—Central deposition of calcium (black) within small epidermal cyst with lining stratified squamous epithelium. Von Kossa; original magnification, ×25. (Courtesy of Akosa AB, Gilliland EA, Ali MH, et al: *Br J Plast Surg* 42:324–327, May 1989.)

Subungual Epidermoid Inclusions: Report of 8 Cases
Fanti PA, Tosti A (Univ of Bologna, Italy)
Dermatologica 178:209–212, 1989 22–11

Subungual epidermoid inclusions (SEI) occur most often on the toes and thumbs. In 8 patients with SEI, previously unreported nail abnormalities were noted. Most of the patients had the condition for about a year before consulting a physician. Usually, only a single digit was affected. Four patients recalled trauma to the nail. Marked subungual hyperkeratosis characterized the clinical appearance, and the nail plate was thickened and usually shortened. The condition was asymptomatic.

The dermis contained small keratin-filled cysts and proliferating epithelial buds. The cyst wall generally had no granular layer. Nail biopsy showed marked hyperplasia of the nail bed in all cases. One type of subungual epidermoid cyst involves the bone and is usually painful. The type described here, SEI, has no bone involvement. The cases described here were classified as type 2 SEI, distinguished by massive nail bed hyperkeratosis and acanthosis. Type 2 SEI can be distinguished from onychomycosis on microscopic and histologic examination.

Subungual epidermoid inclusion often goes unreported and may remain unchanged for years. It has been considered benign, although in 1 instance type 2 SEI was associated with malignant melanoma in situ of the nail.

▶ The authors present a new variant of SEIs and a new subclassification system. They have well illustrated their cases and present convincing arguments that this previously undescribed disease is a real entity.—T.J. Flotte, M.D.

Malignant Peripheral Nerve Sheath Tumors of the Skin
George E, Swanson PE, Wick MR (Univ of Minnesota)
Am J Dermatopathol 11:213–221, 1989 22–12

Two patients were seen with cutaneous malignant peripheral nerve sheath tumors.

Case 1.—Woman, 56, without neurofibromatosis was first seen with a recurrent scalp nodule that had caused pain. Local recurrences developed both 1 year and 4 years after excisional biopsy, and a larger, more painful lesion developed 5 years after diagnosis. The patient had a history of adult polycystic kidney disease and had received a cadaver kidney. A benign-appearing dermal neurofibroma progressed to a highly cellular, pleomorphic neoplasm with prominent mitotic activity and invasion of the subcutis. Ultrastructural study confirmed a nerve sheath origin of the tumor.

Case 2.—Man, 50, with established neurofibromatosis, also was first seen with a scalp mass. Immunohistochemical studies confirmed the nerve sheath origin of the tumor. The patient was well after 11 years without evidence of local recurrence or metastasis.

Malignant peripheral nerve sheath tumors of the skin demonstrate attenuated, overlapping cytoplasmic processes, pericellular basal lamina, and primitive intercellular junctions by transmission electron microscopy. Immunoperoxidase studies may show positive staining for vimentin, S-100 protein, myelin basic protein, and Leu 7. Peripheral nerve sheath tumors should be included in the differential diagnosis of spindle cell neoplasms of the skin. The wider use of immunohistochemical methods will improve the identification of neurogenic sarcomas at cutaneous sites.

▶ This paper presents some well-illustrated examples of malignant peripheral nerve sheath tumors of the skin. Although there are no new findings presented in this paper, it is worth emphasizing the histologic patterns and the special studies that aid in the diagnosis of neurogenic tumors. These tumors are relatively uncommon in the skin and are frequently not included in a differential diagnosis of spindle cell neoplasms. However, if one does not consider this possibility, one will not make the correct diagnosis.—T.J. Flotte, M.D.

Solitary Circumscribed Neuroma of the Skin (So-Called Palisaded, Encapsulated Neuroma): A Clinicopathologic and Immunohistochemical Study
Fletcher CDM (St Thomas's Hosp Med School, London)
Am J Surg Pathol 13:574–580, July 1989 22–13

Solitary, circumscribed neuroma, first described as a palisaded, encapsulated neuroma, is not widely known by histopathologists. Of 824 peripheral nerve tumors reviewed, 39 (4.7%) were this type of neuroma.

The mean age of the 20 male and 19 female patients was 45.4 years. Each patient had a slow-growing, painless nodule for an average of 13.6

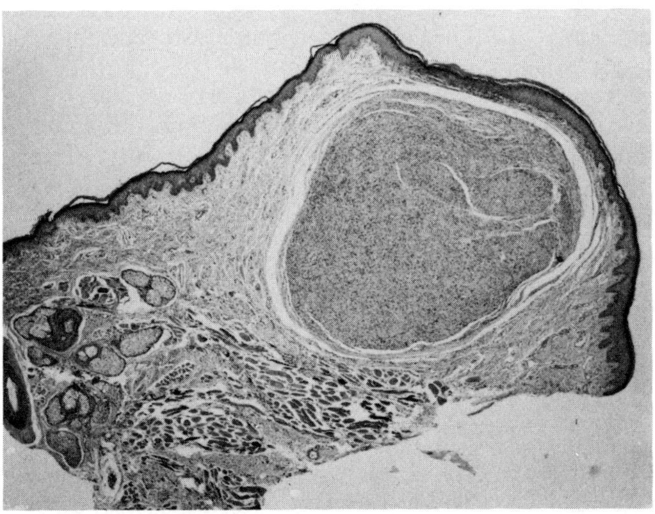

Fig 22–7.—Solitary circumscribed neuroma arising in the dermis and showing typically marked circumscription. (Courtesy of Fletcher CDM: *Am J Surg Pathol* 13:574–580, July 1989.)

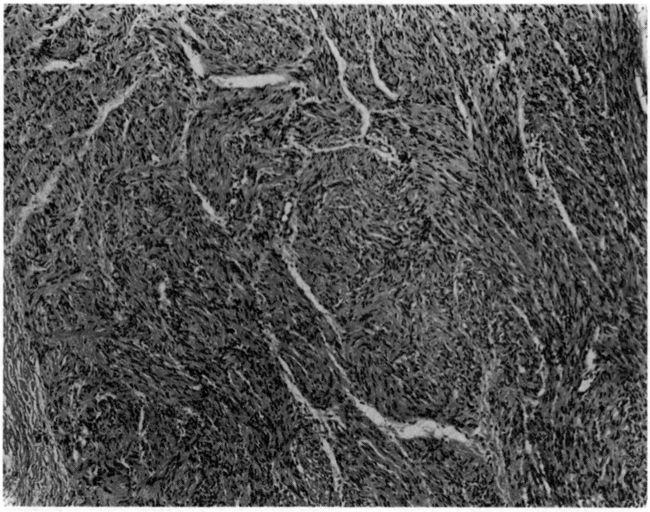

Fig 22–8.—Typical bland, medium-power appearance of solitary circumscribed neuroma. Note the vaguely parallel nuclear array, which is never more marked than here. (Courtesy of Fletcher CDM: *Am J Surg Pathol* 13:574–580, July 1989.)

years before operation. No personal or family history of type II multiple endocrine neoplasia (MEN) syndrome was reported. Most lesions measured ≤5 mm and occurred on the face or near a mucocutaneous junction. The average follow-up period was 5.5 years; all lesions remained solitary and none recurred.

The tumors, which were well circumscribed but not completely encapsulated, arose in the dermis (Fig 22–7). They consisted of bundles of bland Schwann cells with intervening minute axons. The nuclei were sometimes aligned in a parallel manner, but classic palisading was not evident (Fig 22–8). Immunohistochemical tests were positive for epithelial membrane antigen in capsular spindle cells and adjacent nerve perineurium. There was no evidence of previous trauma or inflammation.

This tumor, which warrants greater recognition, is a discrete lesion differing from neurofibroma and benign schwannoma. It is not related to neuroma of MEN type II. The lesion is best designated as a solitary, circumscribed neuroma.

▶ This paper presents a well-illustrated descrpition of the palisaded, encapsulated neuroma. This lesion, although uncommon, is not rare and is underrecognized by many pathologists; therefore, it is worth reviewing the histology of this entity.—T.J. Flotte, M.D.

Immunohistochemical Characterization of Chondroid Syringomas

Argenyi ZB, Balogh K, Goeken JA (Univ of Iowa; New England Deaconess Hosp, Boston; Harvard Med School)

Am J Clin Pathol 90:662–669, December 1988 22–14

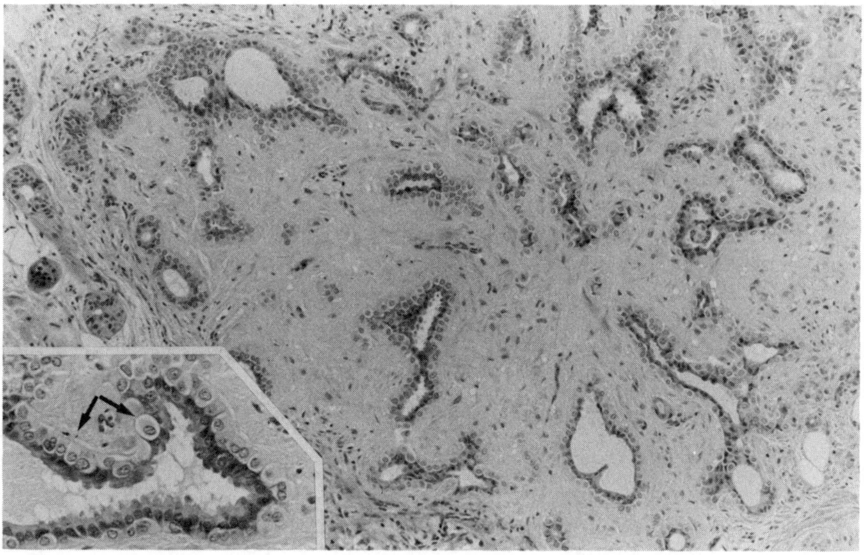

Fig 22–9.—Typical tubuloglandular component embedded in partially hyalinized fibrous stroma. Hematoxylin-eosin; original magnification, ×25. **Insert,** higher magnification of a ductule demonstrating distinct inner- and outer-cell layers (*arrows*). Hematoxylin-eosin; original magnification, ×100. (Courtesy of Argenyi ZB, Balogh K, Goeken JA: *Am J Clin Pathol* 90:662–669, December 1988.)

This histogenesis of chondroid syringomas (CSs), particularly with regard to the role of myoepithelial cells, remains controversial. The lesion was diagnosed in 12 patients. Immunohistochemistry with a broad panel of routinely used antibodies was done to clarify the histogenesis of CS. The cellular elements were classified as tubuloglandular components, stromal cells, and solid nests of epithelial cells.

The immunophenotypes of the inner layer of the tubuloglandular component were characteristic of distinct epithelial lineage, with cytokeratin, carcinoembryonic antigen (CEA), and epithelial membrane antigen (EMA) found almost exclusively in this layer (Fig 22–9). The outer cell layer of the tubuloglandular component showed reactions consistent with both mesenchymal and epithelial differentiation, with S-100 protein, neuron-specific enolase, and vimentin positivity. Glial fibrillary acidic protein also was present in the outer cells of the tubuloglandular components, but muscle-specific actin, desmin, CEA, EMA, and cytokeratin were absent. The stromal cells, and to a lesser extent the solid nests, expressed immunophenotypes similar to those of the outer cell layers (table), but rarely for keratin.

The stromal components may be derived from the outer cells of the tubuloglandular components but do not confirm their exclusive myoepithelial origin.

▶ This paper uses immunohistochemical techniques to attempt to derive information regarding the histogenesis of the cellular elements of chondroid syringomas. This study is interesting because of the detailed panel of antibodies that was used. The presence of glial fibrillary acidic protein in some of the

Cumulative Results of Relevant Immunostains

	Immunostains									
	CK	VIM	CEA	EMA	S-100	DES	MSA	GFAP	NSE	Total No.
Epithelial components										
Outer cells	1	12	1 w	1 w	10	0	0	3	11	
Tubuloglandular component	8%	100%	8%	8%	83%	0%	0%	25%	91%	12
Inner cells	12	3	7	10	3	0	0	1	5	12
	100%	25%	58%	83%	25%	0%	0%	8%	41%	
Solid nests	4 w	5	0	1 w	8	0	0	3	6	9*
	44%	55%	0%	11%	88%	0%	0%	33%	66%	
Stromal cells	4	12	0	0	11	0	0	5	11	12
	33%	100%	0%	0%	91%	0%	0%	41%	91%	

Abbreviations: *w*, weak and variable; *CK*, cytokeratin; *VIM*, vimentin; *DES*, desmin; *MSA*, muscle-specific actin; *GFAP*, glial fibrillary acidic protein; *EMA*, epithelial membrane antigen; *NSE*, neuron-specific enolase.

Myoglobin, chromogranin, A1AT, and UEA-1 were not contributory.

*Three did not contain solid nests.

(Courtesy of Argenyi ZB, Balogh K, Goeken JA: *Am J Clin Pathol* 90:662–669, December 1988.)

cases is interesting, and an explanation for its presence is not obvious.—T.J. Flotte, M.D.

Vulvitis Circumscripta Plasmocellularis: A Report of Four Cases
Woodruff JD, Sussman J, Shakfeh S (Johns Hopkins Hosp)
J Reprod Med 34:369–372, May 1989 22–15

Patients with an irritative or painful lesion of the vulva or adjacent introitus, or both, need to know whether the process is malignant. Clinicians and pathologists must make every effort to identify the specific features of each lesion.

Woman, 73, was first seen at the age of 50 with an irritation of the urethra that had been present for 1 year. There was striking erythema of the urethral meatus and periurethral tissues, suggesting chronic or recurrent infection (Fig 22–10). Local application of silver nitrate provided some symptomatic relief. One year later, the gross characteristics of the lesion had not changed. Silver nitrate was again prescribed, and the patient did not return for 13 years. At that time, the reddish area was more dramatic but still focal. It bled easily on contact. She was treated with local applications of estrogen. Five years later, she returned and

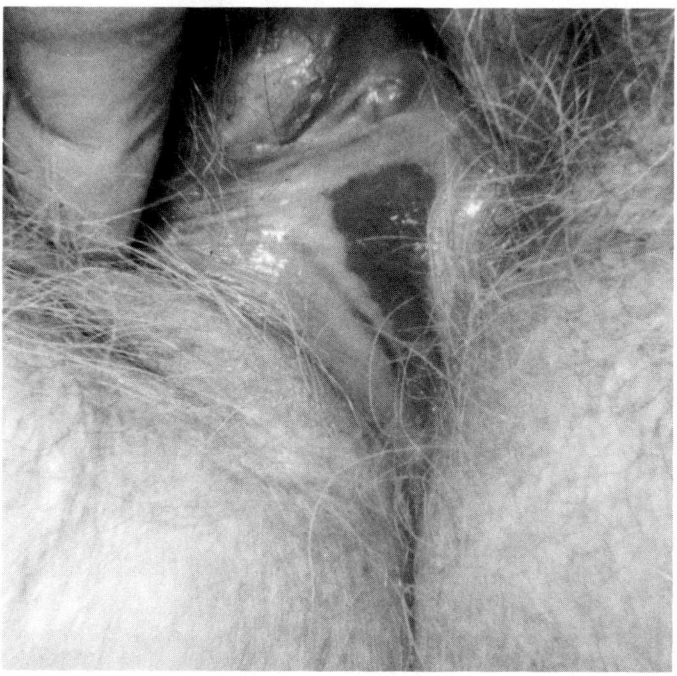

Fig 22–10.—The dark area surrounding the urethra was grossly fiery red. A diagnosis of vulvitis circumscripta plasmocellularis was made by biopsy. (Courtesy of Woodruff JD, Sussman J, Shakfeh S: *J Reprod Med* 34:369–372, May 1989.)

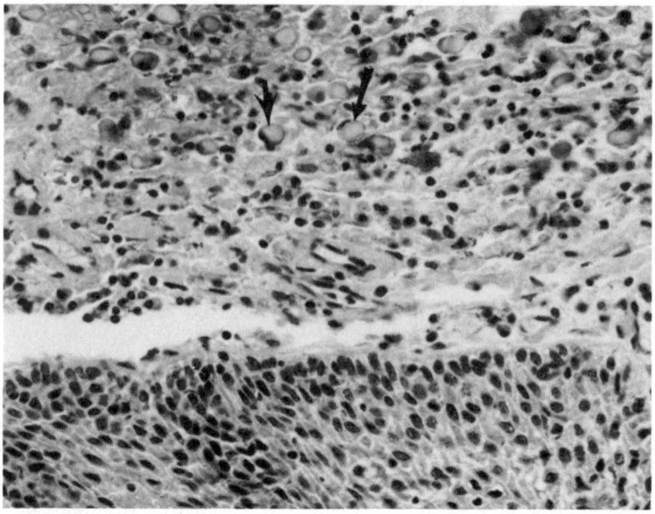

Fig 22–11.—Subcutaneous infiltrate with lymphocytes and plasma cells. Note the Russell bodies (*arrows*). (Courtesy of Woodruff JD, Sussman J, Shakfeh S: *J Reprod Med* 34:369–372, May 1989.)

a biopsy was performed (Fig 22–11). Vulvitis circumscripta plasmocellularis was diagnosed. The area was fulgurated, and the lesion regressed.

Erythematous lesions of the vulva range from acute dermatitis to invasive cancer. A positive diagnosis often can be made only with the use of biopsy. Interpretation of the tissue specimen is very important.

▶ Did you know that Zoon's disease can occur on the vulva? We are familiar with Zoon's balanitis as a circumscribed, solitary, asymptomatic glistening red plaque on the glans. Only biopsy can demonstrate the classic pathology: a dense bandlike or lichenoid plasma cell infiltrate with vascular proliferation. In Zoon's vulvitis there is an acute onset of symptoms (burning, and irritation) involving the labia majora and the adjacent thighs and/or mons veneris. The lesions are often chronic, producing local irritation and involving the introitus and periurethral area. Biopsy of these lesions reveals epidermal separation from the dermis, and a characteristic dermal infiltrate with many plasma cells and the presence of Russell bodies. The latter are somewhat larger than plasma cells and the nuclei stain uniformly with hematoxylin; the cytoplasm is abundant and clear. They are believed to be mucoproteinaceous, with surface gamma globulin, and are thought to be aggregates of immunoglobulins that are made by these cells. To make the diagnosis of Zoon's vulvitis is as satisfying as making the same diagnosis on the penis—one can reassure the patient that malignancy will not develop.—T.B. Fitzpatrick, M.D., Ph.D.

Acantholytic Dermatosis Localized to the Vulvocrural Area
Cooper PH (Univ of Virginia Med Ctr, Charlottesville)
J Cutan Pathol 16:81–84, April 1989 22–16

Clinical Findings in 6 Women With Acantholytic Dermatosis of the Vulvocrural Area

Case	Age (yr)	Anatomic site	Clinical appearance	Duration	Clinical course
1	28	right and left labium majus	multiple isolated and grouped white papules	several years	responded temporarily to topical tretinoin cream (0.05%) but, otherwise, persistent after 12 mo
2	37	right labium majus	scattered 0.1- to 0.3-cm papules	3 mo	lost to follow-up
3	47	left labium majus	0.3-cm raised white papule candidal vaginitis	uncertain*	lesion excised no recurrence after 13 mo
4	83	left inguinal fold	0.4-cm papule with irregular white surface candidal vaginitis	uncertain*	lesion excised no recurrence after 30 mo
5	63	left inguinal fold	0.7-cm raised erythematous keratotic lesion	1 yr	lesion excised no recurrence after 14 mo
6	55	right thigh adjacent to inguinal fold	1.0-cm red roughened area	3 mo	lesion excised no recurrence after 3 mo

*The lesions were apparently noted for the first time during therapy for candidal vaginitis. (Courtesy of Cooper PH: *J Cutan Pathol* 16:81–84, April 1989.)

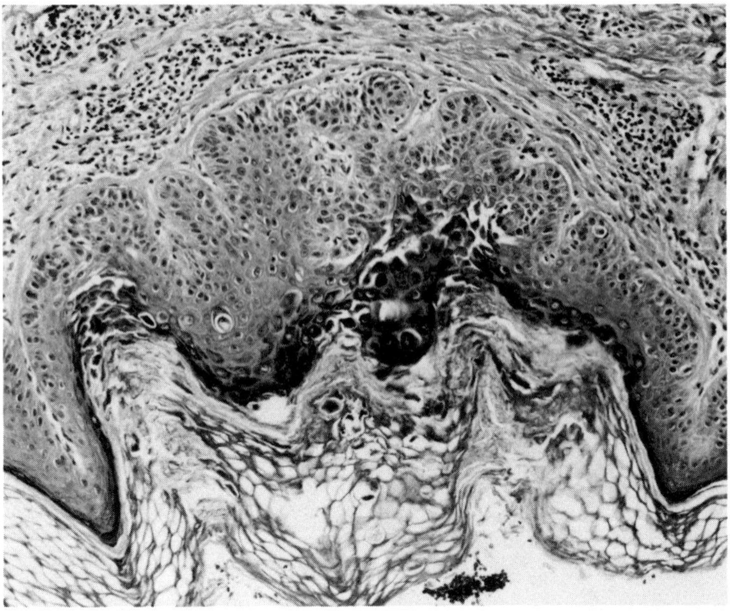

Fig 22–12.—Biopsy specimen shows acantholytic dyskeratosis. (Hematoxylin-eosin; original magnification, ×100). (Courtesy of Cooper PH: *J Cutan Pathol* 16:81–84, April 1989.)

Six women aged 28–83 years had acantholytic lesions localized to the vulvocrural area. The lesions consisted of multiple or solitary papules or plaques situated on the labia majora or adjacent skin (table). None of the patients had similar abnormalities on the body or reported family histories of similar eruptions. Concurrent candidal vaginitis was found in 2 patients.

Microscopically, the biopsy specimens showed either acantholysis with minimal dyskeratosis similar to that in Hailey-Hailey disease or acantholytic dyskeratosis resembling that in Darier's disease (Fig 22–12). In 1 patient, acantholytic dyskeratosis with cuplike configurations resembling warty dyskeratoma was noted. Immunofluorescence microscopy was negative in 1 patient. Localized lesions were cured by excision, whereas the papular eruption in 1 patient was recalcitrant to therapy.

Another 8 reports of acantholytic reactions localized to the vulvocrural area have appeared in the literature. Acantholytic dermatosis localized to the vulvocrural area does not seem to be rare. This lesion needs to be distinguished from other acantholytic dermatoses affecting this area. The lack of a family history or characteristic lesions at other body sites distinguishes this lesion from Hailey-Hailey or Darier's disease.

▶ Dr. Cooper presents 6 cases of a unique acantholytic dermatosis that is limited to the vulvocrural region. He presents the argument that this disease should be recognized as a unique entity and supports his contention with reasonable arguments.—T.J. Flotte, M.D.

White Fibrous Papulosis of the Neck: A New Clinicopathologic Entity?
Shimizu H, Kimura S, Harada T, Nishikawa T (Keio Univ School of Medicine, Tokyo)
J Am Acad Dermatol 20:1073–1077, June 1989 22–17

Sixteen patients were seen with many asymptomatic small papules on the neck. Histopathology showed a relatively circumscribed area of thickened collagen bundles in the papillary to mid-dermis. An additional 16 patients were seen, and a clinical, histologic, and ultrastructural study of the findings was undertaken.

There were 26 (81%) men and 6 (19%) women aged 39–79 years (mean, 62 years). Except for 2 patients with dermatomyositis or lymphoma, no other serious underlying illness was noted. The lesions were multiple, asymptomatic, small (2–3 mm in diameter), nonpedunculated, clearly marginated, white papules around the neck. They were unrelated to hair follicles and ranged in number from a few to 100. Histologically, the epidermis was unaffected, but a relatively circumscribed area consisting of thickened collagen bundles was evident in the papillary to mid-dermis region. Transmission electron microscopy showed tightly compacted collagen fibrils that, except for slight variation in fibrillar diameter, were morphologically normal. There were no significant morphological changes in the elastic fibers.

It has been proposed to call this distinct clinicopathologic entity white fibrous papulosis of the neck.

▶ If white fibrous papulosis of the neck is a new clinicopathologic entity, we still wonder if it might not have more than one cause. The elderly age distribution makes us wonder if some occupational factor or action habitual among the Japanese may play a role. We should be on the lookout for cases here.—J.D. Bernhard, M.D.

Jessner's Lymphocytic Infiltration of the Skin: A Clinical Study of 100 Patients
Toonstra J, Wildschut A, Boer J, Smeenk G, Willemze R, van der Putte SCJ, Boonstra H, van Vloten WA (Univ Hosp, Utrecht; Deventer Hosp, Deventer; Free Univ Hosp, Amsterdam)
Arch Dermatol 125:1525–1530, November 1989 22–18

Jessner's lymphocytic infiltration of the skin is poorly understood. It may be a single entity or a heterogeneous group that can progress to polymorphous light eruption, discoid lupus erythematosus, or even malignant lymphoma.

Fifty-four females and 46 males were studied. The age at onset of the diseased ranged from 16 to 78 years. Most lesions consisted of papules or small plaquelike lesions. In 20 patients, annular lesions also were noted, and in 4 the lesions were annular exclusively. Most patients had more than 1 lesion, ranging from few to many. Lesions were restricted to 1 anatomical area in 50% of the patients. Of 79 patients available for follow-up, 52 still had active lesions and 27 were disease free. Although most patients had been in remission for at least 1 year, some had a short period of follow-up. The disease can recur after a long remission. In most patients the disease ran a cyclic course, with alternating periods of remission and exacerbations. Lesions were exacerbated in 24 patients after sun exposure. The intermittent use of topically applied steroids was sometimes useful but was ineffective in many patients.

Lymphocytic infiltration of the skin appears to be a single entity. In these patients there was no progression to polymorphous light eruption, discoid lupus erythematosus, or lymphoma; however, 10 patients had lymphocytic infiltration of the skin and polymorphous light eruption simultaneously.

▶ This is another interesting paper from the Dutch group on lymphocytic lesions in the skin. The focus of this paper is Jessner's lymphocytic infiltration of skin. This clinical study emphasizes the unique nature of this disease, which would support its being a single entity.—T.J. Flotte, M.D.

Histopathological Discriminant Criteria Between Lichenoid Drug Eruption and Idiopathic Lichen Planus: Retrospective Study on Selected Samples

Van den Haute V, Antoine JL, Lachapelle JM (Catholic Univ Louvain, Brussels)

Dermatologica 179:10–13, 1989 22–19

Many drugs cause skin eruptions that are similar to lichen planus lesions (Table 1), and it can be difficult to distinguish between lichenoid drug eruptions (LDE) and idiopathic lichen planus (ILP) on the basis of clinical examination. Histopathologic sections from 15 patients with

TABLE 1.—Drugs Responsible for LDE in 15 Selected Cases

Case No.	Incriminated drug
1	pyritinol (Encephabol™)
2	methyldopa (Aldomet™)
3	clopamide + pindolol (Viskaldix™)*
4	arsenic (Fowler's solution)
5	doxycycline (Vibramycine™)
6	chlorthalidone + atenolol (Tenoric™)*
7	sodium aurothiopropanol sulfonate (Allochrysine™)
8	auranofin (Ridaura™)
9	atenolol (Tenormin™)*
10	metoprolol (=Seloken™)*
11	clopamide = pindolol (Viskaldix™)*
12	pindolol (Visken™)*
13	atenolol (Tenormin™)*
14	allopurinol (Zyloric™)
15	labetalol (Trandate™)*

*β-Blockers.

(Courtesy of Van den Haute V, Antoine JL, Lachapelle JM: *Dermatologica* 179:10–13, 1989.)

TABLE 2.—Summary of Statistical Features

Histopathological criteria	Lichenoid drug eruptions*	Idiopathic lichen planus*	Significance†
Focal parakeratosis	1.1 ± 1.3 (0–3)	0	p<0.004
Thickness of the granular layer, number of cell layers	1.60 ± 0.920 (0.4–3.2)	4.40 ± 0.901 (2.8–5.8)	p<0.001
Focal interruption of the granular layer	1.2 ± 1.335 (0–3)	0	p<0.004
Epidermal thickness, mm	0.19 ± 0.079 (0.1–0.42)	0.32 ± 0.140 (0.14–0.56)	p<0.01
Vacuolar alteration at the dermo-epidermal interface	2.2 ± 0.8 (1–3)	2.7 ± 0.4 (2–3)	p=0.050
Cytoid bodies			
Cornified and granular layers	1.2 ± 1.2 (0–3)	0	p<0.001
Spinous and basal layers	1.8 ± 0.8 (1–3)	2 ± 0.07 (1–3)	p>0.050 (NS)
Papillary dermis	1.4 ± 0.9 (0–3)	2.2 ± 0.7 (1–3)	p<0.004
Dermal melanophages	1 ± 1.2 (0–3)	1.3 ± 1 (0–3)	p>0.050 (NS)
Infiltrate			
Eosinophils	0.3 ± 0.9 (0–3)	0	p<0.001
Mast cells	1.1 ± 0.8 (0–2)	1.1 ± 0.6 (0–2)	p>0.050 (NS)
Around the deep vessels	0.4 ± 0.6 (0–2)	0.2 ± 0.6 (0–2)	p<0.001
Exocytosis into the upper epidermal layers	1.3 ± 0.8 (0–3)	0.8 ± 0.5 (0–2)	p<0.001

Abbreviation: *NS*, not significant.
*Values are means plus or minus standard deviations with ranges in parentheses.
†Significance corresponds to Mann-Whitney nonparametric U test, except for 2 measured criteria (thickness of granular layer and thickness of total epidermis) for which the unpaired Student's *t* test was used.
(Courtesy of Van den Haute V, Antoine JL, Lachapelle JM: *Dermatologica* 179:10–13, 1989.)

LDE and ILP were studied to determine whether differential criteria exist between the 2 conditions.

For almost all histopathologic criteria significant statistical differences were noted between LDE and ILP (Table 2). However, statistical analysis of results showed that none could be considered a significant criterion that would allow differential diagnosis between the 2 conditions. Nevertheless, several histopathologic signs found in more than 50% of samples of LDE were never seen in samples of ILP: focal parakeratosis, focal interruption of the granular layer, and cytoid bodies in the cornified and granular layers. When these signs are discovered, a drug etiology is strongly suggested.

▶ This interesting paper addresses the problem of the differential diagnosis of lichenoid dermatosis. The authors were unable to provide a significant method of differentiating drug eruptions from other lichenoid dermatoses; however, they do provide a well-reasoned suggestion that we consider parakeratosis, interruption of the granular layer, and cytoid bodies in the granular and cornified layers as suggestive features of drug eruptions.—T.J. Flotte, M.D.

Lichenoid Dermatitis: A Clinicopathologic and Immunopathologic Review of Sixty-Two Cases

Oliver GF, Winkelmann RK, Muller SA (Mayo Clinic and Found, Rochester, Minn)

J Am Acad Dermatol 21:284–292, August 1989 22–20

Lichenoid dermatitis refers to inflammatory tissue reactions in which there is damage to epidermal basal cells. Lichen planus is the prototype for this reaction. The basal cell damage precedes a chain of epidermal events resulting from this damage. Many conditions can produce a lichenoid tissue reaction. Data on 62 patients with microscopically diagnosed lichenoid dermatitis were reviewed to determine whether a characteristic histologic picture develops in the dermatoses that produce this pattern.

The clinical diagnostic groups included contact dermatitis, drug eruption, lupus erythematosus, lichen planus, cutaneous T cell lymphoma, chronic dermatitis or neurodermatitis, and miscellaneous dermatologic conditions (Table 1). Using individual histologic features, it was possible to correlate specific clinical conditions. The clinical groups of dermatitis, drug eruption, lupus erythematosus or lichen planus, and T cell infiltration could be selected histologically. Direct immunofluorescence studies were most helpful in diagnosing lupus erythematosus and atypical lichen planus; these studies should be performed in all patients with lichenoid inflammation (Table 2).

This series of patients with lichenoid dermatitis demonstrates the spectrum of diseases that can produce its histologic picture. Although the non-

TABLE 1.—Clinical Data for 62 Patients With Diagnosis of Lichenoid Dermatitis

Clinical category	No. of patients			Age (yr)	
	Total	Male	Female	Range	Median
Drug reaction					
Definite	4	0	4	56-73	64
Possible	10	5	5	36-78	61
Contact dermatitis					
Definite	4	1	3	43-70	54
Possible	2	0	2	57, 60	58
Lupus erythematosus					
Definite	5	1	4	16-57	41
Possible	1	0	1		65
Probable lichen planus	3	1	2	47-67	58
Cutaneous T cell lymphoma	3	2	1	37-56	47
Chronic dermatitis or neurodermatitis	19	11	8	32-80	59
Miscellaneous disorders	11	5	6	8-72	42
Total	62	26	36	8-80	55

(Courtesy of Oliver GF, Winkelmann RK, Muller SA: *J Am Acad Dermatol* 21:284–292, August 1989.)

TABLE 2.—Results of Direct Immunofluorescence Examination of 16 Patients With Lichenoid Dermatitis

		No. of patients														
		IgG			IgM			IgA			C3			Fibrinogen		
Clinical group	**Total**	**BM**	**Cy**	**BV**	**BM**	**Cy**	**BV**	**BM**	**Cy**	**BV**	**BM**	**Cy**	**BV**	**BM**	**Cy**	**BV**
Lupus erythematosus	4															
Negative		4	4	4	2	1	2	4	3	4	1	4	3	1	3	1
Slight		—	—	—	2*	—	2	—	1	—	—	—	1	—	1	2
Marked		—	—	—	—	3	—	—	—	—	3*	—	—	3†	—	1
Drug reaction	6															
Negative		6	5	6	6	2	6	6	4	6	6	4	6	3	4	6
Slight		—	1	—	—	2	—	—	2	—	—	2	—	2†	2	—
Marked		—	—	—	—	2	—	—	—	—	—	—	—	1†	—	—
Chronic dermatitis or neurodermatitis	4															
Negative		4	3	4	4	4	3	4	3	3	3	4	1	4	4	1
Slight		—	1	—	—	—	1	—	—	1	—	—	3	—	—	3
Marked		—	—	—	—	—	—	—	1	—	1	—	—	—	—	—
Lichen planus	1															
Negative		1	1	1	1	—	1	1	—	1	1	—	1	—	—	1
Slight		—	—	—	—	—	—	—	—	—	—	—	—	—	—	—
Marked		—	—	—	—	1	—	—	1	—	—	1	—	1†	1	—
Miscellaneous (graft-versus-host disease)	1															
Negative		1	1	1	—	—	—	1	1	—	1	—	—	1	1	—
Slight		—	—	—	1*	1	1	—	—	1	—	1	1	—	—	1
Marked		—	—	—	—	—	—	—	—	—	—	—	—	—	—	—

Abbreviations— *BM*, basement membrane; *BV*, blood vessels; *Cy*, cytoid bodies.
*Denotes granular BM.
†Denotes shaggy BM.
(Courtesy of Oliver GF, Winkelmann RK, Muller SA: *J Am Acad Dermatol* 21:284–292, August 1989.)

specific term lichenoid dermatitis has been used previously to classify the histologic features in these cases, a specific diagnosis can be made with careful correlation of histologic, immunodermatologic, and clinical features.

▶ The authors present their findings in a variety of cases of lichenoid dermatitis. This paper reviews some of the histologic findings in the entities, but it presents no new data regarding the differential diagnosis of these processes. The authors suggest that direct immunofluorescence studies should be performed in all cases of lichenoid inflammation. I believe this work presents too sweeping a recommendation. Rather, immunofluorescence studies should be done only on selected cases, particularly in the differential diagnosis of lupus erythematosus.—T.J. Flotte, M.D.

Eosinophils in Skin Lesions of Erythema Multiforme

Patterson JW, Parsons JM, Blaylock WK, Mills AS (Virginia Commonwealth Univ, Richmond)
Arch Pathol Lab Med 113:36–39, January 1989 22–21

There is controversy as to the presence of eosinophils in the dermal infiltrates of erythema multiforme (EM). Some investigators believe that eosinophils are present only rarely, and that lesions containing significant numbers of eosinophils may represent misdiagnosed bullous pemphigoid. Others have the impression that eosinophils commonly occur. To clarify this issue, biopsy specimens from 19 patients who met the clinical and histopathologic criteria of EM were reviewed retrospectively.

Six specimens contained no eosinophils; 9 contained at least some eosinophils, ranging in number from 2 or 3 in an entire microscopic section to 1.3 per high-power field; and 4 specimens contained 3 or more eosinophils per high-power field, representing tissue eosinophilia. With Giemsa stain, mast cells were easily identified in all of the examined sections. Direct immunofluorescence studies in 3 specimens containing eosinophils failed to identify the linear basement membrane zone fluorescence characteristic of bullous pemphigoid.

All 19 patients had clinical features consistent with EM. Drug hypersensitivity reaction and EM were the leading clinical diagnoses in all 19 patients. The 4 patients with tissue eosinophilia were somewhat older than the others, and they also tended to have had the disease longer. Although there were no clear differences in the types of etiologic factors discerned among the 3 groups, all 4 cases of tissue eosinophilia were believed to be drug related.

Eosinophils do indeed occur in the skin lesions of EM, and their number can occasionally be rather high. However, the presence of eosinophils should not be considered a diagnostic feature of EM.

▶ This paper confirms the findings that eosinophils may be present in the lesions of EM, and that their presence suggests the possibility that the EM is drug related.—T.J. Flotte, M.D.

Histiocytic Cytophagic Panniculitis

Alegre VA, Winkelmann RK (Mayo Clinic and Found, Rochester, Minn)
J Am Acad Dermatol 20:177–185, February 1989 22–22

Histiocytic cytophagic panniculitis is a benign, cellular reactive disease of subcutaneous fat that also involves the reticuloendothelial and hematopoietic systems. Cytophagic panniculitis can cause acute destruction of the fatty tissue and may involve the visceral organs. The disorder has also been reported as Weber-Christian disease. The clinical and histopathologic findings of histiocytic cytophagic panniculitis in 19 patients were reviewed.

The 13 women and 6 men aged 23–81 at onset of the disease had skin

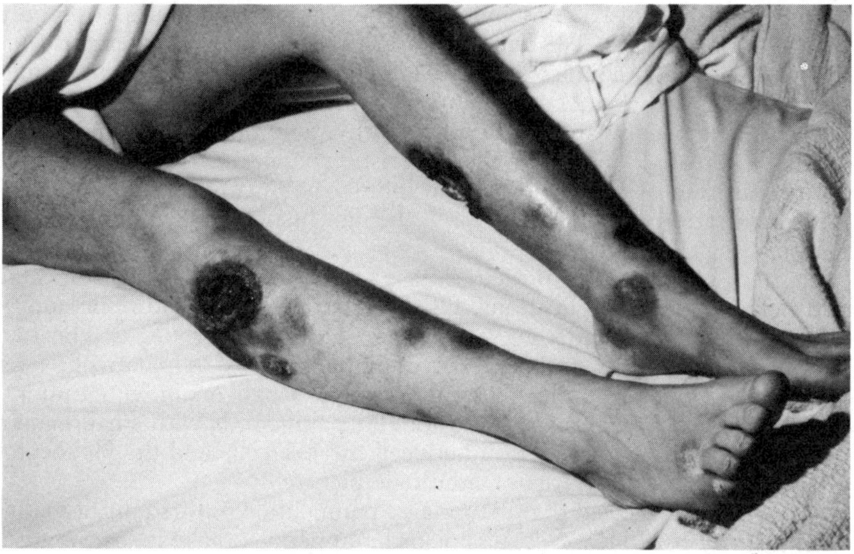

Fig 22–13.—Multiple ulcerated nodules as late lesions. (Courtesy of Alegre VR, Winkelmann RK: *J Am Acad Dermatol* 20:177–185, February 1989.)

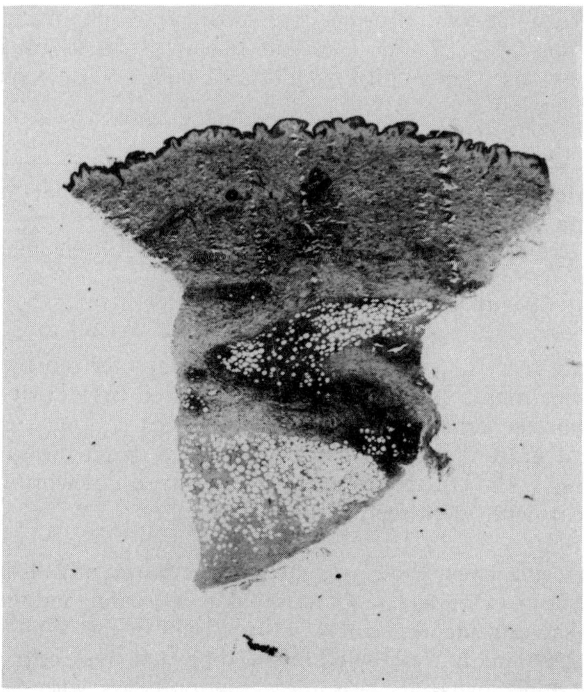

Fig 22–14.—Inflammatory infiltrate predominates in subcutaneous tissue, with septal and lobular involvement. Hematoxylin-eosin stain; original magnification, ×20. (Courtesy of Alegre VA, Winkelmann RK: *J Am Acad Dermatol* 20:177–185, February 1989.)

lesions consisting of large inflammatory subcutaneous nodules or plaques on the arms and legs. The trunk, shoulders, neck, and face were also often involved. Later skin lesions were large and ecchymotic and sometimes became ulcerated (Fig 22–13). Fourteen patients became feverish, 6 had hepatosplenomegaly, and 5 had adenopathy. Skin biopsy specimens were available for all 19 patients. Characteristic changes in the subcutaneous tissue consisted of a deep septal and lobular panniculitis that showed intense infiltration of the fat by large, benign histiocytes with cytophagic features (Fig 22–14).

Thirteen patients died of their disease after a chronic course; 9 of these had hemorrhagic complications. Of the 6 patients who had remission, 4 who had a benign course were being treated with steroids; 2 who had systemic involvement and large ecchymotic plaques of panniculitis responded to aggressive polychemotherapy. The 5 patients in whom immunologic studies were done showed lobular panniculitis with small benign T lymphocytes. The interaction between these T cells and the histiocytes lends the fat its characteristic pathologic picture.

It has been suggested that cytophagic panniculitis is a variant of malignant histiocytosis. However, this disorder appears to have its own pathologic features and dynamics involving a histiocytic response to benign T lymphocytes.

▶ This review of this form of panniculitis adds no new information to the literature; however, it does provide a concise reivew of the clinical and histologic findings as well as a differential diagnosis of cutaneous cytophagia and hemophagocytosis.—T.J. Flotte, M.D.

Clinical, Histological, and Immunohistological Studies of Postoperative Erythroderma

Hidano A, Yamashita N, Mizuguchi M, Toyoda H (Tokyo Women's Med College)

J Dermatol 16:20–30, February 1989 22–23

Postoperative erythroderma, a condition characterized by exanthematous rash after major surgery, has been reported previously. It has been suggested that the cause of the condition, which is almost uniformly fatal, may be a graft-vs.-host reaction to massive fresh blood transfusion. Seven patients with postoperative erythroderma, all of whom died despite intensive treatment, were seen.

Woman, 55, underwent cholecystectomy with removal of gallstones. A lymph node metastasis of carcinoma was discovered at operation, and the patient later underwent pancreaticoduodenectomy with excision of the colon, during which she received 2,400 mL of fresh blood followed by latamoxef, cefotetan, and amikacin. The postoperative course was uneventful for 8 days, when her temperature rose higher than 38°C. A few days later a painless, nonitching morbilliform erythematous rash appeared on most of her body. Prednisolone was given, and antibiotics were discontinued. Fever continued, and the rash became extremely

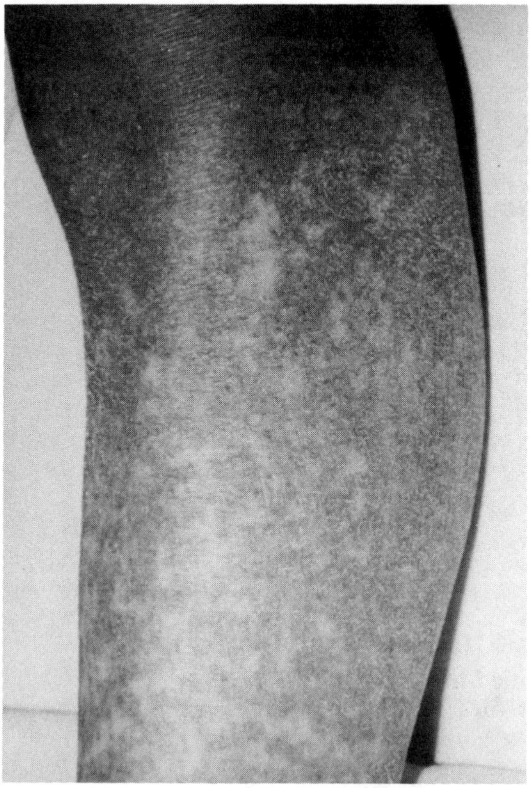

Fig 22–15.—Erythema of the leg. (Courtesy of Hidano A, Yamashita N, Mizuguchi M, et al: *J Dermatol* 16:20–30, February 1989.)

red (Fig 22–15). Steroid pulse therapy with intravenous methylprednisolone was begun and platelets and plasma were transfused. Despite intensive therapy, the patient died 18 days after surgery.

Laboratory findings in this and the other patients showed progressive leukopenia. Examination of biopsy specimens revealed eosinophilic individual necrosis of epidermal cells, basal liquefaction degeneration, satellite cell necrosis, and scanty cell infiltration into the dermis (Fig 22–16, p 424). Langerhans cells disappeared, but T lymphocytes were found in the epidermis.

Findings in these patients were consistent with graft-vs.-host disease after blood transfusion. Other explanations (e.g., drug allergy, toxic shock syndrome, infection, or toxic epidermal necrolysis) seem less plausible.

▶ The authors present a series of 7 patients with postoperative erythroderma. The light microscopic pictures are consistent with graft-vs.-host disease, and the lack of Langerhans cells in their cases strongly supports their point of view. It is interesting that most of the literature on this entity is from Japan. It will be interesting to see the American and European experience with this disease.—T.J. Flotte, M.D.

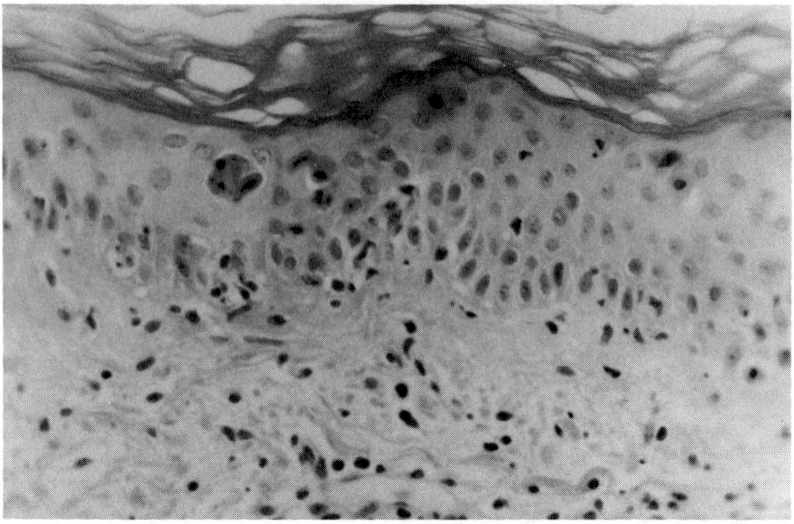

Fig 22–16.—Histologic section of erythema of the thigh (day zero of the eruption). Degenerated cells with pyknotic nucleus and eosinophilic homogeneous cytoplasm are scattered in the prickle layer. A few satellite cell necroses and a slight liquefaction degeneration of the basal layer are noted. Hematoxylin-eosin; original magnification, ×200. (Courtesy of Hidano A, Yamashita N, Mizuguchi M, et al: *J Dermatol* 16:20–30, February 1989.)

Linear Focal Elastosis (Elastotic Striae)

Burket JM, Zelickson AS, Padilla RS (Oregon Health Sciences Ctr, Portland; Univ of Minnesota; Univ of New Mexico, Albuquerque)

J Am Acad Dermatol 20:633–636, April 1989 22–24

Three elderly white men had palpable stria-like yellow lines on the middle and lower back. Symmetric layered lines extended from both sides of the spinal column. The markings were asymptomatic and in each instance were an incidental finding.

Light microscopy showed a deposit of pale-staining material separating collagen bundles. The material was slightly pink and delicately fibrillar. Staining showed the material to be fragmented, agglutinated elastic tissue. Electron microscopy showed fragments of elastic tissue throughout the dermis, with very few normal-appearing fibers. Collagen was unaltered, and fibroblasts appeared structurally intact.

This change may be more frequent than is realized. Two of the patients had vitiligo, considered by some to be an autoimmune process. Results of direct immunofluorescence study were negative in 1 patient.

▶ The authors have described a group of lesions that they believe represent a distinct entity. The cases are well illustrated clinically and by light and electron microscopy. This entity appears to be unique and interesting.—T.J. Flotte, M.D.

23 Miscellaneous Disorders

Influence of Grenz Rays and Psychological Factors on Experimental Pruritus Induced by Histamine and Compound 48/80

Fjellner B, Lindelöf B, Wahlgren C-F, Lengstam I (Karolinska Hosp, Stockholm)

Arch Dermatol Res 281:111–115, April 1989 23–1

Grenz rays are an effective adjunct in the management of certain dermatologic conditions, and they may reduce itch. The influence of grenz rays on experimentally induced pruritus and on concomitant flare reaction was assessed. Experimental pruritus was induced by intradermal injection of histamine and the histamine liberator compound 48/80. Grenz rays were delivered once weekly for 4 weeks on restricted areas of the upper arms, and the results were compared with unconditioned values and with those obtained after placebo treatment. The influence of psychosocial and psychosomatic factors also was evaluated.

Both grenz rays and placebo were equally effective in reducing itch response. Grenz rays had no effect on the flare response and produced slight hyperpigmentation in all participants. Psychosocial and psychosomatic factors were good predictors of individual skin responsiveness. Feelings of tension, depression, and stress were associated with more itch, whereas feelings of relaxation and scores on the Beck's Hopelessness Scale were associated with less itch. Feelings of indolence, tediousness, and impatience correlated negatively with individual cutaneous responses, whereas expectation and relaxation, and scores on the General Health Questionnaire correlated positively.

Grenz rays do not appear to have an ameliorative effect stronger than placebo in histamine-dependent pruritic conditions. Pruritus is a strong placebo-dependent condition, emphasizing the importance of knowing individual characteristics and coping strategies. Feelings of psychological stress are important in predicting cutaneous responses, whereas personality factors play a modulating role. Feelings of distress may activate endogenous opioid pathways, thereby worsening the subjective experience of pruritus.

▶ Although Grenz ray therapy has been used in the treatment of a variety of inflammatory skin disorders, this study documents a lack of effect on the experimental cutaneous flare reaction and pruritus induced by histamine and compound 48/80.—N.A. Soter, M.D.

Granulomatous Perioral Dermatitis in Children

Frieden IJ, Prose NS, Fletcher V, Turner ML (Univ of California, San Francisco; State Univ of New York, Brooklyn; George Washington Univ)

Arch Dermatol 125:369–373, March 1989 23–2

Five children were seen with a distinctive granulomatous perioral, perinasal, and periorbital dermatitis. The children, aged 3–11 years, had a rash consisting of tiny, closely spaced, flesh-colored "micronodules" around the mouth, nose, and eyes; none had a systemic illness. Histopathologic examination in all cases revealed upper dermal and perifollicular granulomas admixed with lymphocytes. The rash resolved spontaneously after months to years, leaving no scars. There was no clear-cut response to the various treatment regimens instituted.

This condition is a variant of perioral dermatitis with granulomatous histologic features. Termed granulomatous perioral dermatitis, the disease is a benign, self-limited condition and is not associated with any systemic manifestation. It can be distinguished clinically and histologically from sarcoidosis and other facial eruptions in childhood.

▶ This report describes 5 children with a long-lasting, spontaneously resolving perioral dermatitis characterized histologically by a predominantly perifollicular granulomatous reaction without caseation necrosis and without systemic evidence of disease. A helpful differential is provided, but the underlying cause (believed to be a contact irritant or allergic response) is often elusive. Potent topical steroid therapy is usually without effect. The occasional response to oral erythromycin is difficult to evaluate. Etiologies to consider include contact with chewing gum, formaldehyde, physical irritants, and fluorinated corticosteroids.—A.R. Rhodes, M.D., M.P.H.

The Perineal Eruption of Kawasaki Syndrome

Friter BS, Lucky AW (Children's Hosp Med Ctr, Cincinnati; Univ of Cincinnati)

Arch Dermatol 124:1805–1810, December 1988 23–3

The occurrence of a distinctive perineal eruption that appears early in the course of Kawasaki syndrome (KS) has had little attention in the medical literature. To evaluate the prevalence of this perineal eruption in KS, the records of 58 patients who were hospitalized during the acute phase of the disease were reviewed. The incidence of this eruption was compared with the other clinical features of KS. The ages of the patients ranged from 2 months to 11 years, 7 months.

Fifty-eight patients met the classic criteria for the diagnosis of KS (table). Of these, 39 (67%) had a distinctive erythematous, desquamating perineal eruption. The eruption began as a confluent, macular to plaque-type erythema, with desquamation occurring concomitantly or soon thereafter. Most eruptions developed within the first 6 days of the first symptoms, with a median day of onset on day 3 of the illness. Age, sex, racial distribution, clinical signs and symptoms, and ultimate cardiac out-

Diagnostic Criteria for Kawaski Syndrome

Fever spiking to temperatures greater than 39.4°C for at least five days' duration
Bilateral conjunctival infection
Erythema and dryness or cracking of the lips
Erythema of the oropharyngeal mucosa, a "strawberry" tongue, or both
At least one of the following
- **Erythema of the palms and soles**
- **Indurative edema of the hands and feet**
- **Desquamation at the tips of the digits or around the nails**

Polymorphous erythematous exanthem
Acute nonpurulent cervical lymphadenopathy

(Courtesy of Friter BS, Lucky AW: *Arch Dermatol* 124:1805–1810, December 1988. Modified from Melish ME: *Ann Rev Med* 33:569–585, 1982; Hicks RV, Melish ME: *Pediatr Clin North Am* 33:1151–1175, 1986; Fuller L, Sutton T, Sullivan B: *Am Fam Physician* 28:219–224, 1983.)

come did not differ between patients with or without perineal rash. Perineal erythema and desquamation appeared more frequently than the typical oropharyngeal changes of KS.

The presence of perineal erythema and desquamation is a valuable early clinical finding that allows a more rapid diagnosis and treatment of KS.

▶ An intensely red, often tender, and scaly rash in the perineum of an irritable and febrile child should suggest the possibility of KS. Approximately two thirds of the 58 cases presented in this report had this finding, usually appearing within the first week of onset of symptoms and frequently in children who were out of diapers. The perineal eruption was not an additional risk factor for coronary artery disease. Early recognition of KS is important so that cardiac evaluation and potentially life-saving therapy with intravenous gamma globulin and aspirin can be instituted at the earliest possible time in an effort to prevent coronary artery complications.—A.R. Rhodes, M.D., M.P.H.

Reflex Sympathetic Dystrophy Syndrome in Children and Adolescents: Report of 18 Cases and Review of the Literature

Silber TJ, Majd M (Children's Hosp Natl Med Ctr, Washington, DC)
Am J Dis Child 142:1325–1330, December 1988 23–4

Reflex sympathetic dystrophy syndrome (RSDS) generally is considered an "adult" disease, but some pediatric cases are documented. Followed were 18 children and adolescents who had RSDS from 1975 to 1985. The median age of the 11 girls and 7 boys was 14 years.

The lower extremity was affected in 11 youngsters and the upper limb in 7. Nearly all patients had sustained mild to moderate trauma 1–6 months previously. Burning, aching, or, occasionally, throbbing pain was the most prominent feature. It often was triggered by manipulation or

Gradations of RSDS

	Grade 1 (Severe)	Grade 2 (Moderate)	Grade 3 (Mild)
Pain	Stabbing, lancinating, burning, not relieved by rest, aggravated by emotional and physical disturbances	Dull, aching, diffuse, mostly aggravated by motion, often relieved by rest	Insidious onset, reluctance to active and passive motion
Vasomotor	Severe vasoconstriction (ice-cold skin, thin, cyanotic, glistening, profuse perspiration), severe vasodilatation (hot, red, dry, scaly skin)	Moderate vasomotor changes: skin can be cold and clammy or hot and dry	Mild changes, but temperature and color are different from the other extremity
Trophic	Fixed, voluntary immobility and firm resistance to motion over time may result in trophic changes of skin and subcutaneous tissue (and eventually of muscles and bones)	The milder course may result in diagnostic delay and consequently osteoporosis may be a finding when initially seen	Usually absent, but may have local edema

(Courtesy of Silber TJ, Majd M: *Am J Dis Child* 142:1325–1330, December 1988.)

stress. Hyperesthesia was a constant feature. Three fourths of the patients had marked vasomotor disorder, and most had persistent edema of the affected extremity. Trophic changes occurred only in the most severe cases. Psychological features included dependency, a low pain threshold, chronic complaining, anxiety, and depression (table).

In pediatric patients who have limb pain and swelling with hyperesthesia and/or vasomotor changes, RSDS is a likely diagnosis. Minor trauma and stress are precipitating factors in children and adolescents who are predisposed. Psychological factors may be important, and psychotherapy is indicated for patients with dysfunctional behavior who are at risk of becoming fixed in the "sick" role.

▶ I had never heard of this disorder, so the article was worth reading for that reason alone. There is no doubt that this is an organic disease, as evidenced by the abnormal bone scan showing vascular changes in the involved extremity. There appears to be a significant psychological overlay, however. As the authors state, it is important to have this taken care of so that these patients don't become "chronically sick."—J.C. Alper, M.D.

Generalized Granuloma Annulare: Clinical and Laboratory Findings in 100 Patients

Dabski K, Winkelmann RK (Mayo Clinic and Found, Rochester, Minn)
J Am Acad Dermatol 20:39–47, January 1989 23–5

Generalized granuloma annulare is an uncommon skin disorder of unknown etiology characterized by predominantly papular primary lesions and a tendency to annular grouping. Any area of the skin may be involved. Generalized granuloma annulare has not been linked to any systemic disease and differs from localized granuloma by its later age of onset, a protracted course with only rare spontaneous resolution, a poor response to therapy, and an increased prevalence of HLA-Bw35. The clinical and laboratory findings in 100 patients with generalized granuloma annulare diagnosed between 1966 and 1986 were reviewed.

The 69 females and 31 males were aged 3 months to 82 years (mean age at onset, 52 years). The mean age at onset in females was 58 years compared with 37 years in males. In 67 patients the skin eruption involved mostly annular lesions, whereas the other 33 had primarily nonannular papules. In 5 patients the predominant distribution of lesions was in sun-exposed areas. One patient had a distribution pattern on the feet that was strongly suggestive of a contact pattern with shoes. Certain

Generalized Granuloma Annulare: Results of Treatment

	No. of patients treated	
Drug or modality	**Ineffective**	**Effective**
Glucocorticosteroids		
Topical	26	8
Systemic	16	7
Intralesional	3	11
Chlorambucil	0	6
Freezing	4	12
Dapsone	3	2
Antimalarials	3	2
Potassium iodide	2	0
Azathioprine (Imuran)	0	1
Antihistamines	3	1
Antifungal		
Topical	3	1
Systemic	3	0
Antibiotics, systemic	3	0
Vitamin E, systemic	2	0
Vitamin A, systemic	1	0
Antituberculosis agents	2	0
Tars	1	0
Colchicine	1	0
X-radiation	1	0
Nonsteroidal anti-inflammatory	2	0

(Courtesy of Dabski K, Winkelmann RK: *J Am Acad Dermatol* 20:39–47, January 1989.)

precipitating factors, including acute sunburn and a direct association with adverse reactions to oral medications, were identified in 16 patients. Sixty-six patients were asymptomatic, 26 complained of pruritus, and 6 described a burning sensation.

The incidence of diabetes mellitus among patients with generalized granuloma annulare was 21%, compared with 9.7% among the 1,350 patients with localized granuloma annulare and 10.3% among the 1,383 patients with all forms of granuloma annulare diagnosed at the Mayo Clinic during the same period. Only intralesional injections of corticosteroids and systemic treatment with low doses of oral chlorambucil offered a success-to-failure ratio of more than 2 (table). Dapsone and antimalarials were effective in some but not all patients.

Follow-up data indicated that generalized granuloma annulare is a chronic disease with a relapsing course and a poor long-term response to treatment. Its pathogenesis is probably immunologic.

Treatment of Angular Cheilitis: The Significance of Microbial Analysis, Antimicrobial Treatment, and Interfering Factors

Öhman S-C, Jontell M (Univ of Gothenburg; Public Dental Service of the City of Gothenburg, Sweden)

Acta Odontol Scand 46:267–272, October 1988 23–6

Although the cause of angular cheilitis is not known, both *Staphylococcus aureus* and *Candida albicans* have been found in lesions. The significance of microbial analysis in the treatment of angular cheilitis, and whether the success of nystatin in this disease results from a specific drug effect or merely from lubrication, were investigated. In an open trial, 50 patients received either nystatin or fusidic acid, or both sequentially, and in a double-blind study, 8 patients with bilateral angular cheilitis (type 2) used placebo or nystatin ointment on the opposite sides.

Eighteen patients with lesions infected only by *C. albicans* were treated with nystatin for 2 or 4 weeks; 17 were cured. Fourteen patients with lesions infected only by *S. aureus* were treated with fusidic acid for 14–42 days; 13 were cured. Patients with angular cheilitis infected by both organisms received either nystatin or fusidic acid first. All 12 patients who received nystatin first were cured within 42 days, compared with only 1 of 6 who received fusidic acid first. The remaining 5 patients were cured after 28 days of nystatin treatment. Patients with persisting angular cheilitis were older, had a more extended length of skinfold, and more frequently had dry skin than patients who were cured after 2 weeks. All 8 sites treated with nystatin were cured after 4 weeks, in comparison with only 1 of 8 treated with placebo ointment.

Nystatin is effective in treating angular cheilitis because of its pharmacologic effect. Retarded healing was associated with advanced patient age, an atopic constitution, and altered mouth corner anatomy. Treatment of lesions in angular cheilitis should be based on microbiological examination.

► Reading this paper aroused nostalgia for the old Mycolog ointment that used to relieve 5 symptoms of angular cheilitis within 24–48 hours and clear the problem within 3–5 days. Recurrences were not uncommon, but response to reinstitution of therapy was rapid and reliable. The authors recommend cultures and appropriate treatment with fusidic acid topically, or nystatin for 4 weeks. They recommend culture for both *Candida* sp. and *S. aureus* to determine which preparation should be preferred. They too yearn for something like the old "Mycolog," which "would make it possible to treat most patients with angular cheilitis without previous microbial analysis."—R. Masters, M.D.

A Survey of Elderly New Patients at a Dermatology Outpatient Clinic
McFadden N, Hande K-O (Ullevaal Hosp, Oslo)
Acta Derm Venereol (Stockh) 69:260–262, June 1989 23–7

Data on 257 new patients older than 70 seen in the dermatology outpatient clinic from January to June 1987 were studied to determine the type of skin diseases and the dermatologic outpatient services needed by the elderly. The most common diagnoses were seborrheic keratosis (15.6%), basal cell carcinoma (13.6%), solar keratosis (13.2%), psoriasis (9.7%), and leg ulcers (9.3%). Allergic contact dermatitis occurred in 3.5% of patients.

The total 68 dermatologic diagnoses were shared by the 257 patients. A skin biopsy was required in 37% of patients and surgical treatment in 31%, compared with 12% and 16%, respectively, of all new patients seen during the period. Overall, 60% needed follow-up and only 10% failed to keep the appointment.

Elderly patients account for 14% of all new dermatologic outpatients. Except for persons aged 1–10 years, those older than 80 years are the most frequent new patients in the clinic.

► This study comes from Oslo, Norway. I think a similar study here would show a higher percent of seborrheic and solar keratoses related to the increased sun exposure of an American population.—R. Masters, M.D.

Late Circumcision and Lichen Sclerosus et Atrophicus of the Penis
Ledwig PA, Weigand DA (VA Med Ctr, Oklahoma City; Univ of Oklahoma Health Sciences Ctr)
J Am Acad Dermatol 20:211–214, February 1989 23–8

Lichen sclerosus et atrophicus is far more common in women than in men, but a link between the disease and late circumcision has been suggested. The disease is characterized by flat, atrophic plaques; its most consistent histologic feature is homogenization of the collagen in the papillary dermis. Lichen sclerosus et atrophicus may be a premalignant disease. Because penile cancer is found most often in uncircumcised men or those circumcised late in life, an association was sought between late circumcision and lichen sclerosus et atrophicus of the penis.

A review of records from 6 medical centers yielded 20 patients; 1 was 14 years, and the remaining patients ranged in age from 34 to 77. None had been circumcised as infants; 14 had never been circumcised. The patients entered the hospital for treatment of other problems or to undergo circumcision. In 75% of the patients, phimosis was the reason for seeking medical attention. Only 1 had the diagnosis of lichen sclerosus et atrophicus before biopsy.

No lichen sclerosus et atrophicus of the glans or prepuce was found among men circumcised in infancy. Of the men in this study, 1 had malignant changes. The association between lichen sclerosus et atrophicus and delayed circumcision should be considered in the decision to withhold or delay circumcision.

▶ The authors have shown a relationship between late circumcision or no circumcision and the development of lichen sclerosus et atrophicus of the penis. The etiology of this disease is unknown, but considering that it occurs almost entirely in uncircumcised males and with 10 times the frequency in females, one wonders whether some urinary metabolite is a contributing factor to genital lichen sclerosus et atrophicus. This would not necessarily explain its presence elsewhere on the body.— R. Masters, M.D.

Massive Necrosis of Fat and Skin as Complication of Obesity

Janigan DT, Prokopetz RD, Chawla S, Durning RG (Victoria Gen Hosp, Dalhousie Univ, Halifax)
Can Med Assoc J 140:665–668, March 15, 1989 23–9

Calcification of the arterial media is common in the extremities of patients with advanced chronic renal failure (CRF). Such changes can also occur in small subcutaneous arteries and may result in ischemic necrosis of the skin and subcutis of the toes, feet, shins, or fingers, or of the thighs, hips, buttocks, or lower abdomen. Six women had severe to morbid obesity and hyperphosphatemia. All 6 had edema. The 5 for whom serum albumin values were available had hypoalbuminemia. Four with CRF reported a 2- to 12-week history of ecchymotic mottling of painfully indurated skin and ulceration, often deep, in the buttocks and perineum.

Despite hemodialysis and other measures, the lesions progressed in 2 patients. Some ulcers enlarged or developed quickly after biopsy and surgical débridement in these 2 patients. The ulcers became infected, and both women died of sepsis. A third patient died of cardiac arrest after 1 week of hospitalization. The fourth patient with CRF recovered after a cadaveric renal allograft and skin autografts. In the 2 women without CRF, lesions identical to those in the CRF patients appeared at 14 weeks and 20 weeks after elective gastroplasty for morbid obesity; 1 woman died of infected ulcers 4 months later. The sixth patient had multiple peritoneal abscesses after gastroplasty that required repeated drainage and total parenteral nutrition, including dibasic potassium phosphate. As the lesions enlarged and progressed, serum levels fell to normal. The necrotic lesions in these patients were secondary to impaired vascular perfusion or to vascular stenosis caused by calcification.

▶ Four deaths occurred in 6 severely obese women who had ecchymotic mottling and painful induration of areas of skin about the buttocks and perineum. Biopsy or surgical débridement in 2 patients led to enlarging ulcers and overwhelming sepsis. The necrosis is caused by small vessel calcification. This may be demonstrated by soft tissue radiography rather than by biopsy.—R. Masters, M.D.

Necrotizing Fasciitis: A Clinical, Microbiologic, and Histopathologic Study of 14 Patients

Umbert IJ, Winkelmann RK, Oliver GF, Peters MS (Mayo Clinic and Found, Rochester, Minn)

J Am Acad Dermatol 20:774–781, May 1989 23–10

Early diagnosis is important in the successful treatment of necrotizing fasciitis, which is associated with significant morbidity and mortality. The histologic features of the dermis, subcutaneous tissue, and fascia are helpful in clinical diagnosis. A clinical, microbiologic, and histopathologic study of 14 patients with necrotizing fasciitis was done. Tissue obtained at autopsy from 6 of these patients also was analyzed.

In all patients the material cultured was positive for multiple organisms, including *Clostridia* and fungi. Organisms were identified by histochemical staining of the tissue sections of 12 patients. The histologic pattern consisted of edema, necrosis, and inflammation of skin, subcutaneous fat, and fascial tissue. Five patients had hyalin necrosis of the sweat glands. Thrombosis of vessels at all levels was prominent, suggesting that examination of coagulation factors may be important (table, p 434; Fig 23–1, p 437).

The findings confirm the necrotic, thrombotic, and infectious nature of necrotizing fasciitis. Although this disease can be diagnosed on the basis of histopathologic findings, decisions about antimicrobial treatment depend on microbiologic assay and culture.

▶ This is an excellent paper that also points out the importance of an adequate biopsy, which should be sufficiently wide and deep to include not only the advancing border but also the necrotic tissue to facilitate recognition of the diagnostic histologic and microbiologic features.—S.L. Moschella, M.D.

Clinical Features and Microbiologic Data of 14 Patients With Necrotizing Fasciitis

Patient No.	Age (yr)	Sex	Site	Previous history	Organism identified: From culture of tissue	Organism identified: With staining of tissue	Outcome
1	26	M	Left leg, left arm, left forearm	Odontogenic oral-pharyngeal abscess, right side	*Bacteroides*, β-hemolytic streptococcus, viridans streptococcus, *Pseudomonas aeruginosa*, *Candida albicans*	Gram-positive organisms, *Candida*	Death
2	67	M	Left hip	Tibiofibular fracture, foreign body	*Enterobacter cloacae*, *Acinetobacter calcoaceticus*, *Clostridium septicum*, *Staphylococcus epidermidis*, *Clostridium perfringens*, *Aspergillus fumigatus*	—	Death
3	55	F	Left arm, left forearm	Diabetes mellitus; chronic active hepatitis; contusion, left elbow (cellulitis)	*Staphylococcus aureus*, *E. cloacae*, *P. aeruginosa*, *C. albicans*, *S. epidermidis*, *Corynebacterium*	Gram-positive organism	Death
4	34	M	Right thigh, perineum, gluteus	Idiopathic anasarca, perirectal abscess	*Escherichia coli*, *Bacteroides*, group D streptococcus, *C. perfringens*, *A. fumigatus*, *Peptostreptococcus*, *P. aeruginosa*, *Acinetobacter* sp., *C. albicans*	Gram-positive organisms	Death

5	67	M	Left side of neck	Neck abscess, diabetes mellitus	*S. aureus,* viridans streptococcus	Gram-positive organisms	Complete recovery
6	5	M	Right arm	Puncture wound	*A. calcoaceticus,* gram-negative bacilli	Gram-negative organisms	Complete recovery
7	66	F	Right midthigh (Fig. 1)	Adenocarcinoma of rectum, meningioma, diabetes mellitus	*Rhizopus, C. albicans*	*Rhizopus, C. albicans*	Death
8	63	F	Abdominal wall	Heminephrectomy, right kidney (as a result of hydronephrosis); partial ureterectomy; diabetes mellitus	*Bacteroides melaninogenicus,* coagulase-negative staphylococcus, *P. aeruginosa, Moraxella* sp., *Candida glabrata*	Gram-positive and gram-negative organisms	Death
9	66	F	Ischiorectal area	Perirectal abscess	*E. coli,* group D streptococcus, *C. perfringens, Bacteroides fragilis*	—	Death
10	62	F	Upper aspect of left thigh	Diabetes mellitus, distal bypass (arterial)	*Proteus mirabilis, E. coli, P. aeruginosa,* group D streptococcus, *C. perfringens,* coagulase-negative staphylococcus, *B. fragilis*	Gram-positive and gram-negative organisms	Amputation, left leg

(Continued)

Table *(continued)*

Patient No.	Age (yr)	Sex	Site	Previous history	Organism identified: From culture of tissue	Organism identified: With staining of tissue	Outcome
11	51	M	Right hand, lower aspect of left leg, right finger	Eosinophilic fasciitis; abscess, right forearm; diabetes mellitus; sporotrichosis	*P. aeruginosa,* coagulase-negative staphylococcus, *Corynebacterium,* β-hemolytic streptococcus	Gram-negative organisms	Complete recovery
12	31	M	Neck	Neck abscess	*Bacteroides, Peptostreptococcus,* β-hemolytic streptococcus, coagulase-negative staphylococcus, viridans streptococcus	Gram-positive organisms	Complete recovery
13	60	F	Left thigh	Diabetes mellitus; abscess, left thigh	*P. aeruginosa, Klebsiella pneumoniae,* group C streptococcus, coagulase-negative staphylococcus, *E. coli, Bacteroides*	Gram-positive organisms	Amputation, left leg
14	64	M	Buttock, scrotum, perineum	Tetanus, perirectal abscess	*E. coli, S. epidermidis,* viridans streptococcus, *Bacteroides, Clostridium innocuum, C. glabrata*	Gram-positive and gram-negative organisms	Complete recovery

(Courtesy of Umbert IJ, Winkelmann RK, Oliver GF, et al: *J Am Acad Dermatol* 20:774–781, May 1989.)

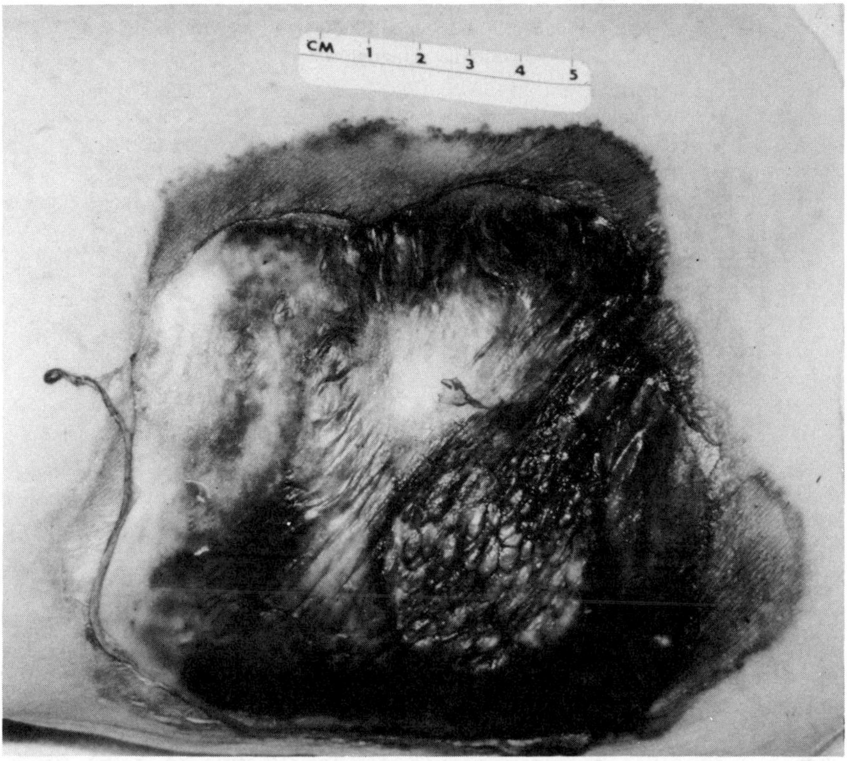

Fig 23–1.—Large hematologic necrotic ulcer with erythematous border in patient with necrotizing fasciitis. (Courtesy of Umbert IJ, Winkelmann RK, Oliver GF, et al: *J Am Acad Dermatol* 20:774–781, May 1989.)

Present Status of Pyoderma Gangrenosum: Review of 21 Cases
Prystowsky JH, Kahn SN, Lazarus GS (Univ of Pennsylvania)
Arch Dermatol 125:57–64, January 1989 23–11

Pyoderma gangrenosum is an uncommon, severe ulcerative condition; about half of the affected patients have an associated systemic disease. A series of 22 patients with this disease and associated diseases, and the results of treatment of 8 patients with high-dose glucocorticoid therapy (pulse therapy), were reviewed.

Eighteen of the 22 patients were examined using the most sensitive routine laboratory technique for detecting monoclonal immunoglobulins, i.e., immunofixation electrophoresis. Four patients were found to have IgA gammopathy (Table 1), confirming previous reports of the incidence of monoclonal gammopathy in patients with pyoderma gangrenosum. Six of 8 patients treated with high-dose glucocorticoid therapy responded favorably; none had serious complications as a result of therapy. The po-

TABLE 1.—Frequently Associated Illness in 22 Patients With Pyoderma Gangrenosum

	No. (%)
Inflammatory bowel disease (IBD)	9 (41)
Ulcerative colitis	7 (32)
Crohn's disease	2 (9)
Arthritis	9 (41)
Rheumatoid arthritis	2 (9)
Associated with IBD	5 (23)
Seronegative	4 (18)
Seropositive	1 (4)
No IBD (seronegative)	2 (9)
Monoclonal gammopathy	
IgA	4 (18)
κ	3 (14)
λ	1 (4)

(Courtesy of Prystowsky JH, Kahn SN, Lazarus GS: *Arch Dermatol* 125:57–64, January 1989.)

tential side effects of pulse therapy include hypertension, petechiae, and hyperglycemia (Table 2).

In the evaluation of patients with pyoderma gangrenosum, it is important to use optimal laboratory techniques for detecting IgA monoclonal gammopathies. Immunofixation electrophoresis was a more sensitive method than immunoelectrophoresis. High-dose glucocorticoid therapy, or pulse therapy, proved to be effective in some severe, refractory cases.

▶ This is an excellent review and update of an uncommon and sometimes very challenging condition. The therapeutically refractory cases mandate aggressive

TABLE 2.—Potential Side Effects of Pulse Therapy

Hypertension
Bitter metallic taste during infusion of corticosteroid
Petechiae
Hyperglycemia
Electrolyte abnormalities
Leukocytosis
Granulocytosis
Lymphopenia
Eosinopenia
Decrease in serum IgG and IgA
Decrease in total hemolytic complement
Decrease in fasting (AM) plasma cortisol levels

(Courtesy of Prystowsky JH, Kahn SN, Lazarus GS: *Arch Dermatol* 125:57–64, January 1989.)

therapies such as pulse therapy (high-dose glucocorticosteroid therapy) and cyclosporine A (1), particularly when vital structures are threatened, such as underlying tendons.—S.L. Moschella, M.D.

Reference

1. Curley RK, et al: *Br J Rheumatol* 113:601, 1985.

Sarcoidosis With Subcutaneous Nodules

Kalb RE, Epstein W, Grossman ME (State Univ of New York, Buffalo; Columbia Univ)

Am J Med 85:731–736, November 1988 23–12

Sarcoidosis is a multisystem granulomatous disease that often is characterized by intrathoracic, dermatologic, or ophthalmologic involvement. There have been several reports of patients with sarcoidosis and subcutaneous nodules.

Six new cases, 3 men and 3 women, had subcutaneous sarcoidosis. All had subcutaneous nodules with no alteration in the overlying epidermis. There were no other specific cutaneous lesions of sarcoidosis. The hospital records of these patients were evaluated for clinical presentation, previous or concurrent illness, and results of chest radiography and laboratory data. Biopsy specimens were obtained in all patients. Some patients also underwent a variety of other tests. Follow-up averaged 17 months.

Patients described the subcutaneous lesions as "bumps" under the skin. The lesions were multiple, painless, firm, mobile, and round. Nodules were distributed over the extremities, being fewer on the face and trunk. Nodules may increase in number and size over weeks or months, but eventually their number remains constant. Some patients have more typical infiltrated papules and plaques. All patients in this series had systemic sarcoidosis. Of 5 patients, all had a positive Kveim test; 5 of 6 had bilateral hilar adenopathy, with or without respiratory symptoms. Three patients had abnormal pulmonary findings, and 2 of 4 patients tested had abnormal eye findings. All 3 patients who underwent intradermal skin testing were anergic (table). The presence of subcutaneous nodules did not predict either the course of disease or the response to treatment.

Most patients had resolution of the disease, including systemic involvement. Some patients had spontaneous resolution, whereas others responded to oral steroid therapy. Only 2 patients progressed to chronic sarcoidosis. These patients often had more typical cutaneous lesions and epidermal changes overlying the subcutaneous nodules.

A possible diagnosis of sarcoidosis should be considered in any subcutaneous lesion if other evidence suggests this disease. Skin or soft tissue

Clinical Findings in 6 Patients With Sarcoidosis and Subcutaneous Nodules

	Patient's Age, Sex, Race	Systemic Symptoms	CXR	OPTH	Kveim	ACE	PFT	Periph-adenopathy	ESR	Serum Calcium	Skin Test	Outcome
1	56 years Hispanic male	None	BHA	Anterior uveitis	+	ND	NL	–	NL	NL	Anergic	Spontaneous resolution, dexamethasone ophthalmologic solution
2	41 years White female	Presented with erythema nodosum and subcutaneous nodules	NL	NL	+	NL	ND	–	ND	NL	ND	Resolved with oral steroid therapy
3	28 years Black female	None	BHA	NL	+	NL	ND	–	ND	NL	ND	Chronic sarcoid; persistent subcutaneous nodules with new cutaneous lesions
4	42 years Black female	Weight loss, mild DOE	BHA, right PTA	ND	+	41 (NL 30)	Mild decrease DC	–	90 (NL 20)	NL	ND	Chronic cutaneous sarcoid
5	34 years Black male	Weight loss, malaise, DOE	BHA with reticular infiltrates	Enlarged lacrimal glands, no uveitis	+	61 (NL 35)	Moderate decrease DC	–	27 (NL 20)	15.7 (NL 10.5)	Anergic	Resolution with oral steroid therapy
6	25 years Black male	Fever, night sweats, weight loss, DOE	BHA	ND	ND	54 (NL 35)	Mild decrease DC	+	NL	NL	Anergic	Resolution with oral steroid therapy

Abbreviations: *ACE*, angiotensin-converting enzyme; *BHA*, bilateral hilar adenopathy; *CXR*, chest x-ray film; *DOE*, dyspnea on exertion; *ESR*, erythrocyte sedimentation rate; *DC*, dilusion capacity; *ND*, not done; *NL*, normal; *OPTH*, ophthalmologic examination; *PFT*, pulmonary function tests; *PTA*, paratracheal adenopathy.

(Courtesy of Kalb RE, Epstein W, Grossman ME: *Am J Med* 85:731–736, November 1988.)

biopsies are the most direct method of determining a diagnosis in any patient with subcutaneous lesions.

► Some 2% to 6% of patients with sarcoidosis reportedly have subcutaneous nodules that histopathologically reveal noncaseating granulomas (1). This type of lesion affects men and women in their third to sixth decades and is usually associated with visceral involvement, especially the lung, liver, or spleen. The nodules may coalesce. The prognosis in these patients is usually good, especially in those with acute disease, who have spontaneous resolution of the subcutaneous and systemic lesions.—S.L. Moschella, M.D.

Reference

1. Maycock RL, et al: *Am J Med* 35:67, 1963.

Acute Febrile Neutrophilic Dermatosis: A Marker of Malignancy?

Clemmensen OJ, Menné T, Brandrup F, Thomsen K, Lange Wantzin G (Gentofte Univ Hosp; Odense Univ Hosp; The Finsen Inst, Copenhagen; Bispebjerg Hosp, Copenhagen)

Acta Derm Venereol (Stockh) 69:52–58, March 1989 23–13

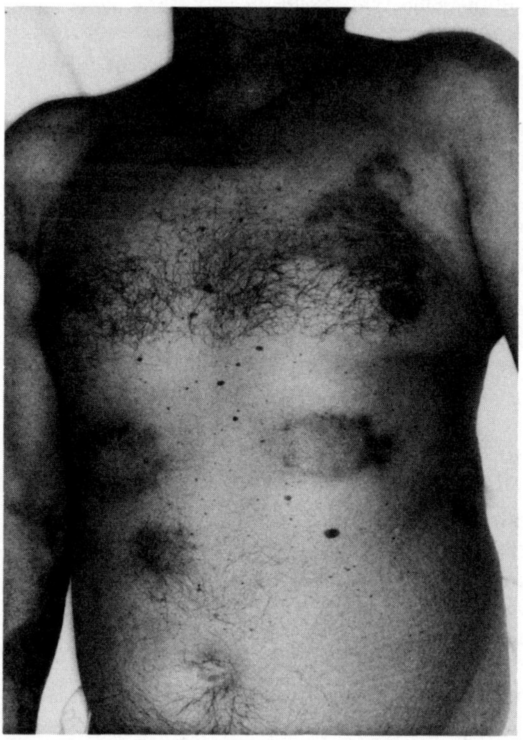

Fig 23–2.—Erythematous, infiltrated somewhat annular plaques of Sweet's syndrome. (Courtesy of Clemmensen OJ, Menné T, Brandrup F, et al: *Acta Derm Venereol (Stockh)* 69:52–58, March 1989.)

Acute febrile neutrophilic dermatosis (Sweet's syndrome) has been associated with myelo- and lymphoproliferative disorders. A retrospective study of 18 patients with Sweet's syndrome was conducted during a 2-year period to determine the features that may indicate associated malignancy (Fig 23–2).

An associated lympho- or myeloproliferative malignancy was found in 6 patients. Sweet's syndrome preceded the diagnosis in 4 patients from 3 months to 6 years. Skin lesions led to diagnosis in only 1 patient. No specific distinguishing feature was found between patients with and without associated malignancy, but those with associated malignancy were generally older and male. They had unexplained anemia, more frequent oral mucosal lesions, and recurring skin lesions.

Sweet's syndrome, a clinical and histopathologic entity, responds promptly to prednisolone therapy. The diagnosis of Sweet's syndrome should be made with increasing awareness of the symptoms of associated malignancy.

▶ The authors used the diagnostic criteria described by Su and Liu (1) for Sweet's syndrome. These are the presence of typical histopathology and of at least 2 typical discrete lesions, or the other, more classic presentation, characterized by the presence of the typical histopathology, 2 typical discrete skin lesions, and fever or blood neutrophilia. In their reported patients the association of myelocytic and lymphocytic neoplasias with Sweet's syndrome was 33%. This figure is high when compared with the 10% reported by Soderstrom (2). One should be aware of the association of Sweet's disease with other types of malignancies such as carcinomas (3).—S.L. Moschella, M.D.

References

1. Su WPD, Liu HH: *Cutis* 37:167, 1986.
2. Soderstrom RM: *Cutis* 28:255, 1978.
3. Green KE, et al: *Arch Dermatol* 111:1461, 1975.

Grey Turner's Sign and Cullen's Sign in Acute Pancreatitis

Meyers MA, Feldberg MAM, Oliphant M (State Univ of New York, Stony Brook; Univ Hosp, Utrecht, The Netherlands; Crouse-Irving Mem Hosp, Syracuse, NY)

Gastrointest Radiol 14:31–37, Winter 1989 23–14

Two clinical signs of cutaneous discoloration have been associated with severe acute pancreatitis—Cullen's sign of periumbilical staining and Grey Turner's sign of flank discoloration. Recently, 4 patients with acute pancreatitis seen on CT and associated with cutaneous discoloration of the abdomen were encountered.

Man, 27, was admitted with recurrent acute pancreatitis. He was a known alcoholic who had 3 episodes of acute pancreatitis in the preceding 3 years. Several days earlier, he had noted cutaneous discoloring in the right paraumbilical area extending around the flank. On admission he was febrile; he had increased abdominal girth with pain in the left upper abdomen and tenderness to palpation in the left flank. Liver function was largely disturbed. Evidence of flagrant pancreatitis with inflammatory spread to the transverse mesocolon and small bowel mesentery, especially toward the right anterior abdominal wall, was revealed by CT. Below the kidneys, extensive pancreatic fluid distention from the anterior pararenal space within the layers of the posterior renal fascia was noted on the left. Treatment with parenteral feeding and antibiotics was begun. Follow-up with CT 3 months later revealed demarcation of a large pancreatic pseudocyst in the left abdomen with exudate and loculated fluid continuing to extend toward the back muscles. A mild stellate appearance of the small bowel mesentery in the right abdomen was still evident. The patient's skin was no longer discolored.

Grey Turner's sign is produced by spread from the anterior pararenal space to the area between the leaves of the posterior renal fascia and later to the lateral edge of the quadratus lumborum muscle. Cullen's sign is secondary to the tracking of liberated pancreatic enzymes to the anterior abdominal wall from the inflamed gastrohepatic ligament and across the falciform ligament.

▶ A thorough review of these 2 classic physical signs. Cullen's sign refers to discoloration of the skin in the periumbilical area, and Grey Turner's sign to discoloration of the skin involving either flank, more often on the left. One or both may develop in about 3% of patients with severe acute hemorrhagic pancreatitis and often presage major complications. The discoloration may vary from slate blue to yellow-brown and is related to extravasation of blood in the subcutaneous tissue. Typically, the color is bluish-black initially and fades through greenish to yellowish tints.

Cullen's sign is usually associated with acute pancreatitis. Less commonly it may occur in patients with perforated duodenal ulcer, ruptured abdominal aortic aneurysm, or ruptured ectopic pregnancy, or after percutaneous liver biopsy. In pregnant patients it may extend from the umbilicus to the pubis.

The authors detail the anatomical pathways through which these signs develop.—R. Masters, M.D.

Pityriasis Rotunda as a Cutaneous Marker of Hepatocellular Carcinoma: A Comparison With Its Prevalence in Other Diseases

Berkowitz I, Hodkinson HJ, Kew MC, DiBisceglie AM (Univ of the Witwatersrand; Baragwanath Hosp, Johannesburg, South Africa)

Br J Dermatol 120:545–549, April 1989 23–15

Pityriasis rotunda is an acquired ichthyosis that is known to occur in association with tuberculosis, malignant tumors, and chronic benign hepatic diseases (Fig 23–3). It was recently observed that South African blacks with hepatocellular carcinoma (HCC) had an increased incidence

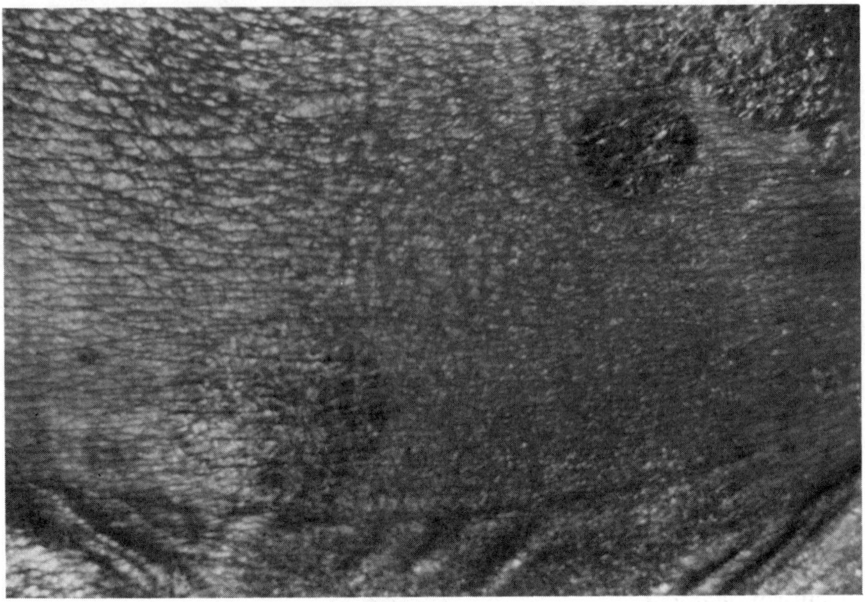

Fig 23–3.—Close-up view of several lesions of pityriasis rotunda. (Courtesy of Berkowitz I, Hodkinson HJ, Kew MC, et al: *Br J Dermatol* 120:545–549, April 1989.)

of pityriasis rotunda skin rash. Whether pityriasis rotunda could be used as a cutaneous marker of HCC was investigated in 63 South African blacks with confirmed HCC and 3 age-matched control groups, including 63 patients with active tuberculosis, 63 with malignant diseases other than HCC, and 63 with chronic benign hepatic disease.

Pityriasis rotunda was present in 10 patients (16%) with HCC, in 3 (5%) with tuberculosis, and in 2 (3%) with chronic benign hepatic disease. None of the patients with malignant diseases other than HCC had pityriasis rotunda. Thus the presence of pityriasis rotunda appears to be a useful cutaneous marker for the diagnosis of HCC in South African blacks.

▶ Pityriasis rotunda refers to acquired pseudo-ichthyotic lesions appearing in discrete circular patterns. It is apparently not uncommon in South Africa and has also been reported in West Indians, Japanese, black Americans, and a Sephardic Jew. The present report shows it to be a cutaneous marker for HCC. Although it may be found in other conditions less frequently, the 16% incidence in HCC patients obliges us to rule out that diagnosis when the cutaneous lesions are present.—R. Masters, M.D.

Tripe Palms and Malignancy

Cohen PR, Grossman ME, Almeida L, Kurzrock R (Columbia Univ; Columbia Presbyterian Med Ctr, New York; Univ of Texas, Houston)

J Clin Oncol 7:669–678, May 1989 23–16

Malignancy-Associated Tripe Palms Without Acanthosis Nigricans

Type of Malignancy	Subtotal	Total	Percent	Median*	Reference
Pulmonary		9	53.0	P3	
Squamous cell	5			C	3, 13, 43, 45, current report (case no. 2)
Adenocarcinoma	1			P2	19
Oat cell	1			P8	3
Unspecified	2			P15	21, 47
Gastric		2	11.7	P5	3, 13
Renal					
Papillary carcinoma		1	5.9	F264	3
Sarcoma		1	5.9	C	8
Tongue					
Squamous cell		1	5.9	C	39
Uterine		1	5.9	C	9
Unspecified		2	11.7	F4	13, 21
Total		17	100.0	C	

*Months that tripe palms either preceded (P) or followed (F) the diagnosis of malignancy. The onset of tripe palms within 1 month of the diagnosis of malignancy is considered concurrent.

(Courtesy of Cohen PR, Grossman ME, Almeida L, et al: *J Clin Oncol* 7:669–678, May 1989.)

Tripe palms, a skin marker of internal malignancy, are characterized by thickened velvety palms with pronounced dermatoglyphics. Tripe palms have been noted as an independent condition or in association with acanthosis nigricans (table).

Man, 62, black, was admitted with thickening and darkening of the palmar and plantar surfaces, as well as progressive enlargement of the distal fingers with concurrent pruritus, burning, and paresthesia for more than 1 year: He reported a 27-kg weight loss and a persistent nonproductive cough of 4 months' duration. He had a 35 pack-year history of cigarette smoking. A chest radiograph revealed a lobulated mass in the posterior aspect of the right upper lobe. Skin biopsy of the right palm showed hyperkeratosis and acanthosis of the epidermis. An endobronchial lesion was biopsied; examination of the specimen revealed a poorly differentiated adenocarcinoma. After surgical resection the pruritus and burning in the hands and feet disappeared, but the cutaneous manifestations were unchanged. The patient was discharged and continued to improve, except for the skin changes on the palmar and plantar surfaces. The patient was readmitted several months later with increasing fatigue, dyspnea, weight loss, hemoptysis, and wheezing. He had lymphadenopathy and digital clubbing. Rugose and hyperpigmented dermatoglyphics on his palms and soles were noted, along with velvet-like, hyperpigmented, papillomatous lesions in the axillae and supraclavicular areas. A large recurrent pulmonary tumor in the right upper lung was noted on chest radiography. Radiotherapy was begun, but the patient died soon after.

A total of 77 patients with idiopathic and malignancy-associated tripe palms have been reported, and 94% had cancer. In cancer patients with tripe palms alone, pulmonary carcinoma was the most common underlying neoplasm. Patients with both tripe palms and acanthosis nigricans often had gastric or pulmonary cancer. Various other solid tumors have been reported as well. Tripe palms were the presenting feature of an undiagnosed malignancy in more than 40% of patients.

▶ Some of the synonyms for this disorder have included acanthosis palmaris, pachydermatoglyphy, palmar hyperkeratosis, palmar keratoderma, and acanthosis nigricans of the palms. Why some paraneoplastic phenomena should affect the palms preferentially is not known. Others include palmar fasciitis in ovarian carcinoma (1) and Burgdorf's reaction (2). Hand and foot aficionados are also reminded of the enormously enjoyable book, *The Palms and Soles in Medicine* by Costello and Gibbs (3). Lastly, look at the hands first!—J.D. Bernhard, M.D.

References

1. Medsger TA, et al: *Ann Intern Med* 96:424, 1982.
2. Burke MC, et al: *Am J Pediatr Hematol Oncol* 11:44, 1989.
3. Costello MJ, Gibbs RC: *The Palms and Soles in Medicine* Springfield, CC Thomas, 1967.

The Accessory Tragus—No Ordinary Skin Tag

Sebben JE (Univ of California, Davis)

J Dermatol Surg Oncol 15:304–307, March 1989 23–17

The accessory tragus, a minor congenital malformation that usually does not present a problem, is sometimes large enough to cause cosmetic concerns. Because of its small, variable appearance it may be confused with other entities. If this structure is incorrectly identified or treated, minor problems can result. Dermatologists must be able to distinguish the accessory tragus clinically and histologically from other abnormalities.

The accessory tragus is most commonly found anterior to the tragus or just anterior to the crus of the helix. Less commonly, it is found on the cheek along the mandible. The accessory tragus is usually single but may be multiple and sometimes bilateral. When excised it is often misdiagnosed. It is usually confused with a skin tag. An accessory tragus is generally easy to identify, however, because it is often a protuberant, fleshy papule in the preauricular region. It is present at birth, unlike skin tags, and histopathologic assessment usually shows hair follicles, sebaceous glands, eccrine glands, elastic cartilage, and adipose tissue. When removing the accessory tragus surgically, the most common mistake is failure to consider the cartilaginous structures. The structure should be excised using a small elliptical incision. Great caution is needed when dissecting deep in the preauricular area.

The accessory tragus is easily treated when correctly diagnosed. Surgical excision is simple and rarely results in complications.

▶ A case of "enslavement via accessory tragus:" One of my most grateful patients was an elderly woman whose mother had told her she should never have her accessory tragus cut off for fear of death. The accessory tragus was one of the mother's main devices for keeping her daughter single and at home with her. After the mother died the patient finally asked about excision, underwent it, and was finally "free."—J.D. Bernhard, M.D.

Papulonodular Demodicidosis Associated With Acquired Immunodeficiency Syndrome

Dominey A, Rosen T, Tschen J (VA Med Ctr; Baylor College of Medicine, Houston)

J Am Acad Dermatol 20:197–201, February 1989 23–18

Demodex folliculorum and *Demodex brevis* are the only species of ectoparasitic mites known to inhaibit humans. These mites commonly inhabit the normal hair follicles and sebaceous glands. Although several skin conditions have been associated with demodectic mites, a number of studies have failed to correlate disease with their presence. Some investigators have proposed that the pathogenicity of *Demodex* is a quantitative matter. A papulonodular variant of demodicidosis developed in 2 men with AIDS.

Man, 49, with AIDS, had a pruritic eruption of the head and neck area of 2 weeks' duration. The lesions had not responded to mild topical steroid application. Physical examination revealed multiple discrete erythematous papules and nodules, some with central microvesiculation and crusting on the upper half of the neck, jawline, and preauricular portion of the cheek bilaterally Analysis of mineral oil preparations of skin scrapings revealed innumerable *D. folliculorum* mites. Treatment consisted of overnight application of a 1% gamma benzene hexachloride (lindane) lotion to the involved areas on 3 consecutive nights. Expression of follicular contents from previously involved areas after treatment demonstrated only a rare *Demodex* mite.

The second case was similar to the first one, except that this patient was treated with daily 10-minute applications of a 1% permethrin cream rinse for some residual pruritic demodectic lesions that were still present when he was hospitalized for unrelated problems after 2 initial applications of lindane lotion.

It has been proposed by other investigators that the development of an unusual hypersensitivity response to *Demodex* can cause disease. In the 2 patients described, alterations of the immune system apparently allowed the normally commensal inhabitants of the skin to proliferate to the extent that they caused the skin disease.

▶ *Demodex folliculorum* lives normally in the human hair follicle and *D. brevis* in the sebaceous gland. *Demodex* has been linked to human cutaneous disease when an excessive number of mites populate the pilosebaceous apparatus and when mites penetrate the dermal tissues. Three skin diseases linked to the mite are *pityriasis folliculorum,* which is manifested clinically as persistent scaling erythematous skin on the cheeks, forehead, and chin and is presumably associated with overpopulation of follicles by mites; a *café au lait-colored plaque* on the face, again related to overpopulation of follicles by the mite; a fine papulopustular *rosacea-like eruption* related to overpopulation and rupture of the follicle by mites. The eruption reported by Dominey et al. in 2 HIV-infected individuals resembles the rosacea-like eruption associated with demodicidosis. Similar hyperinfestation has previously been reported in immunodeficient HIV-infected patients with Norwegian scabies.—R.A. Johnson, M.D.

Pityriasis Folliculorum Revisited

Dominey A, Tschen J, Rosen T, Batres E, Stern JK (Baylor College of Medicine, Houston)

J Am Acad Dermatol 21:81–84, July 1989 23–19

Pityriasis folliculorum is a demodectic infestation characterized by facial erythema and follicular scaling, giving a "frosted" appearance and rough texture. Pityriasis folliculorum was diagnosed in 6 women, all of whom regularly cleansed their faces with water and soap; 5 of the 6 denied using creams, lotions, or heavy make-up.

The women were first seen with uniform facial erythema and follicular plugging, giving the skin a sandpaper-like texture. Numerous *Demodex folliculorum* mites were found in the follicular contents expressed from affected skin. Biopsy showed hyperkeratosis, follicular ostia filled with mites, and a chronic inflammatory infiltrate in the dermis. Five patients had responses to topical tretinoin and lindane; the other had a response to 1% permethrin cream rinse only after oral 13-*cis*-retinoic acid.

The key to the diagnosis of pityriasis folliculorum is finding numerous *Demodex* mites *(D. folliculorum* and *D. brevis)* in material collected from the affected skin. A history of infrequent washing and application of potentially occlusive agents may be useful in making a diagnosis but may be absent from some affected persons. Treatment includes tretinoin and lindane or permethrin cream rinse.

▶ This may not be a medical emergency, but it is a glossologistic one: What's the difference between *pityriasis folliculorum* and *pityrosporum folliculitis?* And if you knew, how could you remember? Such is the stuff upon which the sesquipedalian fame of dermatologists rests. Pityriasis folliculorum is a facial eruption attributed to *Demodex* mites (*D. folliculorum* and *D. brevis* in humans) and is also known as demodicidosis. Pityrosporum folliculitis often affects the upper trunk or upper arms and is caused by the yeasts *Pityrosporum orbiculare* and *Pityrosporum ovale* (1, 2). The twisted etymological (if not entomological) history of these terms goes back to the Greek word *pityron* for bran and the bran-like appearance of the fine scale in certain eruptions. Perhaps the demodectic eruption should be so named (or even better, be renamed *Ayres' demodicidosis*); the yeast-related eruption should retain the *Pityrosporum* term, and we can go back to eating our pityromuffins in peace.—J.D. Bernhard, M.D.

References

1. Back O, et al: *J Am Acad Dermatol* 12:56, 1985.
2. Bufill JA, et al: *Ann Intern Med* 108:560, 1988.

Tungiasis: Report of One Case and Review of the 14 Reported Cases in the United States

Sanusi ID, Brown EB, Shepard TG, Grafton WD (Louisiana State Univ, Shreveport)

J Am Acad Dermatol 20:941–944, May 1989 23–20

Tungiasis is a parasitic skin infestation caused by the *Tunga penetrans* sand flea, which is prevalent in tropical Africa, Central and South America, the Caribbean islands, Pakistan, and the west coast of India. Only 14 cases had been reported in the United States literature (table). One of the authors of this report contracted tungiasis when he worked for 2 months in a missionary hospital in Zaire.

Man, 24, noticed a 3-mm, raised, white, firm papule with a small black speck in the center on the third toe of his right foot 1 week before he was to return to the United States. During his stay he had often walked barefoot along dusty roads. Another physician removed a 2-mm flea, and the lesion healed well. Two weeks after his return, a second similar lesion, 6 mm in diameter, developed on the second toe of his right foot. The pore was enlarged, and the flea was removed in its entirety. Histologic examination showed a flea with a thick outer cuticle and prominent hypodermic cells (Figs 23–4 and 23–5).

Tungiasis can be avoided by wearing shoes in areas where this parasite is endemic.

▶ Differential diagnosis: scabies, tick bites, creeping eruption, dracuncluiasis, myiasis, *Pulex irritans* bites, furuncles.—J.D. Bernhard, M.D.

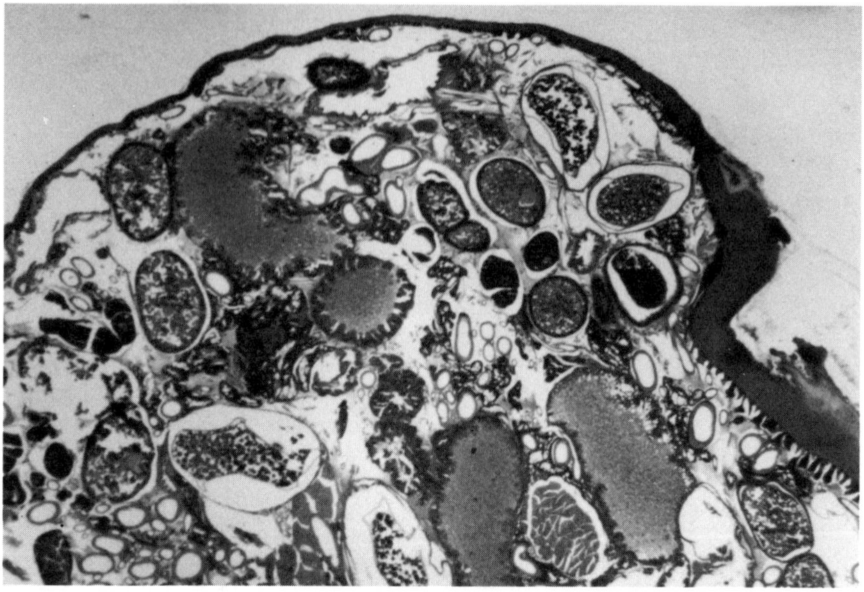

Fig 23–4.—Low-power photomicrograph of *Tunga penetrans* with its thick cuticle, prominent hypodermic cells, tracheal rings, digestive tract, and ovaries containing numerous eggs. Hematoxylin-eosin; original magnification, ×25. (Courtesy of Sanusi ID, Brown EB, Shepard TG, et al: *J Am Acad Dermatol* 20:941–944, May 1989.)

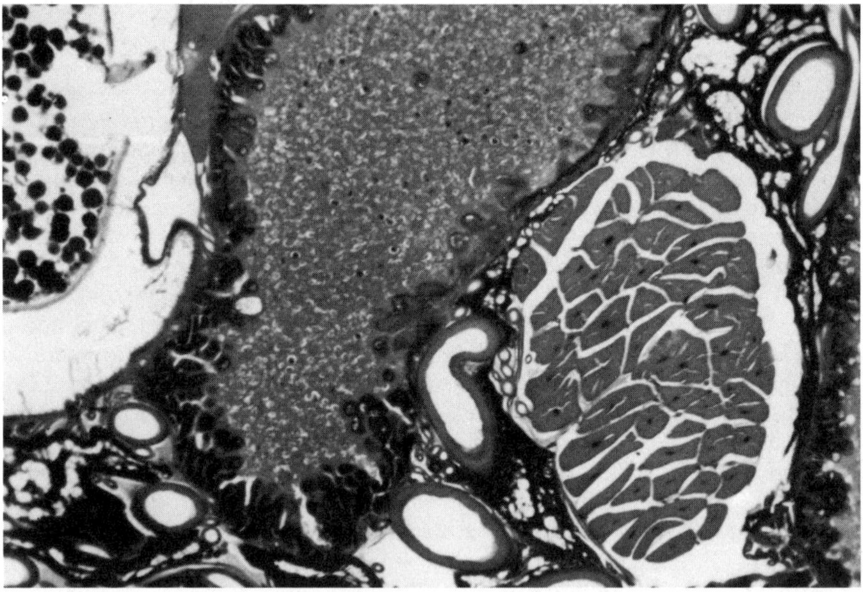

Fig 23–5.—Cross-section of distended digestive tube, *center* of photo, is surrounded by various structures, including tracheal rings and hypertrophied internal muscle band. An ovary containing eggs is seen in *left upper corner*. Hematoxylin-eosin; original magnification, ×100. (Courtesy of Sanusi ID, Brown EB, Shepard TG, et al: *J Am Acad Dermatol* 20:941–944, May 1989.)

Reported Cases of Tungiasis in the United States

Case No.	Reference	Age (yr)	Sex	Number and site(s) of lesion(s)	History of exposure	Treatment and results
1	Faust and Maxwell,[12] New Orleans, La.	Adult	M	Pubic, inguinal, and lower abdomen	Contact with sisal hemp from Mexico	Cured by Whitfield's ointment
2	Reiss,[13] New York City, N.Y.	Adult	M	Numerous lesions on both feet	Recent travel to tropical Africa	Curettage, topical antibiotic; healing in 12 days
3-7	Goldman,[14] Cincinnati, Ohio	Adults	F	Total of 9 lesions: 4 on sole, 3 on back, 1 under breast, 1 on wrist, 1 subungual	Recent travel to Africa	Lesions were debrided; topical antibiotic, healing in 4-5 days
8	Bell et al.,[15] Memphis, Tenn.	63	M	Three lesions on both feet	Recent travel to Brazil; history of barefoot walking	Cured by excision
9	Taubman and Spielman[16]	44	F	Four lesions on toes	Recent travel to Peru; history of wearing open sandals	Curettage, topical antibiotic, and hydrogen peroxide; healing in 3 wk

(Continued)

Table *(continued)*

Case No.	Reference	Age (yr)	Sex	Number and site(s) of lesion(s)	History of exposure	Treatment and results
10	Brothers and Heckmann,[17] Provo, Utah	21	M	Toe	Recent travel to Brazil; history of barefoot walking	Cured by incision, curettage, and topical antibiotic
11	Zalar and Walther,[18] New York City, N.Y.	29	F	Several on toes	Recent travel to tropical Africa; healing in 2 wk	Curettage and topical antibiotic
12	Poppiti et al.,[19] Miami, Fla.	25	M	Nodular lesions on both feet	Recent travel to Brazil; history of barefoot walking	Not mentioned
13	Armin et al.,[20] Maywood, Ill.	70	M	Toe, subungual	Recent travel to Africa	Removal of flea, topical antibiotic; healing in 1 wk
14	Wentzell et al.,[21] Hanover, N.H.	17	M	Toes, periungual	Recent travel to Brazil; history of barefoot walking	Cured by scraping, blunt dissection
15	Sanusi et al., Shreveport, La.	24	M	Two lesions on toes	Recent travel to Africa; history of barefoot walking	Removal of flea by safety pin; healing in a few days

(Courtesy of Sanusi ID, Brown EB, Shepard TG, et al: *J Am Acad Dermatol* 20:941–944, May 1989.)

Ping Pong Patches
Scott MJ Jr, Scott MJ III (Seattle)
Cutis 43:363–364, April 1989 23–21

Ping pong patches result from the skin being struck by a rapidly moving table tennis ball. The lesions are 12–15 mm in diameter, have clear centers, and are uniformly circular in shape. The annular border is 3 mm wide and is generally erythematous, but it may be purpuric. Ping pong patches usually occur on exposed skin areas, but may appear anywhere on the body, even underneath clothing.

When table tennis is played by advanced players, a table tennis ball's velocity may reach more than 100 miles per hour. When a table tennis ball strikes the skin at high velocity, it becomes temporarily indented (Fig 23–6). At the moment of maximum ball indentation, the circular edge of the indented ball impinges with considerable pressure against the skin, producing the typical annular lesion of erythema or purpura. Ping pong

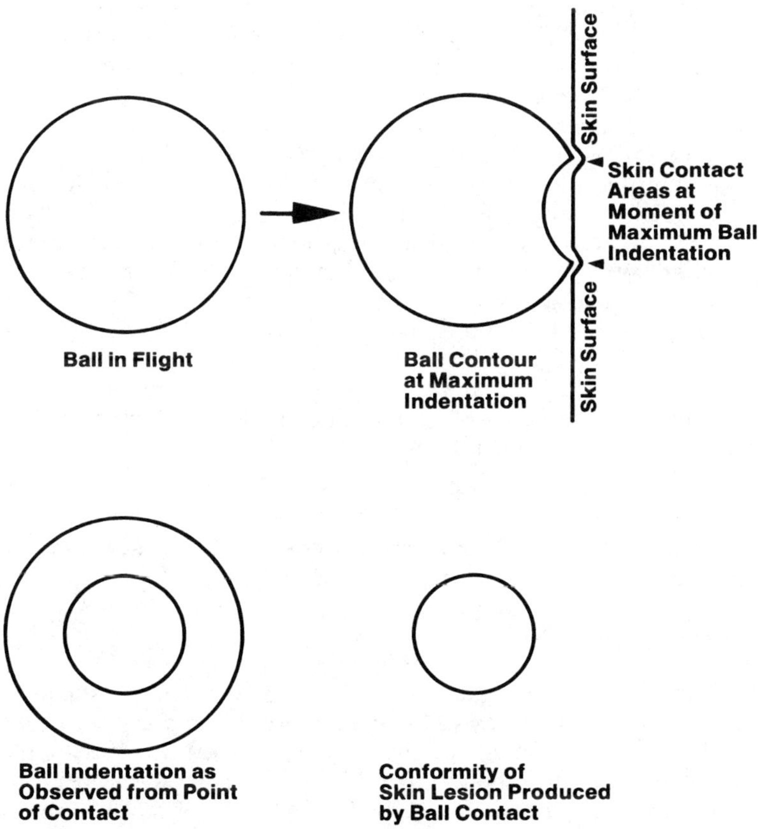

Fig 23–6.—Diagram of impact and indentation made by a ping pong ball. (Courtesy of Scott MJ Jr, Scott MJ III: *Cutis* 43:363–364, April 1989.)

lesions may persist for only a few minutes to several weeks but are usually visible for 2–5 days.

Ping pong lesions are easily misdiagnosed and, in fact, cannot be properly diagnosed without a history. Similar, but larger annular lesions may occur from being hit with a ball used in racketball or squash. Once observed and recognized, ping pong patches are easily diagnosed.

▶ Readers of Clancy's *The Hunt for Red October* will know that 1 ping can make a difference.—J.D. Bernhard, M.D.

Porokeratosis of Mibelli in Transplant Recipients

Komorowski RA, Clowry LJ (Med College of Wisconsin, Milwaukee)

Am J Clin Pathol 91:71–74, January 1989 23–22

Proliferative epidermal lesions are common in transplant recipients. Porokeratosis of Mibelli is an uncommon, inherited, autosomal-dominant dermatosis that usually presents in adolescence as a proliferation of an abnormal clone of epidermal cells. Among the skin biopsy specimens obtained from 602 renal and hepatic transplant recipients, 4 cases of porokeratosis of Mibelli were found.

The lesions developed in the posttransplant period and appeared as single or multiple patches on the legs. Histologic features included the cornoid lamella, which was a thin column of porokeratotic cells rising through the adjacent normal orthokeratotic epidermis, and absence of the granular layer beneath the cornoid lamella. The lesions were persistent and resistant to therapy.

Porokeratosis of Mibelli, although rare, should be added to the list of potential cutaneous complications seen in immunosuppressed organ-transplant recipients. Although cancer developed in none of the patients, the possibility of an increased incidence of malignancy in porokeratotic lesions of transplant recipients should not be discounted.

Disseminated Superficial Actinic Porokeratosis: A Clinical Study

Shumack SP, Commens CA (Skin and Cancer Found, Westmead, New South Wales)

J Am Acad Dermatol 20:1015–1022, June 1989 23–23

Disseminated superficial actinic porokeratosis is an autosomal dominant condition that requires sun exposure for full expression. It is characterized by multiple small lesions on sun-exposed areas with relative sparing of the face. It is commonly mistaken for solar keratoses. It is not a rare condition in Australia and, given the climate of that country, most individuals with an inherited tendency for this condition would have received sufficient actinic radiation to express the disease. An extensive questionnaire and clinical study was undertaken in 29 patients with disseminated superficial actinic porokeratosis.

The mean number of lesions per patient was 268 (range, 15–750). The mean age at recognition of disseminated superficial actinic porokeratosis was 43 years (range, 15–78); 28% of the patients remained unaware of their condition until the time of examination. Clinical evidence of solar damage was seen in 19 patients (66%). The lesions were confined exclusively to sun-exposed areas, being most numerous on the legs and forearms. They were most prominent and usually became more erythematous and scaly during the summer months in 59% of those affected. A slight itch was the only symptom in 38%, occurring mainly during summer or after exposure to heat.

The early lesions of disseminated superficial actinic porokeratosis appear as small, cone-shaped papules, 1–3 mm in diameter, usually follicular in location, and having a small keratotic plug. The papule enlarges centrifugally, with an atrophic central area and a sharply defined, slightly raised fine keratotic border (Fig 23–7). The cornoid lamella is essential for the histologic diagnosis. The frequent occurrence of epidermal atrophy and solar elastosis supports the role of actinic damage in the development of disseminated superficial actinic porokeratosis.

▶ The question in my mind is whether these cases are porokeratosis of Mibelli or actually disseminated superficial actinic porokeratosis (DSAP), which has been seen in transplant patients and other immunosuppressed states. The lo-

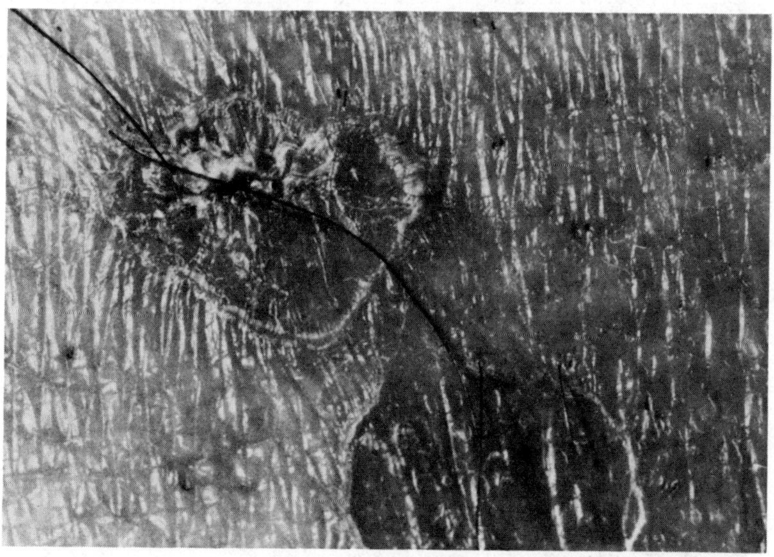

Fig 23–7.—Close-up of lesion of disseminated superficial actinic porokeratosis demonstrating hyperkeratosis around follicular orifice (*upper left*). On histologic examination this follicular hyperkeratosis would be seen as an additional cornoid lamella. (Coutesy of Shumack SP, Commens CA: *J Am Acad Dermatol* 20:1015–1022, June 1989.)

cation on the legs would fit with DSAP (1). The abstract emphasizes the fact that DSAP is not a rare disorder in areas of high solar exposure and a susceptible population (i.e., possesing the dominant gene). Visualizing lesions with tangential lighting and a 7–10× hand lens usually facilitates appreciation of the cornoid lamella.—A.J. Sober, M.D.

Reference

1. Lederman JS, et al: *J Am Acad Dermatol* 13:75, 1985.

Phrynoderma: A Review of 105 Cases

Nakjang Y, Yuttanavivat T (Inst of Dermatology, Bangkok, Thailand)
J Dermatol 15:531–534, December 1988 23–24

Phrynoderma is a follicular hyperkeratosis characterized by large, follicular, keratotic papules at the elbows and knees. The condition occurs predominantly in children and has been associated with a vitamin deficiency. However, controversy remains over which vitamin is involved in its etiology. A recent study found that affected children responded well to vitamin A therapy, suggesting that a fat-soluble vitamin deficiency might be involved in the etiology of phrynoderma.

The clinical and histologic features of phrynoderma were assessed, and the serum vitamin A levels measured, in 67 girls and 47 boys aged 5–17 years with phrynoderma. The average age at onset was 14 years. A group of 82 patients had follicular hyperkeratotic papules limited to the areas around the elbows and knees (Fig 23–8). The other 23 had similar lesions but with extension to other areas. However, the face, hands, and

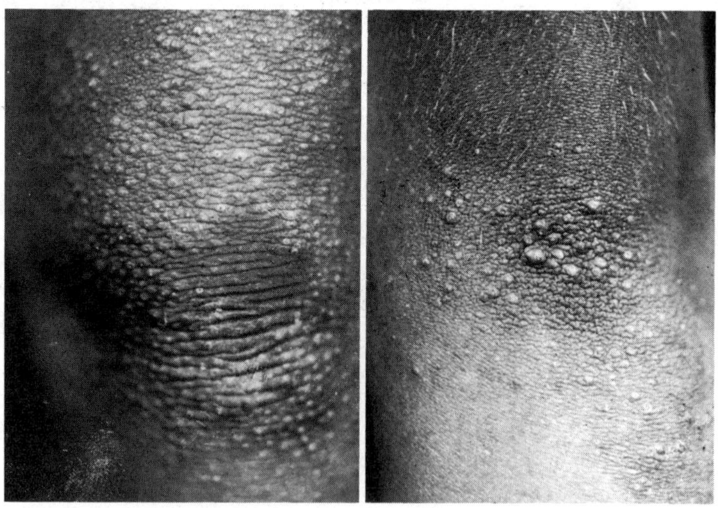

Fig 23–8.—Follicular hyperkeratosis of the knee (*left*) and the elbow (*right*). (Courtesy of Nakjang Y, Yuttanavivat T: *J Dermatol* 15:531–534, December 1988.)

feet were never involved, and lesions in the axillary or genitoanal regions were rare. Skin eruptions were hyperkeratotic, dry, firm, pigmented papules, containing a central, intrafollicular keratotic plug. None of the patients had night blindness or xerophthalmia.

Serum vitamin A levels were normal in 61 patients, higher than normal in 11, and below normal in only 4. The patients with lower-than-normal serum vitamin A levels all had papules limited to the areas around the knees and elbows. All patients with papules extending over the trunk, arms, and legs had normal serum vitamin A levels. Thus, in this study population, no association was found between phrynoderma and vitamin A deficiency.

▶ I think that a more appropriate conclusion for this paper would be that there is no correlation between vitamin A levels and keratosis pilaris. The lesion of phrynoderma is defined as that occurring with vitamin A deficiency, and not isolated follicular hyperkeratotic papules.—J.C. Alper, M.D.

In Vitro Migration of L3T4+ Cloned T Cells to Epidermis: Possible Role for Keratinocyte-Derived Factors

Shiohara T, Moriya N, Gotoh C, Gomi T, Nagashima M (Kyorin Univ School of Medicine, Tokyo)

J Invest Dermatol 92:360–365, March 1989 23–25

The T lymphocytes migrate into the epidermis in certain skin diseases. This affinity of T lymphocytes for the epidermis, called epidermotropism, is not well understood. The migratory behavior of cloned L3T4+ T cells with auto-, allo-, and antigen-reactive specificities was analyzed using an in vitro agar gel assay.

Two epidermotropic T cell lines, the autoreactive BB5 and the alloreactive SK1, demonstrated specific directional migration to the dermis. Nonepidermotropic cloned T cells and freshly isolated lymph node T cells did not demonstrate directional migration to the dermis. Cocultivation with epidermis, but not dermis, inhibited the directional migration of BB5 cells. The latter were attracted to the transformed keratinocyte cell line PAM212, conditioned media from this cell line, and to interleukin (IL)-2, but not to IL-1 or IL-3.

These in vitro results suggest that epidermotropic T cells may be attracted to areas having high concentrations of keratinocyte-derived growth factors and high concentrations of IL-2.

▶ Just think, what if a blocker of IL-2 or keratinocyte-derived growth factor could be developed? We could put an end to the T cell lymphomas. Or would we transform them to typical non-Hodgkin's lymphomas?—J.C. Alper, M.D.

Review Articles

Aging

Badame AJ: Progeria. *Arch Dermatol* 125:540–544, 1989.
Voorhees JJ: Mechanisms and therapy of aging skin. *J Am Acad Dermatol* 21:609–650, 1989.

AIDS

Cohen PR, Grossman ME: Clinical features of human immunodeficiency virus-associated disseminated herpes zoster virus infection—a review of the literature. *Clin Exp Dermatol* 14:273–276, 1989.

Biologic Response Modifiers

Benyon RC: The human skin mast cell. *Clin Exp Allergy* 19:375–387, 1989.
Casto M, Rosenbach T, Grabbe J, et al: Epidermal scales. *Int J Dermatol* 28:86–89, 1989.
Sauder DN: Interleukin 1. *Arch Dermatol* 125:679–682, 1989.
Schaffer HK: Essential fatty acids and eicosanoids in cutaneous inflammation. *Int J Dermatol* 28:281–290, 1989.
Stadler R, Mayer-da-Silva A, Bratzke B, et al: Interferons in dermatology. *J Am Acad Dermatol* 20:650–256, 1989.

Bullous Disorders

Ahmed AR, Rosen, GB: Viruses in pemphigus. *Int J Dermatol* 28:209–217, 1989.
Beutner EH, Chorzelski TP, Wilson RM, et al: IgA pemphigus foliaceus. *J Am Acad Dermatol* 20:89–97, 1989.
Diaz LA, Sampaio SA, Rivitti EA, et al: Endemic pemphigus foliaceus (fogo selvagem). *J Am Acad Dermatol* 20:657–669, 1989.
Frieden IJ: Blisters and pustules in the newborn. *Curr Probl Pediatr* 19:551–614, 1989.
Lin AN, Carter DM: Epidermolysis bullosa: When the skin falls apart. *J Pediatr* 114:349–355, 1989.
Sedano HO, Gorlin RJ: Epidermolysis bullosa. *Oral Surg Oral Med Oral Pathol* 67:555–563, 1989.

Collagen Disorders

Conn DL: Update on systemic necrotizing vasculitis. *Mayo Clin Proc* 64:535–543, 1989.
Jorizzo JL, Solomon AR, Zanolli MD, et al: Neutrophilic vascular reactions. *J Am Acad Dermatol* 19:983–1005, 1988.
Lo JS, Berg RE, Tomecki KJ: Treatment of discoid lupus erythematosus. *Int J Dermatol* 28:497–507, 1989.
Strauss KW, Gonzalez-Buritica H, Khamashta MA, et al: Polymyositis-dermatomyositis: A clinical review. *Postgrad Med J* 65:437–443, 1989.

Cosmctics

Nelson FP, Rumsfield J: Cosmetics, content and function. *Int J Dermatol* 27:665–672, 1988.

Dermatologic Surgery

Colver GB, Dawber RPR: Cryosurgery—the principles and simple practice. *Clin Exp Dermatol* 14:1–6, 1989.
Weber PJ, WEber M, Dzubow LM: Sedation for dermatologic surgery. *J Am Acad Dermatol* 20:815–826, 1989.

Dermatopathology

Cerio R, Wilson-Jones E: New cell markers for routine diagnostic dermatopathology. *Clin Exp Dermatol* 14:177–180, 1989.

Doherty MJ, Russo GG, Jolly HW, et al: Immunoenzyme techniques in dermatopathology. *J Am Acad Dermatol* 20:827–837, 1989.
Jaworsky C, Murphy GF: Special techniques in dermatology. *Arch Dermatol* 125:963–974, 1989.

Eczema

de Groot AC, Young E: The role of contact allergy to aeroallergens in atopic dermatitis. *Contact Dermatitis* 21:209–214, 1989.
Holdiness MR: A review of contact dermatitis associated with transdermal therapeutic systems. *Contact Dermatitis* 20:3–9, 1989.
Thestrup-Pedersen K, Larsen CG, Ronnevig J: The immunology of contact dermatitis. *Contact Dermatitis* 20:81–92, 1989.

Fungal Diseases

Elewski BE, Hazen PG: The superficial mycoses and the dermatophytes. *J Am Acad Dermatol* 21:655–673, 1989.
Lambert DR, Siegle RJ, Camisa C: Griseofulvin and ketoconazole in the treatment of dermatophyte infections. *Int J Dermatol* 28:300–304, 1989.
Radentz WH: Opportunistic fungal infections in immunocompromised hosts. *J Am Acad Dermatol* 20:989–1003, 1989.
Tomecki KJ, Steck WD, Hall GS, et al: Subcutaneous mycoses. *J Am Acad Dermatol* 21:785–790, 1989.

Genodermatoses

Cohen PR, Schneiderman P: Clinical manifestations of the Marfan syndrome. *Int J Dermatol* 28:291–299, 1989.

Insects and Arthropods

Baird JK, Baird CR, Sabrosky CW: North American cuterebrid myiasis. *J Am Acad Dermatol* 21:763–772, 1989.
Gutowicz M, Fritz RA, Sonoga AL: Brown recluse spider bite. *J Am Podiatr Med Assoc* 79:142–146, 1989.
Klenerman P: Mosquitoes: How to be the perfect host. *Int J Dermatol* 28:370–372, 1989.

Internal Medicine

Abel EA: Cutaneous manifestations of immunosuppression in organ transplant recipients. *J Am Acad Dermatol* 21:167–179, 1989.

Kaposi's Sarcoma

Berlin SJ, Clancy JT, Giordano ML: Kaposi's sarcoma of the foot. *J Am Podiatr Med Assoc* 79:311–317, 1989.

Laser

Tan OT, Gilchrest BA: Laser therapy for selected cutaneous vascular lesions in the pediatric population: A review. *Pediatrics* 82:652–662, 1988.

Lyme Disease

Krafchik B: Lyme disease. *Int J Dermatol* 28:71–74, 1989.
Steere AC: Lyme disease. *N Engl J Med* 321:586–596, 1989.

Melanoma

Cascinelli N: Melanoma today. *J Dermatol* 15:355–366, 1988.
Das Gupta TK: Current status of surgical treatment of melanoma. *Semin Oncol* 15:566–568, 1988.

Dracopoli NC, Bale SJ: Genetic aspects of cutaneous malignant melanoma. *Semin Oncol* 15:541–548, 1988.
Elder DE: Dysplastic nevus syndrome—biological significance. *Semin Oncol* 15:529–540, 1988.
Koh HK, Lew RA, Prout MN: Screening for melanoma/skin cancer: Theoretic and practical considerations. *J Am Acad Dermatol* 20:159–172, 1989.
Loggie BW, Eddy JA: Solar considerations in the development of cutaneous melanoma. *Semin Oncol* 15:494–499, 1988.
Tucker MA, Bale SJ: Clinical aspects of familial cutaneous malignant melanoma. *Semin Oncol* 15:524–528, 1988.

Metabolic Disorders

Black MM: The cutaneous hyalinoses: Differential diagnosis. *Australas J Dermatol* 29:73–78, 1988.
Bloomer JR, Bonkovksy HL: The porphyrias. *Disease-a-Month* 35:1–54, 1989.
Cox TM, Lord DK: Hereditary haemochromatosis. *Eur J Haematol* 42:113–125, 1989.
Knobler RM, Becerano S, Gebhart W: Inborn errors of lipid metabolism-dermatological aspects. *Clin Exp Dermatol* 13:365–370, 1988.

Miscellaneous

Cohen PR, Prystowsky JH: Pityriasis rubra pilaris: A review of diagnosis and treatment. *J Am Acad Dermatol* 20:801–807, 1989.
Dinehart SM, Herzberg AJ, Kerns BJ, et al: Acne keloidalis: A review. *J Dermatol Surg Oncol* 15:642–647, 1989.
Ebling FJG: Apocrine glands in health and disorder. *Int J Dermatol* 28:508–511, 1989.
Heymann WR: Noninfectious causes of fever and a rash. *Int J Dermatol* 28:145–156, 1989.
Janssen PA, Vanden Bossche HFA, Van Wauwe JP, et al: The role of cytochrome P-450 in dermatology. *Int J Dermatol* 28:493–496, 1989.
Macauley WL: Lymphomatoid papulosis update. *Arch Dermatol* 125:1387–1389, 1989.
McKay M: Vulvodynia. *Arch Dermatol* 125:256–262, 1989.
Miller SJ: Nutritional deficiency and the skin. *J Am Acad Dermatol* 21:1–30, 1989.
Rogers M, McCrossin I, Commens C: Epidermal nevi and the epidermal nevus syndrome. *J Am Acad Dermatol* 20:476–488, 1989.
Roth RR, James WD: Microbiology of the skin: Resident flora, ecology, infection. *J Am Acad Dermatol* 20:367–390, 1989.
Sardo MJ, Anastasi GW: Dermatofibrosarcoma protuberans: A clinicopathologic review and four case reports. *Contemp Surg* 33:79–83, 1988.
Tremaine RDL, Miller RAW: Lichen sclerosus et atrophicus. *Int J Dermatol* 28:10–16, 1989.
Winkelmann RK: Pruritus. *Semin Dermatol* 7:233–235, 1988.

Mycobacterial Diseases

Kakakhel KU, Fritsch P: Cutaneous tuberculosis. *Int J Dermatol* 28:355–362, 1989.
Sehgal VN, Jain MK, Srivastava G: Evolution of the classification of leprosy. *Int J Dermatol* 28:161–167, 1989.

Occupational Skin Disease

Stevenson CJ: Occupational skin disease. *Postgrad Med J* 65:374–380, 1989.

Panniculitis

Black MM: Panniculitis: Problems with diagnosis. *Australas J Dermatol* 29:79–84, 1988.

Pediatric Dermatology

Bialecki C, Feder HM Jr, Grant-Kels JM: The six classic childhood exanthems: a review and update. *J Am Acad Dermatol* 21:891–903, 1989.

Pregnancy

Black MM: Pregnancy, gynecology, and skin. *Semin Dermatol* 8:1–63, 1989.
Winton GB: Skin diseases aggravated by pregnancy. *J Am Acad Dermatol* 20:1–13, 1989.

Psoriasis

Berardesca E, Maibach HI: Noninvasive bioengineering assessment of psoriasis. *Int J Dermatol* 28:157–160, 1989.
Boyd AS, Menter A: Erythrodermic psoriasis. *J Am Acad Dermatol* 21:985–991, 1989.
Even-Paz Z, Shani J: The Dead Sea and psoriasis. *Int J Dermatol* 28:1–9, 1989.
Seville RH: Stress and psoriasis: The importance of insight and empathy in prognosis. *J Am Acad Dermatol* 20:97–100, 1989.

Skin Cancer

Goldminz D, Scott G, Klaus S: Penile basal cell carcinoma. *J Am Acad Dermatol* 20:1094–1097, 1989.
Myskowski PL, Safai B: The immunology of basal cell carcinoma. *Int J Dermatol* 27:601–607, 1988.

Sweating

Sato K, Kang WH, Saga K, et al: Biology of sweat glands and their disorders. I. Normal sweat gland function. *J Am Acad Dermatol* 20:537–563, 1989.
Sato K, Kang WH, Saga K, et al: Biology of sweat glands and their disorders. II. Disorders of sweat gland function. *J Am Acad Dermatol* 20:713–726, 1989.

Therapy

Barth JH, Cherry CA, Wojnarowska F, et al: Spironolactone is an effective and well tolerated systemic antiandrogen therapy for hirsute women. *J Clin Endocrinol Metab* 68:966–970, 1989.
Czarnetzki BM: Vitamin D_3 in dermatology: A critical appraisal. *Dermatologica* 178:184–188, 1989.
Dover JS, Phillips TJ, Arndt KA: Cutaneous effects and therapeutic uses of heat with emphasis on infrared radiation. *J Am Acad Dermatol* 20:278–286, 1989.
Flowers FP, Araujo OE, Turner LA: Recent advances in antiherpetic drugs. *Int J Dermatol* 27:612–616, 1988.
Gold JA, Shupack JL, Nemec MA: Ocular side effects of the retinoids. *Int J Dermatol* 28:218–225, 1989.
Isseroff RR: Fish again for dinner! The role of fish and other dietary oils in the therapy of skin disease. *J Am Acad Dermatol* 19:1073–1080, 1988.
Jackson DB, Thompson C, McCormack JR, et al: Bioequivalence (bioavailability) of generic topical corticosteroids. *J Am Acad Dermatol* 20:791–796, 1989.
Saurat JH: How do retinoids work on human epidermis? A breakthrough and its implications. *Clin Exp Dermatol* 13:359–364, 1988.
Shalita AR, Armstrong RB, Leyden JJ, et al: Isotretinoin revisited. *Cutis* 42:1–19, 1988.
Shannon RL, Strayer DS: Arsenic-induced skin toxicity. *Hum Toxicol* 8:99–104, 1989.
Shapiro I: Topical estrogens. *Int J Dermatol* 27:673–675, 1988.
Shear NH: Adverse reactions to drugs. *Semin Dermatol* 8:135–226, 1989.
Thiers BH: Antiretroviral therapy. *J Am Acad Dermatol* 21:443–454, 1989.
Witkowski JA: Compliance: The dermatologic patient. *Int J Dermatol* 27:608–611, 1988.
Wozel G: The story of sulfones in tropical medicine and dermatology. *Int J Dermatol* 28:17–21, 1989.

Ulcers

Allman RM: Pressure ulcers among the elderly. *N Engl J Med* 320:850–853, 1989.

Urticaria

Leenutaphong V, Holzle E, Plewig G: Pathogenesis and classification of solar urticaria: A new concept. *J am Acad Dermatol* 21:237–240, 1989.

Vascular Disorders

deGroot WP: Treatment of varicose veins: Modern concepts and methods. *J Dermatol Surg Oncol* 15:191–198, 1989.

Jordaan HF: Acute febrile neutrophilic dermatosis. *Am J Dermatopathol* 11:99–111, 1989.

Picascia DD, Esterly NB: Cutis marmorata telangiectatica congenita: report of 22 cases. *J Am Acad Dermatol* 20:1098–1104, 1989.

Vitiligo

Falabella R: Grafting and transplantation of melanocytes for repigmenting vitiligo and other types of leukoderma. *Int J Dermatol* 28:363–369, 1989.

Koranne RV, Sachdeva KG: Vitiligo. *Int J Dermatol* 27:676–681, 1988.

Warts

Androphy EJ: Human papillomavirus. *Arch Dermatol* 125:683–685, 1989.

Sehgal VN, Koranne RV, Srivastava SB: Genital warts. *Int J Dermatol* 28:75–84, 1989.

Steele K, Irwin WB: Treatment options for cutaneous warts in family practice. *Fam Pract* 5:314–319, 1988.

Subject Index

A

B

C

D

E

F

G

H

I

M

N

O

P

S

T

U

V

W

X

Z

Author Index

A

B

C

D

E

F

G

H

M

S

T

U

V

W

Y

Z

YEAR BOOK READY-ACCESS CARD!

[X] Yes! I'd like to keep current. Please send me a *free* 30-day examination copy of the Year Book(s) checked below:

[ ] *Year Book of Anesthesia*® (20403)	$54.95
[ ] *Year Book of Cardiology*® (20407)	$54.95
[ ] *Year Book of Critical Care Medicine*® (20399)	$51.95
[ ] *Year Book of Dermatology*® (20409)	$54.95
[ ] *Year Book of Diagnostic Radiology*® (20289)	$54.95
[ ] *Year Book of Digestive Diseases*® (20413)	$54.95
[ ] *Year Book of Drug Therapy*® (20398)	$54.95
[ ] *Year Book of Emergency Medicine*® (20301)	$54.95
[ ] *Year Book of Endocrinology*® (20405)	$54.95
[ ] *Year Book of Family Practice*® (20400)	$51.95
[ ] *Year Book of Geriatrics and Gerontology* (20396)	$51.95
[ ] *Year Book of Hand Surgery*® (20306)	$54.95
[ ] *Year Book of Hematology*® (20418)	$51.95
[ ] *Year Book of Health Care Management*® (21145)	$54.95
[ ] *Year Book of Infectious Diseases*® (20420)	$51.95
[ ] *Year Book of Infertility* (20414)	$51.95
[ ] *Year Book of Medicine*® (20402)	$54.95
[ ] *Year Book of Neonatal-Perinatal Medicine* (20410)	$51.95
[ ] *Year Book of Neurology and Neurosurgery*® (20266)	$54.95
[ ] *Year Book of Nuclear Medicine*® (20311)	$54.95
[ ] *Year Book of Obstetrics and Gynecology*® (20315)	$54.95
[ ] *Year Book of Occupational and Environmental Medicine* (20395)	$54.95
[ ] *Year Book of Oncology* (20415)	$54.95
[ ] *Year Book of Ophthalmology*® (20412)	$54.95
[ ] *Year Book of Orthopedics*® (20417)	$54.95
[ ] *Year Book of Otolaryngology – Head and Neck Surgery*® (20401)	$54.95
[ ] *Year Book of Pathology and Clinical Pathology*® (20397)	$54.95
[ ] *Year Book of Pediatrics*® (20286)	$51.95
[ ] *Year Book of Plastic and Reconstructive Surgery*® (20299)	$54.95
[ ] *Year Book of Psychiatry and Applied Mental Health*® (20319)	$54.95
[ ] *Year Book of Pulmonary Disease*® (20406)	$51.95
[ ] *Year Book of Sports Medicine*® (20419)	$54.95
[ ] *Year Book of Surgery*® (20408)	$54.95
[ ] *Year Book of Urology*® (20416)	$54.95
[ ] *Year Book of Vascular Surgery*® (20305)	$54.95

*All Year Books are published annually. For the convenience of its customers, Year Book enters each purchaser as a subscriber to future volumes and sends annual announcements of each volume approximately 2 months before publication. The new volume will be shipped upon publication unless you complete and return the cancellation notice attached to the announcement and it is received by Year Book within the time indicated (approximately 20 days after your receipt of the announcement). You may cancel your subscription at any time. The new volume may be examined on approval for 30 days, may be returned for full credit, and if returned Year Book will then remove your name as a subscriber. Return postage is guaranteed by Year Book to the Postal Service.

NAME/ACCT. NO.

ADDRESS

CITY/STATE/ZIP

CODE: MC-0277

Prepaid orders are shipped postage free; add $3.50 per order to cover handling. Other orders will be billed a shipping and handling charge. Please add applicable sales tax. Prices quoted in U.S. dollars. Canadian orders will be billed in U.S. funds. All prices subject to change without notice.

Mosby-Year Book, Inc. • 11830 Westline Industrial Drive • St. Louis, MO 63146